Handbook of Outpatient Treatment of Adults

Nonpsychotic Mental Disorders

Handbook of Outpatient Treatment of Adults

Nonpsychotic Mental Disorders

Edited by

Michael E. Thase, M.D.
Western Psychiatric Institute and Clinic
Pittsburgh, Pennsylvania

Barry A. Edelstein, Ph.D.
West Virginia University
Morgantown, West Virginia

and

Michel Hersen, Ph.D.
Western Psychiatric Institute and Clinic
Pittsburgh, Pennsylvania

Plenum Press • New York and London

Library of Congress Cataloging-in-Publication Data

Handbook of outpatient treatment of adults: nonpsychotic mental disorders / edited by Michael E. Thase, Barry A. Edelstein, and Michel Hersen.
p. cm.
Includes bibliographical references.
ISBN 0-306-43267-6
1. Psychiatric hospitals--Outpatient services. 2. Psychotherapy. I. Thase, Michael E. II. Edelstein, Barry A., 1945- III. Hersen, Michel.
[DNLM: 1. Mental Disorders--therapy--handbooks. 2. Mental Health Services--United States--handbooks. 3. Outpatient Clinics, Hospital--United States--handbooks. WM 34 H23593]
RC439.4.H36 1990
616.89'14--dc20
DNLM/DLC
for Library of Congress 89-23242
CIP

A Division of Plenum Publishing Corporation
233 Spring Street, New York, N.Y. 10013

Printed in the United States of America

Contributors

GENE G. ABEL, Behavioral Medicine Institute, Atlanta, Georgia 30327–4104; and Emory University School of Medicine, Atlanta, Georgia 30302

JACQUES BARBER, Department of Psychiatry, University of Pennsylvania, Philadelphia, Pennsylvania 19104

THOMAS P. BERESFORD, Michigan Alcohol Program, University of Michigan Medical Center, Ann Arbor, Michigan 48109

GARY R. BIRCHLER, University of California School of Medicine, and Psychology Service, V.A. Medical Center, San Diego, California 92161

JOSEPH E. BIRON, Psychology Department, University of Montana, Missoula, Montana 59812

FREDERIC C. BLOW, Michigan Alcohol Program, University of Michigan Medical Center, Ann Arbor, Michigan 48109

PHILIP H. BORNSTEIN, Psychology Department, University of Montana, Missoula, Montana 59812

BONNIE M. BREKKE, Psychology Department, University of Montana, Missoula, Montana 59812

BENJAMIN BURSTEN, 103 Garnet Lane, Oak Ridge, Tennessee 37830.

JOSEPH R. CAUTELA, Behavior Therapy Institute, Sudbury, Massachusetts 01776

JACK R. CORNELIUS, Western Psychiatric Institute and Clinic, Pittsburgh, Pennsylvania 15213

Paul Crits-Christoph, Department of Psychiatry, University of Pennsylvania, Philadelphia, Pennsylvania 19104

Edward Dengrove, 541 North Edgemere Drive, West Allenhurst, New Jersey 07711

Jeffrey R. Fitzgerald, Western Carolina Center, Morganton, North Carolina 28655

E. B. Foa, Medical College of Pennsylvania, Philadelphia, Pennsylvania 19129

Carolyn Ford, Psychology Department, University of Montana, Missoula, Montana 59812

Charles V. Ford, Department of Psychiatry and Behavioral Sciences, University of Arkansas for Medical Sciences, Little Rock, Arkansas 72205

Minna R. Fyer, Department of Psychiatry, Cornell University Medical College, New York, New York 10021

Alan J. Gelenberg, Department of Psychiatry, University of Arizona College of Medicine, Health Sciences Center, Tucson, Arizona 85724

Madeline Gershwin, University of California School of Medicine, San Diego, California 92161

Joseph R. Haas, Department of Psychology, University of North Carolina at Greensboro, Greensboro, North Carolina 27412–5001

C. V. Haldipur, Richard H. Hutchings Psychiatric Center, Syracuse, New York 13210

Anne K. Hall, Florida Hospital, Orlando, Florida 32803

Kathryn S. K. Hall, Department of Psychiatry, UMDNJ–Robert Wood Johnson Medical School, Piscataway, New Jersey 08854

Richard C. W. Hall, Psychiatric Programs, Florida Hospital, Orlando, Florida 32803

Steven C. Hayes, Department of Psychology, University of Nevada, Reno, Nevada 89557–0062

Dale J. Hindmarsh, Western Psychiatric Institute and Clinic, University of Pittsburgh, Pittsburgh, Pennsylvania 15213

L. K. George Hsu, Western Psychiatric Institute and Clinic, University of Pittsburgh, Pittsburgh, Pennsylvania 15213

Lauren P. Jones, University of California at Berkeley, Berkeley, California 94720

Albert J. Kearney, Maynard Public Schools, Maynard, Massachusetts 01754

Martin B. Keller, Massachusetts General Hospital, Boston, Massachusetts 02114

Michael Kidorf, Department of Psychology, Florida State University, Tallahassee, Florida 32306

Alan R. Lang, Department of Psychology, Florida State University, Tallahassee, Florida 32306

Sandra R. Leiblum, Department of Psychiatry, UMDNJ – Robert Wood Johnson Medical School, Piscataway, New Jersey 08854

Robert C. Long, Benjamin Rush Center, Syracuse, New York 13202

Lester Luborsky, Department of Psychiatry, University of Pennsylvania, Philadelphia, Pennsylvania 19104

Robert S. Marin, Western Psychiatric Institute and Clinic, University of Pittsburgh, Pittsburgh, Pennsylvania 15213

P. R. McCarthy, Biobehavioral Research Institute, Chester Springs, Pennsylvania 19425.

Juan E. Mezzich, Western Psychiatric Institute and Clinic, University of Pittsburgh, Pittsburgh, Pennsylvania 15213

Jerome A. Motto, University of California, School of Medicine, San Francisco, California 94143

Benoit H. Mulsant, Department of Psychiatry, Western Psychiatric Institute and Clinic, University of Pittsburgh, Pittsburgh, Pennsylvania 15213

Pamela E. Parker, Department of Psychiatry and Behavioral Sciences, University of Arkansas for Medical Sciences, Little Rock, Arkansas 72205

B. Ashok Raj, Department of Psychiatry and Behavioral Medicine, University of South Florida College of Medicine, Tampa, Florida 33613

Dennis H. Reid, Western Carolina Center, Morganton, North Carolina 28655

Joanne-L. Rouleau, Behavioral Medicine Institute, Atlanta, Georgia 30327–4104; and Emory University School of Medicine, Atlanta, Georgia 30302

Frances M. Sessa, Massachusetts General Hospital, Boston, Massachusetts 02114

Shawn C. Shea, Monadmock Family Services, Keene, New Hampshire 03431

David V. Sheehan, Department of Psychiatry and Behavioral Medicine, University of South Florida College of Medicine, Tampa, Florida 33613

ANNE D. SIMONS, Department of Psychology, University of Oregon, Eugene, Oregon 97403

PAUL H. SOLOFF, Western Psychiatric Institute and Clinic, University of Pittsburgh, Pittsburgh, Pennsylvania 15213

DAVID B. STUBE, Psychology Department, University of Montana, Missoula, Montana 59812

MICHAEL E. THASE, Department of Psychiatry, University of Pittsburgh School of Medicine, Western Psychiatric Institute and Clinic, Pittsburgh, Pennsylvania 15213

JOE E. THORNTON, Department of Psychiatry, Western Psychiatric Institute and Clinic, University of Pittsburgh, Pittsburgh, Pennsylvania 15213

BICK WANCK, Saratoga Therapy and Training, Saratoga Springs, New York 12866; and Albany Medical College, Albany, New York 12302

Preface

During the past several decades, the field of mental health care has expanded greatly. This expansion has been based on greater recognition of the prevalence and treatability of mental disorders, as well as the availability of a variety of forms of effective treatment. Indeed, throughout this period, our field has witnessed the introduction and the widespread application of specific pharmacological treatments, as well as the development, refinement, and more broadly based availability of behavioral, psychodynamic, and marital and family interventions. The community mental health center system has come into being, and increasing numbers of mental health practitioners from the fields of psychiatry, psychology, social work, nursing, and related professional disciplines have entered clinical practice. In concert with these developments, powerful sociopolitical and socioeconomic forces—including the deinstitutionalization movement of the late 1960s and early 1970s and the cost-containment responses of the 1980s, necessitated by the spiraling cost of health care—have shaped the greatest area of growth in the direction of outpatient services. This is particularly true of the initial assessment and treatment of nonpsychotic mental disorders, which now can often be managed in ambulatory-care settings. Thus, we decided that a handbook focusing on the outpatient treatment of mental disorders would be both timely and useful.

When we first began outlining the contents of this book, the third edition of the American Psychiatric Association's *Diagnostic and Statistical Manual of Mental Disorders* (DSM-III) was in its fourth year of use. Because this classification system had already received acceptance as the official nomenclature for mental disorders in the United States, we decided that our handbook should follow the diagnostic format used by the system. Nevertheless, a number of the conditions covered in this diagnostic system (e.g., a majority of the personality disorder diagnoses) had not received sufficient empirical study to warrant their own chapters in a handbook. In addition, the outpatient management of a variety of special populations could not be comprehensively covered by restricting the content of this handbook to specific diagnostic groupings. Slowly, a structure for this handbook emerged, centering on four major sections. The first, "General Issues," covers topics related to diagnosis and overviews of pharmacotherapy and two major models of psychotherapy: psychodynamic and behavioral therapy. The second section presents coverage of the major specific mental disorders. The publication of a revised edition of the DSM-III midway through this project has been addressed within these specific chapters, as appropriate. The third section provides reviews of the outpatient management of a number of special populations, including adolescents, the elderly, the mentally retarded, Vietnam veterans, and individuals who are comorbid for both a mental disorder and a substance abuse disorder. We have also included in this section a chapter relating the role of marital dysfunction to the overall treatment of specific mental disorders. Finally, in Part IV, special topics related to outpatient clinical practice are addressed: ethical and legal issues, the management of suicidal patients, general office-practice issues, and the conducting of research within an outpatient practice.

As editors, we have grappled with the essential issue of what topics should and should not be covered within the limits of this handbook. We have chosen not to address the specific disorders of alcoholism and drug abuse; rather, we have focused on the impact of alcohol and substance abuse on the assessment and treatment of persons suffering from primary psychiatric disorders. Similarly, we have chosen not to emphasize the role of partial hospital programming because such programming is preferentially used for individuals with psychotic disorders.

Each of us has carried our fair share of the editorial chores. We would like to acknowledge the contributions of the numerous experts whose chapters in their specialty areas appear in this book. Next, we wish to thank our secretaries who typed and retyped many parts of the manuscript. We also thank the editorial staff of Plenum Press for its heroic efforts to translate this long manuscript into its final form. Finally, we appreciate the efforts of our editor, Eliot Werner, whose substantial patience was thoroughly tested in seeing this project through to completion.

Michael E. Thase
Michel Hersen
Barry Edelstein

Contents

Handbook of Outpatient Treatment of Adults

I

General Issues

1

Interviewing and Diagnosis

JUAN E. MEZZICH AND SHAWN C. SHEA

INTRODUCTION

Competent care in outpatient psychiatric settings requires a sensitive and thorough evaluation of the patient's condition. Such an evaluation will furnish the data base crucial to systematically designing a treatment plan that attends to the various problems and needs of the patient. Furthermore, the evaluation constitutes a critical opportunity for engaging the patient in the treatment process by creating in the patient a sense of confidence in and trust of the clinician.

Psychiatric evaluation is a complex process, as is suggested by the following considerations: the involvement in the patient's condition of a plurality of aspects pertinent to understanding the case and to treatment efforts, the diversity of the sources of information that may be available, the different approaches to data gathering that the situation of the patient may demand, and the various ways of organizing the gathered data in order to produce clinical statements suitable to the task at hand. Interviewing and diagnosis are the key elements of a psychiatric evaluation. Interviewing constitutes the centerpiece of both data gathering and contact with the patient, and diagnosis represents the principal informational result (i.e., a summarized and codified statement on the critical features of the patient's condition). Discussions of these two elements, within the framework of a comprehensive psychiatric evaluation, constitute the major sections of this chapter.

INTERVIEWING

Interviewing is the foundation from which all of the outpatient's psychiatric care proceeds. It demands psychopathological knowledge, interpersonal skills, and intuitive abilities. Thus, it is a true blending of science, craft, and art.

JUAN E. MEZZICH • Western Psychiatric Institute and Clinic, University of Pittsburgh, Pittsburgh, Pennsylvania 15213. SHAWN C. SHEA • Monadmock Family Services, Keene, New Hampshire 03431.

Referring to the professional centrality of interviewing, Sullivan (1954) stated, "The psychiatric expert is presumed, from the cultural definition of an expert, and from the general rumors and beliefs about psychiatry, to be quite able to handle a psychiatric interview." The weight of this opinion has been enhanced by a survey of 483 psychiatric educators and practitioners conducted by Langsley and Hollender (1982). They found that 99% of the respondents rated conducting a comprehensive interview as an important requirement for psychiatrists. This represented the highest ranking skill of the 32 listed on the survey form. Furthermore, 7 of the top 10 skills were directly related to interviewing, such as assessing suicide potential, making accurate diagnoses, and recognizing countertranference problems.

The complex task facing the outpatient clinician involves gathering substantial and reliable data, while attending to critical interpersonal issues such as engaging the patient in the process. In the following subsection, we deal with types of interview procedures related to structuring approaches and to the clinician–patient relationship.

The Task-Oriented Perspective

One of the factors significantly influencing interview style is the clinical task at hand. It is important for the outpatient clinician to consider what may be called the *task-oriented perspective,* in which the clinician determines what data are necessary for the assessment of the patient. The required data base may vary according to the clinical situation. For instance, the data base typically obtained in a 30-minute emergency-room interview is quite different from that resulting from a 2-hour comprehensive assessment. Different clinical situations that distinctly influence the interview process and the resulting data include: emergency room assessment, comprehensive diagnostic assessment, consultation and liaison assessment, medication evaluation, psychodynamic assessment, and assessment for behavioral therapy.

The clinician's task is further complicated by the fact that specific interview formats may be pertinent. In this regard, the clinician may be asked to make a determination of competency or to respond to other forensic questions. Another common request made of outpatient clinicians is a basic screening for cognitive deficits as seen in dementia or delirium. A clinician may be asked as a consultant to focus on specific areas of information, such as the patient's psychogenetic history or an exploration of the patient's religious framework or views on meaning of life. Each of these clinical tasks requires a set of flexible skills.

The clinician should also carefully consider the time constraints on completing the evaluation. Each interview becomes a creative attempt to interweave clinical tasks, time constraints, and the unique needs of each patient. Each interview thus represents a unique and dynamic interchange that can never be duplicated. The outpatient clinician must become a master of sorts with regard to the flexible use of specific interviewing techniques.

With regard to clinical setting, Lazare (1979) produced a pivotal text, emphasizing the importance of considering the patient's agenda and needs in the course of the initial intake. He delineated the value of creating a negotiated contract with the patient. This contract, which is either implicit or explicit, allows the clinician and the patient to work together toward the same goals in the initial intake, a shared perspective that can markedly decrease problems that may be encountered with resistance.

The ability to work efficiently and sensitively within various time constraints has been directly addressed by Shea in *Psychiatric Interviewing: The Art of Understanding* (1988). In this text, Shea describes in detail a specific method of conceptualizing the structure of the interview process, a system referred to as *facilics*. Facilics is defined as the study of the transitions and flow of the interview, as well as the structuring of the interview within specific time constraints. This knowledge base provides the clinician with a way of conceptualizing and structuring the interview naturalistically, with an emphasis on the interrelationship of sensitive listening, engagement, and data gathering.

As mentioned earlier, the outpatient clinician may confront specific clinical tasks that require specific technical expertise, such as carrying out a mental status examination for exploring potential cognitive deficits. Strub and Black produced a powerful and easily read book concerning the cognitive examination: *The Mental Status Examination in Neurology* (1977). In this text, the authors delineated comprehensive, practical, sensitive methods to be used by the outpatient clinician in exploring cognitive deficits.

The factors described above, including clinical setting, time constraints, and specific clinical formats, represent key elements of concern in the task-oriented perspective. The contemporary clinician's style of interview must also take into account advances in diagnostic methodology. Indeed, there has been an evolution in interviewing techniques because diagnosis has become intimately related to treatment planning. From a historical perspective, in 1954, when Sullivan wrote his classic text *The Psychiatric Interview,* the need for a specific diagnosis after one interview or shortly after hospitalization was not as significant as it is today. It was not of critical immediate value to treatment to know whether the patient was suffering from schizophrenia or bipolar disorder; neuroleptics were in their infancy; and the use of lithium was an idea just crystallizing in the minds of its proponents. In contrast, if the contemporary clinician can delineate from an interview that a panic disorder is present, then treatment modalities, such as tricyclic antidepressants and specific forms of behavioral therapy, come to mind. The clinician must be aware of pertinent diagnostic criteria and must be able to explore their presence sensitively.

Structural Types

The need for sensitive structuring leads to the second major issue determining the style of a given interview. With regard to the structure of the interview, two concepts outlined by Richardson, Dohrenwend, and Klein (1965) are useful: standardization and scheduling. *Standardization* refers to the extent to which informational areas or items to be explored are specified in the interview procedure. *Scheduling* refers to the prespecification of the wording and sequence of the interview process.

By means of these two concepts, several interview types can be defined. In the freeformat interview, the interviewer can choose fully the areas to be covered and the way of exploring them. A version of this type of interview is frequently used in psychodynamic explorations. At the opposite end of the spectrum is the fully standardized and strictly scheduled interview, in which the required informational areas are specified in detail and the ways of exploring them are also prescribed. An example of this type of interview is the Diagnostic Interview Schedule (Robins, Helzer, Croughan, & Ratcliff, 1981), developed for community surveys conducted by lay interviewers.

Semistructured interviews represent procedures in which the informational areas to be explored are specified, but the sequence and wording to be used in data gathering are only minimally or moderately predetermined. In these interviews, general guidelines for the interview sequence, such as beginning with the chief complaint and following with episodes of the present illness, may be provided, but the clinician is given latitude to move within this framework. The semistructured interview is useful in some research settings and in most patient-care units. Because of the feasibility of its implementation in regular clinical settings, it can lead to the development of rich data bases reflective of realistic clinical-care processes. In these interviews, deliberate attempts are made to obtain a thorough data base while consistently attending to issues of engagement and validity. Because it does not involve specific sequence and wording, the semistructured interview requires a high degree of sophistication of the clinician. An example of this type of interview is the Initial Evaluation Form (Mezzich, Dow, Rich, Costello, & Himmelhoch, 1981; Mezzich, Dow, Ganguli, Munetz, & Zettler-Segal, 1986).

Empathy and Data Gathering

A gracefully structured interview is an empathic interview. The clinician pointedly attempts to understand the world as the patient sees and feels it. The patient may be unaware of the pieces of data that are required in the diagnostic task; it is the clinician's responsibility to guide the patient into pertinent areas of information while consistently providing a safe environment for the sharing of information. Building a strong alliance with the patient will enhance not only the likelihood of obtaining a valid data base, but also the possibility of the patient's agreeing with the recommendations of the clinician and returning for follow-up. This section offers a brief overview of those concepts on which engagement and data gathering are built.

Concerning the engagement process and the concept of empathy, Carl Rogers (1967) remains a powerful pioneer. His concept of unconditional positive regard contains crucial ideas on creating a safe interpersonal environment in which the patient feels accepted. Unconditional positive regard develops if the clinician conveys the feeling that he or she is there not to judge, but to help the patient understand problem behaviors. In his book *The Skilled Helper,* Egan (1975) described in detail various stages of empathy and the methods of attending to the client's needs. He emphasized the term *attending* as the ability to "be with" the other, and to work with the other. He also discussed the importance of appropriate spontaneity and humor as methods of engaging the client. In a similar vein, Benjamin, in his sensitive book *The Helping Interview* (1969), pointed out the need to develop a genuine relationship with the patient, and to avoid the tendency to hide behind rules, position, or sense of authority.

It is from the fields of counseling and clinical psychology that the majority of substantial research on interviewing processes has originated. Such research has frequently focused on issues concerning empathy, including both verbal and nonverbal elements. An excellent review of this literature, far too vast to be summarized in this chapter, was written by Wiens (1976).

Hall (1966), a social scientist, laid a powerful foundation for the study of how humans use space and coined the term *proxemics* to refer to this field of study. His work ties directly in to the concepts of empathy and the methods by which different cultures demonstrate genuineness and caring. Birdwhistell (1952) developed the sister science of kinesics to investigate the ways in which human beings use the movements of their bodies to convey information. These perspectives, which were growing from the field of sociology, were further developed by the work of Scheflin and Scheflin (1972). In their book, *Body Language and Social Order,* an effort was made to demonstrate the various ways in which body movement and the use of space affect human interaction. In particular, they described the concept of "reciprocal behaviors," according to which the nonverbal and verbal behaviors of one human being trigger a corresponding set of movements and behaviors in another. These reciprocal behaviors frequently feed each other until a particular dynamic is fulfilled. By way of example, Scheflin and Scheflin discussed dominance and submission as mechanisms through which human beings may either deescalate or, conversely, increase the potential for violence.

Psychodynamic theorists have also contributed significantly to the literature on the interviewing process. Whitehorn (1944) and Sullivan (1954) emphasized the interpersonal matrix with regard to the interviewing relationship. Both discussed the need to understand how the patient feels about and reacts to the behavior of the clinician. They also pointed out the influence of relationships from the past on the development of current behavior and emotional conflicts. The book written by Sullivan (1954) concerning psychiatric interviewing was published posthumously and became one of the most influential texts on the topic. Concepts such as *participant observation, the self system,* and *parataxic distortion* became part of the basic terminology used by many psychiatrists in the decades that followed.

A key text in the 1970s was *The Psychiatric Interview in Clinical Practice* written by MacKinnon and Michels (1971). It productively explored the role of underlying defense mechanisms and dynamic issues as they relate to the development of the patient's symptoms as well as to behavior during the interview itself.

In past decades, some authors have tended to downplay the role of diagnosis, perhaps feeling that data gathering and empathic listening were antithetical to each other. More recently, authors have reported that, when diagnostic explorations are conducted skillfully, they tend to increase empathy, as the clinician then understands the phenomenology of the patient's experience. More specifically, Shea (1988) attempted to synthesize principles of interviewing from various schools, including counseling, phenomenology, psychodynamics, and descriptive psychopathology. He discussed engagement techniques hand in hand with strategies for eliciting reliable and valid diagnostic data. Understanding the patient's worldview and phenomenology is accorded great significance, as is the clinician's ability to understand and resolve the patient's resistance.

A creative interplay has started to take place among many disciplinary perspectives. Strict disciplinary boundaries are becoming less valued, and greater interest is developing in the sharing of ideas and perspectives by all mental-health fields. This movement appears to be leading to the development of more flexible and sensitive styles of interviewing for the outpatient clinician. These developments also appear to be enhanced by the use of multiaxial diagnostic systems, which tend to view human interaction as an interplay among systems within a holistic framework.

DIAGNOSIS

It should be pointed out at the outset of this section that, although interviewing is the centerpiece of data gathering in a diagnostic evaluation, it is not the only possible source of pertinent information. Also important to keep in mind are other individuals who may accompany the patient or may be available by telephone. Such individuals may include relatives and associates, as well as health professionals, teachers, and other workers. Other valuable sources of information are written documents accompanying the patient and past clinical records stored in paper files or in computerized memories.

Next, we will discuss issues pertaining to the diagnostic organization of the information gathered from interviews and other sources. In order, we will deal with diagnostic definitions or rules for assigning nosological categories to the patient; the architecture of a diagnostic formulation, particularly in the form of multiaxial schemata; and, finally, current and prospective standard diagnostic systems.

Diagnostic Criteria

A major methodological development aimed at reducing undesirable variability or unreliability in the diagnostic evaluation process is the use of explicit or specific diagnostic criteria. Generically, this procedure involves setting clear, denotative, and objective rules for assigning diagnostic categories to individuals under examination. The clinical information used for making these assignments may have been obtained through unstructured, semistructured, or rigidly structured interview procedures.

It appears that the earliest explicit or specific diagnostic criteria published in the international literature was the set developed by Berner (1969) in Vienna for the diagnosis of psychotic disorders.

More recent sets of explicit psychiatric diagnostic criteria are those developed by Feighner, Robins, Guze, Woodruff, Winokur, and Munoz (1972), the so-called Research Diagnostic Criteria (Spitzer, Endicott, & Robins, 1978), and those included in Axes I and II of the third edition of the *Diagnostic and Statistical Manual* (DSM-III; American psychiatric Association, 1980). These three criteria sets were developed in a sequential line, each building on the previous one.

The Feighner criteria were developed "for use in psychiatric research" and pioneered the design of criteria for a substantial set of diagnostic categories. They represented an institutional effort and embodied the descriptive orientation of the department of psychiatry at Washington University in St. Louis. The diagnostic criteria incorporate both inclusion rules (specifying the features required for the diagnosis under consideration) as well as exclusion rules (specifying features that rule out that diagnosis). They cover 15 diagnostic conditions that, in the opinion of the authors, showed adequate evidence of clinical distinctiveness, longitudinal stability, and, in some cases, high familial loading. These 15 disorders are organic brain syndrome, alcoholism, drug dependence, mania, depression, schizophrenia, antisocial personality, hysteria (Briquet's syndrome), anorexia nervosa, obsessive-compulsive neurosis, phobic neurosis, anxiety neurosis, mental retardation, homosexuality, and transsexualism.

Building on the Feighner criteria, Spitzer *et al.* (1978) developed the so-called research diagnostic criteria (RDC), within the framework of a collaborative project on the psychobiology of depression sponsored by the National Institute of Mental Health (NIMH). The scope of psychopathology covered increased over that covered by the Feighner criteria to include the following 23 disorders: schizophrenia, schizoaffective disorder–manic, schizoaffective disorder–depressed, depressive syndrome superimposed on residual schizophrenia, manic disorder, hypomanic disorder, bipolar with manic (bipolar 1), bipolar with hypomanic (bipolar 2), major depressive disorder, minor depressive disorder, intermittent depressive disorder, panic disorder, generalized anxiety disorder, cyclothymic personality, labile personality, Briquet's disorder (somatization disorder), antisocial personality, alcoholism, drug-use disorder, obsessive-compulsive disorder, phobic disorder, unspecified functional psychosis, and other psychiatric disorders. Also included are several non-mutually-exclusive ways of subtyping some of the important categories, such as major depressive disorder. The clinical information required to formulate RDC diagnoses can be obtained through the Schedule for Affective Disorders (SADS), which was developed by Endiott and Spitzer (1978) for this specific purpose.

The third edition of the *Diagnostic and Statistical Manual of Mental Disorders* (DSM-III; American Psychiatric Association, 1980) represented, in terms of explicit diagnostic criteria, one step further in the developmental line initiated by the Feigner criteria. The DSM-III is described as a diagnostic system later in this chapter, but here, the basic features of its explicit diagnostic criteria are mentioned. Most important, given that the main objective of DSM-III was to articulate regular clinical work rather than just to identify homogeneous patient groups for research, its scope includes all forms of psychopathology. This expansion in coverage involved the consideration of a much larger set of categories than those of the RDC and the Feighner criteria as well as some relaxation in the assignment rules for specific diagnostic categories.

Mention also should be made in this section of the so-called polydiagnostic approach, that is, the concomitant use of several diagnostic criteria sets (e.g., Feighner, RDC, and DSM-III) when evaluating an individual. This approach allows the systematic comparison of various criteria sets in terms of their relations to associated events, social functioning, and illness course and treatment (Strauss & Gift, 1977). In fact, some studies have already been reported in the literature comparing different sets of diagnostic criteria for a single category by using outcome as the external validating criterion (e.g., Brockington, Kendell, & Leff, 1978).

Comprehensive Diagnostic Formulation

Models involving comprehensive diagnostic formulations are usually known as *multiaxial schemata.* This approach consists of the systematic formulation of the patient's condition and its etiological and associated factors in terms of several variables, aspects, or axes, which are thought to have high clinical information value, and which are conceptualized and rated quasi-independently. The word *multiaxial* has become the prevalent characterizing term; less frequently, *multidimensional* and *multiaspectual* have been suggested.

In order to examine the possibilities and problems encompassed by the multiaxial model, it seems appropriate to review its historical roots, the specific multiaxial systems proposed in the literature, and some important trends and issues (Mezzich, 1979, 1985).

Although the impact of multiaxial diagnosis is relatively recent, its origins are not. The contrast between the multiaxial and the conventional, uniaxial diagnostic system may perhaps be traced to the old nosological controversy reviewed by Kendell (1975, p. 60) between, on the one hand, the idealized and abstract Platonic disease entity and, on the other, the more clinical, and therefore closer-to-the-patient, Hippocratic approach.

This contrast was revised early in this century by the argument between Emil Kraepelin, who thoroughly endorsed the disease-entity model, and A. Hoche, who proposed the separation of syndrome and etiology in the diagnostic formulation. Kraepelin's position prevailed, and nothing much was heard about this issue until 1947, when Essen-Möller and Wohlfahrt suggested the amendment of the official Swedish classification of mental disorders separating syndrome and etiology.

Increased interest in the use of multiaxial models in psychiatric diagnosis was then prompted by various symposia on the classification of mental disorders sponsored by the World Health Organization and by the American Psychopathological Association. These symposia reviewed a number of fundamental methodological issues in diagnosis and also some germinal multiaxial ideas (e.g., Rutter, Lebovici, Eisenberg, Sneznevskij, Sadoun, Brooke, & Lin, 1969; Stengel, 1959; Zubin, 1961). More recently, in some way building on the diagnostic separation of syndrome and etiology put forward by Essen-Möller and Wohlfahrt (1947) and by Essen-Möller (1961, 1971), a number of multiaxial models have been proposed in various parts of the world, including England (Rutter, Shaffer, & Shepherd, 1975; Wing, 1970); Germany (Helmchen, 1975; von Cranach, 1977); Japan (Kato, 1977); Sweden, (Ottosson & Perris, 1973); and United States (American Psychiatric Association, 1980; Strauss, 1975). Additionally attesting to the significance of the multiaxial model is the incorporation of a transitional form in the *Diagnostic and Statistical Manual of Mental Disorders* (DSM-III), as well as its serious consideration for possible implementation in the future 10th revision of the *International Classification of Diseases*.

The first formal model for multiaxial psychiatric diagnosis was proposed by Essen-Möller and Wohlfahrt (1947) as a suggestion for the amendment of the official Swedish classification of mental disorders. Later, Essen-Möller (1961, 1971) elaborated on the original separation of syndrome and etiology by subdividing the former into specified syndrome and gross syndrome.

Virtually as pioneering as Essen-Möeller and Wolhfahrt's proposal was the triaxial system developed by Leme Lopes (1954) in Brazil. It contains axes on psychiatric syndromes, premorbid personality, and etiological constellation.

Wing (1970), from the institute of Psychiatry in London, reported on a tetraxial diagnostic system, which includes cause (organic or psychological), psychiatric condition, mental subnormality (severity level coded in addition to "intelligence quotient"), and additional physical illness or handicap. This system has been implemented in the Camberwell psychiatric case register.

Ottosson and Perris (1973), from the psychiatry departments of the Universities of Göteborg and Umeå, respectively, proposed a tetraxial system. This system appears to be a significant elaboration on Essen-Möller's proposal. It separates "severity" as an independent axis and adds an axis on "course." A number of papers have appeared more recently reporting experience with a slightly modified version of this multiaxial system (e.g., von Knorring, Perris, & Jacobsson, 1978).

Helmchen (1975), from the Frei Universität in Berlin, building on experience gained using Essen-Möeller's proposal (1961) and Zeh's suggestions (1962), developed a pentaxial diagnostic system, which includes symptomatology, etiology, time frame, intensity, and certainty or ratings on axes. Noteworthy is that etiological factors are classified according to the timing of their psychopathological impact. Also interesting is that the first two axes are further coded according to "intensity," and all of the first three axes according to "certainty," which constitutes an unusual interaxial arrangement.

Child psychiatrists, probably because of the particular complexity of their field, have long been important contributors to the development of multiaxial diagnostic systems. Rutter *et al.* (1969), as participants in the Fifth WHO Seminar on Psychiatric Diagnosis, proposed a triaxial classification of childhood mental disorders that includes clinical psychiatric syndrome, intellectual level, and medical condition. Later, the reliability of a tetraxial system, developed by adding an axis on abnormal psychosocial situations, was evaluated by Rutter, Shaffer, and Shepherd (1975). The most recent version of this classification has five axes, obtained by removing "specific delays of development" from "clinical psychiatric syndrome" in order to constitute a separate second axis (Rutter, Shaffer, & Sturge, 1975).

There were some relatively early suggestions in the United States for a multiaxial conceptualization of psychiatric nosology (e.g., Ziskind, 1965). More recently, Strauss (1975) proposed the first systematic and comprehensive multiaxial model generated in the united States. It includes axes dealing with symptoms, the duration and course of symptoms, associated factors, personal relationships, and work functioning. The last two axes, which cover the area of social functioning, represent a distinct innovation in the history of multiaxial systems.

In 1980, the American Psychiatric Association issued the third edition of the *Diagnostic and Statistical Manual of Mental Disorders* (DSM-III). Major characteristics of the DSM-III are the use of operational or explicit criteria for assigning patients to diagnostic categories, new groupings of syndromes (e.g., all affective disorders are grouped together), and the implementation of a multiaxial framework. This system includes the following five axes: clinical psychiatric syndrome (which is not a purely symptomatological axis, as it has some categories rated according to either severity, periodicity, or chronicity); personality disorders for adults and specific developmental disorders for children and adolescents; nonmental medical or physical disorders; the severity of psychosocial stressors; and the highest level of adaptive functioning in the past year.

Kato (1977), from the Japanese National Institute of Mental Health, proposed an interesting system based mainly on two axes: "illness" (medically evaluated) and "caseness" (culturally evaluated). Additionally, he endorsed the appropriateness of considering axes on symptomatology, etiology, intelligence level, and personality, but he did not elaborate on them.

Von Cranach (1977) reported on a multiaxial model developed and used in the psychiatry department of the Universität München, West Germany. This model includes five axes: symptomatology, acuity of episode, course of illness, etiology (divided into biological and psychosocial), and personality disorder.

The axes considered in the various systems proposed in several parts of the world could be grouped, according to their content, into the following major types or themes:

1. *Phenomenology:* symptomatology, personality disorder, and intellectual functioning.
2. *Etiological or associated factors:* axes on biological and psychosocial factors conceptualized and organized in various ways. Causation may include predisposing, precipitating, and maintaining factors.
3. *Time frame:* axes dealing with onset, duration, and course of psychopathology.
4. *Social functioning:* axes dealing with work performance, interpersonal relations, and other aspects of adaptive functioning.
5. *Other:* psychopathological severity, certainty, and the "illness" versus "caseness" contrast. It should be noted that some axes, such as "certainty," have a "moderator" meaning rather than being conceptually independent axes.

The potential of the multiaxial approach for improving reliability and validity might be facilitated if new axes were to be formulated in a way that is clear and explicit as well as conceptually distinct and differentiable from others. The following specific problems can be identified in regard to the conceptualization of axial content:

1. *Unclear axial definition,* which may be caused by difficulties in neatly conceptualizing a given axis ("psychosocial stressors" is a good example of such a difficult axis) and/or in operationally and explicitly defining it by means of denotative rather than connotative terms.

2. *Interaxis overlap,* which refers to some mixture of the nature of definitions of two or more axes. Two aces that are particularly vulnerable to such an overlap are "social functioning" and "environmental stressors." For example, "experiencing difficulties at work" may, on the one hand, reflect poor social functioning and, on the other hand, represent an environmental stressor.
3. *Variable axial role of a given condition.* For example, alcoholism may be conceptualized both as an overt psychiatric syndrome and as an etiological factor (Wing, 1970). Another example is personality disturbance, which may be considered under symptomatology, characterogenic etiology, and course (Ottosson & Perris, 1973)

The organization of multiaxial systems involves such methodological issues as the selection of the number of axes, and the number and ranking of statements for each axis.

Decisions about the number of axes in a system entail a consideration of the relative importance given to two conflicting objectives in diagnostic development. One objective is greater comprehensiveness and informational richness of the diagnostic formulation, which would promote the inclusion of as many axes or clinical aspects as possible. The other objective is parsimony, that is, limiting the number of axes in order to prevent overloading the clinician cognitively when she or he is trying to conceptualize the patient's problems and to make management decisions. Our review of the multiaxial systems reported in the literature showed that the modal number of axes per system was five.

Another axial organization issue is the number of statements allowed per axis. These statements refer to the same clinical aspect, rather than to different aspects as in the case of subaxes. The axes to which this issue is relevant are those categorical (rather than dimensional) in their scaling, and they are most typically represented by syndrome or symptomatology. In a syndromic kind of axis, the number of statements explicitly allowed ranges from just one (e.g., Rutter, Shaffer, & Sturge, 1975) to three (e.g., von Knorring *et al.,* 1978) and potentially to even more (e.g., DSM-III). Among those multiaxial systems allowing several statements per axis, some systems require a hierarchical organization of the statements by ranking (e.g., DSM-III), and others do not (e.g., von Knorring *et al.,* 1978).

In regard to their scaling, axes can be either typological or dimensional. A typological axis is structured into categories that are qualitatively different from each other and that can be represented by patient clusters or groups. A common example of a typological axis is syndrome description, which involves a set of states, such as generalized anxiety and paranoid schizophrenia. In contrast, a dimensional axis represents continuous, ordered, quantitative variation. The mathematical scale underlying it may be either of the rank type, in which just ordinal information is considered, or of the interval type, in which information about the size of the differences between objects or points is also considered. Individuals are diagnosed according to a dimensional axis on the basis of their standing on the relevant scale. Examples of dimensional axes are chronicity and level of social functioning.

If we compare their diagnostic merits, a typological axis, on the one hand, has the advantage of its traditional and generalized use in standard diagnostic systems, such as the current edition of the *International Classification of Diseases,* and the associated ample familiarity that clinicians have with such a descriptive arrangement. The predilection for the use of categorical labels may extend beyond the clinical area and may respond to deep psychological needs for simplified description, as suggested by Raven, Berlin, and

Breedlove (1971). On the other hand, a dimensional axis or scale, when applicable, involves a fuller use of the available information than that accomplished with a typological scale. Besides the above considerations, the choice between the use of a typological scale or of a dimensional scale to assess a particular clinical aspect may depend on the informational structure of that aspect, as determined by clinical judgment and/or data-based research. For example, the most accepted way of conceptualizing psychopathological symptomatology, as described in established textbooks and most professional journals, is in terms of syndromes or states, which are categories. Probably because of this, all multiaxial proposals reported in the literature use a typological scale for symptomatology. This does not mean, of course, that dimensional scales could not be used in a complementary fashion in the future if adequate research documents their appropriateness and usefulness for at least some specific psychopathological areas, such as personality disorder. Another clinical aspect is social or adaptive functioning, which has been frequently conceptualized in terms of its level. The two multiaxial proposals (DSM-III; Strauss, 1975), which include this clinical aspect, use dimensional axes for it.

According to the scaling of their component axes, multiaxial diagnostic models can be classified into typological, dimensional, and mixed (Mezzich, 1979).

The typological multiaxial model is composed exclusively of typological axes. In its uniaxial version, it corresponds to traditional and standard diagnostic systems such as the DSM-II (American Psychiatric Association, 1968). The proposal by Essen-Möller (1961, 1971) is an example of the typological multiaxial model.

The dimensional multiaxial model is composed exclusively of dimensional axes. It has mathematical appeal and may be quite appropriate for describing some data sets. However, if not parsimonious enough, its application may involve considerable pragmatic difficulties. Although the dimensional multiaxial model is an interesting theoretical option and has been used with reasonable success for personality description (Eysenck, 1960), not much productive research yielding thorough and specific proposals of an exclusively dimensional form for comprehensive psychiatric diagnosis has been published to date.

The mixed multiaxial model is composed of both typological and dimensional axes. It is a more general and powerful model than the pure typological or dimensional models, as both of these could actually be conceptualized as particular cases of the mixed model. Examples implementing this model are the DSM-III, which has three typological axes and two dimensional ones (the severity of psychosocial stressors and level of adaptive functioning); Rutter, Shaffer, and Sturge's system (1975), which has four typological axes and intelligence level as a dimensional axis; and Strauss's proposal (1975), in which the subaxis on duration of symptoms and the axes on personal relationships and work functioning are dimensional, and two axes and one subaxis are typological. This review clearly shows that most multiaxial systems are of the mixed type. This predominance is probably due to the comprehensiveness and flexibility of the mixed model, which includes both typological and dimensional axes and thus reflects, in part, the complexity and the varied informational structure of important clinical aspects.

In addition to its descriptive role (and the related methodological issues), the multiaxial model has the potential of enhancing treatment planning, by identifying a variety of a patient's problems for which specific treatment modalities may be appropriate. For example, an outpatient may be found to have a chronic major depression (for which antidepressant medications may be useful), dependent personality disorder (which may indicate the need for psychotherapy), hypertension (requiring appropriate medication), and a conflictual marital relationship (suggesting a need for family therapy).

Standard Diagnostic Systems

There are official or seimofficial nosological systems that, because of their wide use, deserve to be mentioned. One of these is the currently official ninth revision of the *International Classification of Diseases* (ICD-9; World Health Organization, 1977). It contains some innovations vis-à-vis its predecessor, such as a glossary of diagnostic categories, but its acceptance across the world seems to have been modest.

The third edition of the *Diagnostic and Statistical Manual of Mental Disorders* (DSM-III), developed by the American Psychiatric Association (1980), contains a number of major innovations and has received widespread attention. Its most important features are the use of explicit or operational criteria for the definition of diagnostic categories and the use of a multiaxial framework. These two features, which represent some of the most important methodological developments of recent years, were discussed in the two preceding sections.

The multiaxial system in the DSM-III (American Psychiatric Association, 1980) includes three typological axes (''I: Clinical Psychiatric Syndromes''; II: Personality and Specific Developmental Disorders''; and ''III: Physical Disorders'') and two dimensional ones (''IV: Severity of Psychosocial Stressors'' and ''V: Highest Level of Adaptive Functioning in the Past Year''). Patients are diagnosed in a typological axis through the use of qualitatively distinct categories, whereas in a dimensional axis, patients are described by an indication of their standing on an interval or rank scale.

Axis I: Clinical Psychiatric Syndromes

Axis I of the DSM-III comprises the catalog of mental disorders (other than personality and specific developmental disorders) and related conditions. Most of these disorders have explicit diagnostic criteria—one of the landmarks of the DSM-III. Some overview comments on the broad categories of Axis I follow.

Reflecting an increase in the interest in and the knowledge about child psychopathology, the DSM-III contains a much expanded and much differentiated set of categories for disorders usually starting in infancy, childhood, or adolescence, in contrast to the few categories in the DSM-II.

Organic mental disorders are divided into two parts. One includes two broad categories with a specified etiology or pathophysiology (i.e., dementias arising in the senium and presenium and substance-induced organic mental disorders). The second section corresponds to organic mental disorders described in terms of behavioral syndromes, the etiology or pathophysiology of which either is noted under Axis III (''Physical Disorders'') or is unknown.

Substance-use disorders cover both alcohol and other drugs. They are essentially classified as either abuse or dependence (characterized by manifestations of tolerance and/or withdrawal). Drug-use syndromes newly considered in the DSM-III (in contrast to the DSM-II) are phencyclidine (PCP) abuse and tobacco dependence.

The schizophrenic disorders have a more specific description than that in the DSM-II, including the requirement of a 6-month chronicity. The ''simple'' subtype of the DSM-II is omitted, and schizoaffective disorders are listed separately.

Psychotic disorders not elsewhere classified make up an interesting new broad category. It includes schizophreniform disorder, having all the cross-sectional features of schizophrenia but a chronicity of less than 6 months and more than 2 weeks; brief reactive psychosis, which appears immediately following a recognizable psychosocial stressor;

schizoaffective disorder, which does not have explicit diagnostic criteria and is used whenever a differentiation between affective disorder and either schizophrenic or schizophreniform disorder is not possible; and atypical psychosis, which encompasses two main meanings: a psychosis not fitting the definitions of the specified psychotic disorders or a psychosis unspecified because of inadequate information.

The section on affective disorders constitutes one of the major innovations in the DSM-III. First, major affective disorders are divided principally into bipolar disorder (manic or depressed with a history of mania) and major depression (which has quite an encompassing definition and prevails over concomitant neurotic syndromes of various kinds). Other specific affective disorders (cyclothymic and dysthymic disorders) represent milder and chronic affective conditions. Atypical bipolar and depressive disorders represent unspecified or residual categories.

A number of traditional neuroses are considered next, under the headings of anxiety, somatoform, and dissociative disorders.

Psychosexual disorders are much more differentiated than in the DSM-II and include gender-identity disorders, paraphilias, psychosexual dysfunctions, and the controversial ego-dystonic homosexuality.

Adjustment disorders represent nonpsychotic reactions to stressful situations and are classified according to the predominant affect or behavior shown.

Psychological factors affecting physical condition replace the ''psychophysiological'' or ''psychosomatic'' disorders of traditional systems. Their diagnosis involves both indicating the presence of such psychological factors in Axis I and specifying the corresponding physical conditions in Axis III.

A set of ''V codes'' is provided for conditions not attributable to a mental disorder that are nevertheless a focus of attention or treatment.

Axis II: Personality and Specific Developmental Disorders

This axis tends to represent stable behavioral handicaps. Personality disorders in the DSM-III cover most of the characteristic conditions that appear in the DSM-II. Exceptions are the addition of schizotypal, avoidant, narcissistic, and borderline personality disorders; the deletions of inadequate and asthenic personality disorders; and the transfer to various Axis I sections of cyclothymic and explosive personality disorders. Specific developmental disorders represent an innovation in the DSM-III. It reflects the axis on developmental delays that appear in the multiaxial system for child psychopathology developed by Rutter, Shaffer, and Sturge (1975) under the sponsorship of the World Health Organization.

Axis III: Physical Disorders

Axis III includes any current physical disorders or conditions relevant to the understanding or management of the individual. Such conditions are cataloged in the nonmental disorder sections of the *International Classification of Diseases* adapted for U.S. use (ICD-9-CM; U.S. National Center for Health Statistics, 1978).

Axis IV: Severity of Psychosocial Stressors

Axis IV assesses the psychosocial stressors judged to have been significant contributors to the development or exacerbation of the current disorder.

First, specific psychosocial stressors (e.g., the death of a sister) are identified and listed in order of importance. Then, the overall stressor severity is evaluated on a 7-point scale.

Axis V: Highest Level of Adaptive Functioning in the Past Year

Axis V assesses an individual's highest level of adaptive functioning (for at least a few months) during the past year.

Adaptive functioning is conceptualized mainly as a composite of social relations (the breadth and quality of interpersonal relations with the family, friends, and other people) and occupational functioning (the consistency and quality of performance as worker, student, or homemaker). Use of leisure time is considered accessorily.

A format for facilitating the formulation of DSM-III diagnoses and a description of its use with a large psychiatric population was presented by Mezzich, Coffman, and Goodpastor (1982).

The Revised DSM-III

Recently, the American Psychiatric Association (1987) issued a revision of the third edition of its diagnostic manual. The DSM-III-R represents a moderate modification of the DSM-III, primarily involving an adjustment of the diagnostic criteria in a large number of categories. Less frequent are changes in the diagnostic categories themselves.

The multiaxial system of the DSM-III-R contains some interesting changes. The Axes I and II categories may be further qualified in terms of their severity. Axis II has been expanded by the addition of retardation and pervasive developmental disorders, transferred from Axis I. Personality descriptions may be enriched by use of a catalog of noncoded defense mechanisms. In Axis IV, the clinician is encouraged to list the identified psychosocial stressors, and to classify these into predominantly acute or predominantly chronic, depending on the duration of most stressors' being less or more than 6 months. As before, a global rating of stressor severity is also to be made. In Axis V, there are two major changes. One is the consideration of not only occupational and interpersonal functioning but also symptomatological status, all rated together through the use of a 100-point global functioning scale. The other change involves the time frames of the assessment, including not only the highest level in the past year, but also current functioning.

Development of the ICD-10

Looking to the future, it should be mentioned that the World Health Organization is in the process of developing a 10th revision of the *International Classification of Diseases* (ICD-10), which is expected to be implemented in 1994. In contrast to previous revisions, this one is aimed at helping not only statisticians and public health professionals, but also clinical practitioners and researchers. One of the major features of the revision is the use of two major levels of specificity in diagnostic definitions. One, labeled "Diagnostic Guidelines," which is intended primarily for regular clinical care, is midway between the general and connotative definitions of the ICD-9 and the quite strict criteria of the DSM-III. The other, labeled "Research Criteria," is much more demanding and specific.

SUMMARY

This chapter has reviewed the history, the current status, and promising developments in interviewing and diagnosis, as they apply to outpatient care. In regard to interviewing, the task-oriented perspective, structural types, and the challenge of combining empathy with systematic data-gathering were discussed. Concerning diagnosis, relatively recent methodological developments, such as explicit diagnostic criteria and multiaxial schemata, were considered. Finally, an outline of current and upcoming standard diagnostic systems was offered.

REFERENCES

American Psychiatric Association. (1980). *Diagnostic and statistical manual of mental disorders* (3rd ed.; DSM-III). Washington, D.C.: Author.

American Psychiatric Association. (1987). *Diagnostic and statistical manual of mental disorders* (3rd ed.; DSM-III-R). Washington, DC: Author.

Benjamin, A. (1969). *The helping interview.* Boston: Houghton Mifflin.

Berner, P. (1969). Der Lebensabend der Paranoiker. *Wien Zietschrift Nervenheilkunda, 27,* 115–161.

Birdwhistell, M. L. (1952). *Introduction to kinesis: An annotation system for analysis of body motion and gesture.* Louisville, KY: University of Louisville Press.

Brockington, I. F., Kendell, R. E., & Leff, J. P. (1978). Definitions of schizophrenia: Concordance and prediction of outcome. *Psychological Medicine, 8,* 387–398.

Egan, G. (1975). *The skilled helper: A model for systematic helping and interpersonal relating.* Monterey, CA: Brooks Cole.

Endicott, J., & Spitzer, R. L. (1978). A diagnostic interview: The schedule for affective disorders and schizophrenia. *Archives of General Psychiatry, 35,* 837–844.

Essen-Möller, E. (1961). On classification of mental disorders. *Acta Psychiatrica Scandinavica, 37,* 119–126.

Essen-Möller, E. (1971). Suggestions for further improvement of the international classification of mental disorders. *Psychological Medicine, 1,* 308–311.

Essen-Möller, E., & Wohlfahrt, S. (1947). Suggestions for the amendment of the official Swedish classification of mental disorders. *Acta Psychiatrica Scandinavica Supplement, 47,* 551–555.

Eysenck, H. J. (1960). *The structure of human personality.* New York: Macmillan.

Feighner, J. P., Robins, E., Guze, S. B., Woodruff, R. A., Winokur, G., & Munoz, R. (1971). Diagnostic criteria for use in psychiatric research. *Archives of General Psychiatry, 26,* 57–63.

Hall, E. T. (1966). *The hidden dimension.* New York: Doubleday.

Helmchen, H. (1975). Schizophrenia: Diagnostic concepts in the ICD-8. In M. H. Lader (Ed.), Studies in schizophrenia. *British Journal of Psychiatry, Special Publication, 10,* 10–18.

Kato, M. (1977). *Multiaxial diagnosis in adult psychiatry.* Paper presented at the VIth World Congress of Psychiatry, Honolulu, HA.

Kendell, R. E. (1975). *The role of diagnosis in psychiatry.* Oxford: Blackwell.

Langsley, D. G., & Hollender, M. H. (1982). The definition of a psychiatrist. *American Journal of Psychiatry, 139,* 81–85.

Lazare, A. (1979). *Outpatient psychiatry diagnosis and treatment.* Baltimore: Williams & Wilkins.

Leme Lopes, J. (1954). As dimensões do diagnóstico psiquiátrico. Rio de Janeiro: Agir.

MacKinnon, R., & Michels, R. (1971). *The psychiatric interview in clinical practice.* Philadelphia: Saunders.

Mezzich, J. E. (1979). Patterns and issues in multiaxial psychiatric diagnosis. *Psychological Medicine, 9,* 125–137.

Mezzich, J. E. (1985). Multiaxial diagnostic systems in psychiatry. In H. I. Kaplan & B. J. Sadock (Eds.), *Comprehensive textbook of psychiatry* (4th ed.). Baltimore: Williams & Wilkins.

Mezzich, J. E., Coffman, G. A., & Goodpastor, S. M. (1982). A format for DSM-III diagnostic formulation: Experience with 1,111 consecutive patients. *American Journal of Psychiatry, 1139,* 591–596.

Mezzich, J. E., Dow, J. T., Rich, C. L., Costello, A. J., & Himmelhoch, J. M. (1981). Developing an efficient clinical information system for a comprehensive psychiatric institute: 2. Initial evaluation form. *Behavior Research Methods and Instrumentation, 13,* 464–478.

Mezzich, J. E., Dow, J. T., Ganguli, R., Munetz, J. R., & Zettler-Segal, M. (1986). Computerized initial and discharge evaluations. In J. E. Mezzich (Ed.), *Clinical care and information systems in psychiatry.* Washington, DC: American Psychiatric Press.

Ottosson, J. O., & Perris, C. (1973). Multidimensional classification of mental disorders. *Psychological Medicine, 3,* 238–243.

Raven, P. H., Berlin, B., & Breedlove, D. E. (1971). The origins of taxonomy. *Science, 174,* 1210–1213.

Richardson, S. A., Dohrenwend, B. S., & Klein, D. (1965). *Interviewing: Its forms and functions.* New York: Basic Books.

Robins, L. N., Helzer, J. E., Croughan, J., & Ratcliff, K. S. (1981). National Institute of Mental Health Diagnostic Interview Schedule: Its history, characteristics, and validity. *Archives of General Psychiatry, 10,* 41–61.

Rutter, M., Shaffer, D., & Shepherd, M. (1975). *A multiaxial classification of child psychiatric disorders.* Geneva: World Health Organization.

Rutter, M., Shaffer, D., & Sturge, C. (1975). *A guide to a multiaxial classification scheme for psychiatric disorders in childhood and adolescence.* London: Institute of Psychiatry.

Rutter, M., Lebovici, S., Eisenberg, L., Sneznevskij, A. V., Sadoun, R., Brooke, E., & Lin, T. Y. (1969). A tri-axial classification of mental disorders in childhood. *Journal of Child Psychology and Psychiatry, 38,* 381–389.

Scheflin, A. E., & Scheflin, A. (1972). *Body language and social order.* Englewood Cliffs, NJ: Prentice-Hall.

Shea, S. C. (1988). *Psychiatric interviewing: The art of understanding.* Philadelphia: Saunders.

Spitzer, R. L., Endicott, J., & Robins, E. (1978). Research diagnostic criteria. *Archives of General Psychiatry, 35,* 773–782.

Stengel, E. (1959). Classification of mental disorders. *Bulletin of the World Health Organization, 21,* 601–663.

Strauss, J. S. (1975). A comprehensive approach to psychiatric diagnosis. *American Journal of Psychiatry, 132,* 1193–1197.

Strauss, J. S., & Gift, T. E. (1977). Choosing an approach for diagnosing schizophrenia. *Archives of General Psychiatry, 34,* 1248–1253.

Strub, R. L., & Black, W. (1977). *The mental status examination in neurology.* Philadelphia: Davis.

Sullivan, H. S. (1954). *The psychiatric interview.* New York: Norton.

U.S. National Center for Health Statistics. (1978). *The international classification of diseases* (9th rev.); *Clinical modification (ICD-9-CM)* Ann Arbor, MI: U.S. National Center for Health Statistics.

von Cranach, M. (1977). Categorical vs. multiaxial classification. Paper presented at the VI World Congress of Psychiatry, Honolulu, Hawaii.

von Knorring, L., Perris, C., & Jacobsson, L. (1978). A multi-aspects classification of mental disorders: Experiences from clinical routine work and preliminary studies of inter-rater reliability. *Acta Psychiatrica Scandinavica, 58,* 401–412.

Whitehorn, J. C. (1944). Guide to interviewing and clinical personality study. *Archives of Neurology and Psychiatry, 52,* 197–216.

Wiens, A. M. (1976). The assessment interview. In I. Weiner (Ed.), *Clinical methods in psychology.* New York: Wiley.

Wing, L. (1970). Observations on the psychiatric section of the International Classification of Diseases and the British Glossary of Mental Disorders. *Psychological Medicine, 1,* 79–85.

World Health Organization. (1977). *Manual of the Ninth Revision of the International Classification of Diseases (ICD-9).* Geneva: Author.

Zeh, W. (1962). Bemerkugen zu einem Klassifications vorschlag der psychischen Storungen on Erik Essen-Möller, Lund. *Nervenarzt, 33,* 404–410.

Zubin, J. (1961). *Field studies in the mental disorders.* New York: Grune & Stratton.

2

Differentiating Physical from Psychiatric Disorders

RICHARD C. W. HALL, THOMAS P. BERESFORD, FREDERIC C. BLOW, AND ANNE K. HALL

INTRODUCTION

In 1980, the American Psychiatric Association restated the need for careful medical evaluation of psychiatric patients by incorporating physical disorders as one of three diagnostic axes. In its third edition of the *Diagnostic and Statistical Manual* (DSM-III), the diagnostic criteria further require the exclusion of physical causes of mental symptoms: the clinician must determine that the diagnoses of Axis I are "not due to an organic mental disorder." The impact of these changes is profound: the psychiatrist must consider the effects that an underlying medical disorder may have in producing specific psychiatric symptoms, and he or she must examine and further evaluate patients to rule out such disorders.

The appropriateness and timeliness of these new guidelines cannot be overemphasized. Health care in the United States is undergoing a dramatic transition. As federal cutbacks and limitations increase and support for capitated systems develops, clinicians and hospitals will face increasing pressures to provide fewer diagnostic services. Many patients with chronic psychiatric disorders will find themselves refused access to inpatient diagnostic and treatment facilities. The current insurance-industry trend toward excluding psychiatric disorders wherever possible and toward limiting the benefits payable for their evaluation and treatment will place psychiatric patients and the physicians responsible for them at risk. The danger inherent in this system is that both provider and patient will be

RICHARD C. W. HALL • Psychiatric Programs, Florida Hospital, Orlando, Florida 32803. THOMAS P. BERESFORD and FREDERIC C. BLOW • Michigan Alcohol Program, University of Michigan Medical Center, Ann Arbor, Michigan 48109. ANNE K. HALL • Florida Hospital, Orlando, Florida 32803.

pressured to accept a benign-neglect model of care rather than to engage in an active diagnostic and treatment process. As these constraints become more universal, the need will increase for careful outpatient diagnostic evaluation of patients to rule out associated physical illnesses.

It is our contention that a new standard of practice must evolve requiring the careful medical evaluation of outpatients with specific symptom constellations at the outset of their treatment and annually thereafter. Ongoing research in large population samples will determine the most efficient and most productive systems for such evaluations. This chapter is devoted to a review of these issues and to specific suggestions for the practicing clinician on how best to effect the outpatient evaluation.

HISTORICAL OVERVIEW

In 1912, Bonhoffer wrote of the need to examine carefully patients with psychiatric symptoms. He documented that both morbidity and mortality were higher for psychiatric patients than for the general population. He suggested that psychiatric patients were at particular risk for the presence of concurrent physical illnesses. His observations were later confirmed by others (Alstrom, 1942; Babigiam & Odoroff, 1969; Malzberg, 1952; Odegard, 1951, 1953).

The study by Babigiam and Odoroff (1969) is of particular interest because it defines the mortality found in patients receiving psychiatric treatment both in the hospital and in the clinic, in both public and private sectors. All of the previous studies had suggested that mortality and morbidity rates were higher in psychiatric inpatients. These findings were not surprising when one took into consideration the effects of such variables as overcrowding, poor nutrition, infectious diseases, and the generally low socioeconomic class of state hospital inpatients. In contrast, Babigiam and Odoroff's study dealt with people of all social classes and with individuals seen as outpatients, so that these institutionally determined variables id not come into play. His study, using the Monroe County register from Rochester, New York, permitted a detailed follow-up of any county resident who came in contact with any provider of psychiatric care. The findings were dramatic. Psychiatric patients of all types experienced an increased mortality risk that was 2.5 to 3 times greater than that in a comparable sample of the general population. This report closely matched previous reports of Alstrom (1942) and Odegard (1951, 1953).

The Monroe County study found that white male psychiatric patients were 1.2 times more likely to die of neoplasm than their matched nonpsychiatric counterparts, 2.5 times more likely to die of diseases of the central nervous system, 2.6 times more likely to die of circulatory disease, and 3.5 times more likely to die a respiratory death. The incidence of fatal digestive-system disorders was 3.1 times higher than in a matched population of nonpsychiatric controls. Additionally, the psychiatric population was 8 times more likely to die of suicide and 2.9 times more likely to die of accident (Babigiam & Odoroff, 1969).

White female psychiatric patients were 1.5 times more likely than controls to die of cancer, 2.2 times more likely to experience a fatal nervous-system disease, 3.5 times more likely to develop a circulatory disorder, and 4 times more likely to die of respiratory failure. The investigators concluded:

> All evidence indicates a higher relative risk of death in the register population (i.e., psychiatric patients), than in the general population; the relative risk of death for the registered group when adjusted for age, sex, marital status and socioeconomic status is three times that of the general county population. (Babigiam & Odoroff, 1969, p. 470).

When these figures were adjusted to remove the chronically ill, the aged, and the alcoholic, the relative risk of death for psychiatric patients remained 1.5 to 2 times that of the general population.

The prevalence of physical disorders in psychiatric outpatients seen for routine medical evaluation or in emergency situations is also high. Eastwood and Trevelyan (1972) studied 1,471 patients in a London group practice. They matched 124 cases with psychiatrically well controls and carefully evaluated both groups for physical illness. The psychiatric patients had a significantly greater number of physical diseases of all types than did the controls. Equally important, these researchers observed a clear association between the severity of the psychiatric illness and the number and severity of the physical illnesses present. The patients experiencing the most severe psychiatric dysfunction were those most likely to be suffering from multiple physical illnesses. The severely ill psychiatric patients in this sample comprised only 17% of the total population but were found to suffer from 52.4% of the major physical illnesses diagnosed.

Although physical illnesses are most likely to be found in psychiatrically severely ill patients, their chance of occurrence is also increased in patients presenting with more routine psychiatric complaints. Roessler and Greenfield (1961) evaluated 500 university students seen in the psychiatric outpatient clinic at the University of Wisconsin. These students were matched with a control group of 500 nonpsychiatric, same-sex students. The investigators found that, in 12 of 13 disease categories, the psychiatric patients had a higher incidence of illness than the controls except for the occurrence of malignant tumors. Specifically, psychiatric patients had a higher overall incidence of headache and of gastrointestinal, gynecological, neurological, allergic, inflammatory, upper respiratory, endocrine, and skin disorders than the control group. One of the issues raised was whether these students simply came more frequently to the clinic because they were in need of attention. Review of the records showed that the higher utilization rate was associated with the presence of documented signs and symptoms and that these patients were seen because of an increased need for specific medical treatment.

Summers, Munoz, Read, and Marsh (1981) also demonstrated the utility of physical examinations of psychiatric patients. They examined 75 unselected psychiatric patients admitted to a private hospital. They classified physical findings as "old" if they had been known to the patient or the examiner before the examination. Careful physical examinations of 75 patients yielded a total of 611 findings; 65% were totally new. Each patient averaged 5.3 new physical exam findings and 2.8 old findings. Of the 611 findings, 398 (64%) were considered significant enough to require further medical evaluation. The examination findings led to the consideration of unsuspected physical illness in 42.7% of the subjects, and in 33% of the subjects, they led to the consideration of a medical cause of the psychiatric symptoms. A specific medical cause of the psychiatric symptoms was confirmed in 14 of the 25 patients (18.6%).

In a careful review of the literature, LaBruzza (1981) concluded that 1 of every 20 patients who presents for an initial psychiatric evaluation has psychiatric symptoms that are produced by an underlying medical disorder. Bunce, Jones, Badger, and Jones (1982), in a careful review of the literature, noted that of the 2,395 psychiatric outpatients reported in the literature for whom physical examinations were performed, 50% had a demonstrated physical illness; 52% of the 1,448 inpatients reported on were found to have associated medical disease.

In our study of 658 consecutive psychiatric outpatients who presented for emergency evaluation at a community mental-health center, we found that 9.1% had medically induced psychiatric symptoms. That is, their underlying medical illness either had specifically caused or had exacerbated their psychiatric symptoms to an extent that required intervention. Seventy-seven percent of these patients were unaware that a physical disorder existed. Although many of these patients had a family physician and many had reported that they had been evaluated within the preceding year, a careful review of their records showed that they had received only cursory attention for specific symptoms such as headache or sore throat. Fewer than 1% of the patients who reported having a family doctor had evidence of a careful physical examination during the preceding year. The most important question asked to determine whether they had been carefully examined was, "Did your doctor ask you to remove all of your clothes and place you in a gown before examining you?" (Hall, Popkin, & Devaul, 1977). The psychiatric symptoms that were most likely to be associated with a causal physical disorder were visual hallucinations, distortions, and illusions. We have come to realize that these symptoms indicate organic disease until it is proven otherwise. The most frequent psychiatric presentations caused by underlying medical disorders were organic mental syndromes, anxiety disorders, and depression. Twenty-eight percent of the patients who we believed had developed psychiatric symptoms because of their medical illness presented with symptoms suggesting a diagnosis of a nonspecific acute psychosis (Hall *et al.,* 1977).

In a detailed series of studies, Koranyi (1972) evaluated 2,090 psychiatric clinic patients and was able to demonstrate that 43% suffered from at least one major medical illness. In approximately one half of the cases, this disorder had been unknown to the referring source. After identifying the 902 patients who had associated medical illnesses, koranyi carefully evaluated each case and concluded that the patient's underlying physical illness had produced psychiatric symptoms in 18% of the cases, had aggravated them in 51%, and coexisted in 31%.

In evaluating the response of over 1,000 patients to physical examination, Koranyi noted that only 2 patients refused a physical. The overwhelming majority greeted careful examination with strong positive feelings. Rather than detracting from it, physical examination enhanced the therapeutic relationship and facilitated the work of psychotherapy by making the patient feel that the physician had taken his or her complaints seriously and had carefully considered all diagnostic possibilities.

In another subset, Koranyi (1972) examined 100 patients and found that two thirds had not been evaluated adequately before referral for psychiatric treatment, even though they had been seen at other health-care facilities. One half had not been evaluated at all prior to referral. In this group, unsuspected physical illness was found to be the exclusive cause of the patients' emotional condition in 12% of cases and to have aggravated the psychiatric symptoms in an additional 35%. This study illustrates the necessity of further examining the patient who has been referred by another clinician. In fact, referring physicians expect the patient to be carefully evaluated following their referral.

The impact of this work on an established mental-health system was studied by Koran (1985). Pursuant to California Bill 929, he and his associates undertook a study of the prevalence of undiagnosed and untreated physical diseases in patients under the care of county mental-health systems in four California counties. The study included 529 patients seen at eight mental-health-program sites. Koran and his team obtained a thorough medical history, a comprehensive physical examination, and a panel of laboratory tests for each patient. Five to seven months after initial evaluation, 165 patients were reevaluated. Another 557 mentally ill patients seen at a university psychiatric clinic served as controls. The criteria for inclusion in the study were that the patients were (1) stable and in treatment; (2) had no insurance or financial resources; and (3) were not acutely disturbed.

The inclusion criteria might actually have diminished the incidence of findings, as previous work has shown that the likelihood of associated physical disease increases as the severity of the illness becomes more profound, and that it is higher in acutely distressed patients.

Nevertheless, Koran's team found that 45% of the patients had "acute, important physical disease(s)." Of these patients, 22% had their disease detected at the time of intake into the mental health system, and in 23% of the cases, the disease remained undiagnosed. An interesting note is that the disease was known to the patient in 16% of the cases but was not known to the mental health system, a finding suggesting that a careful medical history had not been obtained. Of the patients studied, 16% had newly detected diseases; 18% of patients were found to have a physical disease that was judged to have caused or exacerbated their mental disorder. Of the diseases that were considered causal, 84% were detected at intake, and 16% were missed. Of those diseases that were felt to have exacerbated the patients' psychiatric symptoms, only 45% were detected at intake, and 55% were missed.

Extrapolating these data to the entire California mental-health system suggests that 23,000 patients have mental disorders produced by physical disease. Of these, 19,200 are known, and 3,800 remain unknown. An additional 24,500 patients have physical illnesses that exacerbate their mental disorders, of which 9,600 are known and 14,900 remain unknown. The investigators further noted that patients whose physical disease was known to the mental health system were as likely to be receiving inadequate or ineffective medical care (36%) as patients whose physical disease was not known to the system. When one considers the amount spent on medically evaluating these patients ($16 per patient at the community mental-health centers and $88 per patient at the state hospitals), the findings are remarkably good. Koran (1985) also demonstrated that patients who had restricted access to a physician were more likely to be physically ill (54% vs. 36%), more likely to have previously undetected physical illnesses, and more likely to suffer from a disease that was specifically related to their mental disease (25% vs. 9%). This study supports the pressing need for the availability of more physicians in such systems.

CURRENT THEORETICAL IMPLICATIONS

Several longitudinal studies have attempted to explore the relationship between mental and physical health and to define psychological correlates for the development of subsequent medical illnesses. A small number of such studies are available at this time for review. Paffenbarger *et al.* in a longitudinal follow-up study design (Paffenbarger, Notkin, Kreuger, Wolf, Thorne, LeBauer, & Williams, 1966), demonstrated an association of early parental loss, only-child status, and "sociophysiologic exhaustion" during late adolescence with subsequent cardiac mortality. In further follow-up, they showed that individuals with a "high emotional index" during late adolescence were more likely to develop cardiac pathology in later life (Paffenbarger, Notkin, Kreuger, Wolf, Thorne, LaBauer, & Williams, 1966). The same investigators demonstrated that subjective concern about physical health, the practice of monitoring one's own heartbeat, and a subjective perception of exhaustion, coupled with secretiveness and seclusiveness, predisposed individuals to the development of subsequent cardiovascular disease and stroke (Paffenbarger & Wing, 1967). Later, these researchers were able to show that the expectations associated with being a firstborn child bore a relationship to the development of subsequent hypertension (Paffenbarger, Thorne, & Wing, 1968). In a prospective study of medical students, Thomas and Duezynski (1974) showed that a correlation exists between lack of family closeness and the later development of malignant tumors. Other work has shown that a similar lack of family bonding is associated with an increased incidence of mental symptoms.

Vaillant's benchmark studies (1978a,b) further defined the relationship between emotional and physical illness. He studied men who suffered from illnesses considered psychosomatic, such as ulcerative colitis, hypertension, and asthma. He compared the psychosomatic group with men who had not experienced any of these illnesses and with a third cohort of men who later developed serious irreversible physical disease. Vaillant showed that psychological factors were more pronounced in the men with serious irreversible physical illnesses than in the group who had no significant illness or in those who had "psychosomatic" disorders. He also demonstrated that men with poor psychological health were more likely to become ill and more likely to consult their physicians because of significant illness.

Physical illnesses can produce or exacerbate mental symptoms through several mechanisms:

1. The underlying disease may produce a direct physical effect on the central nervous system, altering its structure and function. Psychiatric symptoms may thus be produced by such factors as brain tumor, head trauma, central nervous system infection, aneurysm, and penetrating trauma.

2. The disease may produce a metabolic derangement that alters the function of the central nervous system without affecting its structure. Such conditions occur commonly in anorexic and bulimic patients, diabetics, and individuals with endocrine disease.

3. A disease or its treatment can alter or distort sensory input and produce reactive psychiatric symptoms. Conditions such as chronic progressive deafness, cataracts, black-patch psychosis, and slowly progressive spinal-cord lesions can produce symptoms of paranoia, hallucinations, or perceptual delusions.

4. Medicines can produce toxic symptoms resembling psychiatric conditions. The Boston Collaborative Drug Surveillance Study (1971) of 9,000 nonpsychiatric general-hospital patients demonstrated that 3% developed significant psychiatric symptoms as a direct result of drug treatment with nonpsychiatric medications. Hoffman (1982) showed that nonpsychiatric medications often produce psychiatric symptoms that prompt psychiatric hospitalization. Most patients present with delirium or depression, and their drugs are not initially suspected as a cause of symptoms at the time of referral. In Hoffman's study, medications had been previously suspected as a cause of toxic delirium in only 3 of 13 cases. Psychotropic drugs may also produce specific psychiatric symptoms. Examples include the paradoxical agitation and excitement seen in the elderly following the administration of benzodiazepines or barbiturates, reserpine-associated depression and impotence, depression following the administration of other antihypertensives, and agitated psychosis following the administration of bromocriptine, to mention only a few.

5. Medical illnesses may produce discrete psychiatric symptoms as a result of their disrupting or threatening the patient's perception of his or her existence, by impairing his or her ability to cope, or by impairing his or her ability to meet obligations. In this context, illnesses may aggravate unresolved conflicts, produce dysphoric states, or impair the patient's ability to meet economic, social, or sexual demands. The illness may thereby weaken self-esteem and sense of security. Psychotherapy, with careful medical treatment and the mobilization of support systems, is the appropriate treatment strategy in such cases.

6. Similarly, physical illness may disrupt the patient's body image or function and may result in emotional reactions that are delayed or displaced, later appearing as sleep disorders or anxiety. Such displacement reactions are common following radical mastectomy, amputation, spinal injury, and colostomy. An exploration of the impact of these medical changes on the patient and his or her behavior often results in significant improvement in the patient's psychiatric condition.

7. Medical illnesses can disrupt homeostatic regulatory mechanisms and thus lead to specific and discrete symptoms. Examples include the disruption of the normal sleep cycle by medications or by treatment in an intensive-care or burn unit.

The clinician must realize that psychiatric symptoms are *nonspecific* and are significantly influenced by such moderating variables as the patient's constitution, previous experience, specific skills and attitudes, current social situation, emotional state before the onset of the illness, and its rate of progression. The most important variables determining the clinical presentation include the degree of cerebral impairment and the rapidity of changes in the internal milieu. Rapid alterations of brain function are more likely to produce severe disturbances in cognition and behavior than are slowly developing changes. Any illness that disrupts the patient's ability to process incoming information is particularly likely to produce emotional reactions and behavioral symptoms. Reduced sensory input and diminished ability to process information result in disorganized thought patterns and a blending of current and past reality that may simulate a psychotic state.

TECHNICAL METHODS AND STRATEGIES FOR INTERVENTION

The most important element in the detection of physical illness in psychiatric patients is administrative support for the development of a system to evaluate patients. Guidelines for processing and evaluating large number of patients in an efficient manner are easy to establish. Sadly, much of the debate concerning the evaluation of psychiatric patients hinges not on the science or the practical aspects of developing caring systems, but on the willingness of the systems to find illnesses that will require treatment. One administrator in our memory put it bluntly: "We don't want better diagnosis and case finding; if we define disorders, we'll be obligated to treat them." As we move toward a reduced allocation of resources and fewer available inpatient days, we must expend a greater proportion of resources on outpatient diagnostic evaluation and specialty diagnostic units. If we do so, we will not find too little. We may find too much.

The information needed to develop a coherent evaluative process is readily available and can be rapidly implemented by any organization choosing to do so. It is clear that the most common psychiatric presentations for patients with unrecognized physical illnesses include organic mental disorders, depression, anxiety states, schizophreniform psychosis, and agitated, maniclike psychosis. it is also clear that a significant number of patients seen in outpatient psychiatric systems have symptoms produced or exacerbated by underlying physical illnesses, and that, on the basis of the presentation alone, it is difficult to distinguish these physically induced psychiatric symptoms from those that result from purely "functional" causes. Medical symptoms are often incorporated into the patient's psychiatric delusions. Medically ill patients with psychiatric problems often experience difficulty in communicating adequately with their examining physician. It is paramount, therefore, that a detailed physical and laboratory examination be undertaken to evaluate such patients properly.

A careful medical workup is indicated for patients presenting with acute psychosis, anxiety, and mood disorders, and particularly for patients who have their first onset of psychiatric symptoms after the age of 30. Most patients are unaware of the medical illnesses that cause their psychiatric symptoms, although it has been shown that as many as one in six, if carefully questioned, can provide the interviewer with a specific medical cause for her or his symptoms. Cardiovascular, endocrine, central-nervous-system, pulmonary, and infectious disorders are most likely to produce psychiatric symptoms. Endocrine and metabolic disorders are the most frequent causes of medically induced psychiatric symptoms in women, whereas cardiovascular and pulmonary diseases predominate in men. In both men and women, prescribed, over-the-counter, and illicitly obtained drugs are a common cause of such symptoms.

At the time of initial outpatient evaluation, adequate time should be allocated to obtaining a careful history. We routinely provide the patient with a life history questionnaire to be completed before the time of their visit (see Figure 1). This form includes general historical information; two different reviews of systems; measurements of social function, anxiety, and depression; and elements of past social history, past medical history, and family history. It provides an important data base and can serve as a focus for discussion during the interview. The clinician can quickly review this form, and it may call attention to elements not discussed during the interview. A specific symptom-based review of systems is also given to the patient (see Table 1). Previous studies have suggested that four or more positive items on this checklist are associated with a high incidence of positive findings of organic disease (Hall, Popkin, Devaul, Faillace, & Stickney, 1978).

During the course of the interview, several factors are helpful in suggesting the presence of an underlying medical disorder. These conditions are most likely to occur in individuals who develop their initial psychiatric symptoms after the age of 30, and particularly after the age of 40. They are more common in individuals who present with symptoms of major affective disorder, anxiety, or acute psychotic states, as well as in individuals with mental status findings suggestive of organicity. Organic factors should be considered in patients who develop psychiatric symptoms during or shortly after the development of a major medical illness or after being started on medications that are known to produce psychiatric side effects. The onset of psychiatric symptoms in the absence of any apparent life stress or psychic precipitant should also raise concern. Organic factors are more likely in patients with a history of alcohol and substance abuse; in those with a history of physical illnesses that impair organ function, even if the condition is felt to have been remedied (for example, hypothyroidism, congestive heart failure, and compensated emphysema); and in patients taking multiple prescribed or over-the-counter medications (Hall, Beresford, Gardner, & Popkin, 1982; Hall, Gardner, Popkin & LeCann, 1981; Hall *et al.*, 1978; Hoffman & Koran, 1984). A family history positive for degenerative or inheritable brain diseases or metabolic disorders such as diabetes, porphyria, and pernicious anemia should also raise concern.

Certain presentations are characteristic of psychiatric symptoms produced by underlying medical disorders. These include alterations in the level of consciousness; fluctuations in mental status; cognitive impairment; symptoms that have an episodic, recurrent, or cyclical course; and the presence of visual, tactile, or olfactory hallucinations. In addition, impairments of mental status are particularly important.

Our group reviewed CT scan use in psychiatric admissions during a 2½-year period. Scans were positive in 31.4% of the 156 cases in which they were ordered, and they specifically altered the patient's diagnosis in 18% of cases while confirming a suspected

LIFE HISTORY QUESTIONNAIRE

CASE NO. ____________

Name ____

The purpose of this questionnaire is to help us to better understand you and the problems which brought you to the Florida Hospital, Center for Psychiatry. Since some of the information you will be giving us in this questionnaire is of a personal nature, we want to assure you that all case records are held in strict confidence. Unless required by law, your case record will not be released without your permission. Findings from this questionnaire may be used in compiling group data and will never be released in any way that could identify you.

Please read the questions carefully and answer as accurately as you can. The questionnaire will probably take about fifteen minutes to complete, but feel comfortable working at your own pace.

EARLY DEVELOPMENT

Date of Birth ______________________________ Age ____________

1. As a child did you have any of the following?

   Serious Accidents ____ No ____ Yes, please specify ______________________________

   ____

   Serious Illnesses ____ No ____ Yes, please specify ______________________________

   ____

   Surgeries ____ No ____ Yes, please specify ______________________________

   ____

2. Did either parent die during your childhood or adolescence?

   ______ No

   ______ Yes, my mother, when I was ________ years old

   ______ Yes, my father, when I was ________ years old

   ______ Unknown

3. Check the persons with whom you lived **most** of the time while growing up.

   ______ Both my natural parents

   ______ One parent and ______ stepmother or ______ stepfather

   ______ One parent, ______ mother or ______ father

   ______ Other relative (explain) ______________________________

   ______ Foster parent(s)

   ______ Adoptive parent(s)

   ______ An Institution

   ______ Other (explain) ______________________________

4. Were you able to confide in your parents?

   ______ Yes, usually ______ No, not usually ______ Not applicable

5. How well did your parents get along with each other?

   ______ Very well ______ Not very well ______ Don't know

   ______ Fairly well ______ Very poorly ______ Not applicable

6. Check any of the following that you know have applied to your parents or brothers or sisters.

   Specify family member below

   ______ Hospitalization for mental illness ______________________________

   ______ Drinking problem ______________________________

   ______ Drug abuse ______________________________

   ______ Attempted or committed suicide ______________________________

   ______ Don't know ______________________________

7. How many schools did you attend from grades 1 through 12?

   ______ 1-3 ______ 4-7 ______ More than 7 ______ Don't know

8. What kind of grades did you make in school?

   ______ Excellent ______ Good ______ Fair ______ Poor ______ Failing

9. Did you participate in school activities? ______ No ______ Yes, some ______ Yes, many

10. When you were growing up, did you belong to church(es), club(s) or other organized group(s)?

    ______ Yes, many ______ Yes, a few ______ None

Figure 1. Life history questionnaire.

11. Did you have close friends around your own age? ______ Many ______ Few ______ One ______ None

12. Check any of the following that applied to you as a child.

______ nightmares
______ nail biting
______ speech problems
______ daydreaming
______ cruelty to animals
______ scapegoal (picked on)
______ head banging
______ stealing
______ running away
______ bullying
______ sleepwalking
______ bed wetting
______ thumb sucking
______ fire setting
______ accident prone
______ lying
______ temper tantrums
______ loneliness
______ insomnia

13. How would you describe your physical health at present?

______ Excellent ______ Good ______ Fair ______ Poor

14. Have you ever had any of the following?

Yes		Do you still have a problem with this? Yes	Yes		Do you still have a problem with this? Yes	Yes		Do you still have a problem with this? Yes
___	heart trouble	___	___	backache	___	___	hemorrhoids (piles)	___
___	nervous breakdown	___	___	hernia	___	___	jaundice	___
___	epilepsy	___	___	dizziness	___	___	hay fever	___
___	tuberculosis	___	___	blackout	___	___	other allergy	___
___	diabetes	___	___	rheumatism	___	___	venereal disease	___
___	teeth trouble	___	___	chronic cough	___	___	ulcers	___
___	eye trouble	___	___	shortness of breath	___	___	blood in urine	___
___	nose trouble	___	___	fits or convulsions	___	___	sugar in urine	___
___	bladder trouble	___	___	cancer	___	___	varicose veins	___
___	kidney trouble	___	___	asthma	___	___	underweight problem	___
___	bowel trouble	___	___	arthritis	___	___	overweight problem	___
___	stomach trouble	___	___	high blood pressure	___	___	injury to limb(s)	___
___	chest trouble	___	___	low blood pressure	___	___	injury to back	___
						___	injury to neck	___

15. Have you ever had a problem with any of the following?

______ Pep pills, diet pills
______ Tranquilizers, sedatives
______ Marijuana
______ Narcotics
______ Alcohol
______ LSD, or other hallucinogen (exclude marijuana)
______ Other, please specify ______________________
______ No

16. With whom are you living at present?

______ Spouse, or spouse and child(ren)
______ Parent(s)
______ Minor child(ren)
______ Grown child(ren)
______ Other relative(s)
______ Friend(s)
______ Alone
______ Other, explain ______________________

____

17. Check the statement which most closely describes how you are getting along with each of the following persons.

person	very well	fairly well	not very well	very poorly	uncertain	not applicable
Mother						
Father						
Sister(s)						
Brother(s)						
Spouse/Partner						
Female Child(ren)						
Male Child(ren)						

Figure 1 (continued)

18. What is your present marital status?

_______ Single
Living together, how long? _______
Married, how long? _______
_______ Separated
_______ Divorced
_______ Widowed

19. Check the most appropriate response.

Do your hands ever tremble enough to bother you?	____ 3 Often ____ 2 Sometimes ____ 1 Never	Do you smoke?	____ 3 Often ____ 2 Sometimes ____ 1 Never
Are you ever troubled by your hands and feet sweating so that they feel damp and clammy?	____ 3 Often ____ 2 Sometimes ____ 1 Never	Do you ever have loss of appetite?	____ 3 Often ____ 2 Sometimes ____ 1 Never
Have you ever been bothered by your heart beating hard?	____ 3 Often ____ 2 Sometimes ____ 1 Never	Has any ill health affected the amount of work (housework) you do?	____ 3 Often ____ 2 Sometimes ____ 1 Never
Do you tend to feel tired in the mornings?	____ 3 Often ____ 2 Sometimes ____ 1 Never	Do you ever feel weak all over?	____ 3 Often ____ 2 Sometimes ____ 1 Never
Do you have any trouble getting to sleep and staying asleep?	____ 3 Often ____ 2 Sometimes ____ 1 Never	Do you ever have spells of dizziness?	____ 3 Often ____ 2 Sometimes ____ 1 Never
How often are you bothered by having an upset stomach?	____ 3 Often ____ 2 Sometimes ____ 1 Never	Do you tend to lose weight when you worry?	____ 3 Often ____ 2 Sometimes ____ 1 Never
Are you ever bothered by nightmares (dreams which frighten you)?	____ 3 Often ____ 2 Sometimes ____ 1 Never	Have you ever been bothered by shortness of breath when you were not exerting yourself?	____ 3 Often ____ 2 Sometimes ____ 1 Never
Have you ever been troubled by "cold sweats"?	____ 3 Often ____ 2 Sometimes ____ 1 Never	For the most part, do you feel healthy enough to carry out the things that you would like to do?	____ 3 Often ____ 2 Sometimes ____ 1 Never
Do you feel that you are bothered by all sorts (different kinds) of ailments in different parts of your body?	____ 3 Often ____ 2 Sometimes ____ 1 Never	Do you feel in good spirits?	____ 3 Often ____ 2 Sometimes ____ 1 Never
		Do you sometimes wonder if anything is worthwhile anymore?	____ 3 Often ____ 2 Sometimes ____ 1 Never

20. Check any of the following that apply to you at the present time.

___ hallucinating
___ nightmares
___ tense
___ trusting
___ easily hurt
___ don't like vacations or weekends
___ timid
___ headaches
___ calm
___ depressed
___ no appetite
___ fainting spells
___ friendly
___ in conflict
___ talented
___ insomnia
___ horrible thoughts
___ thoughtful
___ aggressive
___ dizzy
___ bad temper
___ affectionate
___ unloved
___ modest
___ well mannered
___ rigid
___ suicidal
___ rejected
___ flexible
___ misunderstood
___ too ambitious
___ helpful
___ bed wetting
___ lonely
___ evil
___ stable
___ inferior
___ forgetful
___ respected
___ confused
___ need help
___ loyal
___ tired
___ unattractive
___ cruel to animals
___ unhappy
___ daydreamer
___ lack of confidence
___ capable
___ open
___ guilty
___ easily influenced
___ unable to have a good time
___ enthusiastic
___ happy
___ shy
___ fire setter
___ indecisive
___ inadequate
___ stupid
___ worthless
___ generous
___ unable to concentrate
___ bored
___ restless
___ lovable
___ regretful
___ panicky
___ soft-hearted
___ ugly
___ agitated
___ cowardly
___ self-confident
___ angry
___ full of hate
___ "can't do anything right"

21. Check any of the following which describe your marriage or sexual partnership.

_______ Not applicable
_______ Stormy
_______ Happy
_______ Insecure
_______ Average
_______ Romantic
_______ Exciting
_______ Friendly
_______ Lack of communication
_______ Good sexual adjustment
_______ Indifferent
_______ Mistake
_______ Good communication
_______ Lack of common interests
_______ Poor sexual adjustment
_______ Mutual respect and love
_______ Perfect
_______ Boring
_______ Secure
_______ Sharing of interest

22. How long did you know your present spouse before marriage? _______ Not married _______ Year(s)

Figure 1 (continued)

23. How many times have you been married? ________________

24. How many close friends do you now have? _______ Many _______ Few _______ One _______ None

25. Are you able to confide in these friends? _______ No _______ Yes _______ Not applicable

26. How comfortable are you with:

	very comfortable	moderately comfortable	moderately uncomfortable	very uncomfortable
Joining a group				
Meeting people				
With persons of same sex				
With persons of opposite sex				
Being a leader				
Being a follower				
Expressing an unpopular opinion				
Being disliked				
Asking for help				
Taking advice				
Accepting criticism				
Competitive situations				
Taking initiative				

27. Does you present work satisfy you? _______ Yes _______ No _______ Unemployed

28. Check any of the following which have been a problem for you.

_______ Gambling _______ Parents _______ Sex _______ Drinking
_______ Trouble with police _______ Temper _______ Marriage _______ Drugs
_______ Men _______ Violence _______ Children _______ Religion
_______ Women _______ Friends _______ Finances _______ Job

29. Here is a picture of a ladder. Suppose the top of the ladder represents the best possible life for you. Where on the ladder do you feel you stand at the present time? (Circle the correct number.)

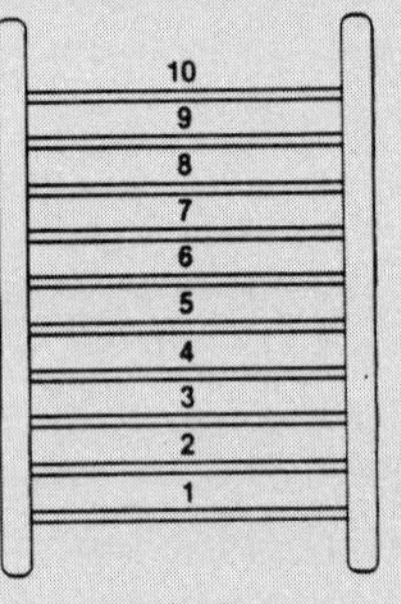

30. Where on the ladder would you say you stood five years ago? (Circle number.)

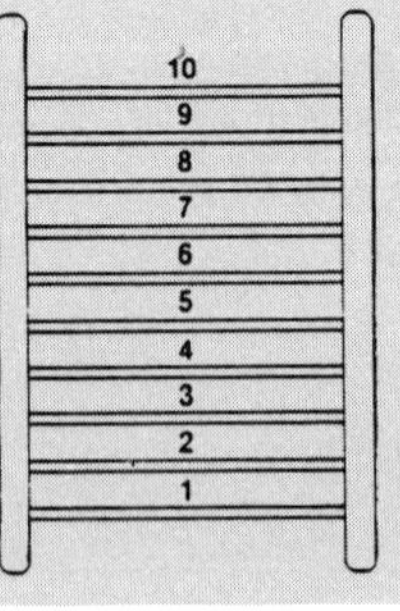

Figure 1 (continued)

31. Where on the ladder would you say you will stand five years from now? (Circle number.)

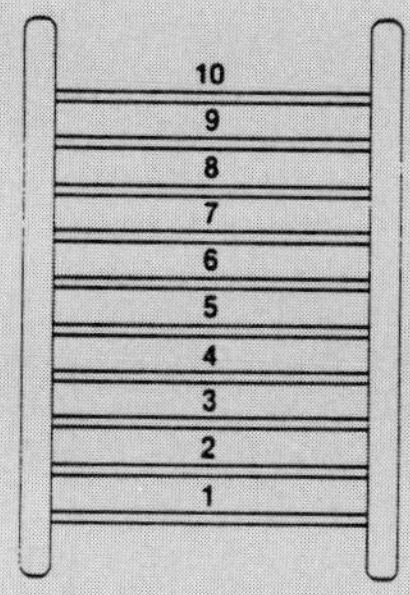

32. Check the most appropriate response.

	None or a little of the time	Some of the time	Good part of the time	Most or all of the time
1. I feel down-hearted and blue				
2. Morning is when I feel the best				
3. I have crying spells or feel like it				
4. I have trouble sleeping at night				
5. I eat as much as I used to				
6. I still enjoy sex				
7. I notice that I am losing weight				
8. I have trouble with constipation				
9. My heart beats faster than usual				
10. I get tired for no reason				
11. My mind is as clear as it used to be				
12. I find it easy to do the things I used to				
13. I am restless and can't keep still				
14. I feel hopeful about the future				
15. I am more irritable than usual				
16. I find it easy to make decisions				
17. I feel that I am useful and needed				
18. My life is pretty full				
19. I feel that others would be better off if I were dead				
20. I still enjoy the things I used to do				

33. Do you know anyone who has come to the Florida Hospital, Center for Psychiatry?
_______ No _______ Yes

34. If so, in your opinion, was the person(s) helped? (Check more than one, if applicable.)
_______ Yes, greatly _______ No, not at all
_______ Yes, moderately _______ No, became worse
_______ Only a little _______ Not applicable

35. Do you think you need help? _______ Yes _______ No _______ Don't know

36. Do others think you need help? _______ Yes _______ No _______ Don't know

37. How long do you think you should be in treatment?
_______ Less than 1 month
_______ More than 1 month, less than 6 months
_______ More than 6 months, less than 1 year
_______ More than 1 year
_______ Don't know

Figure 1 (continued)

PATIENT INFORMATION DATA BASE

NAME: ______________________________

AGE: ______________________________ DATE: ______________

PREVIOUS PHYSICIAN (NAME AND ADDRESS): ______________________________

PAST MEDICAL HISTORY (PLEASE CHECK ALL ITEMS TO THE BEST OF YOUR KNOWLEDGE):

Yes	No	
____	____	Hypertension ____________
____	____	Arthritis ____________
____	____	Diabetes ____________
____	____	Tuberculosis ____________
____	____	Pneumonia ____________
____	____	Venereal Disease ____________
____	____	Thyroid Disease, Goiter ____________
____	____	High Cholesterol or Triglycerides ____________
____	____	Asthma, Hay Fever ____________
____	____	Emphysema ____________
____	____	Bronchitis ____________
____	____	Recurrent Sinusitis ____________
____	____	Skin Disease (Eczema, Psoriasis, Cancer, etc.) ____________
____	____	Heart Attack ____________
____	____	Abnormal Heart Beat ____________
____	____	Heart Failure ____________
____	____	Rheumatic Fever ____________
____	____	Heart Murmur ____________
____	____	Congenital Heart Disease ____________
____	____	Breast Lumps ____________
____	____	Blood Disorders ____________
____	____	Leukemia, Lymphoma ____________
____	____	Anemia ____________
____	____	Peptic Ulcer ____________
____	____	Gall Bladder problems ____________
____	____	Bowel Disorders (Colitis, Spastic Colon, etc.) ____________
____	____	Hernia ____________
____	____	Hemorrhoids ____________
____	____	Liver Disease (Cirrhosis, Hepatitis, etc.) ____________
____	____	Kidney Disease (Cysts, Stones, Infection, etc.) ____________
____	____	Bladder Infections ____________
____	____	Prostate disorders (Males only) ____________
____	____	Female organ disorders ____________
____	____	Stroke ____________
____	____	Paralysis ____________
____	____	Cancer ____________
____	____	Epilepsy ____________
____	____	Serious injuries ____________
____	____	Meningitis ____________
____	____	Encephalitis ____________
____	____	Polio ____________
____	____	Sickle Cell Disease ____________
____	____	Radiation treatments to head or neck ____________
____	____	Emotional problems ____________
____	____	Phlebitis ____________
____	____	Glaucoma ____________
____	____	Cataract ____________
____	____	Gout ____________
____	____	Other (Please list): ____________

Last Hospitalization (date and diagnosis) ______________________________

____

Previous Procedures (approximate date):

Chest X-ray ______________ EKG ______________

Flu Vaccine ______________ Pneumoccal Vaccine ______________

Tetanus Shot ______________ Tuberculosis Skin Test ______________

Figure 1 (continued)

Table 1. Symptom Check List

- General
  - Severe loss of appetite
  - Severe weakness
  - Fever
  - Chills
  - Heavy sweats
  - Heavy night sweats—bed linens wet
  - Extreme fatigue
  - Sudden change in sleep pattern
- Head
  - Struck on head—knocked out
  - Frequent dizziness which makes you stop your normal activity and lasts at least 5 minutes
  - Headaches that are different from those you usually have
  - Headaches that awaken you from sleep
  - Headaches with vomiting
- Eyes
  - Pain in your eyes
  - Suddenly need new glasses
  - Seeing double
  - Loss of part of your vision
  - Seeing flashing lights or forms
  - Seeing solid things become wavy
  - Seeing halos around lights
- Nose
  - Bleeding
  - Pain
  - Cannot breathe well
  - Unusual smells
- Mouth
  - Toothache
  - Soreness or bleeding of:
    - Lips
    - Tongue
    - Gums
  - Unusual tastes
  - Hoarseness
- Ears
  - Pain in ears
  - Ringing in ears
  - Sudden change in hearing
  - Room spins around you
- Neck
  - Pain
  - Lumps
  - Difficulty in swallowing
  - Pain on swallowing
- Nodes
  - Swollen or tender lymph nodes (Kernels)
- Breasts
  - Pain
  - New lumps
  - Discharge from nipple

(continued)

Table 1. (Continued)

Skin
Itching
Easy bruisability that represents a change in the way you normally bruise
Sores
Marked dyness
Hair fragile—comes out in comb
Hair has become fine and silky
Hair has become coarse and brittle
Heart
Pain behind breast bone
Pain behind left nipple
Pain on left side of neck or jaw
Heart racing
Heart "thumps and misses beats"
Short of breath when walking
Need 2 or more pillows to sleep
Legs and ankles swelling (not with menstrual period)
Blue lips and/or fingers or toes when indoors and warm
Lungs
Pain in chest
Pain when you take a deep breath
New cough
Coughing up blood
Green, white, or yellow phlegm
Wheezing
Short of breath (sudden)
Wake up at night—can't catch breath
Unable to climb stairs
Gastrointestinal
Have lost all desire to eat
Food makes you ill
Cannot swallow normally
Pain on swallowing
Food comes halfway up again
Sudden persistent heartburn
Pain or discomfort after you eat
Sharp stabbing pains in shoulder or side after you eat
Gastro-urinary
Stabbing pain in back by lower ribs
Urinating much more frequently
Suddenly awakening at night to urinate
Passing much more urine
Unable to start to urinate
Must go to urinate quickly or afraid of losing urine
Pain on urination
Wetting yourself
Blood in urine
Pus in urine
Facial swelling
Male
Pain in testicles
Swelling of testicles
Swelling of scrotum

(continued)

Table 1. (Continued)

Female
Sudden change in periods
Between-period bleeding
Neurological
Fainting
Fits
Weakness in arms or legs
Change in speech
Loss of coordination
Periods of sudden onset of confusion
Sudden change in personality (i.e., suddenly not the same person)
Loss of ability to concentrate
Seeing things
Hearing things
Loss of touch
Tingling in arms or legs
Unable to chew properly
Memory loss
Tremulous or shaky

diagnosis in 11%. Changes in mental status were more useful in predicting abnormal scan results than were focal neurological findings, and they confirmed the need to obtain careful and detailed mental-status evaluation at the time of the patient's first visit (Beresford, Blow, Hall, Nichols, & Langston, 1985, 1986). A well-documented, standardized mental-status test also provides a data base against which future change can be assessed (Bell & Hall, 1977; Hall, Levenson, & LeCann, 1981), as well as a measure of psychological dysfunction when significant indicators of organ malfunction affecting the brain are present.

Findings such as hypertension, asterixis, focal neurological signs, clonus, needle tracks, diminished breath sounds, and edema may point to specific disorders. Patients with diffuse subcortical dysfunction require detailed evaluation. Signs include impaired speech and mentation, abnormal movement, ataxia, incoordination, tremor, asterixis, chorea, and dysarthria. Patients with specific evidence of cortical dysfunction also require a comprehensive workup. Symptoms include dysphasia, apraxias, agnosias, visual-spatial defects, and defective cortical sensory patterns.

Finally, patients who have been in treatment for some period of time and who are not responding appropriately to either pharmacological or psychotherapeutic interventions require careful review. In these situations, we suggest that the clinician begin as if she or he were seeing the patient for the first time, reformulate a diagnosis, reexamine the patient, and obtain appropriate laboratory, radiographic, and electrophysiological evaluation. If the differential diagnosis is unclear or if suggestions of organic mental disease are present, it is appropriate to obtain consultative advice. The utility of this approach has been demonstrated by Pokorny and Frazier (Hall, Levenson, & LeCann, 1981), who studied 10% of patients admitted to the Texas State Hospital system. They were able to make presumptive diagnoses of neurological disorders in 30% of the patients seen. Of the 1,530 patients, 691 were found to have concurrent medical problems. Similarly, Bunce *et al.* (1982) reported on findings in 102 consecutive female patients admitted to a public psychiatric hospital. They were transferred to a medical-care unit from other wards because of nonspecific changes in either their physical condition or their behavior. The findings suggested that more than 70% of the patients were not able to adequately communicate their physical symptoms to their physicians. Ninety-two percent of the sample were found to have at least one, with an average of three, previously undiagnosed physical diseases that were not predicted by their symptoms at the time of referral. Seventy-eight percent of the medical diagnoses made were unrelated to the patients' descriptions of symptoms, a finding suggesting that the psychiatric illness masked the medical symptoms. Ninety percent of the physical disorders found in these patients were unreported and unsuspected at the time of referral. More than half of the patient population was disoriented or confused, and 27% were either delusional or hallucinating. Of the patients evaluated, 23% were highly agitated; 16% were reported to have been aggressive or assaultive. A careful review and reevaluation of these patients resulted in a significant alteration of their treatment plan and resulting psychiatric improvement.

In our own study of patients who were thought to be free of medical illness, we were able to demonstrate, after careful revaluation, that 46% had an unrecognized medical disorder that had either caused or exacerbated their psychiatric symptoms. Eighty percent of the patients had some form of physical illness that required treatment during their hospital stay. More than 30% of the patients who had disorders causing or exacerbating their psychiatric symptoms had a history of a poor response to treatment appropriate for their initial diagnoses (Hall, Gardner, Stickney, LeCann, & Popkin, 1980).

One of the most common and critical errors made in psychiatric evaluation is the assignment of diagnoses before adequate information has been gathered to define the range of appropriate differential diagnoses. The outpatient evaluation sequence is often aborted because of limitations of time or budgetary constraint, or because the evaluator leaps to a premature conclusion consistent with his or her theoretical beliefs. Ideally, the patient should be carefully evaluated by interview, physical examination, and laboratory study, as appropriate. Data should be obtained from family and other sources with the patient's permission, and old records should be retrieved. A diagnosis can then be made with reasonable certainty, or a further workup can be undertaken.

Two studies show the value of thorough data gathering at the point of admission. Several years ago, our group obtained laboratory evaluations and drug screens on a variety of patients coming to a mental health center. Because we were comparing different laboratory methods for the detection of toxic substances, we did not feel it was appropriate to provide feedback until the laboratory analysis had been completed. This process took several months. The patients, in the meantime, were evaluated by staff and assigned to appropriate therapy modalities. Those patients who were polysubstance abusers and who had not provided their therapist with this information at the time of initial contact were most often diagnosed as suffering from a major mental illness, were often transferred from therapist to therapist, and were seen as treatment-refractory cases. They were usually heavily medicated to control their underlying ''latent'' psychotic disorders, receiving on average more than three times as many medications, usually given at high dose, than comparable patients whose drug use was known. After the drug use data were made available to the treatment staff, the errors of diagnosis became apparent. The treatment was changed, and several of these patients recovered following confrontation and treatment of the actual problem (Hall *et al.*, 1977).

Another illustration of the value of careful data acquisition was provided by Struve

(1980) in a 12-year study at the Long Island Jewish Hospital, where psychiatric patients were routinely given EEGs as part of an ongoing research process. Struve asked the attending physicians whether they felt they would have ordered EEGs on clinical grounds and whether they would have expected the EEG record to be abnormal. Sixty-eight percent of the EEG abnormalities found, excluding controversial diagnoses such as 14-6 spikings, β-mittens, and rare fast, had not been previously expected. That is, the physicians had not felt that their patients were suffering from an organic dysfunction. When the investigator reviewed the records of the most severely disturbed patients, 56% that had been obtained through the protocol would not have otherwise been ordered. Fifty-seven percent of the records showing focal slowing were unsuspected. Overall, 1 out of every 11 patients admitted had an unsuspected, significant EEG abnormality. A retrospective analysis of these cases suggested that elements were present in the history of many of these patients that would have justified further clinical diagnostic study.

The clinician must assemble all of his or her data, evaluate the data carefully, and pursue abnormal findings with appropriate studies. Several excellent textbooks are available to assist the clinician in the elements of specific diagnoses and in understanding how to use specific laboratory tests. Other sources provide information on the types of medical illnesses causing specific psychiatric problems and suggest approaches to their diagnosis and treatment (Dorfman & Christofar, 1985; Hall, 1980; Hall & Beresford, 1983a; Jefferson & Marshall, 1981; Koranyi, 1982; Leishman, 1978).

Information concerning the use of biochemical examinations, the handling of samples, the normative range of laboratory values, alterations of laboratory tests by specific drugs, the choice and interpretation of specific biochemical tests, and the physiological basis of laboratory test abnormalities in psychiatric patients can be found elsewhere (Hall & Beresford, 1983a, 1983–1984).

SPECIFIC APPLICATIONS IN AN OUTPATIENT SETTING

If one is to successfully differentiate physical from psychiatric disorders in an outpatient setting, the following must be present, or available:

1. Administrative support, in institutional settings
2. Interest on the part of the clinician in pursuing all reasonable diagnostic possibilities
3. Time to see, evaluate, and examine the patient and to gain information from important others
4. Personnel and equipment for the drawing of routine blood samples and the examination of patients physically in an appropriate setting or the ability to refer the patient to another clinician having these capabilities
5. An adequate chart-retrieval–data-retrieval system
6. Appropriate consultation
7. Opportunities for case discussions, in institutional settings
8. An ongoing educational process in which both physical and laboratory diagnostic skills can be upgraded
9. The opportunity to follow the patient over time so that the clinician can better understand the impact of the treatment on the patient's psychiatric symptomatology

10. Library facilities
11. An institutional policy that identifies the necessity of and permits the careful reevaluation of difficult or refractory cases
12. Financial support for special diagnostic evaluation (e.g., CT scans, EEGs, heavy-metal screens, and toxicology screens)
13. Opportunities for systemwide follow-up and the ongoing monitoring of cases

As the reader is aware, this list pertains more to the administrative elements of care than to the science of it, but in fact, these are the most important elements determining whether patients will be properly assessed. One additional requirement, which is often overlooked, remains of paramount importance: the availability of appropriately trained psychiatrists.

SUMMARY

The physical and laboratory evaluation of psychiatric outpatients is essential if physical disorders are to be differentiated from the psychiatric symptoms they can produce. A significant number of psychiatric outpatients, between 5% and 10%, present with psychiatric symptoms that are caused by an unrecognized physical illness. It is difficult to distinguish these physically induced psychiatric symptoms from those occurring from a purely "functional" cause on the basis of history alone, although historical elements can be extremely useful in raising the clinician's level of concern. Medical symptoms are often incorporated into the patient's psychiatric symptoms and are frequently unknown to either the patient or the treating clinician.

Patients often experience difficulty in communicating adequately with their examining physicians and often misrepresent or have been trained not to report their physical symptoms. Consequently, detailed physical and laboratory examinations are essential for the proper evaluation of any acutely psychotic patient, patients with impaired mental status findings, and those with indicators of an organic mental syndrome, anxiety, and panic disorders, or depression. The patient should be deemed in need of further physical examination even if seen by a private physician, unless there is evidence that the patient has undergone a recent clothes-off physical examination. Cardiovascular, endocrine, central-nervous-system, pulmonary, and infectious disorders are the diseases most likely to produce psychiatric symptoms, with endocrine and metabolic disorders predominating in females, and cardiovascular and pulmonary diseases predominating in men. Over-the-counter, illicit, and prescribed drugs are also a frequent cause of psychiatric symptoms.

Intake should include a careful history and a detailed mental-status examination. The patient should then have a careful physical and laboratory evaluation. It is suggested that the laboratory examination include a complete blood count, a biochemical panel, urinalysis, urine drug screen, tuberculin skin test, a test for syphilis, and an electrocardiogram and chest X ray for patients over age 30 or if symptomatic. If an organic mental disorder is suspected or determined, further workup should include thyroid function studies, B-12 and folate levels, blood and urine toxicology screens, a plasma determination of current medication levels, an electroencephalogram, and a CT scan. Based on these findings, other studies may be indicated, including heavy-metal testing, lumbar puncture, diagnostic drug challenges, and further specialized X-ray tests. After all of the appropriate information is assembled, the clinician will be in a position to make an adequate diagnosis. A careful workup ensures the patient's physical safety, establishes the baseline knowledge necessary to evaluate the effects of pharmacological treatment, and provides data to assist in the diagnosis of unrecognized physical illness. A negative workup represents a source of reassurance for both the patient and his or her physician, whereas positive findings can be used to direct subsequent diagnostic evaluation and consultation. The workup also indirectly ensures that the patient's civil rights will be appropriately protected and protects the physician from charges of negligence.

Further data defining the yield of routine admission tests in various subpopulations of acutely ill psychiatric patients are desperately needed. Studies similar to those conducted by Koran (1985) will be welcome. The baseline data provided by laboratory and physical examinations of psychiatric patients will also have a significant scientific impact as we evaluate the long-term effects of our medications and treatments and attempt to minimize the complications that they cause. It is essential that, as society moves to further "de-medicalize" the care provided to psychiatric patients because of economic constraints, the intake and evaluation process be "remedicalized" to ensure the long-term adequacy of our diagnosis and treatment.

REFERENCES

Alstrom, C. H. (1942). Mortality in mental hospitals. *Acta Psychiatrica et Neurologica Scandinavica, 17* (suppl. PPL-24).

American Psychiatric Association. (1980). *Diagnostic and statistical manual of mental disorders* (3rd ed.; DSM-III). Washington, DC: Author.

Babigiam, H. W., & Odoroff, C. L. (1969). The mortality experience of a population with psychiatric illness. *American Journal of Psychiatry, 126*(4), 470–480.

Bell, R. C., & Hall, R. C. W. (1977). The mental status examination. *American Family Physician, 16*(5), 145–152.

Beresford, T. P., Blow, R. C., Hall, R. C. W., Nichols, L. O., & Langston, J. W. (1985). Focal signs and brain CT scans in psychiatric patients (Letter to the Editor). *New England Journal of Medicine, 313,* 388.

Bonhoffer, D. (1912). Die Psyhosem im Gefolge von akuten Infektionem Allgemeiner Krankunger. In G. L. Aschaffenbeg (Ed.), *Handbauch der Psychiatrie* (3rd ed., pp. 1–60). Leipzig, Germany: Deuticke.

Boston Collaborative Drug Surveillance Study. (1971). Psychiatric side effects of non-psychiatric drugs. *Seminars in Psychiatry, 3,* 406–420.

Bunce, D. F. M., II, Jones, L. R., Badger, L. W., & Jones, S. E. (1982). Medical illness in psychiatric patients: Barrier to diagnoses and treatment. *Southern Medial Journal, 75,* 941–944.

Dorfman, W., & Christofar, L. (Eds.). (1985). *Psychosomatic Illness Review.* New York: Macmillan.

Eastwood, M. R., & Trevelyan, M. H. (1972). Relationship between physical and psychiatric disorders. *Psychological Medicine, 2* 363–372.

Hall, R. C. W. (Ed.). (1980). *Psychiatric presentation of medical illness: Somatopsychic disorders.* Jamaica, NY: Spectrum.

Hall, R. C. W., & Beresford, T. P. (1983a) Laboratory evaluation of newly admitted psychiatric patients. In R. C. W. Hall & T. P. Beresford (Eds.), *Handbook of psychiatric diagnostic procedures* (pp. 255–314). Jamaica, NY: Spectrum.

Hall, R. C. W., & Beresford, T. P. (1983b). Psychiatric manifestations of physical illness. In J. O. Cavenar, Jr. (Ed.), *Psychiatry* (Vol. 2, Chapter 88, pp. 1–18). New York: Lippincott.

Hall, R. C. W., & Beresford, T. P. (Eds.). (1983–1984). *Handbook of Psychiatric Diagnostic Procedures* (Vols. 1 and 2). Jamaica, NY: Spectrum.

Hall, R. C. W., Popkin, M. K, & Devaul, R. A. (1977). The effect of unrecognized drug abuse on diagnosis and therapeutic outcome. *American Journal of Drug and Alcohol Abuse, 4*(4), 455–465.

Hall, R. C. W., Popkin, M. K., Devaul, R. A., Faillace, L. A., & Stickney, S. K. (1978) Physical illness presenting as psychiatric disease. *Archives of General Psychiatry, 35,* 1315–1320.

Hall, R. C. W., Gardner, E. R., Stickney, S. K., LeCann, A. F., & Popkin, M. K. (1980). Physical illness manifesting as psychiatric disease: 2. Analysis of a state hospital inpatient population. *Archives of General Psychiatry, 37,* 989–995.

Hall, R. C. W., Levenson, A. J., & LeCann, A. F. (1981). Evaluation and assessment of non-functional psychiatric illness in the elderly. In A. J. Levenson & R. C. W. Hall (Eds.), *Neuropsychiatric manifestations of physical disease in the elderly* (pp. 133–149). New York: Raven Press.

Hall, R. C. W., Gardner, E. R., Popkin, M. K., & LeCann, A. F. (1981). Unrecognized physical illness prompting psychiatric admission: A prospective study. *American Journal of Psychiatry, 138*(5), 629–635.

Hall, R. C. W., Beresford, T. P., Gardner, E. R., & Popkin, M. K. (1982). The medial care of psychiatric patients. *Hospital and Community Psychiatry, 33*(1), 25–34.

Hoffman, R. S. (1982). Diagnostic errors in the evaluation of behavioral disorders. *Journal of American Medical Association, 2*(48), 964–967.

Hoffman, R. S., & Koran, L. M. (1984). Detecting physical illness in patients with mental disorders. *Psychosomatics, 25*(9), 654–659.

Jefferson, J. W., & Marshall, R. R. (1981). *Neuropsychiatric features of medical disorders.* New York: Plenum Press.

Koran, L. M. (1985, November). *Physical illness in a sampling of California psychiatric patients.* Paper presented at the Academy of Psychosomatic Medicine 32nd Annual Meeting.

Koranyi, E. K. (1972). Physical health and illness in a psychiatric outpatient department population. *Canadian Psychiatric Association Journal, 17,* SS109–116.

Koranyi, E. K. (1982). *Physical illness in the psychiatric patient.* Springfield, IL: Charles C Thomas.

LaBruzza, A. L. (1981). Physical illness presenting as psychiatric disorder: Guidelines for differential diagnosis. *Journal of Operational Psychiatry, 12,* 24–31.

Leishman, W. A. (1978) *Organic psychiatry.* Oxford, England: Blackwell Scientific Publication.

Malzberg, B. (1952). Rates of discharge and rate of mortality among first admissions to the New York civil state hospitals. *Mental Hygiene, 36,* 104–120.

Odegard, O. (1951). Mortality in Norwegian mental hospitals, 1926–1941. *Acta Genetica et Statistica Medica, 2,* 141–173.

Odegard, O. (1953). The excess mortality of the insane. *Acta Psychiatrica et Neurologica Scandinavica, 27,* 353–367.

Paffenbarger, R. S., Jr., & Wing, A. L. (1967). Characteristics in youths predisposing to fatal stroke in later years. *Lancet, 1,* 753–754.

Paffenbarger, R. S., Jr., Wolf, P. A., Notkin, J., & Thorne, M. C. (1966). Chronic disease in former college students: 1. Early precursors of fatal coronary heart disease. *American Journal of Epidemiology, 83,* 314–328.

Paffenbarger, R. S., Jr., Notkin, J., Kreuger, D. E., Wolf, P. A., Thorne, M. C., LeBauer, E. J., & Williams, J. L. (1966). Chronic disease in former college students: 2. Methods of study and observations on mortality for chronic heart disease. *American Journal of Public Health, 56,* 962–971.

Paffenbarger, R. S., Jr., Thorne, M. C., & Wing, A. L. (1968). chronic disease in former college students: 8. Characteristics in youths predisposing to hypertension in later years. *American Journal of Epidemiology, 88,* 25–32.

Pokorny, A. D., & Frazier, S. H. (1966). *Report of the administrative survey of Texas state mental hospitals.* Austin: Austin Foundation for Mental Health Research, Texas Department of Mental Health and Mental Retardation.

Roessler, R., & Greenfield, N. S. (1961). Incidence of somatic disease in psychiatric patients. *Psychosomatic Medicine, 23*(5), 413–419.

Struve, F. A. (1980). Utilization of clinical electroencephalographic assessment in the psychiatric hospital: Routine vs. selective physician referral. *Journal of Psychiatric Treatment and Evaluation, 2,* 55–62.

Summers, W. K., Munoz, R. A., Read, M. E., & Marsh, G. M. (1981). The psychiatric physical examination: 2. Findings in 75 unselected psychiatric patients. *Journal of Clinical Psychiatry, 42*(3), 99–102.

Thomas, C. B., & Duezynski, W. R. (1974). Closeness to parents in the family constellation in a prospective study of five disease states: Suicide, mental illness, malignant tumor, hypertension and coronary heart disease. *Johns Hopkins Medical Journal, 143,* 251–270.

Vaillant, G. E. (1978a) *Adaptation to life.* Boston: Little Brown.

Vaillant, G. E. (1978b). Natural history of male psychological health: 4. What kinds of men do not get psychosomatic illnesses. *Psychosomatic Medicine, 40,* 420–432.

3

Overview of Drug Treatment

ALAN J. GELENBERG

HISTORY AND OVERVIEW

As the history of medicine goes, the drug treatment of psychiatric outpatients is a comparatively new topic. Before the modern era of pharmacotherapy blossomed around the midpoint of this century, psychiatrists and other physicians had a few classes of drugs available that could serve mostly as adjuncts to various nonbiological approaches. Sedatives—such as barbiturates, bromides, and chloral hydrate—could assist in promoting sleep and could sometimes produce temporary relief of anxiety; stimulants might prompt a temporary surge in energy and sometimes a boost in spirits; but for the most part, psychiatry could expect little help from the pharmacopoeia.

Since 1938, electoconvulsive therapy (ECT) has been an effective treatment for depression and a variety of other conditions. Although primarily applicable to inpatients, ECT is sometimes used for depressed outpatients and, when necessary, for maintenance therapy.

It was the 1950s that primarily saw the birth of psychopharmacology as a modern medical subspecialty. New classes of medications became available that have revolutionized the practice of psychiatry. Inpatients could become outpatients; outpatients could be stabilized and were less likely to need rehospitalization.

By a series of serendipitous discoveries, new drugs brought symptomatic relief where none had been possible before. Phenothiazines and other classes of antipsychotic drugs alleviated many of the acute symptoms of schizophrenic and other functional and organic psychoses. Tricyclic and monoamine oxidase (MAO) inhibitor antidepressants reversed the symptoms of many severe forms of depression and sometimes prevented their recurrence. Lithium successfully treated acute mania and, for many bipolar patients, made recurrences less frequent and/or less severe. And in the 1960s, the benzodiazepine group

ALAN J. GELENBERG • Department of Psychiatry, University of Arizona College of Medicine, Health Sciences Center, Tucson, Arizona 85724.

of anxiolytics and hypnotics represented a class with high efficacy and an enviable safety profile.

Where are we now, in the late 1980s, in our ability to treat psychiatric outpatients with medicine? In this chapter, I will outline the major drug classes, giving a personal perspective on where we have come from and where we now stand on each.

Table 1. Currently Available Antipsychotic Drugs

Nonproprietary name	Trade name	Approximate potency[b]	Available as injectable	Chemical structure/representative agent
Phenothiazines				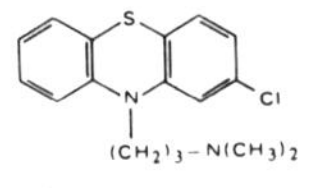 Chlorpromazine
Aliphatic				
Chlorpromazine	Thorazine®	1 : 1	Yes	
Triflupromazine	Vesprin®	4 : 1	Yes	
Piperidine				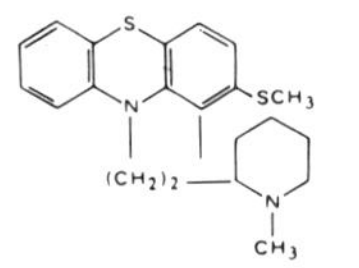 Thioridazine
Thioridazine	Mellaril®	1 : 1	No	
Mesoridazine	Serentil®	2 : 1	Yes	
Piperactazine	Quide®	10 : 1	No	
Piperazine				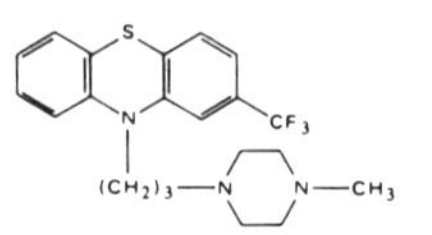 Trifluoperazine
Trifluoperazine	Stelazine®	30 : 1	Yes	
Acetophenzaine	Tindal®	5 : 1	No	
Butaperazine	Repoise®	10 : 1	No	
Carphenazine	Proketazine®	4 : 1	No	
Fluphenazine	Permitil®, Prolixin®	50–100 : 1[c]	Yes[d]	
Perphenazine	Trilafon®	10 : 1	Yes	
Prochlorperazine	Compazine®	7 : 1	Yes	
Thioxanthenes				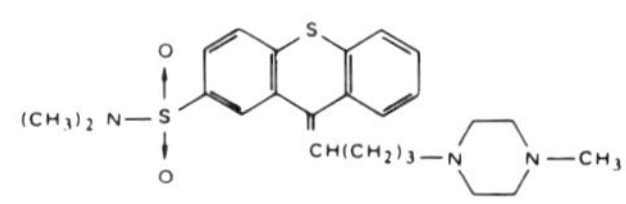 Thiothixene
Chlorprothixene	Taractan®	1 : 1	Yes	
Thiothixene	Navane®	25 : 1	Yes	
Butyrophenone				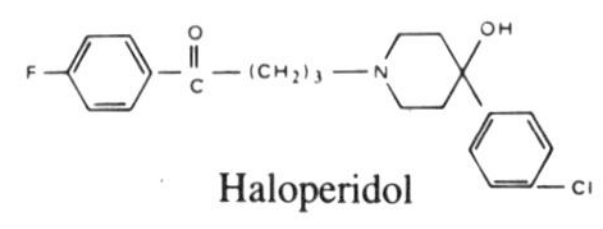 Haloperidol
Haloperidol	Haldol®	50 : 1	Yes	
Dibenzoxazepine				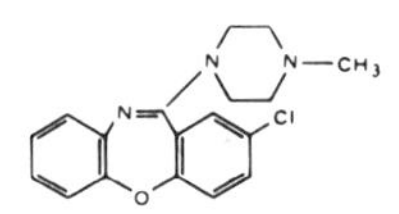 Loxapine
Loxapine	Daxolin® Loxitane®	7 : 1	Yes	
Dihydroindolone				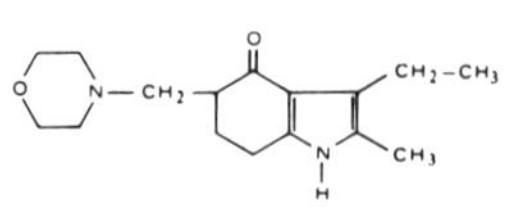 Molindone
Molindone	Lindone® Moban®	10 : 1	No	

[a]Reprinted from Bassuk, Schoonover, and Gelenberg (1983). Copyright 1983. Reproduced by permission.
[b]Milligram equivalence to chlorpromazine.
[c]Oral only. Potency equivalences not established for long-acting injectionable forms. Usual dosage for fluphenazine decanoate is 0.5 to 2.5 ml every 3 to 5 weeks.
[d]Available both as short-acting fluphenazine HCl injection and as long-acting enanthate and decanoate esters.

ANTIPSYCHOTIC DRUGS

Phenothiazines and the other major classes of neuroleptic antipsychotic agents (see Table 1) are of most obvious use in outpatient settings for the maintenance therapy of schizophrenic patients. The major concern regarding the use of these drugs in recent years has been tardive dyskinesia, and probably the most important clinical lesson that has begun to take hold is the effectiveness of comparatively low doses of these compounds.

Fortunately, the concern and the lesson relate to one another: lower maintenance doses of neuroleptics may cause less tardive dyskinesia, as well as fewer side effects across the board (Kane, 1986). Many schizophrenic patients, for example, can be maintained on daily doses of haloperidol below 5 mg—some, perhaps, below 1 mg (McEvoy, 1986). Some patients may avoid schizophrenic relapse on doses of fluphenazine decanoate as low as 1.25–2.5 mg every few weeks (Kane, 1983). And probably some patients can take decanoate injections as infrequently as every few weeks.

A large majority of chronic schizophrenic patients, however, will continue to require some degree of maintenance antipsychotic drug therapy to avoid relapse into psychosis and, often, rehospitalization. But the discovery of the effectiveness of diminishing negative emotional interchange (high expressed emotionality) with close relatives may allow many patients to be maintained on still lower maintenance drug doses (Falloon, Boyd, McGill, Razani, Moss, & Gilderman, 1982).

Antipsychotic drugs are used in outpatients with a wide variety of psychiatric diagnoses, but their efficacy outside of schizophrenia is much less well demonstrated, and the risks of tardive dyskinesia and other hazards persist. In manic-depressive patients, for example (who may be at even higher risk of developing tardive dyskinesia on neuroleptic exposure; Gelenberg, 1984b), the use of maintenance antipsychotic drug therapy requires diligent documentation of effectiveness in that patient (and the lack of effectiveness of other agents, such as lithium). Similarly, the use of these drugs in mentally retarded or brain-damaged individuals (to diminish aggressive behavior) or in patients with borderline personality disorder (to help control emotional lability) should be conducted cautiously and documented clearly. As with schizophrenic patients, the dose for each patient should be titrated to the lowest effective level.

Another shift in practice in recent years is a growing awareness that maintenance antiparkinson drug therapy—to accompany the long-term use of antipsychotic agents—is safe, effective, and often necessary. Although once frowned upon, maintenance (and even sometimes prophylactic) antiparkinson drug use allows patients to be more comfortable, enhances cooperation with treatment, and may even decrease psychopathology (Gelenberg, 1986a).

ANTIDEPRESSANT DRUGS

A patient with a melancholic subtype of major depression deserves a therapeutic trial with a tricyclic antidepressant (see Table 2). Many would argue that virtually any major depression warrants a similar drug trial. MAO-inhibitor antidepressants, once feared because of their association with hypertensive reactions, are now used more widely and with greater awareness of their risks and required cautions (see Table 3). Although still to be answered definitively, there is growing evidence that MAO inhibitors may have special utility in the treatment of certain forms of nonmelancholic depressions (Brotman, Falk, &

Table 2. Preparations and Dosage of Heterocyclic Antidepressants[a]

Heterocyclic	Brand name	Preparations	Initial dosage	Usual therapeutic dosage
Amitriptyline	Elavil®, Endep®, Amitril®	10-, 25-, 50-, 75-, 100-, 150- mg tablets; 25-, 20-mg capsules; vials of 10 ml with 10mg/ml	25–75 mg	150–300 mg
Imipramine	Tofranil®, Presamine®, Imavate®, Janimine®, SK-Pramine®, Philips-Roxane Imipramine®	10-, 25-, 50-, 100-mg tablets; 75-, 150-mg capsules; ampules of 20 ml with 25 mg/2 ml	25–75 mg	150–300 mg
Doxepin	Sinequan®, Adapin®	10-, 25-, 50-, 100-, 150-mg capsules; solution of 10 mg/ml	25–75 mg	150–300 mg
Nortriptyline	Aventyl®, Pamelor®	10-, 25-mg capsules; solution of 10mg/5 ml	20–40 mg	75–150 mg
Desipramine	Norpramin®, Pertofrane®	25-, 50-, 75-, 100-, 150-mg tablets; 25-, 50-mg capsules	25–75 mg	75–200 mg
Protriptyline	Vivactil®	5-, 10-mg tablets	10–20 mg	20–60 mg
Trimipramine	Surmontil®	25-, 50-mg capsules	25–75 mg	75–300 mg
Amoxapine	Asendin®	30-, 100-, 150-mg tablets	50–150 mg	150–600 mg
Maprotiline	Ludiomil®	25-, 50-mg tablets	25–75 mg	75–300 mg
Trazodone	Desyrel®	25-, 50-, 100-mg tablets	50–100 mg	150–600 mg

[a]Reprinted from Bassuk, Schoonover, and Gelenberg (1983). Copyright 1983. Reproduced by permission.

Gelenberg, 1987). Such "atypical" depressions have been variably defined, but they typically involve panic, anxious and phobic features, and/or vegetative symptoms that are in large part the opposite of the "endogenous" cluster (e.g., weight gain or oversleeping).

The newer antidepressants that have been introduced into the United States in the 1980s have, for the most part, not lived up to the original hopes and expectations. They have not brought enhanced efficacy, and in each case, there has been concern about some particular form of toxicity. In at least two instances, the drugs were withdrawn soon after their introduction because of a recognition of unacceptable toxic reactions.

Although traditionally labeled as antidepressants, the tricyclics and MAO inhibitors have recently gained widespread use for a number of other conditions. Both classes appear effective in blocking recurrent episodes of panic attacks, although the latter may enjoy an

Table 3. Preparations and Dosages of Monoamine Oxidase Inhibitors[a]

Generic name	Trade name	Preparation	Usual dosage range (mg/day)
Isocarboxazid	Marplan®	10-mg tablets	10–30
Phenelzine	Nardil®	15-mg tablets	45–90
Tranylcypromine	Parnate®	10-mg tablets	10–30

[a]Reprinted from Bassuk, Schoonover, and Gelenberg (1983). Copyright 1983. Reproduced by permission.

edge in efficacy (Rosenbaum, 1986). Obsessive-compulsive patients sometimes benefit from treatment with one or the other class of antidepressants; the tricyclic clomipramine may have some special advantage for this indication (Jenike, 1986). Other possible indications for these agents include bulimia (Brotman, 1984), cocaine abuse (Brotman, 1985), and perhaps the adult residua of attention deficit disorder (Biederman, 1986).

As with the antipsychotic class, probably the most important recent clinical wisdom about antidepressants also concerns dosage. But unlike the current teaching about the antipsychotic agents, the admonition regarding antidepressants is to use more, rather than less. Probably the greatest cause of treatment nonresponse is using too little or treating for too short a period (Quitkin, 1985). To be considered unresponsive, a patient should have been treated with at least 300 mg daily of imipramine or its equivalent for 4–6 weeks. For the MAOI phenelzine, doses should be "pushed" as high as 90 mg/day.

After the effective treatment of an acute episode of depression, relapse is best prevented by continuing therapy with the drug for approximately six months, and at least four months following total cessation of acute depressive symptoms (Gelenberg, 1985). Many patients with a recurrent unipolar depression are best maintained prophylactically on an antidepressant drug to prevent or ameliorate future episodes (Prien, Kupfer, Mansky, Small, Tuason, Voss, & Johnson, 1984).

One of the greatest disappointments in the 1980s has been the failure of once-heralded biochemical tests—in particular, the dexamethasone suppression test (DST)—to help diagnose depression, select patients for drug therapy, or follow the patients in maintenance treatment (Gelenberg, 1984a). Much investigation continues with a wide range of neuroendocrine and biochemical markers, but to date, none has proved effective and economical for clinical use.

LITHIUM

Lithium remains a strikingly successful and acceptably safe drug for the maintenance treatment of bipolar patients. Again, recent attention has focused on dosing. Some patients appear to be effectively maintained at blood levels lower than previously believed effective (e.g., 0.4–0.6 mEq/L), but this is still an issue in need of rigorous prospective study. Dosing schedules are also being examined: some evidence suggests that once-daily (or even less frequent) dosing can be effective and may be associated with less polyuria and fewer morphologically changes in the kidney (Plenge & Mellerup, 1986).

Although a major concern in the late 1970s, the renal toxicity of lithium appears to be much less a hazard for the millions of patients who receive this treatment than originally believed. Dosage and dosage schedule changes, the use of diuretics and diet adjustment, and other techniques often alleviate the uncomfortable polyuria associated with lithium, and to date, no patient has developed terminal renal failure attributed to lithium treatment (Gelenberg, Wojcik, Falk, Coggins, Brotman, Rosenbaum, LaBrie, & Kerman, 1987).

Alternatives to lithium treatment continue to be evaluated for the 20–50% of patients who are inadequately responsive or who cannot tolerate the ion. The last few years have seen great attention to carbamazepine, but although the recipient of numerous accolades, this anticonvulsant drug remains to be conclusively demonstrated as an effective antimanic therapy (Prien & Gelenberg, 1989). Still, many clinicians turn to it as an adjunct, if not used alone, for patients unresponsive to or intolerant of lithium. Less well studied still are a host of other agents brought forward as possible antimanic treatments in recent years, including the benzodiazepine anticonvulsant clonazepam and the antihypertensive clonidine.

ANXIOLYTICS, SEDATIVES, AND HYPNOTICS

Panic disorder and related conditions have been the focus of much attention in recent years. The first wave of attention led to suggestions that panic and generalized anxiety were two different disorders, but recent study makes this less clear (Rickles & Schweizer, 1986). High-potency benzodiazepines, such as alprazolam and clonazepam, may be effective in preventing panic episodes, as well as in alleviating more general anxiety (Rosenbaum, 1986). There is some possibility that standard benzodiazepines, perhaps in higher doses, may be similarly effective. The benzodiazepine drugs currently in use are summarized in Table 4.

Clearly, many patients with situational, characterological, medically derived, and other causes of anxiety also experience symptomatic relief from benzodiazepine drugs. Although dependence can be a problem in some cases, many patients take stable doses of these drugs for years without ill effects. Providing the physician does not have evidence that the drug is being abused, and providing the physician and the patient are aware of the hazards of abrupt withdrawal, long-term treatment with these agents need not be shunned. Whether benzodiazepines maintain their full efficacy over months and years of use remains an open question, but some indirect lines of evidence suggest that they do; for example, patients withdrawn from long-term use develop reemergent anxiety, even after withdrawal symptoms have ceased, a result suggesting that the drugs had a continuing effect (Schopf, 1983).

The newest entrants into the benzodiazepine arena have been two members of the triazolo subclass: alprazolam and triazolam. Both have been greeted with widespread enthusiasm, but both are associated with some concerns about risks. There is some evidence, still inconclusive, that alprazolam possesses antidepressant and antipanic properties beyond those of other benzodiazepines (Dawson, Jue, & Brogden, 1984). However, many clinicians find patients more reluctant to stop this drug than other benzodiazepines, and withdrawal problems may be more severe with this agent. Some patients develop a ''clock-watching syndrome,'' in which they eagerly await the arrival of the time for their next dose of alprazolam, presumably a same-day withdrawal reaction (Rosenbaum, 1986).

Triazolam is a benzodiazepine hypnotic with a very short half-life. Although this should mean fewer problems of drug accumulation and hangover, problems of rebound insomnia, morning-after anxiety, and profound anterograde amnesia have been associated with this agent (Donaldson, 1983).

The advent of the benzodiazepine drugs and their increasing popularity over the past two decades has led to the welcome retirement of most other classes of anxiolytic and sedative-hypnotic drugs. The many barbiturates and nonbarbiturates (e.g., chloral hydrate, glutethimide, methaqualone, and meprobamate) were certainly no more effective than benzodiazepines (perhaps, less so), were associated with variably more severe (and potentially lethal) withdrawal syndromes, and carried a much greater risk of death by overdose (Gelenberg, 1983).

Table 4. Benzodiazepine Antianxiety Drugs[a]

Drug	Approximate dose equivalents (mg)	Available dosage forms	Rapidity of absorption	Active metabolites	Half-life (hr)
Alprazolam (Xanax®)	0.5	0.25-, 0.5-, and 1.0-mg tablets	Intermediate	α-Hydroxyalprazolam, desmethylalprazolam, 4-hydoxyalprazolam	6 to 20
Chlordiazepoxide (Librium® and others)	10	5-, 10-, 25-mg tablets and capsules, 100-mg/2-ml ampule	Intermediate	Desmethylchlordiazepoxide, demoxepam, desmethyldiazepam, oxazepam	5 to 30
Clorazepate (Azene®, Tranxene®)	7.5	3.75-, 7.5-, and 15-mg capsules (Tranxene®) 3.25-, 6.5-, and 13-mg capsules (Azene®)	Fast	Desmethyldiazepam,[b] oxazepam	30 to 200
Diazepam (Valium®)	5	2-, 5-, 10-mg tablets, 10-mg/2-ml ampules, 50-mg/10-ml vials, 10-mg/2-ml syringe	Fastest	Desmethyldiazepam, oxazepam	20 to 100
Halazepam (Paxipam®)	20	20-, 40-mg tablets	Intermediate	Desmethyldiazepam, oxazepam	Ca. 14 (parent), 50 to 100 desmethyldiazepam 10 to 20
Lorazepam (Ativan®)	1	0.5-, 1-, 2-mg tablets, 2- and 4-mg/ml syringes, 2- and 4-mg/ml vials[c]	Intermediate	None	
Oxazepam (Serax®)	15	10-, 15-, 30-mg capsules, 15-mg tablets	Slower	None	5 to 15
Prazepam (Centrax®, Verstran®)	10	5-, 10-mg capsules, 10-mg tablets	Slowest	Desmethyldiazepam,[b] oxazepam	30 to 200

[a]Prepared with the assistance of Jerrold F. Rosenbaum, M.D.: reprinted from Bassuk, Schoonover, and Gelenberg (1983). Copyright 1983. Reproduced by permission.
[b]These drugs are prodrugs for desmethyldiazepam: the parent compound is rapidly converted to the active metabolite.
[c]As of this writing, approved by FDA only for preanesthetic use.

One of the more important emphases in recent years regarding the pharmacological treatment of insomnia has been the need to diagnose the subtypes of insomnia, particularly those with specific treatments. Thus, physicians have come to recognize the existence of sleep apnea and other syndromes that disturb sleep, yet in which hypnotic drugs may not be effective or may even be hazardous (Gelenberg, 1983).

OTHER AGENTS

Almost everything in the pharmacopoeia has been prescribed, at one time or another, for psychiatric patients. Unfortunately, few have been evaluated systematically, so that we rarely have definitive proof of efficacy or acceptably small "error" limits on lack of effectiveness.

Amino acid precursors of neurotransmitters have been written about for many years as potential psychopharmacological agents. Probably the greatest evidence supports some role for tryptophan as a weak physiological sedative (Hartmann, 1986; Schneider-Helmert & Spinweber, 1986). Its role, alone or as an adjunct, in the treatment of mood disorders remains unproved (Gelenberg, 1989). Similar studies with tyrosine and phenylalanine as antidepressants also have been inconclusive (Gelenberg, 1989).

Another naturally occurring precursor of a neurotransmitter is the phospholipid lecithin. Along with its constituent choline, lecithin has been administered for a variety of conditions that might theoretically be improved by the administration of an agent that can enhance acetylcholine neurotransmission in the brain. Lecithin may have some marginal role in the treatment of tardive dyskinesia (Gelenberg, Dorer, Wojcik, Falk, Brotman, & Leahy, 1988) at least by itself appears to offer little in the treatment of dementia, and seems to produce only marginal clinical benefit as an adjunct in the treatment of mania (Gelenberg, 1988).

The treatment of dementia remains unsatisfactory. Of course, associated symptoms (i.e., psychosis, depression, anxiety, and insomnia) can be treated with the specific classes of agents that alleviate them. However, the only agent with some (limited) suggestion of improving the memory deficits associated with aging is ergoloid mesylates (Hydergine), whose mechanism of action remains unknown but may be related to effects on brain metabolism (Elsasser & Anderson, 1986).

Antihypertensive agents acting on the noradrenergic systems have been used in a variety of states. Physicians have used clonidine to treat akathisia and a variety of psychotic conditions; the evidence at present remains equivocal (Zubenko, Cohen, Lipinski, & Jonas, 1985).

More attention has been focused on the beta-blocker propranolol (Anath & Lin, 1986). There is some evidence that it may alleviate some of the somatic symptoms associated with anxiety and panic (Rosenbaum, 1986) and may counteract akathisia (Adler, Angrist, Pesselow, Corwin, Maslansky, & Rotrosen, 1986; Lipinski, Zubenko, Cohen, & Barreira, 1983). There is contradictory evidence regarding its efficacy, alone or as an adjunct to antipsychotic drugs, for the treatment of psychosis (Gelenberg, 1986b; Manchanda & Hirsch, 1986). Anecdotal data suggest a possible role for propranolol, and perhaps for other beta-blockers, in the treatment of the aggressive behavior associated with various organic brain syndromes (Falk, 1986).

CONCLUSIONS

We have come a long way since the 1940s. The advent and ready availability of safe, effective psychiatric drugs has made the widespread outpatient practice of psychiatry possible—particularly for patients with more severe forms of psychiatric disorder. The last 20 years have seen continuing progress in psychopharmacology—not as dramatic, perhaps, as the original discovery of the primary psychopharmacological classes, but progress that points out routes to greater efficacy and safety with the existing drugs.

Clearly, there is a long way to go. We await greater biochemical sophistication and pharmacological specificity. Clinically, we seek heightened levels of efficacy, together with lower (as well as different) profiles of unwanted effects.

The rest of this book provides abundant detail of our current state in psychopharmacology within the broader context of contemporary outpatient treatment. Clinicians—along with patients and their families—will benefit greatly from the fruits of our science.

REFERENCES

Adler, L., Angrist, B., Pesselow, E., Corwin, J., Maslansky, R., & Rotrosen, J. (1986). A controlled assessment of propranolol in the treatment of neuroleptic-induced akathisia. *British Journal of Psychiatry, 148,* 701–707.

Anath, J., & Lin, K-M. (1986). Propranolol in psychiatry: Therapeutic uses and side effects. *Neuropsychobiology, 15,* 20–27.

Biederman, J. (1986). Desipramine in attention deficit disorder. *Biological Therapies in Psychiatry, 9,* 29–32.

Brotman, A. W. (1984). Antidepressants and anticonvulsants: Magic bullets for bulimia? *Biological Therapies in Psychiatry, 7,* 10–11.

Brotman, A. W. (1985). Antidepressant treatment for cocaine abuse. *Biological Therapies in Psychiatry, 8,* 8.

Brotman, A. W., Falk, W. E., & Gelenberg, A. J. (1987). Pharmacologic treatment of acute depressive subtypes. In H. Meltzer (Ed.), *Psychopharmacology: A generation of progress* (3rd ed.). New York: Raven Press.

Dawson, G. W., Jue, S. G., & Brogden, R. N. (1984). Alprazolam: A review of its pharmacodynamic properties and efficacy in the treatment of anxiety and depression. *Drugs, 27,* 132–147.

Donaldson, S. R. (1983). The benzodiazepine hypnotics. *Biological Therapies in Psychiatry, 6,* 37–40.

Elsasser, G. N., & Anderson, R. K. (1986). Senile dementia: Treatment with vasodilators. *Hospital Formulary, 21,* 197–203.

Falk, W. E. (1985). Carbamazepine (Tegretol) for manic-depressive illness: An update. *Biological Therapies in Psychiatry, 8,* 21–24.

Falk, W. E. (1986). Beta blockers for aggression. *Biological Therapies in Psychiatry, 9,* 41–43.

Falloon, I. R. H., Boyd, J. L., McGill, C. W., Razani, J., Moss, H. B., & Gilderman, A. M. (1982). Family management in the prevention of exacerbations of schizophrenia: A controlled study. *New England Journal of Medicine, 306,* 1437–1440.

Gelenberg, A. J. (1983). Insomnia. In E. L. Bassuk, S. C. Schoonover, & A. J. Gelenberg (Eds.), *The practioner's guide to psychoactive drugs* (2nd ed,, pp. 203–220). New York: Plenum Medical Book Co.

Gelenberg, A. J. (1984a). The DST in even greater perspective. Massachusetts General Hospital Newsletter, *Biological Therapies in Psychiatry, 7,* 1.

Gelenberg, A. J. (1984b). Patients with affective illness: Are they more prone to develop TD? *Biological Therapies in Psychiatry, 7,* 6.

Gelenberg, A. J. (1985). Mood disorders: Preventing recurrences. *Biological Therapies in Psychiatry, 8,* 5–6.

Gelenberg, A. J. (1986a). Prophylactic and maintenance antiparkinson medication. *Biological Therapies in Psychiatry, 9,* 33–35.

Gelenberg, A. J. (1986b). Propranolol (Inderal) for schizophrenia: A review and new data. *Biological Therapies in Psychiatry, 9,* 13–14.

Gelenberg, A. J. (1989). Psychiatric disorders. In D. M. Paige (Ed.), *Manual of clinical nutrition* (2nd ed., pp. 419–428). Pleasantville, NJ: Nutrition Publications.

Gelenberg, A. J., Wojcik, J., Falk, W. E., Coggins, C. H., Brotman, A. W., Rosenbaum, J. F., LaBrie, R. A., & Kerman, B. J. (1987). Effects of lithium on the kidney. *Acta Psychiatrica Scandinavia, 75,* 29–34.

Gelenberg, A. J., Dorer, D., Wojcik, J., Falk, W. E., Brotman, A. W., & Leahy, L. (1988). *Lecithin for tardive dyskinesia.* Unpublished manuscript.

Hartmann, E. L. (1986). Effect of L-tryptophan and other amino acids on sleep. *Nutrition Reviews, Supplement,* 70–73.

Jenike, M. A. (1986). Somatic treatments in obsessive-compulsive disorders. In M. A. Jenike, L. Baer, & W. E. Minichiello (Eds.), *Obsessive compulsive disorder: Theory and management.* Littleton, MA: PSG.

Kane, J. M. (1983). Low dose medication strategies in the maintenance treatment of schizophrenia. *Schizophrenia Bulletin, 9,* 528–532.

Kane, J. M. (1986, March). *Outpatient treatment of schizophrenia.* Paper read before the symposium *Antipsychotic drug therapy: Current Concepts and Future Trends,* Key Biscayne, Florida.

Lipinski, J. F., Zubenko, G. S., Cohen, B. M., & Barreira, P. J. (1983). Propranolol in the treatment of neuroleptic-induced akathisia (letter to editor). *Lancet, 1,* 685–686.

Manchanda, R., & Hirsch, S. R. (1986). Does propranolol have an antipsychotic effect? A placebo-controlled study in acute schizophrenia. *British Journal of Psychiatry, 148,* 701–707.

McEvoy, J. P. (1986). The neuroleptic threshold as a marker of minimum effective neuroleptic dose. *Comprehensive Psychiatry, 27,* 327–335.

Plenge, P., & Mellerup, E. T. (1986). Lithium and the kidney: Is one daily dose better than two? *Comprehensive Psychiatry, 27,* 336–342.

Prien, R. F., & Gelenberg, A. J. (1989). Alternatives to lithium for the preventive maintenance treatment of bipolar disorder. *American Journal of Psychiatry, 146,* 840–848.

Prien, R. F., Kupfer, D. J., Mansky, P. A., Small, J. G., Tuason, V. B., Voss, C. B., & Johnson, W. E. (1984). Drug therapy in the prevention of recurrence in unipolar and bipolar affective disorders. *Archives of General Psychiatry, 41,* 1096–1104.

Quitkin, F. M. (1985). The importance of dosage in prescribing antidepressants. *British Journal of Psychiatry, 147,* 593–597.

Rickles, K., & Schweizer, E. E. (1986). Benzodiazepines for treatment of panic attacks: A new look. *Psychopharmacology Bulletin, 22,* 93–99.

Rosenbaum, J. F. (1986, August). Panic disorder. *Drug therapy,* 113–114.

Schneider-Helmert, D., & Spinweber, C. L. (1986). Evaluation of L-tryptophan for treatment of insomnia: A review. *Psychopharmacology, 89,* 1–7.

Schopf, J. (1983). Withdrawal phenomena after long-term administration of benzodiazepines: A review of recent investigations. *Pharmacopsychiatry, 16,* 1–8.

Zubenko, G. S., Cohen, B. M., Lipinski, J. F., & Jonas, J. M. (1985). Use of clonidine in treating neuroleptic-induced akathisia. *Psychiatry Research, 13,* 253–259.

4

Overview of Psychodynamic Treatment

PAUL CRITS-CHRISTOPH, LESTER LUBORSKY, AND JACQUES BARBER

INTRODUCTION

Dynamic psychotherapies continue to be the most commonly used mode of treatment both in outpatient psychiatric clinics and in private practice (Feldman, Lorr, & Russell, 1958; Henry, Sims, & Spray, 1973). They are the major form of psychotherapy taught in psychiatric residency programs. Among clinical psychologists, a survey by Prochaska and Norcross (1983) showed that 29.2% identified themselves as purely psychodynamic in orientation, and 45% of those who labeled themselves eclectic (30% of the total sample) described dynamic psychotherapy as underlying their eclectic orientations. When compared to surveys conducted during the 1970s (e.g., Garfield & Kurtz, 1976), these figures actually represent an increased interest in dynamic psychotherapy since that time.

The number of specific therapies that fit within the broad dynamic-therapy label is large and ranges from traditional psychoanalysis through neo-Freudian perspectives (Jung, Adler, and Sullivan) to the more recent, time-limited dynamic approaches of Mann, Sifneos, and others. What is common in these perspectives on therapy is a set of concepts that provide the foci for treatment (e.g., conflict, defense, resistance, and transference) and that specify the actions of the therapist (e.g., interpretation). In addition, the dynamic therapies generally emphasize that change occurs, in part, through gains by the patient in self-understanding about conflictual patterns.

What evidence is there that dynamic therapy is effective? In their meta-analysis of

---

PAUL CRITS-CHRISTOPH, LESTER LUBORSKY, and JACQUES BARBER • Department of Psychiatry, University of Pennsylvania, Philadelphia, Pennsylvania 19104.

psychotherapy outcome studies, Smith, Glass, and Miller (1980) reported that the mean effect size ($n = 225$ effect sizes) for dynamic therapy compared to a no-treatment control was .78, a large effect according to Cohen's definitions (1977).

A more recent review (Luborsky, Crits-Christoph, Auerbach, & Mintz, 1988) similarly concludes that the benefits of dynamic therapies are large. These benefits are probably on a par with those of the other main forms of psychotherapy. This conclusion about the comparative equality of benefits is based on several reviews (Lambert, Shapiro, & Bergin, 1986; Luborsky, Singer, & Luborsky, 1975; Smith & Glass, 1977). These reviews convincingly show that comparisons of one form of psychotherapy with another tend to yield nonsignificant difference effects. This is exactly the trend that appeared in a more recent review of all controlled comparisons of dynamic therapies with other therapies (Luborsky, 1986). In this review, there were 16 such comparisons, and all but 2 showed nonsignificant difference effects. The nonsignificant difference effect is especially striking when one considers the probable disinclination to publish nonsignificant difference results, as well as the fact that the majority of these comparative treatment studies were carried out by researchers who were not dynamic psychotherapists themselves.

Despite the generally positive findings reported, more studies are needed, particularly studies of the types of patient populations most suited for dynamic treatment, as well as studies of the effective ingredients of successful treatment. More systematic studies are beginning to appear (e.g., Woody, Luborsky, McLellan, O'Brien, Beck, Blaine, Herman, & Hole, 1983) in which treatment is carefully standardized through the use of treatment manuals and supervision, therapists are carefully selected and trained, and measures especially relevant to the study of dynamic therapy are used.

The purpose of this chapter is to provide an updated overview of the treatment principles of dynamic therapy in its newly described forms. We have chosen to review the relatively recent descriptions of dynamic psychotherapy, as represented in specific published treatment manuals and guides to brief dynamic therapy. This choice reflects our view that, although the early clinical writings in psychoanalysis and psychoanalytic psychotherapy are invaluable sources, the recent treatment manuals provide clear accounts of dynamic techniques, integrating knowledge from the previous clinical and research literatures. Psychotherapy outcome research has begun to be and will become routinely based on these treatment manuals, and therefore, our knowledge about efficacy will be directly tied to these treatment methods. The emphasis in our review of brief treatment is consistent with the trend toward brief therapy in the field. One factor accounting for this trend is the tendency for insurance companies and health maintenance organizations (HMOs) to limit coverage to a fixed number of sessions, which would fall within a brief treatment approach. The major intrinsic factor is that there is more evidence now about the benefits of briefer approaches and more knowledge about the conditions that are helpful and the patients who are appropriate.

Seven different dynamic therapy methods are reviewed here: those of Malan, Sifneos, Mann, Davanloo, Luborsky, Strupp and Binder, and Klerman *et al.* For each, we present the main selection criteria used to screen patients for the treatment, the process of change over therapy, and the major techniques of the method. Although there are strong similarities among the approaches, we have highlighted in our review the unique aspects of each in order to reduce redundancy, and we have provided space for each roughly in proportion to the generality of use of the approach.

Malan, one of Balint's students, has reported his work, including the detailed follow-up of two groups of patients, in two major books (1976a,b). Beginning in the 1950s, the first group of patients was treated by therapists supervised by Balint at the Tavistock Clinic in London. The second group of patients was treated by Malan's own group in the Tavistock Brief Therapy Unit. In his work, Balint tried to develop a short form of treatment based on the principles of psychoanalysis for relatively healthy individuals suffering from acute neurotic conflicts. Even though he found that most of these patients also had more chronic problems, they were accepted into treatment and, surprisingly, were helped by the therapy despite their relatively "weak ego." The long-standing character problems of these patients were somewhat improved after 40 sessions.

Patient Selection

Malan proposed a set of exclusive and inclusive criteria for accepting and rejecting patients for treatment. The excluding factors include serious suicidal attempts, drug addiction, long-term hospitalization, more than one course of ECT, chronic alcoholism, incapacitating obsessional symptoms, chronic phobic symptoms, and gross destructive or self-destructive acting out. In addition to psychiatric criteria, Malan uses the following psychodynamic criteria: quality of interpersonal relationships, degree of emotional openness, response to interpretation of the focal conflict, motivation for therapy, and focality of the complaint.

Process of Change

Malan describes the process of change in the usual psychoanalytic way: Through the skillful interpretation of conflict, defense, and transference, the therapist helps the patient gain self-understanding, which leads to symptomatic change. The specific techniques used by the therapist to accomplish this aim are described below.

Major Techniques

Malan refers to two triangles. One triangle consists of a wish (or derivative of an id impulse), its threat (moral or social), and the defense used to reduce anxiety. The second triangle describes three patterns of interpersonal relationship: one found in the patient's relationship with the therapist (transference), another with important others in the present or the near past, and the third with parental figures of the past. Interpretations that relate these different spheres contribute to the patient's understanding of his or her basic conflict. Most important is the interpretation of the recurrent pattern observed in the transference in light of similar patterns with parental figures. This is called the *transference parent link* (T/P). Malan (1976a) suggested a specific sequence to be followed in the interpretation of the first triangle: the defense is interpreted before the wish and the anxiety. Moreover, the issues involved in the first triangle need to be clarified in one domain before they are generalized to other domains. As to the second triangle, no specific rules are suggested except that the transference needs to be clarified in terms of the wish–defense triangle. Malan advocates that the therapist reserve transference interpretations until the transference has definitely developed, a situation that varies from case to case.

SIFNEOS: SHORT-TERM ANXIETY-PROVOKING THERAPY

In the 1960s, Sifneos developed an interpretive short-term dynamic psychotherapy at the Massachusetts General Hospital in Boston. He challenged the belief that the rapid cure of deep and enduring pathology is mere "transference cure" or "flight into health."

Patient Selection

Sifneos (1972) listed five main selection criteria for his brand of short-term dynamic psychotherapy: (1) above-average intelligence; (2) at least one meaningful relationship in the patient's past history; (3) the ability to express emotion appropriately during the initial interview; (4) the ability to describe one specific chief complaint; and (5) motivation for change. This final criterion includes such factors as the ability to recognize symptoms as psychological, the desire to be an active participant in treatment, active curiosity and the ability to be introspective about oneself, and realistic expectations about therapy.

Process of Change

Preparation of the patient is the first step in the process of change. In particular, during evaluation interviews, a shift occurs in the patient's expectations from a desire for symptomatic relief to a wish for more basic change in attitudes and understanding. Next, the development of a positive therapeutic alliance creates an atmosphere conducive to learning about oneself. The therapist's interpretations then help the patient learn how present-day interpersonal relationships are associated with neurotic conflicts from the past. The patient also learns how his or her attempts to avoid anxiety have created problems. Change also occurs through experimenting with new ways to solve emotional problems. After observing tangible evidence that change has occurred, the therapist considers termination.

Major Techniques

Sifneos (1972) described technique issues as related to five major phases of therapy: (1 the patient–therapist encounter; (2) the early treatment; (3) the height of treatment; (4) the evidence of change; and (5) the process of termination. During the first phase (the patient–therapist encounter), in addition to history taking the therapist uses the patient's positive feelings to set up a therapeutic alliance and begins to formulate a tentative psychodynamic hypothesis that serves to define the goals of treatment. In the early phase of treatment, the therapist begins to look for manifestations of transference. Sifneos believes that the therapist does not have to wait until transference appears as a resistance, and that the confrontation of positive transference does not need to be postponed. During the height-of-treatment phase, the therapist uses confrontation and anxiety-provoking questions concentrated in the areas of unresolved conflict, as seen in the transference relationship, to stimulate the patient to reexamine past conflict and to increase self-understanding. The therapist's role is described by Sifneos (1972) as "one of an unemotionally involved teacher" (p. 117).

After the therapist has demonstrated repeatedly that the patient's conflicts are a repetition of past themes, termination is considered during an examination of whether sufficient changes have occurred in the emotional problems. The criteria that the therapist uses for evidence of change include reduced tension during therapy sessions, decreased symptomatology, and changes in conflict-related interpersonal behavior. When change is evident, the therapist encourages the patient to use the new problem-solving capabilities learned from therapy in other areas of emotional conflict so that the patient will be able to solve future conflicts. When both therapist and patient agree that the goals of treatment have been achieved, a date for termination is set. During this final phase, ambivalent feelings related to termination are handled without exploring all of the implications of the separation. The therapist summarizes and emphasizes what has been achieved. The patient is taught to anticipate future emotional conflicts, and the therapist communicates that she or he trusts the patient to solve future problems on his or her own.

MANN: TIME-LIMITED THERAPY

Mann's approach (1973) is unusual in that he emphasizes the importance of the patient's negative image of herself or himself and the meaning that time has for the patient. Time is viewed on a continuum stretching from an objective perspective of the meaning of time (where needs and wishes can be only partially gratified) to a more infantile perspective (where time has no limit and consequently the person is immortal, and needs are continuously fulfilled). As a consequence, the treatment adheres rigidly to a 12-session limit.

Mann's brief treatment is oriented around a "central issue" related to one of four universal conflict situations that express the different ways in which humans experience loss. These universal conflict situations are (1) independence versus dependence; (2) activity versus passivity; (3) adequate self-esteem versus reduced self-esteem; and (4) unresolved or delayed grief.

Patient Selection

Although Mann's criteria for the inclusion of patients are more flexible than those of Malan or Sifneos, he states that if a central issue or complaint cannot be arrived at in evaluation interviews, time-limited psychotherapy is not the treatment of choice. The lack of a definable central focus is often associated with diagnoses of borderline personality disorder or schizophrenia. Profoundly depressed and acutely psychotic patients are also excluded.

This treatment tends to be most suited to young adults in middle or late adolescence, such as college students. These patients are most likely to be in the midst of a maturational crisis, often related to separation-individuation. Mann (1973) explained:

> The patient in a maturational crisis is best served by treatment that engages all of his own inclinations toward maturity. Hence, a time limit addresses itself to his desire for independence and the confidence that the time is sufficient for him to do the job that must be done. (p. 76)

Process of Change

The process of change is related directly to the time limit of therapy. At the beginning of treatment (approximately Sessions 1–4), knowledge of the termination date increases anxiety about loss, leading to repression of the termination date and activation of defenses against separation. Rapid symptomatic improvement is often seen during this beginning phase as a result of the patient's unconscious wish for union and expectations that past disappointments will be undone. During the middle phase of therapy (roughly Sessions 5–8), the patient's enthusiasm decreases and is replaced with ambivalent feelings and a return of symptoms. Sessions 9–12 constitute the termination phase and are marked by an intensification of the negative transference. The work of the resolution of basic conflicts is done during this phase, which, if successful, includes the patient's coming to some affective understanding of the inappropriate nature of the early unconscious conflict. In addition, the patient internalizes the therapist as a substitute for the earlier ambivalent object.

Major Techniques

The therapist is active in this short-term treatment mode. This active approach begins with an active assessment of the central issue, which is followed by active redirection in order to maintain the appropriate focus. The therapist also encourages and supports the patient to increase self-esteem and engages in a certain amount of education in terms of presenting the facts about sibling rivalry, masturbation, and so on, as they are connected to the central issue. Through the middle and end phases of treatment when the patient's ambivalent feelings are emerging, the therapist acknowledges the patient's feelings of disappointment. The therapist then begins, for the first time, to interpret connections between the therapy and the patient's earlier experiences involving separation without resolution from a significant but ambivalently experienced person. Mann specifically states, however, that these interpretations should not be worded in terms of libidinal and aggressive developmental fantasies.

The difficulty of termination for the therapist is discussed by Mann. Doubts about effectiveness as a therapist and resistance to termination (e.g., by communicating that the treatment might continue beyond 12 sessions) are two ways this difficulty can be manifested. Mann recommends personal psychoanalysis to help the therapist achieve self-knowledge and to improve his or her therapeutic effectiveness.

THE SHORT-TERM DYNAMIC PSYCHOTHERAPY OF DAVANLOO

In several respects, the psychodynamic therapy of Davanloo is different from the other approaches reviewed here. The patient inclusion criteria are more liberal than those advocated by the other schools and depend to a large degree on a unique "trial therapy" period. In addition, Davanloo's techniques are somewhat radical, with a strong emphasis on persistent confrontation of defenses. He is also more optimistic about successful results, claiming a total cure in a high percentage of patients.

Patient Selection

Davanloo (1980) indicated that his therapy has been applied to four major groups of patients: (1) patients with a predominantly Oedipal focus; (2) patients whose focus is a loss; (3) patients with phobic and/or obsessional neuroses; and (4) patients with long-standing characterological problems, including multiple conflicts. Contraindications to treatment include a past history of psychotic decompensation, paranoid conditions, poor impulse control, and serious suicidal attempts. Beyond these contraindications, the assessment of suitability for treatment is accomplished via a pretherapy interview designed to elicit information about the following: (1) the presence of a meaningful past relationship; (2) the ability to become involved in emotional interaction with the interviewer; (3) the presence of a give-and-take relationship; (4) the patient's capacity to tolerate anxiety, guilt, and depression; (5) psychological-mindedness; (6) motivation; and (7) a positive response to interpretation. The last criterion is recognized as the most important, and it is believed to have important prognostic significance in regard to treatment outcome.

Process of Change

Davanloo (1980) described the process of change as follows:

> Within the first few sessions fresh memories usually arise which throw light on the whole development of the patient's neurosis. This on the one hand brings relief, but as the patient is confronted with his painful feelings he often develops negative feelings toward the therapist. Focusing on the patient's anger as soon as it arises is essential. Once more, showing the patient his defense against anger . . . has a potentially powerful therapeutic effect. This leads to other kinds of feelings: grief and loss, and forbidden sexual feelings in the patient's childhood. By about the sixth to eighth session therapeutic effects have already begun to occur, and the patient is beginning to show evidence that he is relating to people in his current life in a new way; and there is also a similar change in the transference situation. I do not consider the therapy successful unless the patient is not only free from symptoms but also from all his previous maladaptive behavior, and unless in addition he shows both cognitive and emotional insight into the core neurosis which has caused all these symptoms and difficulties. When this happens termination is considered. (p. 678)

Major Techniques

The therapist's technique involves the "gentle but relentless questioning and confrontation of the defenses against true feelings" (Davanloo, 1980, p. 46). Active interpretation centers on two triangles similar to Malan's triangles: (1) the triangle of conflict (defense/anxiety/impulse-feeling) and (2) the triangle of person: (transference/significant people in the patient's current life/significant people in the past). These techniques of relentless confrontation and transference interpretation are used both in the trial therapy period and throughout the rest of treatment. Thus, Davanloo advocates active interpretation of transference and of defenses very early in treatment. He does, however, recommend active avoidance of the development of a symbiotic transference relationship and avoidance of inducing regression.

LUBORSKY: SUPPORTIVE-EXPRESSIVE PSYCHOANALYTIC THERAPY

The work of the theorists reviewed above led to what one may call the third generation of short-term psychoanalytically oriented psychotherapies. For our present purposes, the main characteristic of this most recent trend in psychoanalytically oriented psychotherapies is the development of manuals especially designed for teaching, practice, and research in these therapies. Manual-guided therapies represent a prerequisite stage in the move toward a more sophisticated empirical investigation of the therapeutic processes; without them, investigators cannot ascertain that a minimal basis exists for comparing different therapists, patients, or techniques. Moreover, the manuals explicitly describe the techniques used in the therapy, as well as measures of the therapists' compliance with the techniques.

Luborsky's book *Principles of Psychoanalytic Psychotherapy: A Manual for Supportive-Expressive Treatment* (1984) was the first explicit manual for psychoanalytic psychotherapy. In it he described the major principles of this form of treatment as derived from the works of Freud and of therapists from the Menninger Foundation. The manual is addressed to both long- and short-term therapies.

Patient Selection

Unlike the previous set of theorists, Luborsky (1984) did not give a firm list of exclusion criteria. Supportive-expressive (SE) treatment is described as being flexible enough to deal with many kinds of patients, ranging from those with mild situational maladjustments to borderline psychotics. The therapist deals with this broad range of severity by using an appropriate balancing of supportiveness and expressiveness; that is, the greater the psychiatric severity, the more supportive and the less expressive the therapy needs to be. Recent research (Horowitz, Marmar, Weiss, DeWitt, & Rosenbaum, 1984) has supported this position.

Although substance abuse is commonly an exclusion criterion for dynamic therapies, SE treatment has been demonstrated to produce significant improvement beyond treatment-as-usual in opiate addicts (Woody *et al.*, 1983), and therefore, it is recommended in this context as well. Luborsky (1984) also described how SE can be used in combination with pharmocotherapy for more severely disturbed patients.

Process of Change

The SE manual explicity describes what needs to change. The psychological conflicts within the personality, as represented by and contained within the relationship problems, are the most in need of change. During the course of therapy, the patient experiences these vividly in the transference. In SE, these interpersonal manifestations of conflicts are named the *core conflictual relationship theme* (CCRT). The CCRT includes two major components: on one hand, the wish, or need, or intention, and on the other hand, responses from others and responses from the self. The wishes and both sorts of responses theoretically form the basis of the pathology, and therefore, they are expected to change following therapy.

In terms of how change comes about, Luborsky (1984) described three main curative factors: self-understanding, helping alliance, and incorporation of the gains.

Self-Understanding

The theory postulates that understanding represents the main prerequisite for the patient's improvement. The *in vivo* reexperiencing of earlier conflictual relationships in the current relationship with the therapist leads the patient to achieve a better understanding of his or her problems. By "working through" the various editions of the transference (i.e., remembering and repeating them), the patient's sense of mastery and control increases. The patient becomes better able to recognize his or her relationship pattern and the problem areas within it and to find more adaptive ways of behaving, even though "transference potentials remain recognizable" (Luborsky, 1984, p. 23).

Building a Therapeutic Relationship

Luborsky (1984) distinguished two types of "helping alliance." In one, the patient views the therapist as helpful, and in the second, the patient views the treatment as a collaborative endeavor toward achieving the goals of the therapy.

Three main sources contribute to the patient's experience of the helping alliance. The first source is the general form of the therapy, such as regular meetings and the therapist's willingness to help the patient. The second source is the "therapist's attitude of sympathetic understanding" (Luborsky, 1984, p. 25). The third source derives from the therapist's fitting the patient's expectation of a helpful person.

Maintaining the Therapeutic Gains

In psychoanalytic thinking, internalization—that is, the maintenance in memory of the therapist as a helpful person—is viewed as the main mechanism for preserving therapeutic gains. Internalization is thought to be facilitated by the quality of the patient's working through of the termination. For example, the therapist pays close attention to, and even anticipates, the partial relapse of symptoms toward the end of the treatment as the patient's way of confronting the end of this helpful and close relationship.

The decision concerning termination differs, depending on whether the SE psychotherapy is time-limited (TL) or time-open-ended (TO). In TO, the length of the treatment is not decided at the beginning, although the therapist and the patient decide from the outset what achievements will be sought and therefore will lead to termination. In TL, both therapist and patient agree on a termination date at the beginning of treatment. Obviously, when the treatment goals are achieved, termination is considered. Nevertheless, the patient can always decide to work on other goals. When this occurs, the therapist and the patient need to examine whether these new goals are genuine or represent an attempt to deal with the separation by postponing it.

During the termination phase, one often observes the reappearance of symptoms, which reflects the patient's anticipation that the gains will disappear once therapy is ended. The patient's attempt to terminate therapy prematurely may be indicative of the involvement of a transference issue; in some of these instances, interpreting the transference may decrease the patient's pressure to leave.

Major Techniques

The major techniques of supportive-expressive (SE) treatment were extracted from these sources: Bergmann and Hartman (1977); Bibring (1954); Freud (1958a–f); Gill (1951,); Greenson (1967); Hollender (1965); Luborsky, Fabian, Hall, Ticho, and Ticho (1958); Schlesinger (1969); and Stone (1961). The supportive component of SE psychotherapy is made up of those aspects of treatment that are reflected in the patient's experience of the treatment and the relationship with the therapist as helpful.

Under certain conditions, the alliance requires facilitation. Principles that will guide the therapist in facilitating a helping alliance include (1) conveying, through words and manner, support for the patient's wish to achieve the goals of treatment; (2) conveying a sense of understanding and acceptance of the patient; (3) developing a liking for patient; (4) helping the patient maintain vital defenses and activities that bolster the level of functioning; (5) communicating a realistically hopeful attitude that the treatment goals are likely to be achieved; (6) encouraging a "we" bond; (7) conveying respect for the patient; (8) conveying recognition of the patient's growing ability to do what the therapist does in using the basic tools of the treatment; (9) referring to experiences that the patient and the therapist have been through together; and (10) conveying support through an accurate understanding of the patient's communications.

The expressive part of the treatment refers to standard psychoanalytic techniques. These techniques include setting the stage for the patient to express his or her thoughts and feelings; the therapist and the patient subsequently reflect on the expressed thoughts and feelings. The thoughts and feelings gradually expressed make explicit what the patient is doing that is self-defeating and what may, therefore, need to be changed. The most telling revelations about what the patient is doing come from the reexperiencing of early relationship problems in the relationship with the therapist.

The principles that help guide the therapist in understanding the patient's problems include (1) understanding the symptoms in the context of conflictual relationships; (2) attending to shifts in "states of mind"; (3) formulating a core conflictual relationship theme; (4) attending in turn to current relationships, past relationships (especially with parental figures), and the relationship with the therapist; (5) reviewing further, as review tends to produce further understanding; (6) seeing the symptoms as problem-solution or coping attempts; (7) attending to the patient's perception of the therapist's behavior; (8) attending to redundancy; and (9) attending to temporal contiguity. In turn, the nature of the therapist's interpretative responses to the patient are guided by the following principles: (1) the therapist's response should effectively address a facet of the main relationship problem and at times relate that to one of the symptoms; (2) the therapist should recurrently interpret the core relationship theme, as this procedure facilitates the working through; (3) the therapist should recognize the patient's need to test the therapist in transference terms; (4) the therapist recognizes that both therapist and patient find it especially difficult to discuss the patient's relationship with the therapist; (5) the therapist focuses on the main relationship theme in order to further the alliance and maintain a sense of progress; (6) different patients require different degrees of working through the insight; (7) the correspondence between the messages from the patient and the therapist serve as a test of the therapist's response in a session; (8) interpretations should be timed to take into account how near the patient is to being aware of its content; (9) each interpretative statement should be as simple and short as possible; (10) interpretations should be given only when the therapist's understanding is adequate; (11) responses should be timed to take into account the length of the session; (12) the therapist should be alert to countertransference; and (13) recognition of the inclination to respond countertherapeutically provides a good basis for understanding the patient (Luborsky, 1984).

STRUPP AND BINDER: TIME-LIMITED DYNAMIC PSYCHOTHERAPY

In their 1984 book, Strupp and Binder summarized the work done on time-limited dynamic psychotherapy (TLDP) at Vanderbilt's Center for Psychotherapy Research.

Their specific approach to therapy is based, on one hand, on traditional and modern views of psychoanalysis and, on the other hand, on the interpersonal perspective of the neo-Freudian schools.

With respect to etiology, the authors have adopted a Sullivanian-like model of the child's emotional development; that is, they view the adult's restricted ability to create relationship roles as being the consequence of chronic injuries to the child's self-esteem.

Patient Selection

The most important criterion for the selection of patients after one has ruled out major symptomatology (e.g., psychotic disorders) is the patient's ability to form a collaborative relationship with the therapist as exemplified during the "trial intervention." The other criteria are similar to the ones used by Malan, with the exception of the rapid creation of a good therapeutic relationship, as the goal of treatment is to remove the obstacles created by the patient in the process of developing such a relationship. In addition, unlike therapies in which defining the focus of treatment is a prerequisite (e.g., that of Malan), TLDP views the formulation of the "dynamic focus" as the central aspect of the therapy itself.

Theory of Change

Strupp and Binder (1984) introduced the concept of *dynamic focus* (later renamed the *cyclical maladaptive pattern*) as a concept related to Mann's central issue and to Luborsky's CCRT. They conceptualized the dynamic focus as a "heuristic guide to inquiry" (p. 67), which also clarifies and connects behavioral and experiential phenomena that otherwise appear unrelated and discontinuous. The focus is defined as collaboratively as possible, and it serves as a tool for using the limited time of the therapy efficiently. The general form of the focus is a schematic interpersonal narrative, that is, a way of organizing specific meanings into a story. The story describes actions embedded in interpersonal transactions organized in a self-defeating manner. The categories for describing a dynamic focus are as follows: (1) acts of self—these include both private and public actions (i.e., affects, motives, cognitions, and overt behaviors); (2) expectations about others' reactions—these are the anticipated and imagined reactions of others to one's own actions; (3) acts of others toward the self—what others do following acts by the self; and (4) acts of self toward self—how one treats oneself. Parallels between these categories and those of Luborsky's CCRT are evident.

The neurotic repetition is seen as being the result of the creation and maintenance of vicious circles. The best known example of vicious-circle behavior is shyness. The more shy the person, the less he or she will meet and speak with people, and so the lower the probability that he or she will acquire the skills necessary for smooth interpersonal interactions.

The dynamic focus describes a more-or-less unconscious, organizing life script that patients view as an absolute truth. Through telling their life story, patients' awareness of their own script increases, enabling them to begin to make sense of their self-defeating experience. Then, the patients may begin to see new possibilities.

Major Techniques

The techniques of TLDP encompass the goals of the therapist, the manner of understanding the patient, where and how the therapist intervenes, and how the therapist overcomes the obstacles within the therapeutic process.

The Therapist's Goals

Strupp and Binder (1984) presented two important means for the therapist to provide the patient with a constructive experience in living. First, the therapist acts in a consistently mature, reasonably caring manner. An important by-product of the therapist's therapeutic attitude is that some of the false assumptions that patients hold concerning the behavior and motives of others are refuted. Second, the therapist helps the patient to understand that some behavior has symbolic meaning. The patient's maladaptive relationships are best analyzed in the here and now of the transference. The analysis of the transference aims not at merely increasing intellectual understanding, but at providing a kind of experiential learning.

Strupp and Binder (1984), following Sullivan and his students, have emphasized the reciprocal nature of the therapeutic relationship. Both therapist and patient experience their relationship from several perspectives. The patient views the therapist in a flexible and mature manner (observing ego) as well as in a rigid and prejudiced way (transference). The third perspective focuses on the patient's active attempts to make others act in a way that will confirm the patient's expectations.

Therapists are also influenced by several perspectives. They act in a professional way, which is influenced by their personal style. In addition, they are induced into the roles that the patient creates or repeats for them. Finally, therapists may also be influenced by their own unresolved conflicts (countertransference).

The therapist can use those different perspectives to improve his or her understanding of the patient's interpersonal transactions with him or her. These transactions slowly become more explicit because the therapist gently leads the patient to examine them in the actual therapeutic relationship. The patient may then realize their importance and may become aware of the repetitiveness of his or her interpersonal problems.

Where Does the Therapist Intervene?

The therapist examines the patient's actions during therapy and then tries to find some meaning and purpose in them. At times, the therapist will interrupt the patient to reflect, clarify, or interpret the patient's emotional reactions.

As a rule, Strupp and Binder (1984) use T/P (transference-parent) link interpretations less than Davanloo or Malan, because they view T/P interpretation as only one form of intervention (i.e., they also emphasize how patients contribute to their own unhappiness through their rigid expectations). Moreover, they suggest offering T/P link interpretations only after the issue has been sufficiently addressed in the present situation with the therapist. Nevertheless, the realization that similarities exist between present and past relationships broadens the patient's understanding of the continuous influence of her or his history of disappointments, frustrations, and traumas.

The interpretation increases the patient's understanding of a current interpersonal transaction and the complicating factors. Offering an interpretation is a delicate task because of factors such as the patient's selective attention. Thus, an interpretation will be given in an empathic manner when the therapist has, for example, sufficient evidence supporting his or her claim. Then, it remains very important to clarify continuously and empathically how and what the patient understood by the interpretation.

KLERMAN ET AL.: INTERPERSONAL THERAPY FOR DEPRESSION

In contrast to the various therapies described above, interpersonal therapy (IPT; Klerman, Weissman, Rounsaville, & Chevron, 1984; Rounsaville, Klerman, Weissman, & Chevron, 1985) focuses on one disorder: depression. In addition, its roots are mostly in the interpersonal (Sullivanian) school of psychodynamic psychotherapy. This therapy has also received more research attention. Its efficacy has been assessed in comparison to cognitive therapy, medication, and placebo groups in the Collaborative Multi-Center Study for the treatment of depression (Elkin, Parloff, Hadley, & Autry, 1985). Two other clinical trials documenting the effectiveness of IPT for depression have been reported (Klerman, DiMascio, Weissman, Prusoff, & Paykel, 1974; Weissman, Prusoff, DiMascio, Neu, Goklaney, & Klerman, 1979).

Process of Change

IPT focuses on interpersonal functioning because it assumes that impaired social relationships either cause or perpetuate depression. Its goals are limited to the "symptomatic" and "interpersonal" levels, while leaving out the "personality" level.

At first, the symptoms are the center of attention, and no attempt is made to understand all the causes for the onset of the depression. The therapist actively keeps the patient focused on the goals of the treatment. The patient–therapist relationship is not the focus of treatment except when resistance requires it. The therapist presents herself or himself as an ally who focuses mainly on the here and now, despite a recognition of the childhood origins of impaired social behavior. In contrast to most previously described therapies, in IPT the therapist encourages actual practice and even sometimes gives direct advice. The therapist is also more active and less ambitious than in other psychodynamically oriented psychotherapies regarding the range of change to be achieved by the end of treatment.

Major Techniques

Because IPT has two central goals (managing depressive symptoms and improving interpersonal relationships), the techniques relevant to these two domains are separately presented.

Managing Depressive Symptoms

First, the therapist assesses the symptoms and their interpersonal contexts. The patient is then taught the various characteristics of depression and their implications. The need for medication is evaluated. Hope is strengthened by the patient's learning how prevalent depression is and how easily curable it is. Moreover, the patient learns that the syndrome does not indicate that something is basically wrong with him or her. The therapist initially allows the patient to receive the benefits of being diagnosed as sick (the reduction of obligations and the receiving of legitimate help), although the eventual aim is to have the patient give up the "sick role." Suggestions are made to the client to postpone or not to get too involved in activities that increase the depression. In addition, the patient is encouraged to seek situations that bring him or her some relief.

Treatment of the Patient's Interpersonal Functioning

While dealing with the depressive symptoms, the therapist directs the patient toward exploring the interpersonal circumstances surrounding the beginning of the depressive episode. Such exploration leads to the definition of one or more domains that are problems for the patient. Klerman *et al.* (1984) described four domains generally relevant to depression: grief, interpersonal disputes, role transitions, and interpersonal deficits (loneliness and social isolation). A short review of these four problem domains and their treatments follows.

Grief. IPT generally deals with "abnormal" grief reactions. Such abnormal reactions present two forms: delayed and distorted griefs. In delayed bereavement, the patient experiences grief long after the loss. In distorted grief, in contrast, the grieving differs from normal grief and there may be no dysphoria. Nonaffective symptoms may appear (e.g., psychomotor retardation). This reaction can occur directly after the loss or several years later.

In the treatment of abnormal grief, the two main goals are to enable the mourning process to develop and to help the patient regain interest in others to substitute for the loss (Rounsaville *et al.*, 1985). These goals are achieved through thinking about the loss and its implications with the help of the therapist's social support. The therapist needs to reassure the patient that reexperiencing the loss will not lead to a breakdown. In addition, the relationship with the deceased is explored in order to enable the patient to accept his or her contradictory feelings toward the deceased because quite often anger is at the root of the abnormal grief.

Interpersonal Role Dispute. These disputes evolve out of situations where the patient and at least one significant other do not have reciprocal expectations of their relationship (Rounsaville *et al.*, 1985). The treatment of interpersonal disputes consists of identifying the nature of the dispute, helping the patient choose a plan of action, and changing the way of communicating or the expectations of the patient. A first step is to understand the role of the nonreciprocal expectations in such disputes. Then, the patient's options are reviewed, together with redefining and negotiating her or his role. In addition, the therapist looks for parallels in other relationships and, if these are found, tries to understand what the patient's goals are and which assumptions underlie her or his behavior. Finally, the patient has to become more aware of how her or his personality and the significant other person's contribute to the creation and perpetuation of these disputes. As already mentioned, personality changes are not part of the therapeutic agenda, but increasing awareness of the personality style of the participants is often helpful.

Role Transition. Depression related to role transitions is often the result of the patient's difficulties in coping with a specific change. The change is viewed by the individual as a loss. Thus, not only the factual aspects of the transition are important, but also their implications in terms of social support, role definition, and so on.

In the treatment of role transition, two central issues are examined. The first surrounds the loss of a person or a role as a kind of grief reaction. The second issue is the patient's reaction to the role change, which, in general, implies that he or she cannot cope with the change. Therefore, the therapist's goals are to help the patient consider the change in a more positive way and to develop the patient's sense of competence regarding the new demands created by the role transition.

Interpersonal Deficits. The existence of deficits is inferred from a history of inadequate relationships. Because these patients do not have current meaningful relationships, past relationships are emphasized.

In the treatment of interpersonal deficits, the main goal is to reduce the patient's social isolation. While reviewing previous relationships, the therapist pays close attention to recurrent problems to enable the patient to recognize them. As a result, the patient will hopefully change his or her behavior or avoid these situations. For these types of patients, the therapist pays more attention to the patient–therapist relationship, providing a model for the patient to follow in close relationships.

Specific Techniques

We will now turn to some of the specific techniques employed by the IPT therapist. Techniques, in themselves, are not an important part of the therapy (Klerman *et al.*, 1984). They are used in different combinations depending on the patient's needs. The main specific techniques are exploratory techniques, encouragement of affect, clarification, communication analysis, use of the therapeutic relationship, and use of behavior change techniques.

Exploratory techniques can be either direct or nondirect. The nondirect techniques are mainly used with "good" verbal patients who know what their problems are. These techniques include the use of open-ended questions, silence, encouragement to elaborate on a topic, and supportive acknowledgment. Often, direct elicitations follow when the therapist needs more details about a specific issue. Klerman *et al.* (1984) specified that the therapist should ask specific questions only if she or he has something in mind.

Encouragement of affect is used to achieve one or more of the following: (1) to help the patient accept painful emotions that do not need to be changed; (2) to train the patient in the use and the relatively controlled expression of affect in interpersonal relationships in order to change them; and (3) to help the patient develop new or suppressed affects, which will enable the patient to grow and change.

The purpose of clarification is to increase the patient's awareness, which may lead to later discussion of ideas that are suppressed. The main techniques are asking the patient to repeat or rephrase what he or she says, rephrasing what the patient said, and pointing out to the patient the implications of what he or she thinks or the inconsistencies in what he or she says.

Communication analysis is performed to increase the patient's ability to communicate and the effectiveness of such communication. The most common communication failures discussed by Klerman *et al.* (1984) include ambiguous or indirect communication (verbal and nonverbal), the incorrect belief that one has said something to another person that should have been understood and acted upon, and the incorrect belief that one has been understood by another person or has understood another.

The therapeutic relationship is used much as it is in other psychodynamic psychotherapies. As already mentioned, this technique is used when the patient acts in a way that interferes with the therapy. An examination of the relationship enables the patient to receive feedback on his or her impact on others. Klerman *et al.* (1984) suggested interpretation of the therapeutic relationship only after a good therapeutic alliance has been developed.

The three main behavior-change techniques used in IPT are directive techniques, decision analysis, and role playing. Directive techniques such as advice, modeling, education, and problem solving are used more at the beginning of treatment than at the end. They increase the therapeutic alliance as well as allow patients to slowly help themselves. Decision analysis represents a helpful technique toward better problem-solving. It also increases the patients' awareness of their options. Role playing is used to explore patients' feelings toward others, as well as their communication skills. It is also used to allow the patient to rehearse new skills.

DISCUSSION

In this chapter, we have reviewed developments since the late 1960s in dynamic therapies, as exemplified especially by Malan, Sifneos, Mann, Davanloo, Luborsky, Strupp and Binder, and Klerman *et al.* A comparison of these methods is summarized in Table 1, which includes the types of patients selected, the length of treatment, the main focus of treatment, and the major techniques. The table shows considerable convergence in these respects as well as differences in emphases. These are discussed below.

The selection criteria for the short-term therapies reviewed here do not necessarily follow the diagnostic categories in the third edition of the *Diagnostic and Statistical Manual of Mental Disorders* (DSM-III; American Psychiatric Association, 1980), as psychodynamic and personality factors are considered at least as important as the specific diagnosis. Only IPT seriously considers DSM-III definitions, as its targets are clinical diagnoses. Other theorists do not view formal diagnosis as sufficient for selecting patients because their goals consist of improving interpersonal or intrapsychic functioning (or both). The most important criterion seems to be the therapist's appraisal of the patient's potential to create a collaborative relationship with the therapist. This potential is assessed during the first few sessions by an extensive psychiatric (diagnostic) and psychodynamic interview (Sifneos, 1972) and/or by observing how the patient handles trial interventions (e.g., Davanloo, 1980; Strupp & Biner, 1984). One also has to remember that current diagnostic nosology does not assess the severity of a disorder. Moreover, psychological health has been shown to be an important predictor of outcome (Luborsky, 1984), together with similarities between patient and therapist on demographic and attitudinal characteristics. The DSM-III's lack of a severity index may partly explain why these theorists often include criteria in addition to formal diagnoses in selecting patients for their treatment.

The theorists we have reviewed here have different views about the time limitation of their therapy. Some emphasize the limited range of sessions from the outset; others decide on a termination date or the number of sessions only after a therapeutic focus has been agreed upon. Still other theorists offer more open-ended forms of therapy, in which termination is collaboratively decided on once the specific goals have been achieved. In contrast to others, SE, for example, offers both a time-limited and an open-ended version.

Most writers agree that, in addition to the presenting symptoms, a focal problem in

Table 1. A Comparison of Seven Forms of Dynamic Therapy

	Patient selection	Length	Focus	Major techniques
Malan	Strict psychiatric and dynamic criteria	Trainees: limit of 30 sessions Difficult cases: limit of 1 year	Wish–threat–defense triangle, therapist–present-relationship–past (parent) triangle	1. Transference-parent interpretative links 2. Interpretation of wish–defense–anxiety triangle 3. Wait until transference develops
Sifneos	1. Intelligence 2. History of meaningful relationships 3. Appropriate affect 4. One chief complaint 5. Motivation	Usually 12–15 sessions	Unresolved conflict	1. Early transference interpretation 2. Confrontation 3. Anxiety-provoking questions
Mann	Definable central focus Best for young adults	12 sessions	Central issue related to conflict about loss	Interpret connections between therapy and earlier loss
Davanloo	Wide range Pass trial therapy	5–30 sessions	Triangle of conflict Triangle of people	1. Relentless confrontation of defenses 2. Early transference interpretation
Luborsky	Wide range	Time-limited or time-unlimited	CCRT	1. Supportive and expressive techniques 2. Interpretation of CCRT
Strupp	Ability to form collaborative relationship with therapist	25–30 sessions	Cyclical maladaptive pattern	Transference analysis within an interpersonal framework
Klerman	Depression	12–16 sessions	Relief of symptoms Current interpersonal functioning	1. Symptom management 2. Exploration of relationships 3. Directive techniques

interpersonal relationships exists and that its resolution or partial modification is required. Thus, these dynamic therapies have in common the view that the patient's symptoms are the result of conflicts or problems in interpersonal relationships. Different names have been given to the central issue (e.g., CCRT, dynamic focus, and basic conflict) that has to be addressed during treatment. Moreover, these theorists offer different conceptualizations of the patient's perpetuation of the maladaptive behavior. Most writers view it as a repetition or persistence of an underlying structure (schemalike) originating in childhood. Strupp and Binder (1984), following Wachtel (1982), on the other hand, consider the dynamic focus a kind of script narrated by the patient, which, even though it often originates in childhood, is repeatedly used because the individual has not developed better skills. The advantage of the conceptualization advanced by Strupp and Binder over more traditional ones is that it eliminates the need for positing controversial concepts such as repetition compulsion or persisting schemata.

Most theorists agree that the basic conflict influences how the individual creates, maintains, and ends interpersonal relationships. Some view this repeated behavior as influenced more by the intrapsychic pole of the phenomenon (i.e., the interpersonal behavior reflects the balance of forces associated with the triangle of impulse, anxiety, and defense). Others view it from an interpersonal point of view (i.e., the rigid interpersonal relationships are the perpetuation of earlier relationships and are not necessarily the result of the projection of intrapsychic content onto another person).

In regard to techniques, the most commonly discussed procedure is the interpretation of transference. The authors vary, however, in the extent to which they advocate the early interpretation of transference material or waiting for it to develop. Some recommend interpreting transference only when it becomes a resistance to treatment progress. Similarly, most writers would confront defenses to the extent that they impede therapeutic change, whereas other writers confront them as soon as they emerge. These differences are related to the varying amount of confrontation and anxiety induction advocated by the different forms of brief dynamic therapies. IPT is the most dissimilar in technique from the other therapies because it tends to use fewer of the classical psychoanalytic techniques and more of the recently developed techniques (e.g., decision analysis and symptom management). A final difference in the therapies is in the amount of explicit discussion of the supportive techniques to be used in treatment.

SUMMARY

In summary, since the late 1960s, several trends have become apparent within the field of dynamic therapy:

1. More short-term treatments have been developed.
2. A small revolution in practice and research has emerged through the introduction of manuals for delineating the main techniques. Several factors distinguish a manual from the earlier descriptions of treatments. A manual includes representative selections of the main techniques of the treatment, and each technique is exemplified. In addition, the use of each technique is quantified by means of a rating scale, so that judgments about conformity to the manual can be made from samples of treatment. This rating approach is especially useful in research studies, where it is important to document the nature of the treatment provided.

3. The dynamic therapies have made considerable progress in providing additional evidence of effectiveness of the dynamic therapies as compared with other therapies, as well as operational measures of the main concepts of treatment (Luborsky *et al.*, 1988). These operational measures include measures of the helping alliance, of the accuracy of interpretation, of self-understanding, and of relationship patterns (see review by Luborsky, Crits-Christoph, & Mellon, 1986). Through studies using these measures, evidence is now becoming available to support the validity of some of the basic theories underlying dynamic psychotherapies.

REFERENCES

American Psychiatric Association. (1980). *Diagnostic and statistical manual of mental disorders* (3rd ed.; DSM-III). Washington, DC: Author.

Bergmann, M., & Hartman, F. (Eds.). (1977). *The evolution of psychoanalytic technique.* New York: Basic Books.

Bibring, E. (1954). Psychoanalysis and the dynamic psychotherapies. *Journal of the American Psychoanalytic Association, 2,* 402–416.

Cohen, J. (1977). *Statistical power analysis for the behavioral sciences.* New York: Academic Press.

Davanloo, H. (1980). A method of short-term dynamic psychotherapy. In H. Davanloo (Ed.), *Short-term dynamic psychotherapy.* New York: Jason Aronson.

Elkin, I. E., Parloff, M. B., Hadley, S. W., & Autry, A. H. (1985). N.I.M.H. treatment of depression collaborative research program: Background and research plan. *Archives of General Psychiatry, 42,* 305–316.

Feldman, F., Lorr, M., & Russell, S. (1958). A mental hygiene clinic case survey. *Journal of Clinical Psychology, 14,* 245–250.

Freud, S. (1958a). The dynamics of transference. In J. Strachey (Ed.), *The standard edition of the complete psychological works of Sigmund Freud* (Vol. 12, pp. 97–108). London: Hogarth Press. (Original work published 1912)

Freud, S. (1958b). The handling of dream-interpretation in psychoanalysis. In J. Strachey (Ed.), *The standard edition of the complete psychological works of Sigmund Freud* (Vol. 12, pp. 89–96). London: Hogarth Press. (Original work published 1911)

Freud, S. (1958c). Observations on transference-love (further recommendations on the technique of psychoanalysis). In J. Strachey (Ed.), *The standard edition of the complete psychological works of Sigmund Freud* (Vol. 12, pp. 157–171). London: Hogarth Press. (Original work published 1915)

Freud, S. (1958d). On beginning the treatment (further recommendations on the technique of psychoanalysis). In J. Strachey (Ed.), *The standard edition of the complete psychological works of Sigmund Freud* (Vol. 12, pp. 121–144). London: Hogarth Press. (Original work published 1913)

Freud, S. (1958e). Recommendations to physicians practicing psycho-analysis. In J. Strachey (Ed.), *The standard edition of the complete psychological works of Sigmund Freud* (Vol. 12, pp. 109–120). London: Hogarth Press. (Original work published 1912)

Freud, S. (1958f). Remembering, repeating and working-through (further recommendations on the technique of psychoanalysis). In J. Strachey (Ed.), *The standard edition of the complete psychological works of Sigmund Freud* (Vol. 12, pp. 147–156). London: Hogarth Press. (Original work published 1914)

Garfield, S. L., & Kurtz, R. (1976). Personal therapy for the psychotherapist: Some findings and issues. *Psychotherapy: Theory, research, and practice, 13,* 188–192.

Gill, M. M. (1951). Ego psychology and psychotherapy. *Psychoanalytic Quarterly, 20,* 60–71.

Greenson, R. (1967). *The technique and practice of psychoanalysis* (Vol. 1). New York: International Universities Press.

Henry, W., Sims, J., & Spray, S. (1973). *Public and private lives of psychotherapists.* San Francisco: Jossey-Bass.

Hollender, M. (1965). *The practice of psychoanalytic psychotherapy.* New York: Grune & Stratton.

Horowitz, M. J., Marmar, C., Weiss, D. S., DeWitt, K. N., & Rosenbaum, R. R. (1984). Brief dynamic

psychotherapy of bereavement reactions: Relationship of process to outcome. *Archives of General Psychiatry, 41,* 438–448.
Klerman, G. L., DiMascio, A., Weissman, M. M., Prusoff, B. A., & Paykel, E. S. (1974). Treatment of depression by drugs and psychotherapy. *American Journal of Psychiatry, 131,* 186–191.
Klerman, G. L., Weissman, M. M., Rounsaville, B. J., & Chevron, E. S. (1984). *Interpersonal psychotherapy of depression.* New York: Basic Books.
Lambert, M. J., Shapiro, D., & Bergin, A. E. (1986). The effectiveness of psychotherapy. In S. L. Garfield & A. E. Bergin (Eds.), *Handbook of psychotherapy and behavior change.* New York: Wiley.
Luborsky, L. (1984). *Principles of psychoanalytic psychotherapy: A manual for supportive-expressive treatment.* New York: Basic Books.
Luborsky, L. B., Fabian, M., Hall, B. H., Ticho, E., & Ticho, G. (1958). Treatment variables. *Bulletin of the Menninger Clinic, 22,* 126–147.
Luborsky, L. B., Singer, B., & Luborsky L. (1975). Comparative studies of psychotherapy. *Archives of General Psychiatry, 32,* 995–1008.
Luborsky, L., Crits-Christoph, P., & Mellon, J. (1986). Advent of objective measures of transference. *Journal of Consulting and Clinical Psychology, 54,* 39–47.
Luborsky, L., Crits-Christoph, P., Auerbach, A., & Mintz, J. (1988). *Who will benefit from psychotherapy? Predicting therapeutic outcomes.* New York: Basic Books.
Malan, D. H. (1976a). *The frontier of brief psychotherapy.* New York: Plenum Press.
Malan, D. H. (1976b). *Toward the validation of dynamic psychotherapy: A replication.* New York: Plenum Press.
Mann, J. (1973). *Time-limited psychotherapy.* Cambridge: Harvard University Press.
Prochaska, J. O., & Norcross, J. C. (1983). Contemporary psychotherapists: A national survey of characteristics, theories, and practices. *Psychotherapy: Theory, research, and practice, 20,* 161–173.
Rounsaville, B. J., Klerman, G. L., Weissman, M. M., & Chevron, E. S. (1985). Short-term interpersonal psychotherapy (IPT) for depression. In E. E. Beckham & W. R. Leber (Eds.), *Handbook of depression: Treatment, assessment, and research.* Homewood, IL: Dorsey.
Schlesinger, H. (1969). Diagnosis and prescription for psychotherapy. *Bulletin of the Menninger Clinic, 33,* 269–278.
Sifneos, P. (1972). *Short-term psychotherapy and emotional crisis.* Cambridge: Harvard University Press.
Smith, M. L., & Glass, G. V. (1977). Meta-analysis of psychotherapy outcome studies. *American Psychologist, 32,* 752–760.
Smith, M. L., Glass, G. V., & Miller, T. (1980). *The benefits of psychotherapy.* Baltimore: Johns Hopkins University Press.
Stone, L. (1961). *The psychoanalytic situation.* New York: International Universities Press.
Strupp, H. H., & Binder, J. L. (1984). *Psychotherapy in a new key: A guide to time-limited dynamic psychotherapy.* New York: Basic Books.
Wachtel, P. (1982). Vicious circles: The self and the rhetoric of emerging and unfolding. *Contemporary psychoanalysis, 18,* 259–272.
Weissman, M. M., Prusoff, B. A., DiMascio, A., Neu, C., Goklaney, M., & Klerman, G. L. (1979). The efficacy of drugs and psychotherapy in the treatment of acute depressive episodes. *American Journal of Psychiatry, 136,* 555–558.
Woody, G., Luborsky, L., McLellan, A. T., O'Brien, C., Beck, A. T., Blaine, J., Herman, I., & Hole, A. V. (1983). Psychotherapy for opiate addicts: Does it help? *Archives of General Psychiatry, 40,* 639–645.

5

Overview of Behavioral Treatment

JOSEPH R. CAUTELA AND ALBERT J. KEARNEY

INTRODUCTION

The use of behavioral principles and procedures in treating maladaptive behavior has, at various times, been labeled *behavior modification, applied behavior analysis,* or *behavior therapy*. Although these terms have sometimes been used interchangeably, some distinctions can be made. *Behavior modification* is perhaps the broadest of the three terms, encompassing all behavioral procedures. *Applied behavior analysis* refers to applications of operant conditioning procedures to problem human behavior. The applications are very broad, not only encompassing the maladaptive behaviors that are the focus of this book, but also extending into other aspects of human endeavor, such as education, industry, environmental problems, and law enforcement. The term *behavior therapy* focuses on clinically relevant target behaviors. *Behavior therapy* has often been used to suggest the use of respondent procedures such as those developed by Joseph Wolpe (1958).

Although the first use of the term *behavior therapy* is attributed to Ogden Lindsley (Skinner, Solomon, & Lindsley, 1953), the definition set forth by Joseph Wolpe, who is perhaps the most important figure in the history of behavior therapy, is more widely known. According to Wolpe (1969), behavior therapy is essentially applied research based on experimentally established principles of learning. In this chapter, we define behavior therapy as the use of principles and procedures derived from experimental psychology (with an emphasis on conditioning) for the prevention and treatment of maladaptive behavior. Although behavior therapy was originally an approach based on operant and respondent principles and procedures, other approaches based on cognitive and social-psychological principles have recently been included by some proponents.

JOSEPH R. CAUTELA • Behavior Therapy Institute, Sudbury, Massachusetts 01776. ALBERT J. KEARNEY • Maynard Public Schools, Maynard, Massachusetts 01754.

In his book *History of Behavior Modification,* Kazdin (1978b) presented a thorough and excellent account of the development of behavior therapy through the 1970s. In this section, we point out some of the highlights.

The birth of behavior therapy is sometimes said to have taken place in 1924 when Mary Cover Jones published a report on the elimination of children's fears. She treated a 3-year-old boy named Peter who was afraid of a variety of stimuli, including rabbits. Although Jones tried treating Peter's fears and those of several other children in a number of ways, two procedures stood out for their effectiveness. The first was called *social imitation.* Jones grouped Peter with three unafraid children as they played daily in the presence of the rabbit. Eventually, the children played with the rabbit. Before treatment was completed, Peter became ill, and treatment had to be delayed for 2 months. During the interim Peter was frightened by a huge dog and relapsed to a large degree. When treatment was resumed, Jones used the second procedure, called *direct conditioning.* In this procedure, Peter was fed while the rabbit, in a cage, was brought progressively closer to him at a rate that did not elicit fear. This was an *in vivo* application of systematic desensitization, a procedure that will be discussed later. Jones's efforts are also important because they demonstrated that phobic behavior could be treated directly, through the use of learning-based procedures.

In 1938, Mowrer and Mowrer published their now famous report on the use of classical conditioning procedures to treat enuresis. Working with 30 children between the ages of 3 and 13, they developed a pad to place in the children's beds. Dampness served to complete an electric circuit causing a bell to ring, waking the child as soon as urination occurred. Within the classical conditioning model, the response was waking, the unconditioned stimulus was the sound of the bell, and the conditioned stimulus was the physical sensations accompanying a full bladder. The Mowrers reported success in ending all 30 cases of enuresis. Although there were some instances of relapse after the children returned home, many others maintained improvement up to a 2.5 year follow-up, and the researchers found no evidence of symptom substitution. In addition to the development of an effective treatment for enuresis, the Mowrers' work was also important for their conceptualization of the problem as a bad habit that was readily treatable through learning principles. Although the bell-and-pad device was initially used in inpatient settings, parents were soon successfully using it with their children at home with the help of professional supervision. Also of note is the Mowrers' criticism of the medical model, in which symptoms are seen not as the problems to be modified, but as indicating underlying (unconscious) pathological processes.

In 1949, Andrew Salter published a pioneer work in behavior therapy entitled *Conditioned Reflex Therapy.* In his work, Salter relied primarily on classical conditioning principles. He saw hypnosis and emotional conditioning as applications of basic laws of learning, viewing the therapist's words as conditioned stimuli. Salter attributed all psychological problems, not just a small number of very distinct behaviors, to inhibition. According to Pavlov (1927, p. 43), inhibition was a physiological process that prevented a response from occurring. Salter's treatment relied on verbally describing and encouraging more functional ways of behaving and may be thought of as a form of social skills training. Salter is also important for being one of the first to emphasize the importance of dealing with the problem behavior directly rather than trying to modify some underlying unconscious etiology. Salter's book was an important precursor to the development of social skills training.

In the 1940s and 1950s, much operant research was done on verbal behavior. As an operant perspective is functional rather than structural, the effects of a person's verbal behavior on the listener is of particular importance, as is the reciprocal effect of the listener's behavior on the speaker. In now famous experiments, Greenspoon (1951) and other researchers at Indiana University in the early 1950s demonstrated that a person's verbal behavior can be shaped by the response or lack of response of the listener. These studies had tremendous implications for all types of psychotherapy, particularly client-centered therapy. In a later report, Ayllon and Michael (1959) demonstrated how operant procedures could be used to modify a number of maladaptive behaviors in hospitalized mental patients, including psychotic talk. The verbal conditioning work is important not only for its implications for psychotherapy in particular but also for its support of the behaviorist position that the environment is always influencing behavior and that behavior modification, whether intended or recognized, is always occurring.

In 1958, Joseph Wolpe published *Psychotherapy by Reciprocal Inhibition*. Here, Wolpe set forth the reciprocal inhibition principle: An organism cannot simultaneously experience two incompatible physiological responses (such as anxiety and relaxation). This is the principle on which systematic desensitization, which will be discussed in detail later, is based. Wolpe treated a wide variety of behaviors that he labeled neurotic. He reported a 90% success rate in treating over 200 individuals with learning-based procedures, including systematic desensitization, assertiveness training, and therapeutic sexual arousal. It is particularly important to note that, besides the demonstrated effectiveness of systematic desensitization (Paul, 1969), for the first time a psychotherapeutic technique had been derived from already-existing scientific knowledge developed by experimental psychologists.

Interest in behavior therapy was also growing in England. Hans Eysenck (1952), a respected experimental psychologist, suggested that traditional psychotherapy was no more effective than no treatment at all. Later, he published an evaluation of previously reported psychotherapy studies in which he concluded that learning-based procedures resulted in effects superior to those obtainable through other treatments (Eysenck, 1965).

The success of systematic desensitization in using imagery in the treatment of maladaptive avoidance behaviors prompted Joseph Cautela to develop a comparable procedure for treating maladaptive approach behaviors (e.g., overeating, drinking, and smoking). This procedure, which he named "covert sensitization," was first reported in 1966. Several additional covert conditioning procedures, which will be discussed later, followed in the 1970s. Covert sensitization is considered a more humane and practical alternative to aversive conditioning procedures based on electric shock and chemicals. The covert conditioning procedures are considered covert (private) applications of operant conditioning principles.

Currently, there are well over 25 behavioral journals, and the number of texts and other scholarly publications within the field is increasing at an exponential rate.

CURRENT THEORETICAL APPROACHES AND PRINCIPLES AND EMPIRICAL FOUNDATIONS

Originally, the basic underlying theoretical support for behavior therapy came from experimental psychology, particularly the area of learning. Currently, although principles and procedures derived from experimental psychology still characterize a basic component of behavior therapy, behavior therapy now encompasses cognitive variables derived from social and experimental psychology as well as principles and procedures derived from classical and operant conditioning.

Wolpe's assumptions and procedures (1982) were derived primarily from classical (respondent) conditioning. As in classical conditioning, Wolpe emphasized the antecedent conditions that influence behavior. Wolpe's conceptual viewpoint is that anxiety is at the core of all neuroses and that therapy should consist of substituting responses antagonistic to anxiety in the presence of anxiety-provoking stimuli. Wolpe holds not only that maladaptive avoidance behaviors are anxiety-based, but that even maladaptive approach behaviors, such as overeating, smoking, drug addiction, and sexual deviations, are responses to anxiety. Therefore, in both maladaptive approach and maladaptive avoidance behaviors, successful treatment involves eliminating the anxiety components that maintain the maladaptive behaviors. Four of the most widely used antagonistic responses to anxiety are thought stopping, assertiveness training, the use of sexual responses, and desensitization based on relaxation. The desensitization procedure resembles one of Guthrie's interference procedures (1935) for eliminating a response. According to Guthrie, a stimulus is at first presented so weakly that the usual response to that stimulus does not occur. Some other response occurs in its place. Gradually, the stimulus is increased in intensity, the clinician making sure that the steps are so gradual that the original response does not occur. This procedure is continued until a new response replaces the original response.

Wolpe's reciprocal inhibition techniques are analogous to Guthrie's interference procedure. In the use of desensitization, either *in vivo* or in imagination, the aversive stimulus is presented so weakly that it does not elicit the anxiety response. The probability that the anxiety response will not occur in the presence of the aversive stimulus is made stronger by having the individual relaxed when the stimulus is presented. Wolpe has maintained that his procedures are highly effective in dealing with nonpsychotic functional behavior. Indeed, the evidence supports his contention, especially in the use of desensitization in the elimination of phobic responses. Although Wolpe has contended that his procedures are not applicable to the so-called psychotic population, there have been successful attempts to modify some behaviors of institutionalized psychiatric patients (Zeisset, 1968).

It is important to note that Wolpe considers private events, such as thoughts, feelings, and images, behaviors that obey the laws of conditioning. Also, it is often necessary to manipulate these private events to modify overt and covert behavior.

Behavior therapists who have a primarily operant approach to behavior change have focused more on modifying the behaviors of patients in institutional settings, such as psychiatric hospitals, and on modifying the behavior of children in schools and in the home. The operant approach has also been successfully applied to inappropriate behaviors in school settings and to some behaviors in outpatient settings. Whereas the focus of the Wolpe approach is on antecedent conditions, the operant procedure focuses on the consequences of behavior as well as the antecedents. Therefore, if assessment is seen as an ABC process, in which *A* stands for *antecedent, B* stands for *behavior,* and *C* stands for *consequence,* Wolpe focuses on A and the operant approach focuses on C. In practice, most behavior therapists who espouse the learning basis of inappropriate behavior focus both on antecedents and consequences but use a strong emphasis on one or the other.

Although there has been an attempt at some speculation and investigation of the use of private events to modify behavior, most operant conditioners still assume that private events should not be the focus of behavior change. Cautela's covert conditioning approach (Cautela & Kearney, 1986) is an attempt to focus on the manipulation of private events or covert behavior within the operant conditioning framework. Cautela adheres to the homogeneity assumption: Covert and overt behaviors obey the same laws. Cautela assumes *laws* to mean that there are variables that affect learning in a predictable manner. In the covert conditioning approach, the individual is asked to imagine the behavior to be modified, then to imagine the appropriate consequences to modify that behavior. The covert conditioning procedures are analogous to the operant procedures of positive reinforcement (covert positive reinforcement), punishment (covert sensitization), extinction (covert extinction), negative reinforcement (covert negative reinforcement), and response cost (covert response cost). Cautela has also subsumed modeling behavior as described by Bandura (1971) under the operant framework. He assumes that modeling is a behavior that is highly reinforced in children and then maintained throughout life by intermittent reinforcement. Cautela's covert modeling procedure has received empirical validity in a number of investigations, such as those conducted by Kazdin (1974a,b, 1976, 1978a, 1982).

As previously mentioned, there are therapists who label themselves *cognitive behavior therapists* who hold that learning-based procedures are too limited and therefore neglect important cognitive variables such as expectations and attributions. Learning-based procedures such as systematic desensitization and covert conditioning are based on the assumptions that private events obey the same laws as public events, that private events and public events interact with each other, and that the laws according to which these events influence each other are the laws of learning. Proponents of these procedures emphasize the manipulation of imagery, whereas cognitive therapists emphasize the manipulation of thoughts. Cognitivists vary in the extent to which they use behavioral procedures such as overt reinforcement, systematic desensitization, and progressive-muscle-relaxation training.

Cognitive therapists assign the cause and maintenance of maladaptive behaviors to maladaptive cognitions, whereas behavior therapists view the external environment as exerting the most important influence on behavior. It must be added, however, that some behaviorists include internal events as part of the environment (cf. Cautela & Kearney, 1986; Skinner, 1963; Wolpe, 1958). The emphasis of cognitive therapy, then, is on changing irrational beliefs. Rather than basing their approach on learning principles, as do behaviorists, cognitivists rely on hypothetical constructs borrowed from social psychology, such as attitudes, beliefs, and expectations.

The lack of a unifying conceptual basis for some of the current practices in behavior therapy, including cognitive behavior therapy, was recently pointed out by Branch (1987). There are several cognitive therapies receiving considerable attention today, with different degrees of acceptance of behavioral principles, procedures, and terminology. Beck's cognitive therapy (1976) seems mostly limited to dealing with the problem of depression. He has attributed depression to distorted thinking, which focuses more on failures and misinterpretations of events than on successes. Treatment includes helping the patient to recognize these distortions and encouraging the patient to engage in activities that will have successful results and to practice positive thinking styles. Meichenbaum's self-instructional training approach (1977) deals largely with anxiety. Behavior is governed by instructions or rules once learned on a conscious level. Eventually, the instructions become unconscious, while the behavior patterns continue. If the instructions were abnormal, the resulting behavior is often inappropriate, thus leading to anxiety. Treatment involves using modeling procedures to teach new instructions.

Although there has been a great deal of enthusiasm for cognitive behavior therapy, the level of empirical support found for behavior therapy has not yet been reached by cognitive therapy researchers. The use of the cognitive procedures has often been confounded by the additional use of behavioral procedures (Latimer & Sweet, 1984). It must be remembered, however, that behavior therapy puts a greater emphasis on empirical support than many other approaches, and cognitive behavior therapy is a relatively new development.

TECHNICAL METHODS AND STRATEGIES

Assessment

Whatever approach to therapy is used, the early stages are devoted to assessment. In behavior therapy, the therapist's assessment is often called a *behavioral* or *functional analysis,* which is a method of determining the behavior to be modified and of discovering the current antecedents and consequences that control that behavior. Most behavior therapists have enough in common to proceed in a somewhat similar way in assessment. For example, there is little interest in past history except as it may shed light on current events in the patient's life. Also, some contemporary behavior therapists use a variety of norm-referenced objective psychological tests. Although some use personality tests such as the Minnesota Multiphasic Personality Inventory and feel that they are appropriate, others feel that the model on which they are based is inappropriate and that those instruments do not provide useful information.

Although behavior analysis can be conducted in a variety of ways, we outline here a 10-step system that we described in greater detail in *The Covert Conditioning Handbook* (Cautela & Kearney, 1986, pp. 23–28).

1. *Operationalize the target behavior.* The first task in behavioral analysis is to operationalize the target behavior, that is, to identify as far as possible the concrete specific behaviors to be modified rather than attempt to modify a psychological abstraction such as shyness, being aggressive, or feeling depressed. Sometimes, the presenting problem is very clear-cut and includes the target behavior: "I want to cut down on my drinking"; "I want to get over my fear of flying"; "I want to stop hitting my husband." Often the target behavior or behaviors are not as clearly described: "I feel depressed"; "I'm anxious all the time." The therapist first must try to identify in objective terms what behaviors are included in those terms: Does the patient cry a lot? Does the patient think over and over again that the future is hopeless? Does the patient avoid socializing and talking to people? In an outpatient setting, the target behaviors can usually be operationalized by careful questioning of the patient, by the administration of a variety of self-report questionnaires (Cautela, 1977), and by talking with significant others in the patient's life.

2. *Establish a baseline.* Before actually beginning treatment, it is helpful to have the patient record the frequency, intensity, duration, and latency of the target behavior. This record provides objective data for comparison with future trends and evaluations of treatment effectiveness. When behaviors occur at such a high frequency that a total count is not practical (e.g., stuttering, eye blinking, or seemingly constant obsessional thoughts), sampling procedures can be used to estimate the total frequency. Although data collection ordinarily begins before treatment, it should continue during direct treatment and into the follow-up stage to help in monitoring the effectiveness of the treatment approach used.

3. *Look for antecedents.* What else is going on just before the target behavior occurs? Is binge eating regularly preceded by an argument with the patient's spouse, or are anxiety

attacks preceded by invitations to upcoming social events? In searching for possible antecedent events, the therapist must consider both overt and not so obvious covert events, such as bodily states and recurring thoughts that may influence subsequent behavior.

4. *Determine the consequences.* What happens immediately after the target behavior? The behavior may be maintained by a variety of consequences; for example, avoidance of school may be due to fear of punishment (academic failure) and positive reinforcement for staying home (watching TV and receiving special attention).

5. *Identify the setting.* In what setting does the target behavior occur most frequently (and least frequently)? Does the problem occur in the home but not in more public settings such as at work and school? Does it occur when more than three or four persons are present but not in small groups? Does it occur in formal circumstances but not in recreational circumstances?

6. *Note the time.* When does the target behavior occur with the greatest (and least) frequency? If a pattern based on time can be established, it may be possible to recognize events regularly occurring at these times as important antecedents or consequences.

7. *Identify positive reinforcers and aversive stimuli.* What can the therapist use to shape the patient to act in more appropriate ways? There are a variety of ways in which reinforcers and aversive stimuli might be determined: (1) the interview; (2) the use of self-report inventories such as the Reinforcement Survey Schedule (Cautela & Kastenbaum, 1967) and the Fear Survey Schedule (Wolpe & Lang, 1964); (3) direct observation; and (4) information from significant others.

8. *Plan and implement the program with the help of the patient.* Not only must the patient help to select which potential target behaviors will be increased or decreased, but particularly when aversive procedures such as covert sensitization are being considered, the patient should be consulted regarding his or her willingness to accept their use. In addition, the patient can also provide practical suggestions about the best ways of adapting particular techniques to his or her lifestyle. If a particular procedure is not practical or is unacceptable for any reason, there are usually a variety of alternatives from which to choose.

9. *Monitor the program.* Is the patient's behavior changing? The therapist must always be on the lookout for changes in the frequency, intensity, and duration of the patient's behavior. Whatever system is established during the baseline period can usually be extended through treatment and follow-up.

10. *Evaluate and adjust the program as needed.* Is the treatment acceptably effective? Is it clinically relevant—that is, is the patient functioning better (e.g., the patient may have gone from smoking 20 cigarettes a day to smoking 10 cigarettes a day, which may be statistically significant but not clinically significant)? If not, what changes can be made to improve the treatment's effectiveness? One of the advantages of the continual monitoring of target behaviors is that the information can be used to evaluate and modify the treatment program. If the patient is not making satisfactory progress, it may be necessary to review the earlier steps of the behavior analysis. Adjustments could include anything from minor modifications in treatment to totally abandoning the procedures in use and developing an entirely new treatment program.

Treatment Procedures

Behavior therapists have two primary endeavors: (1) working with the patient to eliminate the maladaptive behaviors that are interfering with the patient's quality of life and (2) teaching the patient coping skills to deal with daily living as well as any conflicts or environmental stresses that may arise.

Although we will briefly mention some of the major therapy techniques in the behavior therapist's arsenal, an exhaustive or in-depth discussion of the numerous techniques available is beyond the scope of this chapter. For greater detail on specific behavioral procedures, we refer the reader to such books as *Behavior Modification* (Redd, Porterfield, & Andersen, 1979), *Clinical Handbook of Psychological Disorders* (Barlow, 1985), *Clinical Procedures for Behavior Therapy* (Walker, Hedberg, Clement, & Wright, 1981), *The Covert Conditioning Handbook* (Cautela & Kearney, 1986), *The Dictionary of Behavior Therapy Techniques* (Bellack & Hersen, 1985), *Outpatient Behavior Therapy: A Clinical Guide* (Hersen, 1983), and *The Practice of Behavior Therapy* (Wolpe, 1982).

The following procedures can readily be used in outpatient settings:

1. *Assertiveness training.* Wolpe reported using assertiveness training as a reciprocal inhibition procedure in his 1958 book *Psychotherapy by Reciprocal Inhibition,* and Andrew Salter (1949) was the first to discuss assertive behavior within the learning perspective. It was Wolpe's inclusion of assertive behavior under reciprocal inhibition therapy that propelled the use of assertive behavior as an important treatment modality for many problem behaviors, such as extremely aggressive overt behavior, temper tantrums, alcoholism, antisocial behavior, and social anxiety.

The therapist explains that the patient should properly assert himself or herself in personal situations with acquaintances, friends, and family members. If it is clear that the patient does not assert himself or herself appropriately in any of these situations, the therapist asks why not: "What are you afraid will happen?" The patient may respond, "I don't know"; "I never thought of it"; "I don't want to be pushy"; or "I don't want to be yelled at." The therapist can respond with, "Well, it is important that you speak up as tactfully as possible when an injustice is done, for a number of reasons":

1. The other person will respect you more.
2. You will lose some of your resentment toward that person, who is preventing you from reaching a goal. It is not fair to that person to resent him or her without giving the reason.
3. Asserting yourself whenever an injustice is done will give you confidence in all social situations. You will feel in control and have less anxiety.
4. You will respect yourself more.
5. If done properly, at least 50% of the time, you will get what you want.

After the rationale is made clear, the therapist gives some examples of injustices and how to behave assertively. The therapist might say, "Now I would like to see you assert yourself as much as you can until I see you the next time. Keep a record of how many times you were assertive and how many times you were not assertive and should have been, as well as a record of the times you're not sure whether you should have been assertive or not."

If the patient has some difficulty in behaving assertively, techniques such as behavior rehearsal and desensitization may be used.

2. *Behavior rehearsal.* Behavior rehearsal is a kind of role playing in which special attention is paid to the consequences of the targeted behaviors. It is frequently used in assertiveness training and other forms of social skills training to allow the patient a chance to practice new behaviors with and under the supervision of the therapist. Usually, the therapist first instructs the patient in the appropriate behavior and then acts out with the

patient a series of scenarios including the desired outcome. Shaping involves successive approach interactions to the target behavior. Shaping may begin with simple social interactions and lead toward much more complex true-to-life situations. As the patient becomes more skilled in performing these behaviors, the therapist may add unplanned complications to the situation to help the patient learn to behave appropriately in a wider range of situations. Modeling, positive reinforcement, shaping, and, in cases involving anxiety, counterconditioning are the major learning principles underlying behavior rehearsal.

3. *Behavioral group therapy.* Although the early use of token economics in institutionalized settings may be considered a kind of group therapy, behavioral group therapy that involves group interaction (BGT) has been relatively neglected until recently (Rose, 1976; Upper & Ross, 1985). A distinction must be made between administering basically individual treatments to a group of individuals (e.g., systematic desensitization or covert conditioning) and actually using the group as a therapeutic agent. The primary purpose of BGT is to have the group members and the therapist modify the target behaviors by the use of behavioral strategies. The ultimate goal of BGT is to have the group members continue to assess their behaviors and to continue to use their newly acquired behavioral strategies as self-control procedures within the group, outside the group, and when BGT is terminated.

Bennett (1984) described group psychotherapy as "the application of psychotherapeutic principles with a group of people simultaneously" (p. 81). Conventional group therapy is less structured and focuses on clarification, confrontation, catharsis, and social support. Although BGT is more structured, it still uses some of the conventional strategies. In addition to these concerns, BGT places a greater emphasis on assessment, which includes record keeping by group members as well as gathering baseline data on specified target behaviors.

The interaction among group members is used to assess the target behaviors for the individuals and to provide appropriate contingencies within the group to modify the target behaviors. In BGT, the group members and the therapist work together to specify the target behaviors for the group. Then, various behavioral strategies are discussed that could be used to modify the target behaviors. Some of the commonly used behavioral strategies are discussed that could be used to modify the target behaviors. Some of the commonly used behavioral strategies include modeling, behavioral rehearsal, problem solving, cognitive restructuring, progressive muscle relaxation, desensitization, and social skills training. Homework, in terms of record keeping and practicing various strategies, is frequently assigned in BGT.

The therapist focuses on shaping individual target behaviors and helping the individuals shape each other's behavior to achieve the target goals. (Shaping involves reinforcing successive approximations of the target behavior, e.g., reinforcing successive approximations of acting assertively within the group and the patient's reports of having acted assertively outside the group.) The members of the group shape each other's behavior in the desired direction by applying the appropriate contingencies. For example, if one of the members recounts how assertive he or she has been during the week, the therapist and other group members socially reinforce the report of assertive behavior by complimenting the group member. In another example, a group member might report that he or she has eaten inappropriately during the night. The member is reminded by the group what strategies could have been used to avoid that behavior. As a third example, a usually timid patient may speak up in the group, asking the therapist not to reschedule the time of the session to an inconvenient hour. The patient's assertive behavior would be reinforced by the support of the other group members and the therapist's agreeing to a mutually convenient time.

4. *Cognitive restructuring.* Cognitive restructuring includes three cognitive approaches to therapy: Beck's cognitive therapy (Beck, 1976); Ellis's rational-emotive therapy (Ellis & Greiger, 1977); and Meichenbaum's self-instructional training (Meichenbaum, 1977). It appears that the common thread of these procedures is that the patient's thoughts or self-talk mediates the external environment and his or her response to it. If those self-statements are inaccurate, the patient's response is likely to be inappropriate. Treatment consists of helping the patient to examine his or her cognitions and, when they are found to be inaccurate, helping him or her to replace them with more accurate ones that should lead to more appropriate observable behavior. For example, a patient said to "have" agoraphobia may report fear of getting lost in a major city such as Boston. Treatment might include helping him to realize that, although he may become temporarily disoriented, there are plenty of people to ask for directions, and he would never be lost in the same sense as if he were in a jungle or desert. Because discussions of more appropriate behavior in this context may occasionally include descriptions of contingencies, some successes may be explained in operant terms.

5. *Contingency contracting.* A contingency contract is an agreement between two or more individuals specifying what behaviors, performed by whom, will result in what consequences. Contingency contracts usually take one of two forms: (a) "If you do X, then you may do Y," or (b) "If you do X, then I will do Y." Contingency contracts should be written as specifically as possible for a limited amount of time. If the contract is rigidly adhered to, it is more apt to be effective. Both reinforcing and punishing consequences may be used. It is helpful to allow all parties concerned to be involved in negotiating the contract and to sign it when it is complete. For example, in a family situation, an agreement might be that one spouse will prepare X number of meals in return for being freed of child-care responsibilities on X number of occasions. Sometimes, the data indicate that it is necessary to change the terms of the contract. Contingency contracting is particularly useful when a significant other is available to assist in the treatment program. For more information, see DeRisi and Butz (1975).

6. *Covert conditioning.* Covert conditioning is a family of behavior therapy procedures that combines the use of imagery with the principles of operant conditioning. It is based on a firm learning-theory foundation, from which it derives procedures and relevant parameters.

In covert conditioning procedures, the patient is asked to imagine the target behavior and then to imagine appropriate consequences that will modify that behavior. For example, if covert positive reinforcement (CPR), the covert analogue of positive reinforcement, were to be used to help a patient who has a cardiovascular problem to increase his adherence to his exercise regimen, that patient might be instructed to imagine a series of scenes in which he goes for a walk or uses an Exercycle during his lunch break. Each scene presentation would then be followed by a reinforcing scene, such as a scene of attending his child's college graduation.

Other covert conditioning procedures include covert negative reinforcement, covert modeling, covert extinction, covert sensitization (punishment), and covert response cost. The most recent addition to the covert conditioning family is the self-control triad (SCT). The SCT combines thought stopping, relaxation, and a reinforcing scene in a procedure that, unlike the other covert conditioning procedures, is designed to be used when troublesome situations occur in the natural environment rather than when one is preparing in advance for those situations.

Covert conditioning has been used to treat a wide range of problems, including phobias, social skills deficits, sexual dysfunctions, addictive behavior, and organic dysfunctions, and it is ideal for use in outpatient settings. Because it involves teaching the patient to practice covert conditioning trials on his or her own, covert conditioning is well suited to self-control applications. A more thorough discussion of covert conditioning, its empirical support, and its theoretical underpinnings can be found in *The Covert Conditioning Handbook* (Cautela & Kearney, 1986).

7. *Flooding.* Flooding is a procedure in which an individual with an anxiety disorder is intentionally exposed to a high level of the fear-provoking stimulus until the anxiety decreases. This exposure can take place *in vivo* or in imagery (Bellack, 1987). One of the potential problems with the flooding procedure based on imagery is a lack of cooperation, as it is so aversive. *In vivo* flooding may result in greater cooperation.

Flooding is an application of classical extinction and should be used in a manner consistent with basic classical-conditioning principles. Unlike systematic desensitization, relaxation training is not used in flooding. However, a hierarchical approach to stimuli presentation is sometimes used. *In vivo* sessions lasting 1½ to 3 hours are apparently the most effective. Although the evidence is inconclusive, it is a theoretical possibility that too brief exposure may result in negative reinforcement of the flight response, thereby actually increasing the fear. A patient with a fear of elevators might, for example, be instructed to spend several hours riding up and down in an elevator in a large office building. In a recent review of the behavioral treatment of posttraumatic stress disorder (PTSD), Fairbank and Brown (1987) pointed out that flooding and implosive therapy are increasingly being used in the treatment of this disorder. For more information, see Michelson (1985).

8. *Imaginal systematic desensitization.* Systematic desensitization is used primarily in the treatment of anxiety disorders. There are three components in systematic desensitization: First, in progressive muscle relaxation, the patient is taught to relax the major muscle groups step-by-step by tensing and then relaxing the appropriate muscles. After three or four sessions, most patients are able to relax in non-anxiety-provoking situations in a matter of seconds. Second, an anxiety hierarchy is constructed by organizing fear-related stimuli in ascending order of their increasing anxiety-producing potential. Patients are instructed to assign hierarchy items a rating according to how disturbing they find each item. The therapist helps to develop new items to bridge the gaps so that the steps between hierarchy items are not too great. Third, the first two components are combined in desensitization itself, by having the patient imagine each step of the hierarchy while maintaining a state of deep relaxation. In using systematic desensitization, there is often a time lag between feeling comfortable while exposed to the anxiety-provoking stimulus in imagination and in overt exposure.

Systematic desensitization is probably the most widely used method for treating phobias. Although there is some controversy regarding the necessary components for the success of systematic desensitization, it is probably the most widely investigated and highly supported therapeutic strategy ever used. For more information, see Wolpe (1982).

9. *Implosive therapy.* Implosive therapy is a procedure that relies on the intentional induction of high levels of anxiety in the short run as a means of reducing anxiety in the long run. In this procedure, the patient usually imagines extremely aversive scenes related to the fear stimuli until the anxiety is diminished. Implosive therapy appears to have been

based originally on two major assumptions. The first is the acceptance of Mowrer's two-factor learning theory (1960) as the basis of anxiety problems. According to this theory, the fear is initially classically conditioned. Avoidance behaviors are then strengthened and maintained through negative reinforcement as the individual acts to avoid and escape from fear-related situations in day-to-day life (Hansen, 1987). The second assumption, as originally proposed by Stampfl and Levis (1967), is that many anxiety cues are learned from unpleasant childhood experiences. According to the original psychoanalytic formulation of implosive therapy, psychodynamic cues related to these experiences must be included in the description of images that the client is instructed to form. These cues ostensibly raise the client's anxiety level, which dissipates over time. Some more recent accounts of implosive therapy do not include psychoanalytic interpretations and associated stimuli and are more like flooding in imagery. For more information, see Stampfl and Levis (1967).

10. *In vivo desensitization*. In *in vivo* desensitization, the patient is exposed gradually to the fear-provoking items from the anxiety hierarchy in real life rather than in imagery or other symbolic forms. Although not always practical to use, this technique can be both a useful adjunct to other procedures and an effective treatment in its own right. It is recommended that *in vivo* desensitization be used together with imaginal systematic desensitization or covert positive reinforcement so that the patient practices approaching the formerly fear-evoking stimuli as soon as they have been mastered in imagery. For example, an individual afraid of water might go to a beach and, near a lifeguard, gradually wade into deeper and deeper water. Like imaginal desensitization, *in vivo* desensitization is based on the reciprocal inhibition principle and also involves extinction. For more information, see Wolpe (1982, pp. 199–201).

11. *Modeling*. Modeling is sometimes referred to as *imitation, observational learning,* or *vicarious learning*. In modeling, an individual's behavior changes as a result of observing a model's behavior. Although several explanations of the modeling process have been offered, two of the most prominent are the behavioral (Skinner, 1953) and the cognitive (Bandura, 1971). In addition to live modeling, other mediums such as films and imagery have been used successfully. Modeling is particularly useful in teaching social and self-help skills and in treating maladaptive avoidance behaviors. Although it appears that modeled behaviors may be acquired without the inclusion of reinforcing consequences, reinforcement is apparently needed for the performance of those behaviors. In general, the more similar the model is to the observer (e.g., same sex and same age), the more effective the modeling will be. Through the inclusion of aversive consequences, modeling can also be used to teach adaptive avoidance behaviors (e.g., avoidance of drinking and driving). Complex skills that would require a lengthy shaping process to teach are especially appropriate for modeling. For example, a swimming instructor may demonstrate the breast stroke before asking her students to attempt to do it. For more information, see Bandura (1971).

12. *Rational-emotive therapy*. Rational-emotive therapy (RET) is a type of cognitive restructuring developed by Albert Ellis. The primary tenet of RET is that patients' irrational and overgeneralized beliefs cause most of their problems. If the therapist can successfully dispute these beliefs and replace them with more rational beliefs, the patient will act more rationally and overcome his or her problems. Although many procedures are used by RET therapists, including some behavioral procedures, the major procedure is disputing. It involves confronting the patient's irrational beliefs, often by challenging the patient to provide empirical evidence for those beliefs, and helping the patient to arrive at

more rational realistic self-statements to replace the irrational ones. For more information, see Ellis and Greiger (1977).

13. *Relaxation.* In *Psychotherapy by Reciprocal Inhibition* (1958), Wolpe presented a shortened version of Jacobson's progressive muscle relaxation procedure (1938). Since Wolpe introduced relaxation as a specific behavior-therapy procedure, relaxation has been one of the most widely used therapeutic strategies of behavior therapy. Wolpe used progressive muscle relaxation as a component of systematic desensitization, in which relaxation became a substitute response for anxiety.

Besides being used as part of the desensitization procedure, progressive muscle relaxation has been used to reduce general stress levels and also as a self-control response that is cued by particular internal or external stimuli.

In addition to progressive muscle relaxation, behavior therapists have used other methods of relaxation, such as imagery-produced relaxation, relaxation by hypnotic induction, meditation, and Benson's relaxation response (1975). Benson contended that, whatever method is used, similar results are produced. We have found that progressive muscle relaxation appears particularly suited to use in cued relaxation. In cued relaxation, the patient is instructed to relax when particular stimuli or situations occur. For example, if the patient usually becomes agitated when criticized, the patient is instructed to immediately relax when criticism is expected or begins to occur. In work with patients with developmental disabilities, these cues are usually provided by the therapist or staff workers.

Sometimes, the particular form of relaxation has to be tailored to suit individual differences. For example, some patients report that, although their bodies seem fully relaxed, their minds are racing. For these individuals, imagery-produced relaxation may be the best relaxation procedure. Athletes appear to respond better to progressive muscle relaxation. Some patients who have been taught yoga exercises or meditation prefer the Benson relaxation procedure.

Benson's relaxation procedure involves the following components:

1. Sit in a quiet place in a comfortable position with the eyes closed.
2. Breathe in and out slowly and, upon exhaling, say a particular word, preferably one with religious significance (Benson, 1975).
3. If any interfering thoughts come in, passively receive them and then again focus on the breathing and the word.

In almost all relaxation procedures, the patient is instructed to practice two times a day for 10–20 minutes. Benson (1975) claimed that relaxation has to be practiced every day for psychological gains to be maintained.

Relaxation-induced anxiety has been reported by a number of investigators. Apparently, some patients feel that they become more vulnerable if they let their guard down by relaxing. With these patients, we have found it useful to tape imagery relaxation in the office and have the patients practice the procedures at home. Even though they indicate some anxiety while the relaxation procedure is taped in their presence, most patients who use this method of relaxation gradually become desensitized to feeling vulnerable.

14. *Self-instructional training.* Self-instructional training is a treatment package designed to teach patients more appropriate ways of behaving in a variety of situations. The components of self-instructional training include cognitive modeling, rehearsal (overt and covert), graded practice, and feedback. The goal is to teach patients to recognize their own inappropriate ways of handling specific situations, to stop them as they occur, and to

replace them with more appropriate, effective ways of acting. For more information, see Meichenbaum (1977).

15. *Social skills training*. Behavior therapy has been particularly effective in teaching appropriate social skills to patients with social skills deficits. Many of the procedures listed, such as modeling, behavior rehearsal, assertiveness training, and covert conditioning (particularly covert modeling), have been successfully used both alone and in combination to treat patients with a variety of social skills difficulties. Giving the patient feedback (which includes social reinforcement) on his or her efforts is also a common and important component of social-skills training-programs. Behaviors targeted in social skills training might include motor behaviors, such as eye contact, proper social distance, and appropriate grasp when shaking hands, or vocal behaviors in terms of content, pitch, volume, and the like. The recently expanded availability of relatively low-cost and easy-to-use video equipment has provided many social-skills trainers with a very valuable tool, particularly in providing feedback to patients.

There is, of course, a distinction to be made between situations in which the appropriate social behavior is in the patient's behavioral repertoire but not appropriately emitted and situations in which the behavior has never been acquired. Some patients appear to have already acquired the appropriate social skills, but other factors such as the fear of the consequences of demonstrating those skills may block or inhibit their use. Other patients may simply never have learned those skills. For example, some patients may very nicely demonstrate an appropriate way of introducing themselves to a stranger when role playing with the therapist but may be overcome by anxiety when in real-life situations; others may feel reasonably calm but may not know what to say to the stranger. Recent research by Stravynski, Grey, and Elie (1987) has attempted to investigate the relative importance of anxiety reduction and skill acquisition in social skills training; it may be necessary to explore the anxiety components that may be inhibiting the performance of appropriate behavior and to use techniques such as systematic desensitization or covert conditioning to reduce the anxiety. Two of the most frequently reported applications in the social-skills-training literature, dating behavior and assertiveness training, commonly involve anxiety components that should not be overlooked. For more information, see Sprafkin (1984).

16. *Thought stopping*. Thought stopping is a self-control procedure used to eliminate unwanted and/or dysfunctional thoughts by thinking or yelling, "Stop!" to oneself. From an operant perspective, thought stopping appears to be a punishment procedure when applied by a therapist. When used by the patient, thought stopping may just interrupt a chain of behavior and preclude emission of the "thought." Training usually involves having the patient, at the therapist's direction, begin to imagine the troublesome thought. As soon as it is begun, the patient signals to the therapist, who then shouts, "STOP!" thereby startling the patient and interrupting the thought. A second step involves having the patient begin to imagine the thought himself or herself; then the patient shouts, "STOP!" out loud, again stopping the thought. In the third step, the patient imagines the thought and covertly shouts, "STOP!" This procedure may be practiced 10–20 times, after which the patient is instructed to use it as needed as a self-control device.

Most patients report that, when they remember to use the procedure, it is quite effective. A few patients report that, when they use thought stopping on an intense thought or image, it has little immediate effect, so they give up on it. They are then told to keep using thought stopping for as many times as it is necessary to decrease the thought's intensity enough so that it does not interfere with their functioning or until the thought goes away. When the patient reports difficulty with the thought-stopping procedure, the therapist should practice thought stopping with the patient in the office until the procedure can be used effectively. For more information, see Cautela and Wisocki (1977).

SPECIFIC APPLICATIONS IN OUTPATIENT SETTINGS

Selection of the appropriate treatment procedure for the patient depends on a number of factors: (1) the experience of the therapist; (2) the documented evidence that a treatment is useful for a particular kind of problem; (3) the nature of the problem (e.g., its severity and/or the degree to which it interferes with present functioning); (4) the probability of imminent danger to the patient and others; and (5) the face validity of the procedure as perceived by the patient. Although the factors that influence treatment selection are somewhat similar in behavioral approaches and in other approaches, there are two important differences. First, the behavioral approaches are generally more specific and well defined than some other possible treatment approaches, such as manipulating the transference, indicating warmth and acceptance, and working through. Second, behaviorists gather data and monitor progress continually, using relatively objective methods and measures.

Throughout the therapeutic process, the behavior therapist consistently, in a teaching, cooperative role with the patient, uses such phrases as, "Let us look at . . ."; "We should consider . . ."; "Our best bet is to . . ."; "What do you think?" These phrases emphasize the cooperative endeavor.

As in other treatment approaches, the developing of rapport is an essential step in getting client cooperation.

Behavior therapists assume that, during the course of treatment, the therapist does more than simply apply a series of treatment procedures to patients' problems. Over 20 years ago, Krumboltz (1966, pp. 7–8) pointed out that, although certain generally accepted elements of the therapeutic relationship, such as understanding, empathy, and regard for the patient, are necessary for change, they are not sufficient. New learning must also take place. Kanfer and Grimm (1980) conceptualized the behavior therapy process as taking place in seven phases, beginning with establishing the therapeutic alliance and ending with planning for generalization and termination.

Developing a good relationship with a patient may be conceptualized as establishing oneself as an effective social reinforcer. Often, the therapist, because of his or her relatively prestigious status, begins the relationship as an effective social reinforcer. This position allows the therapist to make great use of verbal conditioning procedures to strengthen successive approximations of desired patient behavior throughout treatment. Especially when the therapist indicates disapproval through verbal and nonverbal communication, it is important that the therapist make a distinction between the patient's behavior, which may be unacceptable, and the patient, who is always accepted. In addition to rapport, the presentation of the rationale and the description of the possible procedure to be used encourage cooperation.

Occasionally, techniques may be used in an outpatient setting to encourage cooperation. Covert or overt reinforcement may be used for the completion of record-keeping forms. The patient may be asked to imagine he or she is filling out the records or forms and then to imagine a pleasant scene. Covert reinforcement may also be used to encourage reinforcer sampling. The patient may be instructed to imagine a number of scenes in which he or she is making steps toward enrolling in some appealing class at a center for adult studies. The selection of a problem treatment procedure is likely to produce beneficial results and is a good strategy for gaining the confidence and cooperation of the patient.

It has been our experience that, if patients are under a low level of general reinforcement (Cautela, 1984), the few reinforcing events that do occur are much more reinforcing than they would be if the patients had a higher number of reinforcers in their lives. Therefore, it follows that highly reinforcing maladaptive approach behaviors, such as addiction or inappropriate sexual behavior, are difficult to modify, as removing them would take away more powerful reinforcers than if the patient had other reinforcing activities in life. Therefore, in order to overcome the ''resistance'' that one might encounter in attempting to remove sources of reinforcement, it is often necessary for the therapist to assist the patient by increasing the general level of reinforcement by providing encouragement, increasing reinforcer sampling, and encouraging significant others to increase their reinforcement of the patient.

SUMMARY

Behavior therapy can be defined as the use of principles and procedures derived from experimental psychology (with an emphasis on conditioning) for the prevention and treatment of maladaptive behavior. Historically, behavior therapy has its roots in traditional learning theory, specifically classical and operant conditioning. Watson and Rayner (1920) and Mary Cover Jones (1924) demonstrated how conditioning procedures could be applied to the development and elimination of maladaptive behavior.

Eysenck's attack (1952, 1965) on the efficacy of traditional therapeutic approaches set the stage for the reception of Wolpe's book *Psychotherapy by Reciprocal Inhibition* (1958). In his book, Wolpe presented a learning-theory model for the assessment and treatment of neurotic behavior. Wolpe's claims of therapeutic success prompted investigations that used and experimentally tested many of his assumptions and procedures. Although learning theory provided the roots of behavior therapy for a number of years, more recently proponents of other approaches emphasizing cognitive factors based on social-psychological principles have claimed to provide a way of remedying some of the perceived deficiencies of a behavioral model based solely on learning theory.

What the behavioral approaches appear to have in common is their focus on present internal and external factors affecting the individual, the use of principles and procedures derived from experimental psychology, and their insistence on the experimental verification of theory and procedures.

One of the major contributions of behavior therapy has been its approach to the assessment of problem behaviors. The behavioral approach emphasizes operationally defining the target behaviors and identifying the antecedents and consequences of the target behaviors. Record keeping by the patient and data collection by the therapist are considered essential in assessment.

Treatment is based on continual assessment throughout the therapeutic endeavor. A number of procedures have wide use among behavior therapists: relaxation, cognitive restructuring, contingency contracting, contingency management, and covert conditioning.

It has been emphasized that behavioral approaches view the nature of the relationship between the patient and the therapist as an important determinant of therapeutic outcome.

It is essential in the behavioral approach to teach the patient self-control and coping strategies for use throughout life. Although the early enthusiasm of behavior therapists has been dampened somewhat by experimental data, there is sufficient evidence to indicate that the behavioral approach is at least equal in efficacy to other approaches in general and superior in dealing with specific problems and populations, such as anxiety, stress-related disorders, addictive behavior, and the treatment of the developmentally disabled. The number of textbooks, articles, and books focusing on the behavioral approach appears to be increasing every year. The number of articles on applying the behavioral approach in mainstream clinical journals has been steadily increasing over the years. Although some behavioral ideology and procedures may change in the future, behavior therapy seems assured of a lasting place among various therapeutic approaches primarily because of its emphasis on an experimental analysis of the effective components of behavior change.

REFERENCES

Ayllon, T., & Michael, J. (1959). The psychiatric nurse as a behavioral engineer. *Journal of the Experimental Analysis of Behavior, 2,* 323–334.

Bandura, A. (1971). *Psychological modeling: Conflicting theories.* New York: Aldine Atherton.

Barlow, D. H. (Ed.). (1985). *Clinical handbook of psychological disorders: A step-by-step treatment manual.* New York: Guilford Press.

Beck, A. T. (1976). *Cognitive therapy and the emotional disorders.* New York: International Universities Press.

Bellack, A. S. (1987). Flooding. In R. J. Corsini (Ed.), *Concise encyclopedia of psychology* (pp. 433–434). New York: Wiley.

Bellack, A. S., & Hersen, M. (1985). *The dictionary of behavior therapy techniques.* New York: Pergamon Press.

Bennett, T. S. (1984. Group psychotherapy. In R. J. Corsini (Ed.), *The Wiley encyclopedia of psychology* (Vol. 2, p. 81). New York: Wiley.

Benson, H. (1975). *The relaxation response.* New York: Morrow.

Branch, M. N. (1987). Behavior analysis: A conceptual and empirical base for behavior therapy. *The Behavior Therapist, 10*(4), 79–84.

Cautela, J. R. (1966). Treatment of compulsive behavior by covert sensitization. *Psychological Record, 16,* 33–41.

Cautela, J. R. (1977). *Behavior analysis forms for clinical intervention.* Champaign, IL: Research Press.

Cautela, J. R. (1984). General level of reinforcement. *Journal of Behavior Therapy and Experimental Psychiatry, 15,* 109–114.

Cautela, J. R., & Kastenbaum, R. (1967). A reinforcement survey schedule for use in therapy, training, and research. *Psychological Reports, 20,* 1115–1130.

Cautela, J. R., & Kearney, A. J. (1986). *The covert conditioning handbook.* New York: Springer.

Cautela, J. R., & Wisocki, P. A. (1977). The thought-stopping procedure: Description, application, and learning theory interpretations. *Psychological Record, 1,* 255–264.

DeRisi, W. J., & Butz, G. (1975). *Writing behavioral contracts.* Champaign, IL: Research Press.

Ellis, A., & Greiger, R. (Eds.). (1977). *Handbook of rational-emotive therapy.* New York: Springer.

Eysenck, H. J. (1952). The effects of psychotherapy: An evaluation. *Journal of Consulting Psychology, 16,* 319–324.

Eysenck, H. J. (1965). The effects of psychotherapy. *International Journal of Psychiatry, 1,* 99–144.

Fairbank, J. A., & Brown, T. A. (1987). Current behavioral approaches to the treatment of posttraumatic stress disorder. *The Behavior Therapist, 10*(3), 57–64.

Greenspoon, J. (1951). *The effect of verbal and non-verbal stimuli on the frequency of members of two verbal response classes.* Unpublished doctoral dissertation, Indiana University.

Guthrie, E. R. (1935). *The psychology of human learning.* New York: Harper & Bros.

Hansen, F. W. (1987). Implosive therapy. In R. J. Corsini (Ed.), *Concise encyclopedia of psychology* (p. 569). New York: Wiley.

Hersen, M. (1983). *Outpatient behavior therapy: A clinical guide.* Orlando, FL: Grune & Stratton.

Jacobson, E. (1938). *Progressive relaxation.* Chicago: University of Chicago Press.

Jones, M. C. (1924). The elimination of children's fears. *Journal of Experimental Psychology, 7,* 382–390.

Kanfer, F. H., & Grimm, L. G. (1980). Managing clinical change: A process model of therapy. *Behavior Modification, 4,* 419–444.

Kazdin, A. E. (1974a). Covert modeling, model similarity and the reduction of avoidance behavior. *Behavior Therapy, 5,* 325–340.

Kazdin, A. E. (1974b). Effects of covert modeling and model reinforcement on assertive behavior. *Journal of Abnormal Psychology, 83,* 240–252.

Kazdin, A. E. (1976). Effect of covert modeling, multiple models, and model reinforcement on assertive behavior. *Behavior Therapy, 7,* 211–222.

Kazdin, A. E. (1978a). Covert modeling: The therapeutic application of imagined rehearsal. In J. L. Singer & K. S. Pope (Eds.), *The power of human imagination* (pp. 255–278). New York: Plenum Press.

Kazdin, A. E. (1978b). *History of behavior modification.* Baltimore: University Park Press.

Kazdin, A. E. (1982). The separate and combined effects of covert and overt rehearsal in developing assertive behavior. *Behavior Research and Therapy, 20,* 17–25.

Krumboltz, J. D. (1966). *Revolution in counseling.* Boston: Houghton-Mifflin.

Latimer, P. R., & Sweet, A. A. (1984). Cognitive versus behavioral procedures in cognitive-behavior therapy: A critical review of the evidence. *Journal of Behavior Therapy and Experimental Psychiatry, 15,* 9–22.

Meichenbaum, D. (1977). *Cognitive-behavior modification: An integrative approach.* New York: Plenum Press.

Michelson, L. (1985). Flooding. In A. S. Bellack & M. Hersen (Eds.), *Dictionary of behavior therapy techniques* (pp. 126–131). New York: Pergamon Press.

Mowrer, O. H. (1960). *Learning theory and behavior.* New York: Wiley.

Mowrer, O. H., & Mowrer, W. M. (1938). Enuresis—A method for its study and treatment. *American Journal of Orthopsychiatry, 8,* 436–459.

Paul, G. L. (1969). Outcome of systematic desensitization, Part 2. In C. M. Franks (Ed.), *Behavior therapy: Appraisal and status* (pp. 105–159). New York: McGraw-Hill.

Pavlov, I. P. (1927). *Conditioned reflexes.* Humphrey Milford, London: Oxford University Press.

Redd, W. H., Porterfield, A. L., & Andersen, B. L. (1979). *Behavior modification.* New York: Random House.

Rose, S. (1976). *Group therapy: A behavioral approach.* Englewood Cliffs, NJ: Prentice-Hall.

Salter, A. (1949). *Conditioned reflex therapy.* New York: Farrar, Strauss.

Skinner, B. F. (1953). *Science and human behavior.* New York: Macmillan.

Skinner, B. F. (1963). Behaviorism at fifty. *Science, 140,* 951–958.

Skinner, B. F., Solomon, H. C., & Lindsley, O. R. (1953, November 30). *Studies in behavior therapy,* Metropolitan State Hospital, Waltham, MA, Status Report I.

Sprafkin, R. P. (1984). Social skills training. In R. J. Corsini (Ed.), *The Wiley encyclopedia of psychology* (Vol. 3, pp. 343–344). New York: Wiley.

Stampfl, T. G., & Levis, D. J. (1967). Essentials of implosive therapy: A learning theory-based psychodynamic behavioral therapy. *Journal of Abnormal Psychology, 72,* 496–503.

Stravynski, A., Grey, S., & Elie, R. (1987). Outline of the therapeutic process in social skills training with socially dysfunctional patients. *Journal of Consulting and Clinical Psychology, 55,* 224–228.

Ullmann, L. P., & Krasner, L. (Eds.). (1965). *Case studies in behavior modification.* New York: Holt, Rinehard, & Winston.

Upper, D., & Ross, S. M. (Eds.). (1985). *Handbook of behavioral group therapy.* New York: Plenum Press.

Walker, C. E., Hedberg, A. G., Clement, P. W., & Wright, L. (1981). *Clinical procedures for behavior therapy.* Englewood Cliffs, NJ: Prentice-Hall.

Watson, J. B., & Rayner, R. (1920). Conditioned emotional reactions. *Journal of Experimental Psychology, 3,* 1–14.

Wolpe, J. (1958). *Psychotherapy by reciprocal inhibition.* Stanford, CA: Stanford University Press.

Wolpe, J. (1969). Foreword. In C. M. Franks (Ed.), *Behavior therapy: Appraisal and status* (pp. ix–xiii). New York: McGraw-Hill.

Wolpe, J. (1982). *The practice of behavior therapy* (3rd ed.). New York: Pergamon Press.

Wolpe, J., & Lang, P. (1964). A fear survey schedule for use in behaviour therapy. *Behavior Research and Therapy, 2,* 27–30.

Zeisset, R. M. (1968). Desensitization and relaxation in the modification of psychiatric patients' interview behavior. *Journal of Abnormal Psychology, 73,* 18–24.

II

Specific Disorders

6

Mood Disorders

ANNE D. SIMONS AND MICHAEL E. THASE

INTRODUCTION

The term *mood disorders* refers to a variety of clinical conditions in which alterations of mood constitute the primary disturbance. These disorders include conditions in which mood is predominantly depressed, as well as those less frequent conditions in which mood is abnormally elated or euphoric. Although the adjectives *depressed* and *euphoric* are part of everyday speech, they mean very different things when used as clinical descriptors. Thus, although almost everyone experiences fluctuations in mood over a given period of time, these feelings are usually appropriate emotional responses to the immediate psychosocial circumstances. For example, when one is confronted with disappointments or negative events, a limited period of sadness and self-doubt is natural. Similarly, joy and renewed confidence following a promotion, a vacation, or some new opportunity are an appropriate response to these happy circumstances. Such normal "highs" and "lows" are distinguished from clinical conditions not by whether there is an event that can be found that explains the response, but by the mood state's (1) intensity; (2) duration; (3) coexistence with other clinical signs and symptoms; and (4) impact on an individual's functioning.

For mental health professionals, the importance of understanding the diagnosis and treatment of mood disorders cannot be overestimated. Mood disorders are the most common set of conditions for which individuals seek help from either mental health or general medical practitioners (Blacker & Clare, 1987). This observation reflects the large numbers of people who suffer from these disorders, as well as the significant distress and dysfunction that are the result of these conditions. Although population estimates vary, recent epidemiological investigations suggest that, at any given time, 5% of the U.S.

ANNE D. SIMONS • Department of Psychology, University of Oregon, Eugene, Oregon 97403.
MICHAEL E. THASE • Department of Psychiatry, University of Pittsburgh School of Medicine, Western Psychiatric Institute and Clinic, Pittsburgh, Pennsylvania 15213.

population is suffering from clinical depression, with an expected lifetime prevalence of 20% (Boyd & Weissman, 1981). Further, depression is associated with an increased risk of suicide. Again, the true rates are impossible to ascertain, but estimates suggest that the risk of suicide is approximately 30 times as high for those with an affective disorder as for the general population (Guze & Robins, 1970).

HISTORICAL OVERVIEW

Conceptualization of Mood Disorders

Mood disorders have been recognized and described since antiquity. Interestingly, over the course of history, the accounts of the experience and manifestations of mood disorders, particularly depression, have changed very little. The profound sadness, helplessness, and hopelessness that are the core of the experience of depression are a common thread that runs throughout both historical and contemporary descriptions (Jackson, 1986). However, the conceptualization, classification, and treatment of these disturbances have changed dramatically.

Explanations of mood disorders and their treatment have varied markedly with the times. Even today, there are many points of confusion and controversy surrounding the question of what causes mood disorders and how best to treat them. According to forerunners of the Hippocratic school (fourth century B.C.), mental disorders were determined by natural causes, specifically the balance (or imbalance) of the body's "humors." These humors (blood, phlegm, yellow bile, and black bile) were thought to be located in specific organs (the heart, the brain, the liver, and the spleen, respectively) and to reflect the four basic elements of the earth: fire, water, air, and the earth itself. Black bile, thought to be manufactured in the spleen, was held to be responsible for causing depression (Jackson, 1986). Hippocrates maintained the belief in such natural causes but focused on the idea that black bile and phlegm resulted in brain dysfunction, causing darkening of the spirit and melancholy.

The Middle Ages ushered in a period when the Church was the most influential source of explanations for mental disorders. At this time, it was widely believed that supernatural factors (i.e., witchcraft or diabolic possession) were the basis for many forms of mental disorders. Such thinking, and the barbaric treatment that went with it, held sway for many years. Not until the Renaissance did explanations of mental illness return to a focus on natural causes and the consequent development of more humane treatments. The ideas of Descartes (17th century) regarding the independence of mind and body helped to clear the way for an objective, empirical, and humane approach to mental disorders. So, from the fourth century B.C. to the early 1900s, conceptualizations of mood disorders—indeed, of mental illness in general—can be seen as "a pendulum swinging between two poles: the supernatural and the empirical" (Whybrow, Akiskal, & McKinney, 1984, p. 24).

Modern views of psychopathology can be traced to the end of the 19th century and the careful observations and descriptive studies of Kraepelin (1921). Kraepelin was the first to dichotomize mental illness into manic-depressive insanity and dementia praecox (schizophrenia, today). The full range of affective disturbances, from mild to severe manifestations of mania and depression, was encompassed by "manic-depressive illness." The highs and lows were seen as opposite faces of the same unknown underlying biological disturbance. Interestingly, Kraepelin's thinking that the fundamental causes of psychiatric disorder are biologically based is very much in evidence in current conceptualizations of mood disorders.

Not all of Kraepelin's original ideas have stood the test of time. In particular, the concept of mania and depression as opposite poles of a single disorder has been largely replaced by nonunitary conceptualizations of affective disturbance. Although disagreement remains on just how many different types of mood disorder there may be, the prevailing opinion is that there is more than one type. This idea of a heterogeneous group of disorders appears to be particularly true of depressions. Over the years since Kraepelin, numerous ways of dividing depression have been suggested. Dichotomous pairings have represented a popular approach to sorting out the depressions. Among these are the unipolar-bipolar, neurotic-psychotic, reactive-endogenous, and primary-secondary distinctions.

The *unipolar-bipolar* dichotomy is based on the essential distinction of whether or not episodes of depression are interspersed with episodes of mania or hypomania. This fundamental distinction appears to be generally, though not universally, accepted (Depue & Monroe, 1978). Interestingly, the bipolar group appears far more homogeneous than the unipolar group. Early reports of differences in the family history of affective disorder in bipolar and unipolar patients encouraged the view that these were two different disorders (Perris, 1966). More recent studies have indicated that bipolar and unipolar disorder can also be distinguished on the basis of differences in genetic transmission, female–male incidence ratio, age of onset (earlier for bipolar), and response to lithium (see, for example, Goodwin & Jamison, in press). Further, it has been observed that, in a number of bipolar depressions, the administration of tricyclic antidepressants can induce hypomania, an uncommon occurrence in unipolar depressions (Akiskal, Rosenthal, Rosenthal, Kashgarian, Khani, & Puzantian, 1979). Finally, there may be subtle difference in the symptom profiles of bipolar and unipolar depressions. For example, the depressed phase of bipolar disorder appears to be more likely to be characterized by hypersomnia, psychomotor retardation, and/or weight gain (Akiskal, 1983a; Kupfer, Foster, Detre, & Himmelhoch, 1975a). By contrast, such symptoms are less common in unipolar disorder and, when present, form the basis for descriptions of atypical depressive states (Davidson, Miller, Turnbull, & Sullivan, 1982; Liebowitz, Quitkin, Stewart, McGrath, Harrison, Rabkin, Tricamo, Markowitz, & Klein, 1984).

The *neurotic-psychotic* and *reactive-endogenous* pairings have been a fundamental part of much of the controversy and confusion regarding the classification of depression for the past 50 years. Part of the problem stems from the terms themselves and the different meanings that have been attached to them. Indeed, Kendell (1976) commented that these terms have produced so much misunderstanding that "we might be well advised to abandon all four terms and start afresh" (p. 18). Although often used interchangeably, the terms originally described different aspects of depression. The psychotic-neurotic distinction referred to clinical symptomatology. Although a narrow definition of psychotic depression based on the presence of delusions and/or hallucinations has remained of considerable interest, the term unfortunately has also been used in this country to refer to severe depressions. The term *neurotic depression* has been used to refer to milder depressive syndromes, with only an inferred descriptive connection with coexistent neurotic conflict or character pathology.

The endogenous-reactive distinction, on the other hand, originally concerned a classification based on presumed etiology. Originally, endogenous depressions were presumed to have a biological origin and to be relatively autonomous, or independent of stressful events. The concept of *reactivity* was used to refer to the ability to respond, affectively, to environmental events during an episode of depression (Gillespie, 1929). Later, the term *reactive* was used to refer to depressive syndromes presumed to be *precipitated* by particular psychosocial circumstances. Although such a view has obvious intuitive appeal, depressions that occur with no preceding life stresses are actually quite rare (see, for example, the discussion of van Praag, 1982). Moreover, episodes of both depression and mania in bipolar disorder (i.e., a presumably endogenous condition) are often associated with adverse life events (Akiskal, 1983a). Recently, the *endogenous* term has come to be used to describe depressions that fit a particular symptom profile, such as that defined by research diagnostic criteria (RDC; Spitzer, Endicott, & Robins, 1978). The absence of a psychosocial precipitant no longer is required for such an atheoretical diagnosis. Similarly, the ancient term *melancholia* was selected for use in the third edition of the American Psychiatric Association's *Diagnostic and Statistical Manual* (DSM-III; APA, 1980) to describe this type of depression in order to avoid the confusion described above. The question of whether endogenous depression represents a distinct diagnostic entity remains controversial. Clinically, of course, the crucial concern is whether patients in this subgroup are more likely to respond to one particular form of treatment as opposed to another. This point will be discussed further in the "Outpatient Treatment Application" section.

The *primary-secondary* distinction represents an attempt to sort out those depressions (and, more rarely, manias) that emerge following the onset of any of the other major psychiatric disorders. The rationale for this distinction is that a mood disorder that occurs *after* (although not necessarily *as a result of*) another *nonaffective* illness would be expected to follow the clinical course of the first illness (Andreasen, 1982). This subgrouping is used primarily for research purposes and helps to yield more homogeneous patient samples. Some investigators and clinicians also include mood disorders that are associated with medical conditions within the secondary-affective-disorder classification.

Treatment

It was not until the middle of the 20th century that any form of effective treatment for mood disorders was demonstrated. Before this time, a variety of treatments, ranging from the "bizarre to the whimsical," had been used. For example, in the 16th century, the arsenal against "melancholic humors" included blood letting, the application of aromatic poultices, and even the attachment of leeches around the anus. Later therapeutics included arsenic, emetics, and purges. Less unpleasant remedies included baths (warm for mania, cold for melancholia), music, and rubbing the belly with flannel for half an hour each morning and evening (Jackson, 1986). As recently as 1934, Lewis concluded that "of the factors potent to heal, *time* is more important than any kind of interference so far attempted" (p. 35). This state of affairs changed dramatically shortly after Lewis's words were published. Somatic treatments, as well as nonbiological forms of treatment, were introduced and thus challenged the claim that time was the most potent healing factor.

Somatic Treatments

Electroconvulsive Therapy

One of the earliest successes in the treatment of mood disorders was electroconvulsive therapy (ECT). Following the observation (subsequently shown to be inaccurate) that epileptic patients did not seem to suffer from schizophrenia and the accidental findings that seizures could be induced with insulin, convulsive therapy was initially induced with insulin and was used successfully with patients then diagnosed as schizophrenic. (Some of these patients probably now would be diagnosed as having affective disorders owing to differences in the classification of psychotic symptoms; Noll, Davis, & DeLeon-Jones, 1985). Later, electrical current was used to induce seizures with fewer problems than had been associated with insulin induction (Cerletti, 1956). Since then, electroconvulsive treatment has spread quickly as a specific treatment for severe affective disturbance, including both depressions and mania.

The use of ECT, however, was (and is) not without considerable controversy. The procedures used in the early days of ECT left much to be desired. Anesthesia and muscle-relaxing drugs were not used then, as they are now to minimize the physical and psychological impact of the procedure. Negative sequelae, such as broken bones as a result of the convulsions, were common. Worse, however, was the retrograde amnesia experienced by many recipients of this treatment. Much has been done to eliminate these problems, and ECT is now a safer and less disturbing experience (Fink, 1979). First, it is used more selectively. A number of studies have shown that this procedure is remarkably effective in well-selected samples (particularly with delusional depression), often in a short period of time (Avery & Lubrano, 1979; Brown, Frances, & Kocsis, 1982; Markowitz, Brown, Sweeney, & Mann, 1987; National Institutes of Health, 1985). Patients with a lower chance of improvement (i.e., individuals with chronic schizophrenia or personality disorders) are not as frequently treated and are therefore not subjected to repeated ECT treatments that cannot be expected to be beneficial. Second, as noted above, anesthetizing and muscle-relaxing drugs are now used to prevent damage to bones and muscles. Finally, unilateral treatment, in which current is passed through only the nondominant hemisphere, is often selected to decrease the problem of memory loss. In spite of these improvements, patient groups have been vocal in their opposition to the procedure. Their concerns center on the memory defects brought on by the procedure, as well as on the possibility (unproven) that more enduring neurological damage may occur. Largely as a result of lobbying efforts by patient groups, the use of ECT has been legally curtailed and regulated in some communities (Kramer, 1985).

Lithium

Lithium is a naturally occurring ion that was first used for medical, rather than psychiatric, purposes. Animal studies had shown that excitement in guinea pigs, remotely resembling psychotic behavior in humans, could be produced by injecting the animals with urea. These effects were reversed with the administration of lithium salts. The first reported use of lithium for the treatment of mood disorders was in Australia shortly after World War II (Cade, 1949). Lithium was subsequently found to produce symptom remission in manic patients, with rapid relapse on its discontinuation. Since these early studies, lithium has been shown to be an unequivocally effective treatment for acute mania. It also has some degree of efficacy as an antidepressant, particularly in bipolar depressions (Klein, Gittelman, Quitkin, & Rifkin, 1980; Schoonover, 1984).

Antidepressants

Two serendipitous discoveries in the 1950s revolutionized the treatment of affective disorders: the nearly simultaneous identification of two major classes of antidepressants, the tricyclics (so named because of their three-ring molecular structure) and monoamine oxidase inhibitors (MAOIs). The first of the tricyclics (TCAs) shown to treat depression was imipramine. Its antidepressant properties were discovered in the process of research for improved antipsychotic compounds. In a parallel development, iproniazid (the first MAOI) was shown to have antidepressant action during the treatment of institutionalized mental patients with tuberculosis. Consequently, trials as potential antidepressants were begun with other drugs that inhibit the enzyme monoamine oxidase.

Since the time of these discoveries, newer treatments and succeeding generations of antidepressant agents have been developed. However, the majority of the currently used somatic treatments for mood disorders still derive from these original four biological interventions; electroconvulsive therapy, lithium salts, tricyclic antidepressants, and monoamine oxidase inhibitors.

Psychological Treatments

Psychoanalysis was the first form of psychotherapy to be specifically recognized as such. Although one can find earlier roots of what we now call psychotherapy, it did not take on its more contemporary form until the work of Freud (1959). The impact of the psychoanalytic approach on contemporary approaches to abnormal human behavior is substantial and, with particular relevance to the affective disorders, heralded the advent of contemporary outpatient practice. Nevertheless, in 1952, Eysenck published the now famous report in which he concluded that there was no evidence to support the efficacy of psychotherapy. Since then, a large number of new forms of psychotherapy have been developed that have challenged the prevailing psychoanalytic schools of thought and the findings of Eysenck. Of particular relevance to mood disorders are the therapies for depression based on behavioral principles (Costello, 1972; Ferster, 1966; Lewinsohn, 1975) and interpersonal difficulties (Klerman & Weissman, 1982) and those emphasizing the role of cognitions in emotional disorders (Beck, 1976; Ellis, 1962). Since the introduction of these approaches to the understanding and treatment of depression, there has been a burgeoning of clinical and research activity using these treatments, many of which have been shown to be effective in the alleviation of depressive symptoms. Moreover, the practice of selectively combining somatic and psychotherapeutic modalities in the treatment of depressed patients has both considerable intuitive appeal and some empirical support (Blackburn, Bishop, Glen, Whalley, & Christie, 1981; Hollon, DeRubeis, Evans, Tuason, Wiemer, Garvey, & Grove, 1988). These treatments will be more thoroughly discussed later in an ''Outpatient Treatment Applications'' subsection.

In contrast to the successful development of psychosocial treatments for depression, nonsomatic treatments for mania have not been developed. Though not commonly used as the primary form of intervention, psychotherapy has been, and continues to be, used as an adjunct to the medical treatment of mania, particularly with respect to the secondary aspects of the illness (e.g., the disruptive effects of a manic episode, compliance with medication) (Jamison, 1987).

SPECIAL DIAGNOSTIC CONSIDERATIONS

The diagnosis of the particular symptoms, complaints, and difficulties expressed by an individual serves many purposes. A diagnosis allows a vast array of complex patient information to be captured by a single concept. This concept then provides a basis for the communication and exchange of descriptive and predictive information regarding the possible etiology, course, treatment selection, and prognosis associated with the condition. Classification facilitates diagnosis by providing a systematic framework of different types and subtypes of disorders.

The most recent classificatory system of mental disorders, the DSM-III (APA, 1980) and its revised form, the DSM-III-R (APA, 1987), reflects the current psychiatric zeitgeist of a descriptive approach to classification. The descriptive approach to diagnosis does not follow from any particular theoretical persuasion. In contrast to earlier versions of the DSM, the current edition and its revision assume that, for most major psychiatric disorders, etiology is still largely theoretical speculation. Although such speculations and hypotheses will hopefully yield to empirical findings and will be replaced by specific causes of biological, psychological, or interactive origins, there are currently too many reasonable etiological theories for each disorder to use etiology as a defining feature. Instead, the DSM-III (and the DSM-III-R) define disorders in terms of observable clinical data, specifying operationalized criteria regarding particular behavioral signs and symptoms with hierarchical decision rules necessary for arriving at a diagnosis. Diagnostic criteria were developed as part of an effort to develop a reliable and objective system for diagnosing patients for research purposes. Forerunners of the DSM-III and the DSM-III-R include the Feighner criteria (Feighner, Robins, Guze, Woodruff, Winokur, & Munoz, 1972) and the research diagnosis criteria (RDC; Spitzer *et al.*, 1978).

The major psychiatric disorders are grouped and further subtyped according to shared clinical features (e.g., mood disorders, anxiety disorders, and personality disorders). In order to increase the utility of the diagnostic system for treatment planning and prediction, the DSM-III-R uses a multiaxial system that extends beyond the psychiatric disorder by providing additional axes for the inclusion of information that may color the diagnostic picture, inform treatment, and bear on prognosis (see Table 1). This information includes physical disorders, the severity of the psychosocial stressors, and an assessment of overall psychological, interpersonal, and occupational functioning.

The full DSM-III-R diagnostic system for mood disorders is summarized in Figure 1. Mood disorders have replaced the DSM-III term *affective disorders* for this diagnostic class. The complexity of Figure 1 reflects the fact that the term *mood disorders* subsumes many clinical forms and that there is considerable variation within each of these forms. As can be seen, the most fundamental division is the time-honored dichotomy of bipolar and nonbipolar depressive disorder, a categorization based of the presence or absence of a history of an episode of mania or hypomania. The presence of such a history defines the bipolar disorders, whereas the absence of a prior manic or hypomanic episode in the presence of depression defines the nonbipolar (presumably unipolar) depressive disorders. Of course, some caution is necessary in the diagnosis of unipolar conditions, as the

Table 1. DSM-III-R Multiaxial System

Axis I	Clinical syndrome
Axis II	Personality disorders
Axis III	Physical disorders
Axis IV	Psychosocial stressors
Axis V	Global assessment of functioning

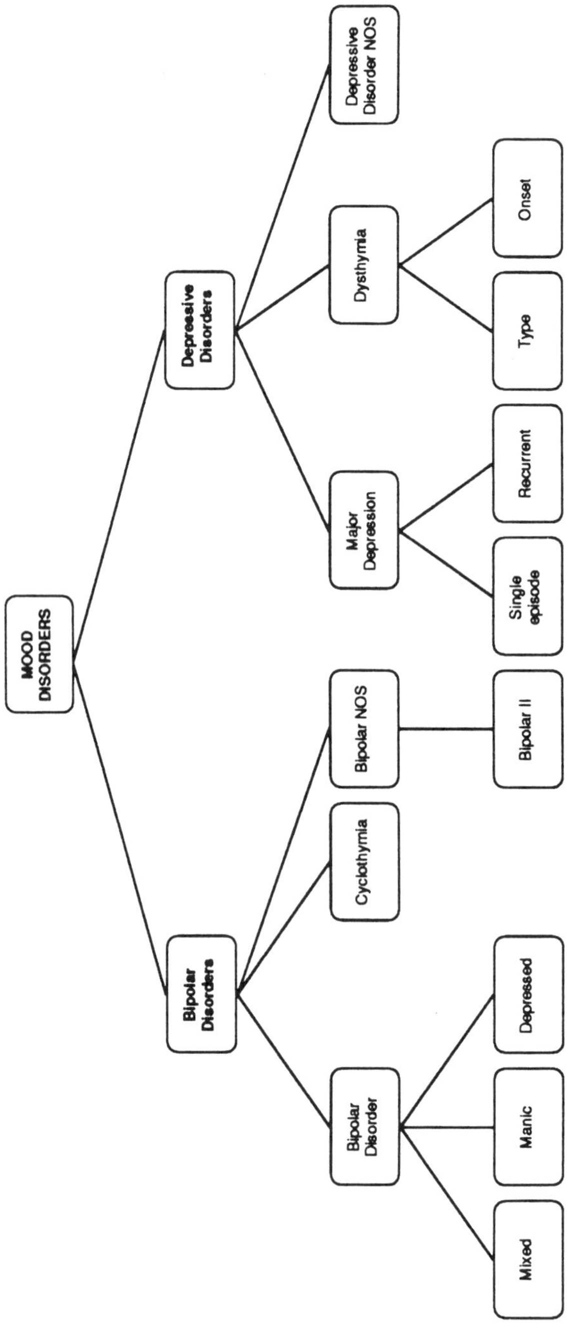

Figure 1. DSM-III-R mood disorder diagnoses.

classical manic-depression syndrome may often be initiated by an episode of depression. In current practice, a useful compromise is to withhold use of the term *unipolar* until an individual has suffered at least three episodes of depression. Even then, there still is some chance (i.e., 5%–15%) that the person will subsequently experience a manic episode during longitudinal follow-up (Akiskal, 1983a).

Within these two broad categories are several further subcategories. The bipolar disorders are subclassified into three groups: bipolar, cyclothymia, and bipolar not otherwise specified (NOS). The first category is further divided according to the nature of the current clinical state (i.e., manic, depressed, or mixed). Further specification of severity, presence of psychotic symptoms, and adherence to a seasonal pattern can also be made. The category cyclothymia is used for subsyndromal conditions in which neither the elated nor the depressed episodes are ever sufficiently severe or persistent to reach syndromal criteria for a full episode of mania or depression. Finally, the category bipolar NOS is used to refer to conditions that follow a different pattern of depression and elation from standard bipolar disorders. Further descriptive specifications regarding severity, psychotic features, and seasonal pattern may also be made.

Like bipolar disorders, depressive disorders are first subdivided into "standard," subsyndromal, and atypical forms. The standard forms are further divided according to whether the condition is making its first appearance (single episode) or there have been prior depressive episodes (recurrent). Further specifications include whether the disorder is chronic (has lasted at least 1 year) and whether the symptoms fit the description of melancholia (lack of reactivity to environmental events and pervasive inability to experience pleasure even when something good happens, and associated neurovegetative features). As for the bipolar disorders, specifications regarding severity, psychotic features, and seasonal pattern may also be made. The subsyndromal form dysthymia is subdivided according to onset (early or late) and type (primary or secondary).

Unipolar Disorders

Major Depression

Major depression is the diagnostic classification used to refer to periods of "prominent and relatively persistent" (APA, 1987) low mood, which may be experienced and presented as sadness, irritability, or loss of the capacity for feelings, especially feelings of pleasure. This term is used for the full syndrome of depression whether the episode is part of a unipolar or bipolar picture. In order to reach criterion for this diagnosis, the mood state must be accompanied by a constellation of at least four other symptoms, which may include disturbances in sleep (sleeping either much more or much less than would be "normal" for the individual, i.e., hypersomnia or insomnia), in appetite (again, either more or less than usual, i.e., hyperphagia or anorexia), or in psychomotor activity (moving more quickly or more slowly, i.e., agitated or retarded). Additional symptoms often include fatigue, feelings of worthlessness or guilt, loss of interest in usually enjoyable activities, decreased ability to concentrate, and thoughts of suicide. (Table 2 describes the full diagnostic criteria for major depression.)

As the list of symptoms in Table 2 suggests, there is considerable variability in how major depression is manifested. Although both unipolar and bipolar depressions are included in this category, there is some evidence that the symptom profile of these two groups differs. Depressed bipolars tend to present with anergia, hyperphagia, and hypersomnia; unipolar depressives tend to cluster toward insomnia, agitation, and decreased appetite (Akiskal, 1983a; Davidson *et al.*, 1982). Although the data are incomplete on this point, further research may reveal that bipolar and unipolar types of depressions respond differently to treatments of depression. It may be useful to look beyond the diagnosis and to attend to these symptom profiles (Himmelhoch & Thase, in press).

The "checklist" approach to the diagnosis of major depression (also the syndromal classification of depression) is rather easy to achieve and therefore may "catch" more people than it should. Examples of "false-positive" patients include those with long-standing personality problems and those whose symptoms can be seen as representing a demoralized state in reaction to a prolonged "siege" of difficult life circumstances (Akiskal, 1983a; Nelson & Charney, 1981). More stringent criteria for a type of depression are those for melancholia (i.e., the subform of depression in the DSM-III-R most closely linked to classical definitions such as vital, endogenous, or autonomous depressions). As can be seen in Table 3, these criteria are met by a much smaller group of people, particularly in outpatient settings. The question of whether the melancholic type truly represents a distinct subtype remains controversial. There are some family data and biological data to support the validity of a separate type (Feinberg & Carroll, 1982; Leckman, Weissman, Prusoff, Caruso, Markiangas, Pauls, & Kidd, 1984; Thase, Frank, & Kupfer, 1985). Another point that remains inadequately tested is whether, as suggested by some (Nelson & Charney, 1981), this type of depression is refractory to psychosocial intervention and requires somatic treatment. Chronic depressive syndromes are discussed in detail in Chapter 7 of this book.

Dysthymic Disorder

Significant numbers of people suffer from chronic depression. The National Institute of Mental Health (NIMH) epidemiological catchment-area study reported prevalences of 3%–4% of the adult population. This rate makes chronic depression the third or fourth most common psychiatric disorder in the United States (Regier, Myers, Robins, Blazer,

Table 2. DSM-III-R Diagnostic Criteria for Major Depression

A. At least five of the following present for 2-week period:
   1. Depressed mood
   2. Loss of interest or pleasure
   3. Appetite/weight loss or gain
   4. Insomnia or hypersomnia
   5. Psychomotor agitation or retardation
   6. Fatigue; loss of energy
   7. Feelings of guilt/worthlessness
   8. Decreased concentration; indecisiveness
   9. Recurrent thoughts of death or suicide or suicide attempt

B. Not due to organic factors nor to bereavement

C. Delusions or hallucinations not present in absence of mood symptoms

D. Not superimposed on schizophrenia, schizophreniform or paranoid disorder

Hough, Eaton, & Locke, 1984; Robins, Helzer, Weissman, Orvashel, Burke, & Regier, 1984). In studies of depressed patients, rates of chronic depression have been as high as 25%–36% (Keller & Shapiro, 1982; Rounsaville, Sholomskas, & Prusoff, 1980). Dysthymic disorder was introduced as a diagnosis in the DSM-III for the categorization of mild chronic depressions. The original DSM-III diagnosis proved to be overly inclusive, encompassing an extremely broad spectrum of depressions. The DSM-III-R, therefore, retained this new diagnostic category within mood disorders but modified the diagnostic criteria in an attempt to better discriminate it from major depression and to provide for subtyping within this heterogeneous group.

In spite of these modifications, the validity of dysthymic disorder (and its subtypes) as a distinct diagnostic entity remains a somewhat controversial point. Major issues include the relationship between chronic mild and acute episodic forms of depression, factors that influence the clinical course of chronic depressions, and the nature of the relationship between chronic depression and personality disorders.

Double Depression

One of the more frequent presentations of depression is so-called "double depression," This term refers to major depressions that occur on top of a preexisting baseline of low-grade, chronic depression, or dysthymia (Keller & Shapiro, 1982; Keller, Lavori, Endicott, Coryell, & Klerman, 1983; Kocsis & Frances, 1987). Indeed, it has been argued that most, if not all, patients who at one time meet the criteria for dysthymic disorder either have had an episode of major depression in the past or will develop one (Kocsis & Frances, 1987). This observation reinforces the question of whether a separate diagnosis of dysthymic disorder is necessary. The double-depression combination is seen as particular "pernicious" as patients seem to be at particular risk for repeated episodes of major depression (Keller *et al.*, 1983), although treatment may be quickly effective in relieving the more acute exacerbation.

Chronic depressive syndromes are discussed in detail in Chapter 7.

Table 3. DSM-III-R Diagnostic Criteria for Dysthymic Disorder

A. Depressed mood for most of the day, more days than not, for at least 2 years

B. Presence of at least two of the following:

1. Poor appetite or overeating
2. Insomnia or hypersomnia
3. Low energy or fatigue
4. Low self-esteem
5. Poor concentration or difficulty making decisions
6. Feelings of helplessness

C. During the 2-year period of the disturbance, never without the symptoms of A for more than 2 months at a time

D. Has never had a manic episode, or an unequivocal hypomanic episode

E. Not superimposed on a chronic psychotic disorder

F. Cannot be established that an organic factor initiated and maintained the disturbance

As stated, bipolar disorders are defined by the presence of manic episodes in addition to episodes of major depression. (See Table 4 for the DSM-III-R diagnostic criteria for episodes of mania.) Rarely, an individual will present with manic episodes and no history of depression. Such individuals are classified as "bipolars" (i.e., rather than unipolar mania) because they do not appear to differ in terms of manic symptomatology or family history from patients who have had depressions as well as manic episodes (Akiskal, 1983a).

Intervals between episodes of mania or depression may be relatively symptom-free, or there may be oscillation (i.e., rapid cycling) between the two kinds of disturbance, with little or no asymptomatic intervals. Cycle length may range from as long as several decades to documented cases "running" on a 48-hour cycle (Wehr, Sack, Rosenthal, & Goodwin, 1987). In current practice, individuals suffering from four or more episodes of mania and/or depression with 1 year are said to have rapid-cycling bipolar disorder. Such cases often have profound impairments in social, vocational, and interpersonal functioning associated with a poor response to treatment. A relatively modest percentage (10%–20%) of individuals with mood disorders are classified as bipolars. Epidemiological studies indicate that relatively equal numbers of men and women develop this disorder, at the average age age of 24–32 years, and that approximately 0.4%–1.2% of the adult U.S. population have had this disorder (Keller, 1987). Bipolar affective disorder has generally been found to have an earlier age of onset than nonbipolar disorders (see, for example, Depue & Monroe, 1978). Moreover, as bipolar disorder is now readily diagnosed in adolescents, future studies will undoubtedly yield an earlier age of onset. It occurs more frequently in individuals whose first-degree biological relatives have this disorder.

Table 4. DSM-III-R Diagnostic Criteria for Mania

A. Elevated, expansive, or irritable mood

B. Three (if mood elevated) or four (if mood irritable) of following:
   1. Inflated self-esteem or grandiosity
   2. Decreased need for sleep
   3. Talkative; pressure to keep talking
   4. Flight of ideas of racing thoughts
   5. Distractibility
   6. Increased activity level or psychomotor agitation
   7. Excessive involvement in pleasurable activities with high potential for painful consequences

C. Mood disturbance sufficiently severe to cause marked impairment in functioning

D. Delusions or hallucinations not present in absence of mood symptoms

E. Not superimposed on schizophrenia, schizophreniform, or paranoid disorder

F. Not due to organic factors

Mania

Manic episodes are characterized by profound changes in mood, behavior, and cognition. Although a patient may present as intensely irritable, mood is characteristically elated, even euphoric or ecstatic. Individuals in a manic episode are behaviorally accelerated, moving and talking more rapidly than usual. Thinking is also markedly quick, tangential, and overly inclusive. Though these patients may become psychotic and cognitively disorganized, rationality and logic are often intact. When present, psychotic features are usually mood-congruent, taking the form of grandiose schemes or special powers and abilities. Marked creativity and productivity may be part of the symptom picture. Needing little sleep and possessing tremendous energy and confidence, some manic individuals experience these episodes as positive and enjoyable. Understandably, such features decrease an individual's desire for compliance with treatment. However, because patients' grandiosity and poor judgment can lead to ruinous behavior, such as sexual promiscuity, overspending, and dangerous risk-taking, treatment is indicated. Indeed, involuntary inpatient treatment is usually necessary in such cases. Diagnosis may be difficult, especially when sleep deprivation or intercurrent drug or alcohol abuse is reflected in increased irritability, confusion, or paranoia, or if the patient develops mixed features of elation and depression. Manic episodes may develop slowly, over several weeks or even months, or quite precipitously. Several lines of research have recently been brought together to implicate sleep loss as a potential final common pathway (Wehr *et al.*, 1987).

Hypomania

The term *hypomania* is used to classify the less severe forms of mood elevation and the associated symptoms. Such episodes are seldom diagnosed in isolation. They rarely compel an individual to seek treatment, as the increased energy, self-confidence, increased productivity, and heightened sense of pleasure are typically welcomed and, indeed, are often adaptive for people in certain occupations (Akiskal, 1983a). More often, hypomanic episodes are detected in the longitudinal course of a bipolar disorder or during the treatment of a presumed "unipolar" depression. Hypomania occurs both in the course of syndromal bipolar disorder and in its subsyndromal analogue: cyclothymia. Individuals who experience depression and hypomanic, but not manic, episodes are often categorized as having bipolar II or cyclothymic disorder, depending on the severity of the depression (Keller, 1987). It is currently questioned whether the research diagnosis of bipolar II affective disorder should be grouped together with, or separately from, classical bipolar I affective disorder (Coryell, Andreasen, Endicott, & Keller, 1987; Endicott, Nee, Andreasen, Clayton, Keller, & Coryell, 1985).

Cyclothymia

Cyclothymia can be viewed as a less severe and debilitating form of bipolar disorder. It is similar to bipolar disorder in that it includes periods of both elevated and depressed mood and associated symptoms. Cyclothymia is distinguished from bipolar disorder by its comparative mildness. (See Table 5 for the DSM-III-R diagnostic criteria.) The symptom severity and the associated social and occupational improvement are less marked than in bipolar disorder. The onset of cyclothymia typically occurs when the individual is in his or her late teens or 20s. It has been found that, often, these individuals subsequently develop a full bipolar disorder (Akiskal, 1983a). The hypomanic phase of the disorder rarely brings people to the offices of mental health professionals. Rather, it is almost always the depressed phase of this disorder that brings these individuals to seek help.

Other Related Conditions

Bereavement and Adjustment Reactions

Depression that is experienced after the death of a significant figure in an individual's life is not usually classified as a depressive disorder. Although sadness, combined with the other symptoms which together compose the criteria for clinical depression, is found in approximately 35% of recently bereaved individuals, few such individuals view themselves as abnormally depressed or seek professional help (Clayton, 1983). The experience of bereavement is often experienced differently from depression and usually resolves itself with time and without treatment. In cases where the grieving process assumes a protracted and severe course, a diagnosis of major depression may be made, and treatment may be indicated. Useful clinical clues that bereavement is becoming "complicated" by major depression would include the development of suicidal ideation, profound neurovegetative disturbance, and/or psychotic features.

Other clearly distressing events (besides the death of a loved one) often trigger maladaptive behavior and dysphoria. Divorce, a child's illness, or sudden unemployment are just a few events that often result in short-lived episodes with some of the clinical manifestations of a major depression. If the clinical picture actually meets full criteria for major depression, then this diagnosis is appropriate, independent of whether a clear-cut cause can be identified. If, on the other hand, the profile or duration of symptoms falls short of a major depression, the diagnosis of adjustment reaction with depressed mood is made. Thus, neither the patient's, nor the evaluator's, assessment of a causal link between a life event and the development of an episode of depression is relevant *if* the syndromal criteria are met. Such an approach differs markedly from that of earlier eras.

Table 5. DSM-III-R Diagnostic Criteria for Cyclothymia

A. During last 2 years, presence of numerous hypomanic episodes (all of criteria for manic episode except C: marked impairment) and numerous periods with depressed mood or loss of interest or pleasure that does not meet criteria for major depression

B. During a 2-year period of the disturbance, never without hypomanic or depressive symptoms for more than 2 months at a time

C. No clear evidence of major depressive episode or manic episode during the first 2 years of the disturbance

D. Not superimposed on a chronic psychotic disorder, such as schizophrenia or delusional disorder

E. Not initiated or maintained by an organic factor

Comorbidity

Depression often occurs in tandem with, or superimposed on, other disorders. Such comorbidity complicates the diagnosis and treatment of depression and may also alter the prognostic picture. Some of the most frequent dual diagnoses are briefly discussed in this section.

Depression and Anxiety

Concurrent depression and anxiety are frequently seen (Barlow, DiNardo, Vermilyea, Vermilyea, & Blanchard, 1986). This is not surprising given the considerable overlap between the symptoms of both disorders (e.g., fatigue, tension, insomnia, and irritability). The co-occurrence of anxiety and depression takes many forms. Some patients with an anxiety disorder, such as obsessive-compulsive disorder or panic disorder, later develop an episode of major depression (Grunhaus & Birmaher, 1985). A larger number of individuals with both sets of symptoms are those with distinct mood disorders who experience anxiety symptoms or panic attacks in the context of their depressions (Leckman, Weissman, Merikangas, Pauls, & Prusoff, 1983). Indeed, the presence of panic attacks is considered by some a good prognostic sign (in terms of response to antidepressant medications), although the coexistence of other of the anxiety disorders (generalized anxiety disorder) changes the prognostic picture for the worse (Thase & Kupfer, 1987). Interestingly, although both classes of antidepressants (monoamine oxidase inhibitors and tricyclics) have been shown to be effective in treating certain of the anxiety disorders (Grunhau & Birmaher, 1985), the converse does not seem to hold; that is, anxiolytic medications are not particularly useful in treating major depression (Klein, Gittelman, Quitkin, & Rifkin, 1980).

Eating Disorders

It has been suggested that eating disorders may be a symptom expression of a biologically mediated affective disorder. Evidence offered in support of this hypothesis comes from several sources. First, symptom profiles in eating- and mood-disordered patients have been found to be similar (Hudson, Laffer, & Pope, 1982; Pyle, Mitchell, & Eckert, 1981). Second, there may be a high incidence of major affective disorder among first- and second-degree relatives of eating-disorder patients (Hudson *et al.,* 1982; Strober, Salkin, Burroughs, & Morrell, 1982). Third, there is some preliminary evidence indicating the presence of similar biological markers in both diagnostic groups (Gwirtsman, Roy-Byrne, Yager, & Gerner, 1983; Katz, Kuperberg, Pollack, Walsh, Zumoff, & Weiner, 1984; Walsh, Lo, Cooper, Lindy, Roose, Gladis, & Glassman, 1987). Finally, antidepressant medication has been found to be effective in treating both groups of patients (Hughes, Wells, Cunningham, & Ilstrip, 1986; Pope, Hudson, Jonas, & Yurgelun-Todd, 1983; Walsh, Stewart, Roose, Gladis, & Glassman, 1984).

Organic Affective Syndromes

Many medical illnesses may cause an affective syndrome (see, for example, Thase, 1987). These so-called organic affective disorders (i.e., affective syndromes caused by medical conditions) more often take the form of depression than of mania. Clinically, organic affective disorders may look identical to major mood disorders. Certain medications (as well as alcohol and other drugs of abuse) may also induce an affective syndrome. Consequently, the initial evaluation of an individual presenting with a disturbance in mood and related symptoms should routinely include a physical examination and appropriate laboratory studies. Indeed, fully 10% of the patients referred to our mood-disorders inpatient unit subsequently are found to be suffering from an organic affective disorder. In contemporary practice, the most common causes of these problems are hypothyroidism and depressogenic reactions to antihypertensive medication (Kathol, 1985). When mood disorders are caused by medical illness, treatment of the causative disease should result in improvement in the affective symptomatology. In clinical practice, however, the severity of the affective syndrome often dictates whether or not psychotropic treatment is used. For example, the symptomatic treatment of a maniclike episode associated with Cushing syndrome or systemic lupus erythematosis may be necessary in conjunction with medical treatment. In less severe organic affective syndromes, a more passive "wait-and-see" approach to thymoleptic treatment may suffice. Mood disorders and medical illness may also coexist, however, in a noncausative relationship, which suggests a different treatment approach. For example, a patient may have two unrelated conditions (a mood disorder and a medical disorder), in which case both disorders are treated independently.

Quite commonly, mood symptoms, especially depression, are seen as a psychological reaction to the illness and the adjustments required by the medical condition. Unfortunately, dysphoria in these cases is often seen by the patient, significant others, and health professionals as both a reasonable and a normal reaction ("Who wouldn't be depressed if they had this illness?"), and the major depression goes untreated. Common sense and compassion dictate that these patients be offered treatment. At minimum, treatment can improve the quality of life for a medically ill person. At best, improvements in mood may positively impact immune-system functioning and the biology and subsequent course of the disease itself (Cousins, 1977; Kiecolt-Glaser, Stephens, Lipetz, Speicher, & Glaser, 1985; O'Leary, 1985; Scheier & Carver, 1987; Visintainer, Volpicelli, & Seligman, 1982).

Diagnostic Biological Tests for Depression

Much work in the last decade has focused on the development of biological tests for the diagnosis of depression. Among numerous parameters studied, the dexamethasone suppression test, the thyroid-releasing-hormone stimulation test, and all-night electroencephalographic (EEG) sleep studies have received the most vigorous investigation (Thase, 1987; Thase *et al.*, 1985). As we have reviewed elsewhere (Thase, 1987; Thase *et al.*, 1985), there is compelling evidence of the existence of a number of biological disturbances in depression, but less optimism that any of these disturbances will prove universal or specific enough to major depression for practical application as diagnostic tests. Indeed, the very heterogeneity of depressive syndromes may preclude the development of such general "tests" for depression.

FREQUENT CLINICAL PROBLEMS

Suicide

Suicide is the most compelling of the clinical problems that a mental health practitioner can be expected to encounter when working with individuals with mood disorders. Depression is one of the diagnostic categories associated with the highest risk for suicidal behavior (alcoholism and schizophrenia similarly have high suicide rates). Indeed, suicide is the most common cause of death in follow-up studies of formerly hospitalized mood-disordered patients. Studies indicate that as many as 15% of individuals with recurrent major affective disorders ultimately die by suicide (Guze & Robins, 1970). Therefore, it is imperative that anyone working with this population be well versed in assessing the risk of suicide and implementing the appropriate intervention strategies. Although it is currently impossible to accurately predict who will commit suicide, studies of completed suicides are helpful in identifying certain demographic and clinical characteristics associated with this behavior. For example, although women are more likely to make attempts, men are more likely to be successful in their attempts. It has been suggested that this may be due to the methods chosen by men as compared to women, and that this sex difference in completed suicides has been decreasing as women have begun to use more lethal methods (Linehan, Goodstein, Nielson, & Chiles, 1983). The suicide rate has also been shown to increase with age. Thus, completed suicide is most common in elderly men. Moreover, since the mid-1960s in the United States, each successive cohort (group of people within same 5-year age range) appears to have been more at risk for suicide than the same age cohort of the previous generation (Murphy & Wetzel, 1980). A family history of suicide is associated with increased risk, particularly when a family history of depression is also present (Murphy & Wetzel, 1982). Chronic medical illness is also a risk factor for suicide (Fawcett, 1972; Isherwood, Adam, & Hornblow, 1982). Clinically, one of the major associations with suicidal behavior is previous attempts (Hirsch, Walsh, & Draper, 1982; Pokorny, 1983). Feelings of hopelessness have also been implicated as a strong contributor to suicidal behavior (Kovacs, Beck, & Weissman, 1975). Recently, biochemical assessment methods have been investigated with an eye toward the possible future development of tools for the identification of at-risk individuals. For example, studies have shown that suicide attemptors have lower cerebrospinal fluid levels of 5-hydroxy-indoleacetic acid (5-HIAA), a serotonin metabolite (Brown, Goodwin, & Bunney, 1982; van Praag, 1982).

Different approaches have been advocated for intervening with a suicidal individual, including a strong emphasis on early prevention. Obviously, attention must first be paid to decreasing access to means that could be used to hurt oneself. In some cases in which the risk is seen as unacceptably high, hospitalization may be necessary. Most treatment approaches advocate an active orientation aimed at quickly decreasing the social isolation that is characteristic of suicidal individuals. An active approach also combats hopelessness by conveying the idea that something can be done about how the individual is feeling, because impulsivity is often a part of suicidal behavior; therefore, it can be useful to teach alternative strategies for controlling, tolerating, and living through such self-destructive impulses. Finally, as suicidal individuals often see killing themselves as the only solution to their problems, a focus on problem solving and the generation of alternatives other than suicide can be beneficial (Boyer & Guthrie, 1985).

Drug and Alcohol Abuse

There is substantial overlap between the clinical presentation of a depressive disorder and the manifestations of acute withdrawal from alcohol, sedatives, and/or psychostimulants. Indeed, as reported in Keller's review (1988), approximately one half of alcoholic patients in treatment have a clinical depressive syndrome. There are similarly high associations between suicidal behavior and a family history of alcoholism and affective disorder (Schuckit, 1983b). In clinical practice, it is often difficult to differentiate whether the depressive syndrome is a consequence of the physiological effects of prolonged alcohol use and/or its sudden withdrawal, or whether a depressed individual has been using drugs or alcohol to self-medicate an affective syndrome. A careful review of the history, as well as interviews of significant others, often helps to clarify comorbidity. Thus, it is essential to carefully interview each new patient presenting with an affective syndrome to ascertain the nature and extent of her or his drug and alcohol abuse. Moreover, it is not uncommon to find that patients initially conceal such a history and only later reveal the extent of their self-medication effort. One implication of this observation is the importance of periodically reassessing the issue of concurrent use of alcohol and drugs, including both medications prescribed by other practitioners and illicit drugs. We have also found it useful to recommend that all patients receiving acute treatment abstain from alcohol or other drug use, as there appears to be an additive or synergistically negative interaction between alcohol use and mood disorder.

Chronicity

Approximately 10%–20% of patients with a major depression or mania do not recover during their initial year of treatment (Keller, 1988). Clinical risk factors for chronicity generally include the presence of a second major psychiatric syndrome (e.g., an anxiety disorder), intercurrent drug or alcohol abuse, and, unfortunately, inadequate treatment (Thase & Kupfer, 1987). Of course, the more chronic an episode of affective illness is before treatment, generally the greater the likelihood of persistent chronicity. Thus, prompt recognition of the affective syndrome and aggressive treatment, coupled with the appropriate treatment of other major psychiatric and/or medical conditions, are the best clinical approach to minimizing the risk of chronicity. Nevertheless, even in our setting, we still find that between 5% and 10% of patients with major mood disorders do not recover. Further, following clinical recovery from an index episode, there is a substantial risk (perhaps 40%–50%) of relapse during the initial year or two after achieving remission (Prien, 1988). Because chronicity and relapse are strongly demoralizing factors, it must be assumed that such patients are at even higher risk for suicide. Therefore, a longitudinal approach appears preferable for the management of recurrent major affective disorders, both unipolar and bipolar, and such longitudinal support and treatment may represent one of the cornerstones of outpatient mental-health practice.

Personality Disorders

As many as 40% of patients who meet the criteria for major depression also simultaneously meet the criteria for a personality disorder diagnosis on Axis II (Pilkonis & Frank, 1988; Shea, Glass, & Pilkonis, 1987). The diagnosis of dependent, avoidant, borderline, or narcissistic personality disorder (and various combinations) are the most common Axis II diagnoses made in conjunction with major depression (Pilkonis & Frank, 1988). A substantial early literature posits that certain temperaments may actually predispose an individual to the development of an affective illness (see, for example, Akiskal, Hirschfeld, & Yerevanian, 1983). Conversely, clinical evaluation often indicates that such dysfunctional personality styles may emerge in adult life as a consequence of depression (Akiskal *et al.*, 1983). Indeed, in our work with chronically depressed or treatment-resistant patients, we have noticed a strong tendency for clinicians to rediagnose patients with personality disorder diagnoses when mood-altering treatments have failed to be rapidly effective (Thase & Kupfer, 1987). Although such a practice may appear justified and even defensible, it is also important to recognize that this may be an attempt to "blame the patient" for his or her lack of success in treatment. The longitudinal study of acutely depressed patients will be the key to documenting and establishing the relative risks of the development of "postdepressive" personality changes. In the meantime, it is important to exercise a high level of caution in making personality disorder diagnoses in affectively disordered patients, as the mood and cognitive changes in both depression and mania may color or exaggerate descriptions of personality. Indeed, in our experience, family members may also distort or misperceive personality in depressed patients.

OUTPATIENT TREATMENT APPLICATIONS

Treatment of Nonbipolar Depression

Differential Therapeutics

The decision about which form of treatment is most appropriate for a given depressed individual is based on a number of factors. Although research has provided some guidelines for which treatment can be expected to produce the greatest improvement in patients with specific diagnoses and clinical profiles, there is still a great deal of missing information that the clinician must fill in based on professional training, clinical judgment, and experience. This seems to be particularly true with respect to nonbipolar depression. A major treatment decision concerns adherence to either a pharmacological or a psychological model. Until relatively recently, medication represented the treatment of choice for major forms of depression. Then, in 1977, a study was published demonstrating for the first time that a form of psychotherapy, cognitive therapy, was as effective as medication in relieving the symptoms of depression (Rush, Beck, Kovacs, & Hollon, 1977). This study had some methodological weaknesses that may have reduced the success rate for the medication group. Subsequent studies with improved methods have demonstrated that at least two forms of psychotherapy (cognitive therapy and interpersonal therapy, discussed in a later section of this chapter) are effective treatments for major depression (Beck, Hollon, Young, Bedrosian, & Budenz, 1985; Blackburn, Bishop, Glen, Whalley, & Christie, 1981; Elkin, Shea, Watkins, Shaw, Docherty, Imber, Pilkonis, Leber, Collins, & Glass, 1986; Hollon *et al.*, 1988; Murphy, Simons, Wetzel, & Lustman, 1984; Teasdale, Fennell, Hibbert, & Amies, 1984; Weissman, 1979; Wilson, 1982). The current zeitgeist discourages conceptualizing treatment in terms of "which one is best." With any form of intervention, a proportion of patients will respond, will fail to respond, or will fall somewhere in between. Therefore, the more clinically meaningful endeavor becomes the pursuit of identifying factors that will aid in the appropriate matching of patients and treatments. Unfortunately, there are currently few consistent data bearing on this issue. Recent research and investigations in progress focus on the possible discriminating role of many diverse factors. These include the coexistence of other Axis I (especially anxiety disorders) and Axis II diagnoses (Pilkonis & Frank, 1988), different depressive subtypes and the presence of biological "markers" of depression (Jarrett, Rush, & Roffwarg, 1987; Thase & Simons, 1989), and differences in psychosocial circumstances (Monroe, Thase, Hersen, Bellack, & Himmelhoch, 1985).

The combination of a psychosocial approach and a pharmacological approach is often used in outpatient practice. Although this practice often gives the psychological benefit of a feeling that the depression is being attacked on all levels, it also carries the possibility that neither the psychotherapy nor the pharmacotherapy will be pursued as aggressively as when it represents the sole form of intervention. The results of research on the combined treatment of major depression are inconsistent, perhaps because of a ceiling effect; that is, because the effects of each of the treatments alone is quite strong, further improvement is difficult to document.

As both the psychosocial and the pharmacological approaches to the treatment of depression have proved efficacious, unless medical factors contraindicate the use of antidepressants the basis of the decision often becomes the personal preference of the clinician and the patient. Having outlined these preliminary considerations, we now present general guidelines for the treatment of nonbipolar mood disorders, followed by guidelines for specific somatic and psychological treatments.

Although patients usually seek professional consultation with treatment in mind, such treatment should always follow careful assessment. Thus, in outpatient practice, the decision to initiate a particular form of treatment may be legitimately deferred (unless an emergency exists) for one or even several visits while a complete evaluation is made of the nature of the mood disturbance.

A comprehensive pretreatment evaluation should normally include (1) a precise description of the current presenting signs and symptoms, as well as the chronology of their emergence; (2) an assessment of lethality, *always* including specific questions on hopelessness, suicidal thoughts and/or plans and, when indicated, thoughts of homicide; (3) a description of the current psychosocial context, including the presumed precipitants and the availability of social support; (4) a past history of psychiatric disorders, including questions regarding phasic or episodic changes in mood and affect; (5) a past treatment history, especially focusing on helpful and ineffective aspects of prior therapies and including the dosages and duration of prior medications, as well as the side effects experienced, even if only as approximations; (6) medical history and current medical status (which generally should include a recent physical examination, an EKG, and screening laboratory studies); and (7) questioning regarding the use of alcohol, illicit drugs, and prescription sedatives, sleeping pills, and stimulants. Collateral contact with the spouse or a family member is preferred, but it must be kept in mind that permission for such contact must be given by the patient in all but the most urgent (i.e., life-threatening) circumstances.

On completion of an assessment, the first decision made about treatment (either implicitly or explicitly) involves the appropriateness of providing outpatient treatment. Each clinician develops a "threshold" for the recommendation of hospitalization, and such a threshold is shaped by training, the availability of inpatient services, and personal philosophy. Pertinent patient characteristics that need to be weighed in this decision-making process include the risk of lethality, the severity and degree of impairment of day-to-day life, the availability of social support, and past responsivity to treatment. Our own threshold includes the elective use of hospitalization in cases that are diagnostically difficult or nonresponsive to aggressive outpatient treatment. Mental health commitment laws (the criteria of which vary from state to state) provide an external source of support for clinicians to obtain emergency involuntary hospitalization for patients who present an immediate danger to themselves or others because of a depressive or manic disorder.

Currently available somatic treatments for nonbipolar major depressive disorders fall into four general categories: antidepressant medications, lithium, antipsychotic medications, and electroconvulsive therapy.

Antidepressant Medications. There are three major classes of antidepressant drugs: tricyclics (TCAs), monoamine oxidase inhibitors (MAOIs), and the more recently introduced second-generation heterocyclic antidepressants (HCAs). The general principles that apply to each of these drugs are reviewed before we go into the specifics of the individual classes of drugs.

First, the use of any medication involves an assessment of its relative costs and benefits. Several factors should be considered in this equation. This type of treatment is not undertaken lightly; the mood disorder should be of sufficient severity to warrant the initiation of such treatment. Medication must be taken regularly and over an extended period of time for therapeutic benefit. As a general rule, these medications require a trial of several (3–6) weeks at adequate dosages before the optimal response can be expected. During the first weeks of treatment, the benefits may not be immediately apparent, whereas the side effects often are. Therefore, the patient may need considerable support and reassurance during this time. This is especially true as the appropriate dose may not be achieved without some "tinkering" because of individual differences in metabolism, weight, tolerance of discomfort, and health habits (such as smoking and exercise) (Klein *et al.*, 1980). Finally, the ratio of toxic dose to therapeutic dose for these medications is low, meaning that an overdose of as little as a week's worth of medication may have serious, even fatal, consequences. Therefore, cautious prescription practices must be followed with depressed patients, especially those with suicidal ideation.

The psychology of taking medication is also worth attention. Many patients have implicit, if not explicit, sets of beliefs, attitudes, and fears about medication that can affect their willingness to take medication, their tolerance of side effects, and their compliance. For some patients, an explanation of their symptoms as being the result of an illness that medication can alleviate is received with relief. Such an explanation can impart the message that the patient is not responsible for the depression. The advantage of this model is that it allows patients to seek and accept help without being blamed or blaming themselves for their difficulties. For other patients, however, these messages (not so much the attribution of symptoms but the attribution of responsibility for their alleviation) are disadvantageous, as they can serve to undermine already sagging feelings of self-efficacy and can reinforce feelings of helplessness (Brickman, Rabinovitz, Karuza, Coates, Cohn, & Kidder, 1982).

Systematic reviews of a multitude of clinical trials of antidepressants indicate that approximately 60%–70% of depressed patients can be expected to respond to antidepressant medication (e.g., Klein *et al.*, 1980; Morris & Beck, 1974). This proportion contrasts with the 0%–50% improvement rate that can be expected from the administration of a placebo (Klein *et al.*, 1980; Morris & Beck, 1974). The wide range in placebo response rates reflects both the heterogeneity of depressions *and* variations in research methods. Nevertheless, a useful rule of thumb in interpreting the results of a study is that the global drug-response rate should be about two times greater than the placebo response rate.

Many studies have attempted to identify which depressed patients are most likely to respond to these medications. The following features generally are found to be positive predictors of TCA response: the presence of "typical" (i.e., melancholic) neurovegetative symptoms (i.e., weight loss, diminished libido, or the presence of sleep disturbance, especially middle and terminal insomnia), diurnal variation (mood worse in the morning), acute onset, short duration (i.e., $\geq$ 1 year), a family history of good response to somatic treatment for depression, and previous response by the patient to somatic treatment (Bielski & Friedel, 1976; McNeal & Cimbolic, 1986; Nelson & Charney, 1981). It is not clear whether these indicators of response apply specifically to TCAs or are strong predictors of response to all treatments of depression (Thase & Kupfer, 1987). Conversely, predictors of poor response seem to include chronicity, a family history of schizophrenia, previous antidepressant medication failure, and mood-incongruent psychotic features (Bielski & Friedel, 1976; Nelson & Charney, 1981). Global severity may bear a curvilinear relationship to TCA response (relative to placebo), so that both mild and very severe depressions are less likely to respond than those in the middle range of severity (Thase & Kupfer, 1987). Indeed, it is difficult to differentiate the effects of active antidepressant therapy from placebo in very mild depressions (Stewart, Quitkin, Liebowitz, McGrath, Harrison, & Klein, 1983).

It is not clear how antidepressant medications achieve their effects. The most widely researched explanation has been the monoamine hypotheses, which were introduced over 20 years ago by Schildkraut (1965) and Bunney and Davis (1965). Briefly, the idea is that depression is a result of reduced biogenic amine (e.g., serotonin or norepinephrine) activity in the brain. Through different mechanisms, both TCAs and MAOIs increase the activity of monoaminergic systems. TCAs block the reuptake of amines released from the neuron, and MAOIs prevent their degradation. Both types of drugs thus increase the availability of monoamines in the neuronal synapse. However, relatively simplistic explanations of antidepressant action based on the increased availability of biogenic amines at the synapse do not appear justified, as some agents exert powerful synaptic effects without enduring antidepressant action (i.e., cocaine) and because the time course of TCA-mediated synaptic effects precedes clinical improvement by weeks (McNeal & Cimbolic, 1986). Recently, attention has focused on changes in complex amine and regulator recep-

Table 6. Tricyclic Antidepressants[a]

		Daily dosage (mg)	
Generic name	Brand name(s)	Range[b]	Usual[c]
Amitriptyline	Elavil, Endep	25–300	150–200
Desipramine	Norpramin, Pertofrane	25–300	100–200
Doxepin	Adapin, Sinequan	25–300	150–200
Imipramine	Janimine, SK-Pramine, Tofranil	25–300	150–200
Nortriptyline	Aventyl, Pamelor	20–200	50–150
Protriptyline	Vivactil	10–60	20–40
Trimipramine	Surmontil	25–300	150–200

[a]Adapted from Thase (1987).
[b]Minimum dosages generally apply to debilitated or geriatric populations: dosages higher than the listed maximum are sometimes used for individuals who are not responding to treatment.
[c]The usual dosage values are the daily amount needed to achieve a therapeutic response in a majority of individuals.

tor systems. Such changes include the down-regulation of the inhibitory feedback of $alpha_2$ presynaptic receptors and a reduction in sensitivity to norepinephrine at brain noradrenergic beta receptors (McNeal & Cimbolic, 1986; Sulser, 1983).

Tricyclic Antidepressants. Tricyclic antidepressants (TCAs) have been widely used for over 25 years. Currently, a number of members of this drug family are available (see Table 6). These drugs differ somewhat in chemical structure and, to a degree, in their side-effect profiles. Overall, they seem about equally effective when tested in groups of depressed patients. Therefore, the prescription of one versus another of these medications is based on individual factors, such as past response, family history of response, particular concerns about individual side effects (e.g., sedation), or, perhaps most commonly, the preference of the pharmacotherapist.

Many of the side effects of tricyclics stem from anticholinergic effects. Dry mouth, blurry vision, constipation, and urinary hesitance are examples. Other side effects (weight gain and sedation) are most likely related to the drugs' antihistaminic properties. One of the more troublesome side effects is orthostatic (postural) hypotension, which is experienced as severe light-headedness upon rising. Severe orthostatic blood pressure changes (i.e., a drop of $\geq$ 20 mm Hg in systolic or diastolic blood pressure) can lead to fainting spells and injuries associated with falling, especially in older patients. The substitution of a different antidepressant medication may sometimes be useful in these cases. TCAs can also accelerate heart rate and change cardiac conduction patterns. Careful monitoring with serial electrocardiograms is essential in treating elderly patients and persons with known cardiac conditions. In some cases, the use of these drugs is simply contraindicated. Plasma blood levels of antidepressant medication can also be used to guide dosage and to help to achieve a dose that is sufficient for the expected benefit to occur, although it should be noted that reliable and standardized assays are not available for all of the TCAs (Perel, 1983).

Since the late 1970s, a number of "second-generation" nontricyclic antidepressants have been tested and introduced into clinical practice. These agents are summarized in Table 7. Such drugs have, of course, been developed with the dual aim of lessening the annoying side effects of the TCAs and of identifying effective pharmacological treatment for patients who do not respond to TCAs. To some extent, the introduction of these drugs has achieved both goals (Blackwell, 1987a; Cole & Schatzburg, 1983). This is particu-

Table 7. Heterocyclic Antidepressants[a]

Generic name	Brand name(s)	Daily dosage (mg)	
		Range[b]	Usual[c]
Amoxapine	Asendin	50–600	200–400
Maprotiline	Ludiomil	25–400	100–150
Trazodone	Desyrel	50–600	150–300
Fluoxetine	Prozac	20–80	20

[a]Adapted from Thase (1987).
[b]Minimum dosages generally apply to debilitated or geriatric populations: dosages higher than the listed maximum are sometimes used for individuals who are not responding to treatment.
[c]The usual dosage values are the daily amount needed to achieve a therapeutic response in a majority of individuals.

larly true of trazodone, which is sedating, and fluoxetine, which is nonsedating. What is of particular note is that neither of these drugs is strongly anticholinergic. However, as clinical experience mounts with these relatively new agents, some specific hazards in their routine clinical use are noted. For example, maprotiline is now known to have an increased risk of causing seizures; amoxapine may convey the risk of tardive dyskinesia with prolonged treatment because of its dopamine-blocking properties; trazodone has been associated with priapism; and fluoxetine may cause an intolerable increase in anxiety and agitation in sensitive patients (Cole & Schatzburg, 1983; Thase, 1987). Thus, although the clinical use of each of these agents was initially high, many practitioners have returned to the selection of a "classical" tricyclic as the treatment of first choice, largely on the basis of the longer track record of efficacy and safety. Further, there is no compelling evidence that any of the second-generation agents has antidepressant efficacy superior to that of the standard tricyclic in unselected populations (Blackwell, 1987a).

Further research is needed to identify particular subgroups of patients who may not do well on tricyclics but who respond nicely to a second-generation agent. In our own practices, one such subgroup appears to include those patients who cannot tolerate the anticholinergic side effects of the standard tricyclics, including the relatively better tolerated desipramine. Such patients are often able to tolerate and benefit from treatment with trazodone or fluoxetine, the clinical selection being based on whether the patient would benefit from a sedating antidepressant or a nonsedating one.

In outpatient practice, the prescription of these antidepressants differs somewhat from inpatient approaches. For example, the initial starting dosage of a standard tricyclic (such as imipramine) is usually relatively low (i.e., 50 mg at bedtime), and the dosage is titrated at a somewhat slower pace. It is common after an initial visit to have the patient check back in (via telephone or in person, depending on his or her clinical status) within 3 or 4 days and to increase the dosage by 50 mg if the medication has been well tolerated. Further increases then proceed by 50–100 mg each week up to a target dose of approximately 200 mg of imipramine. The slowness of this pace is, of course, dictated by the fact that outpatients cannot be frequently monitored for blood pressure changes or other side effects and because only a minority of patients tolerate a full tricyclic dose (i.e., 200 mg of imipramine) at the initiation of treatment. Titration of the dose thus allows the medication level to be slowly built over the first several weeks of treatment and permits desensitization of the patient to the various side effects that may be experienced. The pace of dosage adjustment is slowed, or the dosage strength is halved, in patients who are sensitive to side effects and in older patients. The one exception to this general rule appears to be fluoxetine, which seems to be as effective at the initial starting dose (20 mg) as at higher doses (e.g., 40–80 mg each day) (Blackwell, 1987a). Thus, it is reasonable to hold the dose of fluoxetine at the initial level until the patient has had 4–6 weeks to respond.

Several options for use in clinical practice include whether or not to prescribe the tricyclic in divided dosages or in a single daily dose and whether or not to monitor antidepressant blood levels frequently. The single daily bedtime dose may be preferred because of its convenience and because of its facilitating effects on treatment adherence. There also are some advantages in concentrating the period of the highest likelihood of annoying side effects (i.e., the first several hours after dosing) to a time when the person is asleep. One practical implication is that patients with significant sleep disturbance related to the depression often get the early benefit of improved sleep efficiency. Nevertheless, some patients simply cannot tolerate a full daily dose of tricyclic given all at once.

These patients do better on a divided-dose schedule. Similarly, other patients with prominent anxiety report a "smoother" response throughout the day when taking a divided dose. Although it is clear that a single daily dose is as effective as a divided dose, such decisions are part of the art of clinical practice and represent one way in which the prescription of medication should be matched to the patient's complaints and symptoms.

After a period of several weeks on what is usually an "adequate" dose, it is necessary to evaluate the efficacy of the agent. Some clinicians prefer to document such evaluations by using a depression rating scale such as the one developed by Hamilton (1960) or the self-report Beck Depression Inventory (Beck, Ward, Mendelson, Mock, & Erbaugh, 1961). Whether or not such a scale is used, virtually all treating clinicians and their patients use (either explicitly or implicitly) some form of global outcome evaluation that is scaled along a continuum from worse through no change to well. Research ratings of significant improvement correspond quite well to global evaluations of at least a moderate level of improvement. Therefore, when a patient reports no improvement or even minimal improvement, further increase in the antidepressant dosage, if tolerable, is indicated. Such increases are then evaluated at 1- or 2-week intervals, up to the maximum tolerable or maximum clinically appropriate dosage of the antidepressant.

At this stage, the clinical use of antidepressant blood levels is important, as the blood level can give independent information about the amount of medication in the patient's system. Therefore, a further reason to use a standard TCA in the initial treatment of a patient is the ability to obtain accurate and reliable plasma drug levels (Thase, 1987). For this reason, imipramine, amitriptyline, nortiptyline, and desipramine would appear to be the drugs of choice. Nonresponse associated with extremely low antidepressant blood levels would suggest the possibility of prescribing dosages above the normal range (i.e., $>$ 300 mg of imipramine each day). However, such low blood levels may be more likely to indicate unsuspected noncompliance than a condition of poor absorption or increased metabolism. Accordingly, critical discussion with the patient is necessary to ensure that treatment adherence is not an issue. When supranormal dosages of antidepressants are used, the treating clinician is obliged to provide careful documentation of the rationale for the higher dose, the patient's current side-effects profile, and, usually, repeated documentation of the absence of cardiovasular effects with serial electrocardiograms (Klein *et al.*, 1980).

Undertreatment of major depression with tricyclic antidepressants remains a major problem, even among psychiatrists. Although there is no exact consensus on what constitutes an adequate trial of a tricyclic antidepressant, it is generally agreed that a period of 6 weeks of treatment, including several weeks at the maximally tolerated, clinically appropriate dosage, increases the confidence in and adequacy of treatment (Thase & Kupfer, 1987). Documentation of the antidepressant blood level, when available, increases the confidence that the antidepressant trial has been adequate. In addition, the use of nortriptyline may present the additional problem of nonresponse due to excessive blood level. For example, several studies have documented lower response rates when blood levels of nortripytline exceed 150–200 ng/ml (see, for example, the review by Perel, 1983). These findings are strengthened by the clinical observation that antidepressant response develops when the dosage of nortriptyline is lowered to bring the blood level within the range of 50–150 ng/ml.

Monoamine Oxidase Inhibitors. The currently available MAOIs are included in Table 8. After a period of relative underuse, this class of antidepressant medications has regained popularity for treating patients who do not respond to TCAs and for patients with certain types of atypical depressions. These include depressions with phobic features or panic attacks and those with other atypical aspects such as increased appetite, hypersomnia, and mood worsening late in the day (Davidson *et al.*, 1982; Liebowitz *et al.*, 1984; Nies & Robinson, 1982; Quitkin, Rifkin, & Klein, 1979). In our recent experience, about 60% of TCA nonresponders will benefit from a trial of MAOI, including about 80% of those patients with reversed vegetative symptom profiles (Thase & Kupfer, 1988).

MAOIs produce a number of side efects, ranging in severity from mild and merely annoying to potentially life-threatening (Blackwell, 1987b). Common annoying side effects include weight gain, chills, insomnia, anorgasmia, and orthostatic hypotension. Although the MAOIs are only weakly anticholinergic, dry mouth, blurry vision, and constipation all occur more often than would be expected from a placebo. Such side effects are sufficiently troublesome so that about 10%–20% of patients will not be able to tolerate a therapeutic trial.

The most serious side effect is the hypertensive crisis caused by the effects of intake of foods with high tyramine content (e.g., cheese and other foods with fermented protein, red wine) or drugs with sympathomimetic activity (e.g., diet pills and many cold remedies) in individuals with high levels of monoamine oxidase enzyme inhibition. This enzyme system normally degrades and neutralizes these substances as part of the digestive process. Adherence to dietary restrictions prevents this dangerous elevation in blood pressure. It therefore is imperative that all patients prescribed MAOIs receive thorough instruction about the necessary dietary precautions. (See Chapter 3 for detailed dietary information.)

Following an infraction of the dietary restrictions (either volitional or inadvertent), the hypertensive reaction is experienced initially by sensations of flushing, pounding pulse, palpitations, autonomic arousal, and headache. In severe cases, a distinctive occipital headache and visual disturbances may develop. Although emergency medical treatment is required, the hypertensive crisis can be readily controlled with slow intravenous administration of phentolamine (5 mg). Some clinicians prescribe several tablets of chlorpromazine (25 mg or 50 mg) for interim use, as this agent's alpha-adrenergic blocking effects may also forestall a hypertensive crisis. In our own practices, we insist on emergency-room evaluation for documentation and treatment of all suspected reactions. A card explicitly detailing emergency treatment instructions is provided for use in settings where the management of such crises is uncommon.

Given the potential for serious side effects and the nuisance of following an MAOI

Table 8. Monoamine Oxidase Inhibiting Antidepressants[a]

Generic name	Brand name(s)	Daily dosage (mg) Range[b]	Daily dosage (mg) Usual[c]
Isocarboxazid	Marplan	10–60	20–40
Phenelzine	Nardil	15–90	30–75
Tranylcypromine	Parnate	10–60	20–40

[a]Reprinted with permission from Thase (1987).
[b]Minimum dosages generally apply to debilitated or geriatric populations: dosages higher than the listed maximum are sometimes used for individuals who are not responding to treatment.
[c]The usual dosage values are the daily amount needed to achieve a therapeutic response in a majority of individuals.

diet, these drugs are often withheld until after a trial of one of the TCAs or second-generation drugs has proved to be unsuccessful. Moreover, particular caution must be exercised in prescribing MAOIs to patients with poor impulse control.

The outpatient prescription of monoamine oxidase inhibitors follows the general pattern discussed for the tricyclics. For example, the initial prescription of phenelzine would begin at 15 or 30 mg a day or tranylcypromine at 10 or 20 mg a day. The dosage is similarly titrated upward over several weeks to the average standard dose (i.e., 60 mg of phenelzine or 40 mg tranylcypromine). MAOIs differ substantially from tricyclics in that MAOIs have relatively short half-lives and are generally nonsedating (or even activating). Thus, a divided daily dosage is generally favored; the dosages are usually given in the morning and the mid-afternoon rather than at bedtime. Of course, a bedtime dosage can be used for the occasional patient who develops oversedation. Some patients do fine on a twice-a-day dosage schedule (i.e., 7:00 A.M. and 1:00 P.M.), whereas others require more intricate regimens.

Unlike for several of the tricyclics, blood levels for the MAOIs are not available to guide clinical treatment. Although assays exist to determine the degree or percentage of monoamine oxidase enzyme inhibition (Type B), this strategy is generally restricted to research. Moreover, platelet MAO inhibition has not been established as being related to the efficacy of at least one of the MAOIs, tranylcypromine. Indeed, our group has collected preliminary evidence to suggest that the acute antidepressant effects of tranylcypromine may not be related to platelet monoamine oxidase inhibition (Thase, Himmelhoch, & Mallinger, 1988). This important observation certainly requires more definitive study. For those individuals fortunate enough to have reliable and inexpensive platelet MAO inhibition assays available, it is important to remember that these levels must be taken from the initiation of treatment, as the inhibition of MAO is a relative, not an absolute, value.

Following several weeks at a standard adequate dose, further increases in increments of one pill per week or per two weeks should be initiated if the patient is not receiving the benefit of an adequate response. Again, conventional practice places a ceiling on the maximum dose. Currently, this ceiling appears to be 90 mg for phenelzine and 60 mg for tranylcypromine. As with the tricyclics, occasional patients may require and benefit from even larger doses. Again, it is important to document the lack of effect for the standard maximum dose, the patient's current side-effect profile, and the relative safety of the higher-than-normal dosage.

Lithium. The support for the efficacy of lithium salts in treating nonbipolar depression is less compelling than that for bipolar disorders (Klein *et al.*, 1980), although it may benefit those patients with mild recurring depression or those whose depressions are linked (familially) to bipolar disorder (Coppen, Metcalfe, & Wood, 1982; Prien, Kupfer, Mansky, Small, Turson, Voss, & Johnson, 1984; Worrall, Moody, Peet, Dick, Smith, Chambers, Adams, & Naylor, 1979). Lithium salts may also have a place as an adjunctive treatment in depressions that show only partial remission with TCAs or MAOIs (deMontigney, Cournoyer, Morissette, Langlois, & Caille, 1983).

A more detailed description of the side effects of lithium treatment is given in the subsection on bipolar disorder. It is important to keep in mind, however, that lithium, like TCAs, has a small dosage range in which it can be considered both therapeutic and safe. A dosage of only two to four times the therapeutic amount may be sufficient to result in serious adverse effects. The long-term use of lithium is also suspected of producing functional and structural kidney abnormalities, such as impaired concentration of urine and, after many years of treatment, interstitial changes. Such findings clearly support the use of tests of these functions at regular intervals during long-term treatment with lithium (Coppen *et al.*, 1982).

When lithium carbonate is selected as the primary antidepressant agent for a patient with nonbipolar affective disorder, the starting dose is generally 300 mg either twice a day or three times a day. Dosages, again, are titrated upward in keeping with the patient's clinical response, side-effect profile, and plasma lithium levels. Although guidelines for the most effective lithium blood level for treating depression are not clear-cut, many clinicians initially use lower levels (i.e., 0.5–0.8 mEq/l) for several weeks before pushing the dose higher. Clinical signs and symptoms of toxicity variably present when blood levels exceed 1.0 mEq/l and are usually present when the blood level is greater than 1.5 mEq/l (Jefferson & Griest, 1987). It is commonly observed in clinical practice that many depressed patients cannot tolerate or do not benefit from the same dosages and levels of lithium required to treat mania. Such anecdotal observations, however, do not necessarily apply to a given individual. The necessary time-frame for evaluating the response to lithium is again approximately 6 weeks, including a period of at least 2 weeks at the highest clinically appropriate and well-tolerated level.

Continuation and Maintenance Treatment. Antidepressant therapy should be continued for at least 4 months past the resolution of an episode of depression; earlier withdrawal of treatment appears to be associated with a 50% rate of relapse (Prien & Kupfer, 1986). The provision of treatment during this 4-month period has been termed *continuation* therapy, and the resurfacing of depression during the continuation period is called, arbitrarily, a *relapse* (Prien & Kupfer, 1986). Although continuation therapy is routinely recommended, it is particularly important in cases with naturally high rates of relapse. These would include psychotic depression, "double" depression, and depressions that have required ECT. Continuation treatment generally uses the same dosage of antidepressant that was necessary initially, although occasional dosage reductions may be made because of changes in side-effect tolerance. Patient appointments are generally shifted to biweekly, then monthly intervals during this time.

Following the successful completion of a period of continuation therapy, decisions must be made regarding the need for ongoing maintenance therapy. Obviously, patients who have experienced a single, or infrequent, mild episode(s) of depression usually do not receive maintenance therapy. Conversely, patients who have experienced multiple severe episodes of incapacitating depression are routinely provided maintenance therapy. A risk–benefit equation should be developed for each individual patient, and, if possible, the decision should be made collaboratively. This process ideally includes the spouse or a significant other as well. Some patients opt for an "early-detection" program, in which maintenance treatment is not pursued and antidepressant therapy will be resumed at the first signs of a recurrence of depression. (We recommend the use of a period of 2 weeks of depressed mood with a minimum of four associated symptoms before reinitiating treatment in order to prevent "false starts.") For others, the anticipated pain and suffering of a new episode of depression is so aversive that maintenance treatment is a small price to pay. In such cases, we do not address the issue of "lifetime" treatment, and we focus instead on discrete periods of 1, 2, or 3 years.

The best available evidence indicates that maintenance antidepressant therapy reduces the risk of recurrence by 50%–70% (Prien, 1988; Prien *et al.*, 1984). Many practitioners reduce the dosage of the antidepressant to approximately one-half the level used during acute treatment. We suspect that this practice may undertreat a number of patients and thus increase the risk of recurrence in such patients. In the absence of convincing data to support the value of "minidosing," we recommend maintenance therapy at the same dosage as acute treatment unless changes in side-effect tolerance dictate otherwise. Other clinicians discontinue the heterocyclic antidepressant in favor of lithium carbonate. This practice is more common in Europe than the United States and does appear justified in milder recurrent depressions (Prien *et al.,* 1984).

Side effects are generally not a major problem during maintenance treatment because many patients have accommodated to minor side-effects, and intolerant patients have not continued the therapy. Occasionally, patients will complain for the first time of erectile or orgasmic difficulties because the prospect of prolonged periods of sexual disability is not appealing. Dosage reduction or the substitution of an alternate antidepressant is generally necessary if the sexual dysfunction appears to be caused by the antidepressant. Excessive weight gain may become a progressively more vexing problem during extended anti-depressant treatment, affecting up to 25%–30% of patients (Fernstrom, Krowinski, & Kupfer, 1987). Further research is necessary to ascertain if such weight gain is the simple result of increased caloric intake, or whether it also may reflect specific effects of anti-depressant on basal metabolism. Monitoring the patient's weight at each visit and providing vigorous attention to exercise and diet (including recommending the use of dieting support groups) appear useful to prevent weight gain from becoming an unspoken problem that undermines the treatment alliance.

Discontinuation of antidepressants following a prolonged period of continuation or maintenance therapy never should be abrupt. There is an uncomfortable, anticholinergic withdrawal syndrome associated with tricyclic discontinuation (Dilsaver & Greden, 1984), which may be difficult at first to differentiate from the recurrence of depression. Moreover, most antidepressants suppress rapid-eye-movement (REM) sleep, and their sudden withdrawal will induce REM rebound. Accordingly, a slow taper of about 20%–25% of the dosage each week will minimize the symptoms and provide a smoother transition.

ECT. Electroconvulsive therapy is seldom used in contemporary outpatient practice. Reviews of existing studies, however, indicate that, for severe depressions, those accompanied by delusions, or those that have been refractory to pharmacotherapy, ECT is not only effective but more effective than other treatments (Fink, 1979; Scovern & Kilmann, 1980). Moreover, ECT may be a life-saving treatment of serious depression in patients who cannot safely tolerate pharmacotherapy. Therefore, we recommend reserving the acute use of ECT to inpatient settings for refractory, severe, or complicated cases. In conventional practice, a therapeutic dose of a previously effective or well-tolerated anti-depressant or lithium is resumed following the completion of ECT. In our experience, switching antidepressant classes (i.e., from a TCA to a MAOI) is sometimes useful when a patient has previously failed to respond to a particular agent. The use of maintenance ECT on an outpatient basis after a successful inpatient course of treatment is generally not required. Nevertheless, this understudied approach does appear useful in patients with severe, relapsing affective disorders that cannot be maintained with pharmacotherapy. Such treatments often begin weekly and are switched to biweekly and then monthly as remission lengthens. The maximum duration of maintenance ECT is unknown.

The major issue concerning the use of ECT is its effects on cognitive functioning, particularly memory. Much has been written about this, and disentangling transient from permanent effects is important to the evaluation of this question. Research indicates that transient effects on retrograde and anterograde memory are very real. Whether or not these, or other brain disturbances, endure beyond the first few months after treatment remains a topic of debate (American Psychiatric Association, 1978; Pettinati & Bonner, 1984).

Other Somatic Therapies. The outpatient pharmacotherapy of nonbipolar depression sometimes necessitates the use of medications that fall outside a strict grouping of thymoleptic drugs. In particular, we briefly consider here the selected use of three other classes of medication: (1) benzodiazepines; (2) neuroleptics, (3) anticonvulsants, and (4) psychostimulants.

Benzodiazepines, of which diazepam (Valium®) and chlordiazepoxide (Librium®) are prototypes, are safe and broadly effective anxiolytics and hypnotics (sleeping pills). Benzodiazepines can be quite effective initially in lessening the tension, psychic distress, and insomnia associated with depression. They range in efficacy from equivalently to somewhat more effective than placebo when used as primary antidepressants, and they exert their effects on anxiety and insomnia more rapidly than standard antidepressants (Klein *et al.,* 1980). Benzodiazepines are generally well-tolerated, and their fairly immediate positive effects make them quite acceptable to distressed patients. Unfortunately, these very effects often make the benzodiazepines drugs the first choice of busy primary-care providers, even though their ultimate efficacy as antidepressants is not robust. Further, the hypnotic and anxiolytic effects of these agents may habituate and, after several months of regular use, there is some risk of tolerance and physical dependence. Accordingly, we do not routinely use benzodiazepines as an adjunct to antidepressant therapy, even though we recognize that this practice is relatively common in the community. (A proprietary fixed-dosage combination of amitriptyline and chlordiazepoxide is even available.) Beyond the worries of habituation and dependence (which are minimal when care is supervised by a physician "sensitized" to such problems), we are concerned that the routine use of adjunctive benzodiazepines may obscure a true assessment of the primary antidepressant's efficacy. From this standpoint, relief of sleep disturbance and anxiety secondary to a major depression is a critical criterion in evaluating the utility of the initial antidepressant, and an alternate agent should be tried if the initial choice is ineffective.

Perhaps one exception to this general strategy is alprazolam, a triazolobenzodiazepine. This agent appears to have more robust antidepressant efficacy than other benzodiazepines, particularly in outpatient depressives with features of anxiety (Rickels, Chung, Csanalosi, Hurowitz, London, Wiseman, Kaplan, & Amsterdam, 1987). Some recent evidence, however, suggests that alprazolam is less effective than the standard tricyclics in patients with more classical endogenous features (Goldberg, Ettigi, Schultz, Hamer, Hayes, & Friedel, 1986; Rush, Erman, Schlesser, Roffwarg, Vasavada, Khatami, Fairchild, & Giles, 1985). It is generally used in dosages of 1.0–6.0 mg per day. Alprazolam is fast becoming a cornerstone of the treatment of panic disorder and thus may be quite useful (when tricyclics and MAOIs fail) in mixed anxiety–depression or secondary-depression syndromes. Of course, concerns about habituation, tolerance, and physical dependence must be addressed, especially if long-term therapy is considered.

Neuroleptics (antipsychotics) have been similarly used as adjunctive agents, particularly in the treatment of agitated and anxious depressions. Further, there is an older literature (from the 1960s) to support the efficacy of several neuroleptics as primary antidepressants (see Klein *et al.*, 1980). Although physical dependence is not a concern, these "major" tranquilizers have a significant number of acute side effects and convey the long-term risk of tardive dyskinesia, a disfiguring and potentially irreversible neurological disorder.

The major current indication for the use of neuroleptics in depression is in severe syndromes characterized by psychotic features. In this circumstance, some antipsychotics offer the additional advantage of raising the plasma levels of selected antidepressants. The results of a controlled inpatient study at our institute document the utility of an antidepressant–neuroleptic (amitriptyline–perphenazine) combination in psychotic depression when compared with the use of either component alone (Spiker, Weiss, Dealy, Griffin, Hanin, Neal, Perel, Rossi, & Soloff, 1985). Given the severity, the incapacity, and the risk of suicide associated with psychotic depression, we generally prefer to hospitalize such patients. Nevertheless, some delusionally depressed patients refuse hospitalization and do not meet the criteria for involuntary admission. These patients must be managed as outpatients. Dosages should be titrated rapidly, with a simultaneous adjustment of both the antipsychotic and the antidepressant. We favor the use of the amitriptyline–perphenazine combination on the basis of both clinical experience and empirical support. Perphenazine is initiated at 8 mg or 16 mg per day and is increased, as tolerated, until relief of psychotic symptoms is achieved. Dosages of 64 mg or even 80 mg per day (i.e., comparable to the dosages used in acute schizophrenia) are sometimes necessary. Generally, second-generation heterocyclics and MAOIs should not be chosen in this situation (unless standard tricyclics cannot be tolerated), given the lack of experience in using these agents in psychotic depression.

Anticonvulsants have a long and checkered history of use as treatments for depression. Although their use has received some powerful personal testimony (Dreyfuss, 1981), there is little evidence to support the use of anticonvulsants in most cases of depression unless virtually all other viable strategies have failed. One exception to this observation involves the use of standard anticonvulsants, such as phenytoin sodium, in combination with antidepressants in patients with suspected subclinical (subictal) cerebral dysrhythmias. Such patients may have low-grade focal or generalized EEG disturbances (which may be accentuated by sleep deprivation or antidepressant pharmacotherapy), and/or they may manifest clinical features such as mood lability, auras, or migrainelike phenomena without frank convulsions (Himmelhoch & Thase, in press). Clinical suspicion is often suggested by an atypical response to one or more standard antidepressants. A related usage of anticonvulsants involves the agent carbamazepine (Tegretol®). This anticonvulsant is particularly effective in temporal lobe epilepsy and trigeminal neuralgia and, as will be discussed later, is being increasingly used in the treatment of bipolar affective disorder. Some recent work has evaluated the antidepressant efficacy of carbamazepine when other standard agents have failed, and although the results are not striking, occasional patients show excellent results (Post, 1987). In our own practices, we do not use carbamazepine in nonbipolar depression unless there is suspicion of a temporal-lobe cerebral dysrhythmia.

Psychostimulants have been available for the treatment of depression for over four decades, and their inconsistent clinical effects are well established (Klein *et al.*, 1980). Moreover, the psychostimulants are strongly addictive and habituating and thus are monitored closely as controlled substances. Drugs such as dextroamphetamine and methylphenidate may produce transient improvement or worsening in mood states but have not appeared to surpass placebo in controlled clinical trials. Thus, the use of psychostimulants in the treatment of depression should be restricted to cases in which the standard treatments have been ineffective or cannot be tolerated. In this regard, some investigators and clinicians have had particular success using stimulants in combination with tricyclic antidepressants (see, for example, Klein *et al.*, 1980). Some evidence suggests the possible value of brief trials (i.e., 1–3 days) on a psychostimulant, particularly dextroamphetamine, as a prognostic test for tricyclic responsivity (Little, 1988), although this practice is hardly common.

Several recent studies indicate that recurrent depressions that follow a seasonal pattern (i.e., fall–winter depression or seasonal affective disorder) may be responsive to treatment with bright white light (see, for example, Rosenthal, Sack, Skewerer, Jacobsen, & Wehr, 1988). Such phototherapy is generally provided during the fall and winter months, in 1- to 2-hour periods of exposure to bright (2,500–10,000 lux), full-spectrum fluorescent light. During this time, patients may read or watch television but should remain within 6–10 feet of the light source. Early-morning exposure to light is preferred over evening or midday exposure, with the conceptual appeal of expanding the photoperiod during the short fall and winter days. However, it should be noted that evidence favoring a photoperiodic effect is scanty (Terman, 1988), and the time of day for phototherapy may not be critical for some patients.

Phototherapy is currently recommended for patients who desire a nonpharmacological treatment and who manifest a clear pattern of fall–winter depressions. Light "boxes" are available from several reputable commercial sources, and the treatment should be supervised by a competent professional, just as any other somatic therapy is. Some investigators report a disproportionate number of bipolar II cases in samples with seasonal effective disorder, and most studies document an increased prevalence of reversed vegetative symptoms in such patients (see Thase, 1989). It remains to be seen if phototherapy has any efficacy in nonseasonal depressions and if it is equally effective in winter depressions characterized by the more classical features of melancholia.

Treatment-Resistant Depression. Despite the good prognosis of most forms of mood disorders, a substantial minority of patients do not respond to the initial choice of treatment. The topic of treatment-resistant depression has received extensive review elsewhere (see, for example, Zohar & Belmaker, 1987), and a myriad of strategies exist for tricyclic nonresponders. Our preferred approach is summarized in Table 9. There are clear regional and idiosyncratic differences in various experts' approaches to resistant depression. Nevertheless, the common themes include (1) establishing the adequacy (i.e., dosage and time) of one treatment before trying another; (2) more aggressive use of MAOIs and ECT; (3) reserving "exotic" medication combinations for patients who fail to respond to virtually all standard strategies; (4) continuously reevaluating the psychiatric diagnosis, the psychosocial support system, and the medical status of treatment nonresponders; and (5) not giving up on such patients.

Psychosocial Treatments for Nonbipolar Depression

As noted earlier, the DSM-III-R makes very few assumptions about what causes and/or maintains various mood disorders. The somatic treatments discussed above can be reasonably applied following this atheoretical descriptive approach. It can be argued, however, that psychosocial treatments are typically derived from some set of implicit or explicit hypotheses about the nature of the problem and what processes ought to constitute the focus of intervention. Such proposed psychosocial variables include unresolved dynamic conflicts, social skill deficits, ongoing interpersonal disputes (particularly marital discord), biased information-processing, deficient self-reinforcement strategies, and maladaptive personality styles. Given the variation in depressive disorders, it is not surprising that there are many models for understanding it and many therapies available to treat it. A comprehensive review of all psychosocial treatments for depression is beyond the limits of this chapter. Instead, the focus is on two of the more extensively researched and widely practiced therapies: cognitive behavior therapy and interpersonal psychotherapy. (See Jarrett & Rush, 1986, for a review of additional psychotherapies for depression.)

Cognitive Approach to Depression. It is most accurate to view the cognitive model of depression as several different, though overlapping, frameworks that provide conceptualizations of the etiology, the cross-sectional psychopathology, and the treatment of depression. It has been developed since the mid-1960s by A. T. Beck and colleagues (Beck, 1976; Beck, Rush, Shaw, & Emery, 1979). At the simplest level of conceptualization, the cross-sectional view holds that depression and its associated symptoms can be understood and described in cognitive terms. The term *cognition* refers to the content, process, and structure of thinking. *Cognitive content* refers to the spontaneous thoughts and images that run through people's minds. These thoughts are experienced as involuntary and automatic. The cognitive content of depressed individuals is seen as revolving

Table 9. Outpatient Management of Treatment-Resistant Depression

Step 1:	A. Establish adequacy of TCA trial: Check compliance and blood level. Titrate dosage higher (if tolerated) to provide at least 3 additional weeks at an adequate level. Recheck thyroid axis using Thyroid releasing hormone (TRH) stimulation test: supplement with thyroid hormone if indicated by elevated thyroid-stimulating-hormone response or low thyroid indices. Monitor EKGs and drug plasma levels if supranormal dosages of TCA are used.
	B. Switch to a TCA with measurable (and validated) blood levels if necessary: imipramine, amitriptyline, desipramine, or nortriptyline.
Step 2:	A. If no response, add Li_2CO_3 (300 mg b.i.d. or t.i.d.). Titrate Li^+ blood level to 0.6–1.0 mEg/l range. Provide 4- to 6-week Li^+ augmentation trial. Proceed to Step B if no response.
	B. If intolerant, withdraw TCA and initiate an alternate HCA (or MAOI) after appropriate washout. Regional preference will determine whether fluoxetine, trazodone, or an MAOI is selected. If no response (after 6 weeks), reimplement Step 2A as described above.
Step 3:	A. Reevaluate diagnosis and indications for psychosocial treatment.
	B. Consider elective admission and possible ECT.
	C. Provide MAOI trial if not used above. Allow at least 5 weeks for fluoxetine washout. Ensure adequate MAOI treatment by advancing to maximum appropriate dose (i.e., 60 mg/day of tranylcypromine or 90 mg/day of phenelzine).
	D. Li^+ augmentation of MAOI as described above.
Step 4:	A. Strongly consider elective admission and ECT.
	B. Combined TCA (HCA) and MAOI treatment if 4A is refused or ineffective: The combination of amitriptyline and phenelzine has had the greatest use.
	C. Experimental therapeutics (see Zohar & Belmaker, 1987, for alternate options).

around negative and often inaccurate views of themselves, their future, and their world (the so-called cognitive triad). Examples of such negative automatic thoughts include, "I am a failure"; "there is no hope"; and "The world is against me." Hypothetically, this type of thinking is traceable to faulty or idiosyncratic processing of incoming information. For example, depressed individuals often seem to misinterpret situations, attaching the most negative meanings and reaching the most negative conclusions about the situation. For example, depressed people are very good at reading rejection into situations where none was intended and at attaching an inordinately negative meaning to an objectively benign event. Theoretically, cognitions and the characteristic symptoms of depression are viewed as being in a reciprocal relationship (Teasdale, 1983). Negative thoughts affect how a person feels and behaves. If, for example, one is thinking and believing, "I am no good" and "My life is a mess," then symptoms of depression such as crying and feeling sad are logical reflections of these thoughts. By the same token, negative mood affects thinking. Research is accumulating to show that mood states may prime certain types of thoughts (Bower, 1987; Singer & Salovey, 1988).

An important component of the cognitive model is the hypothetical existence of relatively stable cognitive structures or schemata. Schemata are viewed as filters or templates for incoming information, or the "software" used for the processing and interpreting of life's circumstances. It is these schemata that theoretically make a person vulnerable to depression. In other words, depression is seen as the result of an interaction between a preexisting diathesis or vulnerability (schema) and a particular stress confronting the individual. For example, many depressed patients can be seen as having schemata that make them exquisitely sensitive to rejection and disruptions in interpersonal relationships. Such schemata may develop from early experiences with parental disapproval or loss. Situations that activate these themes are highly stressful and difficult for such vulnerable individuals. Conversely, these same individuals may not be at risk for the development of depression in situations that would indeed affect others with different vulnerabilities. This notion of *specific vulnerability* helps to explain why there is not a one-to-one correspondence between certain life events and the subsequent development of depression. Depending on a person's life circumstances, certain potentially depressogenic schemata remain quiescent, and depression may never develop. Not all aspects of the cognitive model of depression have received consistent empirical support (for review and critique, see Coyne & Gotlib, 1983, 1986; Segal & Shaw, 1986a,b). Hypotheses regarding the vulnerability factor, the schemata, and the role of cognitions in the etiology of depression are perhaps the least well supported, as well as the most difficult to test (Segal, 1988).

The potential clinical usefulness of cognitive therapy for depression, however, does not depend on the validity of the etiological model. The therapy model holds that, once one is depressed, the symptoms can be alleviated by intervention at the cognitive level. Cognitive therapy is usually practiced as a short-term, structured approach (Beck *et al.*, 1979). The thrust of the therapy is problem-oriented. The therapist and the patient work together according to a principle of "collaborative empiricism." Working as a team, the patient and the therapist break down the patient's distress into specific target problems. These problems are then translated into cognitive terms and are analyzed with respect to the dysfunctional thinking, beliefs, and assumptions that may be mediating the problem or interfering with its solution. Having identified the cognitive culprits, the therapist and the patient treat these thoughts and assumptions as hypotheses to be empirically tested and evaluated. Using exercises and homework assignments, patients learn to collect evidence that either supports or contradicts the hypothesis in question. Once the evidence is collected, the patient is encouraged to logically evaluate the data and reach his or her own conclusions regarding the validity and utility of the hypothesis.

The efficacy of this treatment has been subjected to a number of systematic tests. Recent clinical trials support the efficacy of cognitive behavior therapy (CBT) with patients diagnosed as having nonpsychotic, nonbipolar depression (Beck *et al.*, 1985; Beutler, Scogin, Kirkish, Schretier, Corbishley, Hamblin, Meredith, Potter, Bamford, & Levenson, 1987; Blackburn, Eunson, & Bishop, 1986; Elkin *et al.*, 1986; Murphy *et al.*, 1984; Rush *et al.*, 1977; Teasdale *et al.*, 1984). Although other data caution against seeing this treatment as a panacea (Fennell & Teasdale, 1982; Harpin, Libermen, Marks, Stern, & Bohannon, 1982), the cumulative results indicate that cognitive therapy has reduced symptoms in samples of depressed outpatients compared to no treatment or to other control conditions. Importantly, cognitive therapy also achieves results generally equivalent to those of other empirically established forms of somatic and psychosocial treatments for depressed patients. The results of follow-up studies of patients who have been treated with cognitive therapy have generated some enthusiasm in that preliminary findings indicate that it provides some protection against relapse (Blackburn, Eunson, & Bishop, 1986; Kovacs, Rush, Beck, & Hollon, 1981; Simons, Murphy, Levine, & Wetzel, 1986). Theoretically, such "prophylaxis" is a consequence of two processes: changing the factor that made the individual vulnerable to depression (i.e., the schemata or underlying assumptions) and teaching the patient skills for coping with challenges and problems and for minimizing his or her dysfunctional emotional sequelae.

Interpersonal Approach to Depression. The interpersonal model of depression draws heavily on the earlier writing of Harry Stack Sullivan, Adolph Meyer, and others who emphasized the role of interpersonal relationships in the development of depression. The conceptualization of Klerman and Weissman and associates (Klerman, Weissman, Rounsaville, & Chevron, 1984) targets interpersonal difficulties as important contributors to the development and maintenance of depression. These difficulties can be seen as being influenced by early developmental experiences, especially early attachments. Early bonds are seen as important determinants of whether an individual will be vulnerable and respond with depression in the face of environmental and psychosocial stressors and disruptions in relationships (Kleiman, Weissman, Rounsaville, & Chevron, 1984).

Interpersonal psychotherapy (IPT) is a short-term treatment that focuses on and intervenes in depressive symptoms and social and interpersonal relations. Although it shares many features with the brief insight-oriented psychotherapies (i.e., Davanloo, 1980; Malan, 1963; Sifneos, 1972), it differs in that it is more active and sets more limited goals. For example, interpersonal psychotherapy does not attempt to change long-standing and enduring personality traits, even though these may be recognized as potential contributors to the patient's depression. Instead, the goals are to alleviate the depressive symptoms and to improve interpersonal functioning, with particular reference to dealing with the problems associated with the development of the depressive symptoms. These two goals are achieved in two general ways: education and problem solving. The educational component involves teaching the patient about the syndrome of depression and helping him or her to understand that such distress is part of a well-known syndrome with a good prognosis. Problem solving involves defining the interpersonal problems that may be at the source of the depression and developing strategies for their resolution. These problems usually fall into one of four areas: (1) grief; (2) interpersonal role disputes (e.g., a disagreement between the patient and an important other person regarding the expectations each has about the nature of their relationship); (3) role transitions (i.e., difficulty in adapting to a new role in life); and (4) interpersonal deficits (i.e., lack of the skills necessary for forming and maintaining meaningful relationships). Because of the short-term nature of IPT, the focus of therapy is typically limited to one or two problem areas.

The efficacy of interpersonal psychotherapy has been researched in several comparative outcome studies. All of these studies indicate that interpersonal psychotherapy decreases depressive symptoms in a proportion of patients (Elkin *et al.*, 1986; Klerman, DiMascio, Weissman, Prusoff, & Paykel, 1974; Rounsaville, Klerman, & Weissman, 1981; Weissman, Prusoff, & DiMascio, 1979). The most recent of these studies indicates that interpersonal psychotherapy and cognitive therapy achieve approximately the same results when one is comparing groups of patients (Elkin *et al.*, 1986). As discussed earlier in this chapter, however, the important question of which individuals respond best to this particular form of therapy remains relatively unanswered.

Treatment of Bipolar Disorder

Somatic Modalities for the Treatment of Bipolar Disorders

It is difficult to manage full-blown manic episodes in an outpatient treatment setting; individuals experiencing a manic episode often makes this difficulty explicitly clear with noncompliance, alcohol and substance abuse, and/or refusal to attend scheduled appointments. Manic episodes may worsen precipitously, and dire financial and psychosocial consequences often follow the behavioral escapades of the manic individual. Even worse, when manic patients become psychotic (particularly when the delusions are paranoid) they may present a clear danger to themselves, their family, or the community. Strong treatment alliances with the patient (predating the manic episode) and the patient's family are necessary to achieve the level of collaboration required for outpatient management. Fortunately, mental-health commitment laws permit an additional source of external control (i.e., involuntary hospitalization) when less restrictive options are ineffective.

Lithium carbonate is, of course, the cornerstone of the pharmacotherapy of mania and hypomania. Milder episodes of mania and hypomania that develop when the patient is off psychotropic medication should be treated first with lithium alone; alternate strategies should be held in reserve. The correct dosage may be surmised from past treatment experience or may be titrated from a standard starting point (i.e., 300 mg three times each day). Blood lithium levels should be checked weekly until the dosage is stabilized; generally, a blood level of 0.8–1.2 mEq/l is associated with antimanic efficacy. Some individuals require even higher levels (i.e., 1.2–1.5 mEq/l) to achieve response, and other patients benefit from lower levels (e.g., 0.4–0.7 mEq/l). Adjusting the dosage to achieve the best possible balance of response and minimal side effects is part of the art of pharmacotherapy. Lower starting dosages are recommended for older persons, persons taking diuretics, and individuals with a past history of poor tolerance of lithium therapy.

The decision to start lithium therapy in a never-medicated individual should include considerable education about the presumed illness (bipolar disorder or cyclothymia) and its treatment. This should include likely outcomes and the potential benefits and risks of the treatment. The risks of treatment must also be offset against the risks of not receiving treatment. We prefer to compare the mood swings of bipolar disorder to a very frightening roller-coaster ride; the goal of initial treatment is to level out, or stabilize, the most unpleasant aspects of the mood swings. Individuals who experience productive hypomanias generally require some sincere reassurance that therapy is not intended to "rob" them of their productive periods. Other individuals find it reassuring that lithium is a natural element or that lithium does not exert its effects via tranquilization. In any event, careful instruction regarding the importance of compliance, of maintaining good hydration status, of blood-level monitoring, and of restriction of alcohol use is necessary. A recent physical examination, including routine blood work and an electrocardiogram, are also required. The blood work should include white blood cell differential, electrolytes, blood urea nitrogen, creatinine, serum calcium, and thyroid indices (including TSH level), as lithium treatment may alter these parameters. Given the evidence of the long-term effects of lithium on the kidney, a baseline 24-hour urine collection is often recommended for a determination of creatinine clearance and an estimation of renal concentrating capacity. Thus, although it is important to emphasize the relatively benign nature of lithium treatment, it is also important to temper such reassurances by conveying the importance of compliance and medical monitoring.

The common side effects of acute lithium therapy include nausea or upset stomach, diarrhea, tremors, polyuria, excessive thirst, sedation, and a metallic taste (Jefferson & Greist, 1987). Tremor may be controlled by the addition of propanolol (or another beta-blocker), although we prefer to try dosage reduction if possible. Weight gain and acnelike skin eruptions may present more problems during extended treatment. Confusion, ataxia, and slurring of speech suggest CNS toxicity and are usually encountered when the blood lithium level exceeds the therapeutic range. Nevertheless, some sensitive individuals may experience these unacceptable side effects at usually "therapeutic" levels. The development of such signs of toxicity should generally lead to dosage reduction, unless it is clear that the person inadvertently took too large a dosage or was transiently dehydrated.

In a majority of cases, the unpleasantness of such side effects can be mitigated by patient education and dosage adjustment. For example, nausea can be lessened by shifting dosing to mealtimes, whereas sedation can be dealt with by a consolidation of the dosage at bedtime. Several delayed-absorption forms of lithium carbonate are available and may be well tolerated when the standard preparations are not. Ultimately, the ability to tolerate unpleasant side effects is modulated to some extent by the perceived therapeutic benefit.

The therapeutic effects of lithium may take several weeks to develop fully, and close follow-up (i.e., weekly at a minimum) is required. Patients with marked insomnia or agitation must be monitored ever so closely for the worsening of mania. As noted earlier, hospitalization may be necessary. Although treatment with lithium alone is preferred, the adjunctive use of either benzodiazepines or neuroleptics may be necessary until the full effects of lithium are achieved. In practice, it is useful to reserve the use of neuroleptics for those patients with a past history of psychotic mania or for when prodromal signs of impending psychosis are apparent. In such cases, the choice of nonsedating (e.g., haloperidol or fluphenazine), sedating (e.g., chlorpromazine or thloridizine), or intermediate (e.g., thiothixene or perphenazine) antipsychotics is based more on the clinician's familiarity with them or attempts to match side-effect profiles than on empirical data. Similarly, the selection of a particular benzodiazepine for "nonspecific" sedation or hypnotic effects is generally based on clinical experience. Some data support the antimanic effects of one benzodiazepine, clonazepam (Chouinard, Young, & Annable,

1983). Until definitive evidence is available, some clinical researchers have adopted this agent when a benzodiazepine is to be used, because, at worst, it is equivalent to other agents and, at best, may offer a specific advantage (Janicak & Boshes, 1987).

Carbamazepine provides another option for patients who do not respond to lithium or who cannot tolerate this agent (Goodwin & Jamison, in press). Although carbamazepine is being increasingly used in the treatment of bipolar affective disorder, it has not yet been approved for such use by the Food and Drug Administration. Preliminary evidence, however, indicates that it is about as effective as lithium in uncomplicated cases (Lerer, Moore, Meyendorff, Cho, & Gershon, 1987), although the clinical pharmacology of carbamazepine continues to relegate it to a second-line role. Accordingly, many clinicians use carbamazepine in combination with lithium when monotherapy has not been effective. Interestingly, this anticonvulsant agent does not appear to be selectively effective in manic patients with EEG abnormalities, nor are its antimanic effects reliably related to anticonvulsant blood levels (Post, 1987).

Carbamazepine is generally initiated at 200 mg twice each day, and the dosage is titrated against clinical response and side effects. Dosage is increased by units of 100, 200, or 300 mg per day on a weekly basis if the medication is well tolerated. Some individuals require a dosage in excess of 2,000 mg each day, whereas others do well on as little as 200 mg each day. Like lithium, carbamazepine must be monitored closely. A dosage yielding blood levels within the "anticonvulsant" range (i.e., 6–12 mcg/ml) is first sought, and complete blood counts (including platelets) and liver function studies are checked weekly (Jefferson & Greist, 1987). Fortunately, although carbamazepine is a relatively new addition to psychopharmacology, its long track record as an anticonvulsant provides useful guidelines for clinical practice. Bone marrow suppression is the most worrisome side effect, and rarely, agranulocytosis and aplastic anemia have been reported (Jefferson & Greist, 1987). Should the white-blood-cell or platelet counts fall dramatically (i.e., a total white-blood-cell count < 2,000 or a platelet count < 100,000), carbamazepine should be discontinued immediately. Less precipitous and transient reductions in blood cell counts occur relatively frequently during carbamazepine therapy and serve to keep the physician vigilant, without necessitating drug discontinuation.

Other common side effects of carbamazepine include dry mouth, blurry vision, lightheadedness, constipation, and ataxia (Jefferson & Greist, 1987). Accommodation to such side effects often occurs; dosage reduction is sometimes necessary when such side effects are intolerable. Carbamazepine also induces the liver enzymes which metabolize a number of drugs (including haloperidol and warfarin), and its metabolism is slowed by the standard antibiotic erythromycin. Therefore, carbamazepine should be used cautiously in combination with medications other than lithium.

Acute Treatment of Bipolar Depression. The pharmacotherapy of the depressed phase of bipolar illness depends, in part, on whether the person has been maintained on lithium carbonate (and/or carbamazepine) before the onset of the depressive episode. If the patient has been off maintenance pharmacotherapy, then the first step is simply to resume the mood stabilizer, usually lithium carbonate. This resumption is justified because both lithium and carbamazepine may be effective primary antidepressants in some bipolar patients *and* because it is likely that a resumption of prophylactic treatment will be recommended (Goodwin & Jamison, in press). Following several weeks of treatment at lower blood levels (i.e., 0.5–0.8 mEq/l of lithium), titration to higher levels is indicated if the drug has been well tolerated.

Bipolar depressions that "break through" despite maintenance treatment, or that fail to respond following the resumption of the mood stabilizer, should be considered for additional treatment with a heterocyclic antidepressant or an MAOI. The virtual absence of controlled empirical data relating directly to the antidepressant treatment of bipolar depression is surprising (see, for example, Goodwin & Jamison, in press). Moreover, recommendations based on clinical experience vary widely, so that expert opinions range from the extreme positions of virtually never using a tricyclic, to using tricyclics exactly as in nonbipolar depression.

Concern about the use of tricyclic (and heterocyclic) antidepressants in bipolar depression stems from evidence that tricyclics may reduce cycle length and, in the most dramatic cases, may induce a pattern of rapid cycling (Wehr & Goodwin, 1987). Such concerns do not appear to be justified when attention is restricted to bipolar cases with long cycle lengths and are not universally shared (e.g., Angst, 1985). Thus, in an uncomplicated case of bipolar depression that has not responded to lithium alone, the selection of a standard tricyclic (such as imipramine) and the titration of the dosage upward, as described earlier, appear justified if tricyclics have not failed in the past. Nevertheless, if a pattern of rapid cycling emerges, heterocyclic treatment (particularly in brief 2- to 4-week "pulses") should be avoided. Alternate treatments for rapid cycling include thyroid augmentation, low-dose neuroleptics, MAOIs, carbamazepine, lithium plus carbamazepine, and ECT (Potter, 1983). In our practices, we prefer an elective hospitalization, a vigorous workup of the metabolic and endocrine systems, and, if necessary, a "fresh start" on treatment with a course of ECT to try to break a pattern of rapid cycling.

The use of MAOIs in the pharmacotherapy of bipolar depression has been an overlooked topic. Some preliminary work by our group suggests that the MAOI tranylcypromine may be particularly useful in bipolar depressions characterized by anergia, motor retardation, and hypersomnia and/or weight gain (Himmelhoch & Thase, in press; Thase, Himmelhoch, & Mallinger, 1988). These interesting findings, which require extension and replication, further indicate that tranylcypromine (average dosage: 40 mg/day) may be nearly twice as effective in anergic bipolar depression as the standard tricyclic imipramine under double blind conditions (82% response rate versus 46% response rate), without any increased induction of manic or hypomanic episodes (Thase, Himmelhoch, & Mallinger, 1988). Moreover, 75% (9/12) of the imipramine failures in this study subsequently responded when crossed over to tranylcypromine (Thase, Himmelhoch, Mallinger, Safer, & McKnight, 1988). It remains to be seen whether the other available MAOIs (phenelzine and isocarboxazid) are similarly effective in bipolar depression *and* whether such efficacy extends to bipolar depression syndromes characterized by more classical "endogenous" features, such as insomnia, agitation, or weight loss.

Continuation and Maintenance Treatment in Bipolar Disorder. Continuation therapy is almost always recommended after the resolution of any episode of bipolar affective disorder. Continuation antidepressant therapy (in addition to lithium) should be tapered off after a 20-week period, or sooner if there is evidence of cycling into hypomania. Continuation therapy with neuroleptics or benzodiazepines can be tapered off more quickly after the resolution of mania, in deference to minimizing the risk of tardive dyskinesia or drug dependence. However, these agents should be reinstituted promptly if evidence of a manic relapse surfaces.

Maintenance treatment with lithium and/or carbamazepine is recommended in all but the most mild cases of bipolar disorder, or in those with extremely long cycle lengths (i.e., with episodes occurring years apart). Some investigators have also recommended withholding routine maintenance treatment until after the second major episode of depression or mania, because some individuals will experience only a single episode without subsequent recurrence (Dunner & Clayton, 1987). Although the approach has conceptual appeal (and is popular with patients), we note that early-onset bipolar disorders hold a high risk of both recurrence and development of chronicity (Akiskal, 1983a). Thus, we suggest that such medication-free periods be conducted under the most careful medical supervision possible and in collaboration with a supportive and informed family.

Maintenance therapy with lithium and/or carbamazepine is usually provided monthly or every other month, with laboratory profiles obtained before each visit (Jefferson & Greist, 1987). Annual physical examinations, electrocardiograms, and monitoring of renal and thyroid status are strongly recommended. The infrequency of such appointments makes the early detection of manic episodes unlikely. Determination of the characteristic early-warning signs (i.e., a decrease in sleep requirement, seasonal trends, a change in spending habits, or increased libido) and incorporation of the family as independent monitors help reduce the risk of serious untreated relapses. The availability of the pharmacotherapist to see the patient on short notice so as to modify the medication may forestall a number of recurrences.

Maintenance therapy with neuroleptics and/or antidepressants are also sometimes necessary in more severe or chronic forms of bipolar disorder. Maintenance antidepressant therapy generally follows the guidelines reviewed earlier, with an added concern regarding monitoring to avoid an induction of mania or rapid cycling. Neuroleptic maintenance treatment should be well documented, both in terms of its indications and for the development of signs of tardive dyskinesia. Informed consent probably should be obtained, and patients must be informed of the risk of tardive dyskinesia. As is now the case in the treatment of schizophrenia, reduction of the dosage to minimal levels (i.e., perphenazine dosages < 8 mg per day) should be tried before committing the patient to ongoing treatment at higher dosages.

Psychosocial Treatment of Bipolar Disorders

As has been discussed in the previous sections, the effectiveness of medication in the management of bipolar affective disorders is well documented. Psychotherapy has generally been used as an adjunct to medication in the treatment of bipolar patients. In particular, cognitive therapy has been reported to be helpful in increasing compliance with lithium treatment (Cochran, 1984). A significant proportion of lithium patients have been found to be noncompliant with their treatment; estimates range from approximately 20% to 50% (Cochran, 1984; Jamison, Gerner, & Goodwin, 1979). Therefore, methods of decreasing this rate would be welcome additions to the available treatments.

To our knowledge, psychotherapy is rarely used or recommended as the sole form of treatment for bipolar patients. There is one case report in the literature that discusses the use of cognitive therapy with a patient who desired to discontinue lithium in anticipation of becoming pregnant. The use of lithium by pregnant women is of concern, particularly in the first trimester (Ackerman, Jefferson, Greist, Baudhuin, & Vukovich, 1984). In general, the same techniques of cognitive therapy were used for treating mania as for treating depression. Specifically, these included the careful monitoring of automatic thoughts, and the subsequent identification of possible distortions, and the development of more accurate responses.

SUMMARY

The last several decades have witnessed a tremendous growth in the information about the diagnosis and treatment of depression. Research into this significant public-health problem continues to yield additional data to guide mental health professionals' efforts to help individuals suffering from these disorders. Specific areas of investigation include considerable work on the biological bases of at least some forms of mood disorders. In terms of treatment, research is focusing on addressing the all-important question of matching patient to treatment and understanding the mechanisms by which both somatic and psychosocial treatments achieve their results. Another area that is generating much interest is the recurring nature of depression. Identifying treatments that may alter (favorably) the longitudinal course and that may interrupt the pattern of repeated bouts of depression would represent a significant therapeutic advance.

REFERENCES

Ackerman, D. L., Jefferson, J. W., Greist, J. H., Baudhuin, M. G., & Vukovich, J. (1984). The Lithium Index: An innovative approach to consultation by computer. *American Journal of Psychiatry, 141,* 415–417.

Akiskal, H. S. (1982). Factors associated with incomplete recovery in primary depressive illness. *Journal of Clinical Psychiatry, 43,* 266–271.

Akiskal, H. S. (1983a). The bipolar spectrum: New concepts in classification and diagnosis. In L. Grinspoon (Ed.), *Psychiatry update* (Vol. 2). Washington, DC: American Psychiatric Association.

Akiskal, H. S. (1983b). Dysthymic disorder: Psychopathology of proposed chronic depressive subtypes. *American Journal of Psychiatry, 140,* 11–20.

Akiskal, H. S., Rosenthal, R. H., Rosenthal, T. L., Kashgarian, M., Khani, M. K., & Puzantian, V. H. (1979). Differentiation of primary affective illness from situational, symptomatic and secondary depressions. *Archives of General Psychiatry, 36,* 635–643.

Akiskal, H. S., Rosenthal, T. L., Haykal, R. F., Lemmi, H., Rosenthal, R. H., & Scott-Strauss, A. (1980). Characterological depression: Clinical and sleep EEG findings separating "subaffective" dysthymias from "characterspectrum" disorders. *Archives of General Psychiatry, 37,* 777–783.

Akiskal, H. S., King, D., Rosenthal, T. L., Robinson, D., & Scott-Strauss, A. (1981). Chronic depression: Part 1. Clinical and familial characteristics in 137 probands. *Journal of Affective Disorders, 3,* 297–315.

Akiskal, H. S., Hirschfeld, R. M. A., Yerevanian B. I. (1983). The relationship of personality to affective disorders: A critical review. *Archives of General Psychiatry, 40,* 801–809.

American Psychiatric Association (APA). (1978). Electroconvulsive therapy, *Task Force #14.* Washington, DC: Author.

American Psychiatric Association (APA). (1980). *Diagnostic and statistical manual of mental disorders (3rd ed.;* DSM-III). Washington, DC: Author.

American Psychiatric Association (APA). (1987). *Diagnostic and statistical manual of mental disorders* (3rd ed., rev.; DSM-III-R). Washington, DC: Author.

Andreasen, N. C. (1982). Concepts, diagnosis, and classification. In E. S. Paykel (Ed.), *Handbook of affective disorders.* New York: Guilford Press.

Angst, J. (1985). Switch from depression to mania—a record study over decades between 1920 and 1982. *Psychopathology, 18,* 140–154.

Avery, D., & Lubrano, A. (1979). Depression treated with imipramine and ECT: The DeCarolis study reconsidered. *American Journal of Psychiatry, 136,* 559–562.

Barlow, D. H., DiNardo, P. A., Vermilyea, B. B., Vermilyea, J., & Blanchard, E. B. (1986). Comorbidity and depression among the anxiety disorders: Issues in diagnosis and classification. *Journal of Nervous and Mental Disease, 174,* 63–72.

Beck, A. T. (1976). *Cognitive therapy and the emotional disorders.* New York: International Universities Press.

Beck, A. T., Ward, C. H., Mendelson, M., Mock, J., & Erbaugh, J. (1961). An inventory for measuring depression. *Archives of General Psychiatry, 4,* 561–571.

Beck, A. T., Rush, A. J., Shaw, B. F., & Emery, G. (1979). *Cognitive therapy of depression: A treatment manual.* New York: Guilford Press.

Beck, A. T., Hollon, S. D., Young, J. E., Bedrosian, R. C., & Budenz, D. (1985). Treatment of depression with cognitive therapy and amitriptyline. *Archives of General Psychiatry, 42,* 142–146.

Beutler, L, Scogin, F., Kirkish, P., Schretler, D., Corbishley, A., Hamblin, D., Meredith, K., Potter, R., Bamford, C. R., & Levenson, A. I. (1987). Group cognitive therapy and alprazolam in the treatment of depression in older adults. *Journal of Consulting and Clinical Psychology, 55,* 550–556.

Bielski, R. J., & Friedle, R. O. (1976). Prediction of tricyclic antidepressant response. *Archives of General Psychiatry, 33,* 1479–1489.

Blackburn, I. M., Bishop, S., Glen, A. I. M., Whalley, L. J., & Christie, J. E. (1981). The efficacy of cognitive therapy in depression: A treatment trial using cognitive therapy and pharmacotherapy, each alone and in combination. *British Journal of Psychiatry, 139,* 181–189.

Blackburn, I. M., Eunson, K. M., & Bishop, S. (1986). A two year naturalisitic follow-up of depressed patients treated with cognitive therapy, pharmacotherapy, or a combination of both. *Journal of Affective Disorders, 10,* 67–75.

Blacker, C. V. R., & Clare, A. W. (1987). Depressive disorder in primary care. *British Journal of Psychiatry, 150,* 737–751.

Blackwell, B. (1987a). Newer antidepressant drugs. In H. Y. Meltzer (Ed.), *Psychopharmacology: The third generation of progress* (pp. 1041–1049). New York: Raven Press.

Blackwell, B. (1987b). Side effects of antidepressant drugs. In R.E. Hales & A. J. Frances (Eds.), *American Psychiatric Association annual review* (pp. 724–745) (Vol. 6). Washington, DC: American Psychiatric Press.

Bower, G. (1987) Mood and memory. *Behavior Research and Therapy, 25,* 443–455.

Boyd, J. H., & Weissman, M. M. (1981). Epidemiology of affective disorders: A reexamination and future directions. *Archives of General Psychiatry, 38,* 1039–1046.

Boyer, J. L., & Guthrie, L. (1985). Assessment and treatment of the suicidal patient. In E. E. Beckham & W. R. Leber (Eds.), *Handbook of depression: Treatment, assessment, research.* Homewood, IL: Dorsey Press.

Brickman, P., Rabinowitz, V. C., Karuza, J., Coates, D., Cohn, E., & Kidder, L. (1982). Models of helping and coping. *American Psychologist, 37,* 368–384.

Brown, G. L., Goodwin, F. K., & Bunney, W. E. (1982). Human aggression and suicide: Their relationship to neuropsychiatric diagnoses and serotonin metabolism. In B. T. Ho, J. C. Schoolar, & E. Usdin (Eds.), *Serotonin in biologic psychiatry: Advances in biochemical psychopharmacology* (Vol. 34). New York: Raven Press.

Brown, R. P., Frances, A., & Kocsis, J. H. (1982). Psychotic vs. nonpsychotic depression: Comparison of treatment response. *Journal of Nervous and Mental Disease, 170,* 635–637.

Bunney, W. E., & Davis, J. M. (1965). Norepinephrine in depressive reactions: A review. *Archives of General Psychiatry, 13,* 483–494.

Burns, D. (1980). *Feeling good: The new mood therapy.* New York: William Morrow.

Cade, J. F. J. (1949). The use of lithium salts in the treatment of psychotic excitement. *The Medical Journal of Australia, 2,* 349–356.

Carroll, B. J. (1982). The dexamethasone suppression test for melancholia. *British Journal of Psychiatry, 140,* 292–304.

Cerletti, U. (1956). Electroshock therapy. In F. Marti-Ibanex, A. M. Sackler, M. D. Sackler, & R. R. Sackler (Ed.). *The great physiodynamic therapies in psychiatry* (pp. 91–120). New York: Hoeber-Harper.

Chor, P. N., Mercier, M., & Halper, I. S. (1988). Use of cognitive therapy for treatment of a patient suffering from a bipolar affective disorder. *Journal of Cognitive Psychotherapy: An International Quarterly, 1,* 51–58.

Chouinard, G., Young, S. N., & Annable, L. (1983). Antimanic effect of clonazepam. *Biological Psychiatry, 18,* 451–466.

Clayton, P. J. (1983). Epidemiologic and risk factors in suicide. In L. Ginspoon (Ed.), *Psychiatry update* (Vol. 1, pp. 428–434). Washington, DC: American Psychiatric Association.

Clayton, P. J., & Lewis, C. E. (1981). The significance of secondary depression. *Journal of Affective Disorders, 3,* 25–35.

Cochran, S. (1984). Preventing medical noncompliance in the outpatient treatment of bipolar affective disorders. *Journal of Consulting and Clinical Psychology, 52,* 873–878.

Cole, J. O., & Schatzburg, A. F. (1983). Antidepressant drug therapy. In L. Grinspoon (Ed.), *Psychiatry update* (Vol. 2). Washington, DC: American Psychiatric Association.

Coppen, A., Metcalfe, M., & Wood, K. (1982). Lithium. In E. S. Paykel (Ed.), *Handbook of affective disorders.* New York: Guilford Press.

Coryell, W., Andreasen, N. C., Endicott, J., & Keller, M. (1987). The significance of past mania or hypomania in the course and outcome of major depression. *American Journal of Psychiatry, 144,* 307–315.

Costello, C. G. (1972). Depression: Loss of reinforcers or loss of reinforcer effectiveness? *Behavior Therapy, 3,* 240–247.

Cousins, N. (1977). Anatomy of an illness. *Saturday Review, May 28,* 48–51.

Coyne, J. C., & Gotlib, I. H. (1983). The role of cognition in depression. *Psychological Bulletin, 94,* 472–505.

Coyne, J. C., & Gotlib, I. H. (1986). Studying the role of cognition in depression: A critical appraisal. *Psychological Bulletin, 94,* 472–505.

Davanloo, H. (1980). *Short-term dynamic psychotherapy.* New York: Jason Aronson.

Davidson, J. (1983). MAO inhibitors: What have we learned? In F. J. Ayd, I. J. Taylor, & B. T. Taylor (Eds.), *Affective disorders reassessed: 1983.* Baltimore: Ayd Medical Communications.

Davidson, J. R. T., Miller, R. D., Turnbull, C. D., & Sullivan, J. L. (1982). Atypical depression. *Archives of General Psychiatry, 39,* 527–534.

deMontigney, C., Cournoyer, G., Morissette, R., Langlois, R., & Caille, G. (1983). Lithium carbonate addition in tricyclic antidepressant-resistant unipolar depression. *Archives of General Psychiatry, 40,* 1327–1334.

Depue, R. A., & Monroe, S. M. (1978). Learned helplessness in the perspective of the depressive disorders: Conceptual and definitional issues. *Journal of Abnormal Psychology, 87,* 3–20.

Dilsaver, S. C., & Greden, J. F. (1984). Antidepressant withdrawal phenomena. *Biological Psychiatry, 19,* 237–256.

Dreyfus, J. (1981). *A remarkable medicine has been overlooked.* New York: Dreyfus Medical Foundation.

Dunner, D. L., & Clayton, P. J. (1987). Drug treatment of bipolar disorder. In H. Y. Meltzer (Ed.), *Psychopharmacology: The third generation of progress* (pp. 1077–1083). New York: Raven Press.

Elkin, I., Shea, T., Watkins, J., Shaw, B. R., Docherty, J., Imber, S., Pilkonis, P., Leber, W., Collins, J., & Glass, D. (1986, June 19). *NIMH treatment of depression collaborative research program.* Presented at the 17th annual meeting of the Society for Psychotherapy Research, Wellesley, Massachusetts.

Ellis, A. (1962). *Reason and emotion in psychotherapy.* New York: Stuart.

Endicott, J., & Spitzer, R. L. (1978). A diagnostic interview: The schedule for affective disorders and schizophrenia. *Archives of General Psychiatry, 35,* 837–844.

Endicott, J., Nee, J., Andreasen, N., Clayton, P., Keller, M., & Coryell, W. (1985). Bipolar II: Combine or keep separate. *Journal of Affective Disorder, 8,* 17–28.

Eysenck, H. J. (1952). The effects of psychotherapy: An evaluation. *Journal of Consulting Psychology, 16,* 319–324.

Fawcett, J. (1972). Suicidal depression and physical illness. *The Journal of the American Medical Association, 219,* 1303–1306.

Feighner, J. P., Robins, E., Guze, S. B., Woodruff, R. A., Winokur, G., & Munoz, R. (1972). Diagnostic criteria for use in psychiatric research. *Archives of General Psychiatry, 26,* 57–63.

Feighner, J. P., Herbstein, J., & Damlouji, N. (1985). Combined MAOI, TCA, and direct stimulant therapy of treatment-resistant depression. *Journal of Clinical Psychiatry, 46,* 206–209.

Feinberg, M., & Carroll, B. J. (1982). Separation of subtypes of depression using discriminant analysis: Separation of bipolar endogneous depression from nonendogenous ("neurotic") depression. *Journal of Affective Disorders, 5,* 129–139.

Fennell, M., & Teasdale, J. D. (1982). Cognitive therapy with chronic, drug refractory depressed outpatients: A note of caution. *Cognitive Therapy and Research, 6,* 460–485.

Fernstrom, M. H., Krowinski, R. L., & Kupfer, D. J. (1987). Appetite and food preference in depression: Effects of imipramine treatment. *Biological Psychiatry, 22,* 529–539.

Ferster, C. B. (1966). Animal behavior and mental illness. *Psychological Record, 116,* 345–356.

Fink, M. (1979). *Convulsive therapy: Theory and practice.* New York: Raven Press.

Freud, S. (1959). Mourning and melancholia. In *Collected papers* (Vol. 4). New York: Basic Books (Original work published 1917).

Gillespie, R. D. (1929). The clinical differentiation of types of depression. *Guy's Hospital Report, 9,* 306–344.

Goldberg, S. C., Ettigi, P., Schulz, P. M., Hamer, R. M., Hayes, P. E., & Friedel, R. O. (1986). Alprazolam versus imipramine in depressed out-patients with neurovegetative signs. *Journal of Affective Disorders, 11,* 139–145.

Goodwin, F. K. (1979). The lithium ion. *Archives of General Psychiatry, 38,* 8.

Goodwin, F. K., & Jamison, K. R. (in press). *Manic depressive illness.* New York: Oxford University Press.

Goodwin, F. K., & Zis, A. P. (1979). Lithium in the treatment of mania: Comparisons with neuroleptics. *Archives of General Psychiatry, 36,* 840–844.

Grunhaus, L., & Birmaher, B. (1985). The clinical spectrum of panic attacks. *Journal of Clinical Psychopharmacology, 5,* 93–99.

Guze, S., & Robins, E. (1970). Suicide and primary affective disorder. *British Journal of Psychiatry, 117,* 437–438.

Gwirtsman, H. E., Roy-Byrne, P., Yager, J., & Gerner, R. H. (1983). Neuroendocrine abnormalities in bulimia. *American Journal of Psychiatry, 140,* 559–563.

Hamilton, M. (1960). A rating scale for depression. *Journal of Neurology, Neurosurgery and Psychiatry, 23,* 56–62.

Harpin, R. E., Liberman, R. P., Marks, I., Stern, R., & Bohannon, W. E. (1982). Cognitive therapy for chronically depressed patients: A controlled pilot study. *Journal of Nervous and Mental Disease, 170,* 295–300.

Himmelhoch, J. M., & Thase, M. E. (in press). The vagaries of atypical depression. In J. E. Howells (Ed.), *Modern perspectives in the psychiatry of depression.* New York: Brunner/Mazel.

Hirsch, S. R., Walsh, C., & Draper, R. (1982). Parasuicide: A review of treatment intervention. *Journal of Affective Disorders, 4,* 299–311.

Hollon, S., DeRubeis, R. J., Evans, M. D., Tuason, V. B., Wiemer, M. J., Garvey, M. J., & Grove (1986). *Cognitive therapy, pharmacotherapy, and combined cognitive-pharmacotherapy in the treatment of depression: Differential outcome.* Unpublished manuscript, University of Minnesota and the St. Paul–Ramsey Medical Center, Minneapolis–St. Paul, Minnesota.

Hudson, J. I., Laffer, P. S., & Pope, H. G. (1982). Bulimia related to affective disorder by family history and response to the dexamethasone suppression test. *American Journal of Psychiatry, 137,* 695–698.

Hudson, J. I., Pope, H. G., & Jonas, J. M. (1983). Phenomenologic relationship of eating disorders to major affective disorder. *Psychiatry Research, 9,* 345–354.

Hughes, P. L., Wells, L. A., Cunningham, C. J., & Ilstrip, D. M. (1986). Treating bulimia with desipramine: A double-blind placebo-controlled study. *Archives of General Psychiatry, 43,* 182–186.

Isherwood, J., Adam, K. S., & Hornblow, A. R. (1982). Live event stress, psychosocial factors, suicide attempt, and auto accident proclivity. *Journal of Psychosomatic Research, 26,* 371–384.

Jackson, S. W. (1986). *Melancholia and depression.* New Haven, CN: Yale University Press.

Jamison, K. R. (1987). Psychotherapeutic issues and suicide prevention in the treatment of bipolar disorders. In R. E. Itales and A. J. Frances (Eds.), Review of psychiatry (Vol. 6, pp. 108–124). Washington, DC: American Psychiatric Press.

Jamison, K. R., Gerner, R. H., & Goodwin, F. K. (1979). Patient and physician attitudes toward lithium: Relationship to compliance. *Archives of General Psychiatry, 36,* 866–869.

Janicak, P. G., & Boshes, R. A. (1987). Advances in the treatment of mania and other acute psychotic disorders. *Psychiatric Annals, 17,* 145–149.

Jarrett, R. B., & Rush, A. J. (1986). Psychotherapeutic approaches for depression. In J. O. Cavenar (Ed.), *Psychiatry* (pp. 1–35). Philadelphia: Lippincott and Basic Books.

Jarrett, R. B., Rush, A. J., & Roffwarg, H. P. (1987). *Biological measures and cognitive therapy for depression.* Paper presented at the 21st Annual AABT Convention, Boston.

Jefferson, J. W., & Greist, J. H. (1987). Lithium carbonate and carbamazepine side effects. In R. E. Hales & A. J. Frances (Eds.), *American Psychiatric Association Annual Review* (Vol. 6) (pp. 746–780). Washington, DC: American Psychiatric Press.

Kathol, R. G. (1985). Depression associated with physical disease. In E. E. Beckham & W. R. Leber (Eds.), *Handbook of depression: Treatment, assessment, research.* Homewood, IL: Dorsey Press.

Katz, J. L., Kuperberg, A., Pollack, C. P., Walsh, B. T., Zumoff, B., & Weiner, H. (1984). Is there a relationship between eating disorder and affective disorder? New evidence from sleep recordings. *American Journal of Psychiatry, 141,* 753–759.

Keller, M. B. (1988). Diagnostic issues and clinical course of unipolar illness. In A. J. Frances & R. E. Hales (Eds.), *Review of psychiatry* (Vol. 7) (pp. 188–212). Washington, DC: American Psychiatric Press.

Keller, M. B., & Shapiro, R. W. (1982). "Double depression": Superimposition of acute depressive episodes on chronic depressive disorders. *American Journal of Psychiatry, 139,* 438–442.

Keller, M. B., Lavori, P. W., Endicott, J., Coryell, W., & Kleman, G. L. (1983). "Double depression": Two year follow-up. *American Journal of Psychiatry, 140,* 689–694.

Kendell, R. E. (1976). The classification of depressions: A review of contemporary confusion. *British Journal of Psychiatry, 127,* 305–315.

Kiecolt-Glaser, J. K., Stephens, R. E., Lipetz, P. D., Speicher, C. E., & Glaser, R. (1985). Distress and DNA repair in human lymphocytes. *Journal of Behavioral Medicine, 48,* 311–320.

Klein, D. F., Gittelman, R., Quitkin, F., & Rifkin, A. (1980). *Diagnosis and drug treatment of psychiatric disorders: Adults and children (2nd ed.).* Baltimore: Williams & Wilkins.

Klerman, G. L., DiMascio, A. Weissman, M. M., Prusoff, B. A., & Paykel, E. S. (1974). Treatment for depression by drugs and psychotherapy. *American Journal of Psychiatry, 131,* 186–191.

Klerman, G. L., Weissman, M. M., Rounsaville, B. J., & Chevron, E. (1984). *Interpersonal psychotherapy of depression.* New York: Basic Books.

Kocsis, J. H., & Frances, A. J. (1987). A critical discussion of DSM-III dysthymic disorder. *American Journal of Psychiatry, 144,* 1534–1542.

Kovacs, M., Beck, A. T., & Weissman, A. (1975). Hopelessness: An indicator of suicide risk. *Suicide, 5,* 98–103.

Kovacs, M., Rush, A. J., Beck, A. T., & Hollon, S. D. (1981). Depressed outpatients treated with cognitive therapy or pharmacotherapy: A one year follow-up. *Archives of General Psychiatry, 38,* 33–39.

Kraeplin, E. (1921). *Manic depressive insanity and paranoia.* Edinburgh: E. S. Livingstone.

Kramer, B. A. (1985). Use of ECT in California, 1977–1983. *American Journal of Psychiatry, 142,* 1190–1192.

Kupfer, D. J., Foster, F. G., Detre, T. P., & Himmelhoch, J. M. (1975a). Sleep EEG and motor activity as indicators in affective states. *Neuropsychobiology, 1,* 296–303.

Kupfer, D. J., Pickar, D., Himmelhoch, J. M., & Detre, T. P. (1975b). Are there two types of unipolar depression? *Archives of General Psychiatry, 32,* 866–871.

Leckman, J. F., Weissman, M. M., Merikangas, K. R., Pauls, D. L., & Prusoff, B. A. (1983). Panic disorder and major depression: Increased risk of depression, alcoholism, panic and phobic disorders in families of depressed probands with panic disorder. *Archives of General Psychiatry, 40,* 1055–1060.

Leckman, J. K., Weissman, M. M., Prusoff, B. A., Caruso, K. A., Merikangas, K. R., Pauls, D. L., & Kidd, K. K. (1984). Subtypes of depression: Family study perspective. *Archives of General Psychiatry, 41,* 833–838.

Lerer, B., Moore, N., Meyendorff, E., Cho, S. R., & Gershon, S. (1987). Carbamazepine versus lithium in mania: A double-blind study. *Journal of Clinical Psychiatry, 48,* 89–93.

Lewinsohn, P. M. (1975). The behavioral study and treatment of depression. In M. Hersen, R. M. Eisler, & P. M. Miller (Eds.). *Progress in behavior modification* (Vol. 1, pp. 19–64). New York: Academic Press.

Lewis, A. L. (1934). Melancholia: A historical review. *The Journal of Mental Science, 328,* 1–42.

Liebowitz, W. M., Quitkin, F. M., Stewart, J. W., McGrath, P. J., Harrison, W., Rabkin, J., Tricamo, E., Markowitz, J. S., & Klein, D. F. (1984). Phelzine *v* imipramine in atypical depression. *Archives of General Psychiatry, 41,* 669–677.

Linehan, M. M., Goodstein, J. L., Nielson, S. L., & Chiles, J. A. (1983). Reasons for staying alive when you are thinking of killing yourself: The reasons for living inventory. *Journal of Consulting and Clinical Psychology, 51,* 276–286.

Little, K. Y. (1988). Amphetamine, but not methylphenidate, predicts antidepressant efficacy. *Journal of Clinical Psychopharmacology, 8,* 177–183.

Malan, D. H. (1963). *A study of brief psychotherapy.* London: Tavistock.

Markowitz, J., Brown, R., Sweeney, J., & Mann, J. J. (1987). Reduced length and cost of hospital stay for major depression in patients treated with ECT. *American Journal of Psychiatry, 144,* 1025–1029.

McNeal, E. T., & Cimbolic, P. (1986). Antidepressants and biochemical theories of depression. *Psychological Bulletin, 99,* 361–374.

Monroe, S. M., Thase, M. E., Hersen, M., Bellack, A. S., & Himmelhoch, J. M. (1985). Life events and the endogenous-nonendogenous distinction in the treatment and post-treatment course of depression. *Comprehensive Psychiatry, 26,* 175–186.

Morris, J. B., & Beck, A. T. (1974). The efficacy of antidepressant drugs. *Archives of General Psychiatry, 30,* 667–674.

Murphy, G. E., & Wetzel, R. D. (1980). Suicide by birth cohort in the United States. *Archives of General Psychiatry, 37,* 519–523.

Murphy, G. E., & Wetzel, R. D. (1982). Family history of suicidal behavior among suicide attempters. *Journal of Nervous Disease, 170,* 86–90.

Murphy, G. E., Simons, A. D., Wetzel, R. D., & Lustman, P. J. (1984). Cognitive therapy and pharmacotherapy: Singly and together in the treatment of depression. *Archives of General Psychiatry, 41,* 33–41.

National Institutes of Health. (1985). Electroconvulsive therapy: Consensus development. *Conference statement, 5,* 11.

Nelson, J. C., & Charney, D. S. (1981). The symptoms of major depressive illness. *American Journal of Psychiatry, 138,* 1–13.

Nies, A., & Robinson, D. S. (1982). Monamine oxidase inhibitors. In E. S. Paykel (Ed.), *Handbook of affective disorders.* New York: Guilford Press.

Nolen-Hoeksema, S. (1987). Sex differences in unipolar depression: Evidence and theory. *Psychological Bulletin,* 259–282.

Noll, K. M., Davis, J. M., & DeLeon-Jones, F. (1985). Medication and somatic therapies in the treatment of depression. In E. E. Beckham & W. R. Leber (Eds.), *Handbook of depression: Treatment, assessment, research.* Homewood, IL: Dorsey Press.

O'Leary, A. (1985). Self efficacy and health. *Behavior Research and Therapy, 23,* 437–451.

Perel, J. C. (1983). Tricyclic antidepressant plasma levels, pharmacokinetics, and clinical outcome. In L. Grinspoon (Ed.), *Psychiatry update* (Vol. 2). Washington, DC: American Psychiatric Association.

Perris, C. (1966). A study of bipolar (manic-depressive and unipolar recurrent depressive psychoses. *Acta Psychiatrica Scandinavica, 42*(Supplement 194), 1–188.

Pettinati, H. M., & Bonner, K. M. (1984). Cognitive functioning in depressed geriatric patients with a history of ECT. *American Journal of Psychiatry, 141,* 49–52.

Pilkonis, P. A., & Frank, E. (1988). Personality pathology in recurrent depression: Nature, prevalence, and relationship to treatment response. *American Journal of Psychiatry, 145,* 435–441.

Pokorny, A. D. (1983). Prediction of suicide in psychiatric patients. *Archives of General Psychiatry, 40,* 249–257.

Pope, H. G., Hudson, J. I., Jonas, J. M., & Yurgelun-Todd, D. (1983). Family history study of anorexia nervosa and bulimia. *British Journal of Psychiatry, 142,* 133–138.

Post, R. M. (1987). Mechanisms of action of carbamazepine and related anticonvulsants in affective illness. In H. Y. Meltzer (Ed.), *Psychopharmacology: The third generation of progress* (pp. 467–576). New York: Raven Press.

Potter, W. Z. (1983). Rapid cycling bipolar disorder. In F. J. Ayd, I. J. Taylor, & B. T. Taylor (Eds.), *Affective disorders reassessed: 1983* (pp. 138–150). Baltimore: Ayd Medical Communications.

Prien, R. (1988). Somatic treatment of unipolar depressive disorder. In A. J. Frances & R. E. Hales (Eds.), *Review of psychiatry* (Vol. 7) (pp. 213–234). Washington, DC: American Psychiatric Press.

Prien, R. F., & Kupfer, D. J. (1986). Continuation drug therapy for major depressive episodes: How long should it be maintained? *American Journal of Psychiatry, 143,* 18–23.

Prien, R., Kupfer, D., Mansky, P., Small, J., Turson, V., Voss, C., & Johnson, W. (1984). Drug therapy in the prevention of recurrences in unipolar and bipolar affective disorder. *Archives of General Psychiatry, 41,* 1096–1104.

Pyle, R. L., Mitchell, J. E., & Eckert, E. D. (1981). Bulimia: A report of 34 cases. *Journal of Clinical Psychiatry, 42,* 60–64.

Quitkin, F. M., Rifkin, A., & Klein, D. F. (1979). Monamine oxidase inhibitors: A review of antidepressant effectiveness. *Archives of General Psychiatry, 36,* 749–760.

Regier, D. A., Myers, J. K., Kramer, M., Robins, L. N., Blazer, D. G., Hough, R. L., Eaton, W. W., & Locke, B. Z. (1984). The NIMH epidemiologic catchment area program. *Archives of General Psychiatry, 41,* 934–941.

Rickels, K., Chung, H. R., Csanalosi, I. B., Hurowitz, A. M., London, J., Wiseman, K., Kaplan, M., & Amsterdam, J. D. (1987). Alprazolam, diazepam, imipramine, and placebo in outpatients with major depression. *Archives of General Psychiatry, 44,* 862–866.

Robins, L. N., Helzer, J. E., Weissman, M. M., Orvaschel, H., Burke, J. D., & Regier, D. A. (1984). Lifetime prevalence of specific psychiatric disorders in three sites. *Archives of General Psychiatry, 41,* 949–958.

Rosenthal, N. E., Sack, D. A., Skewerer, R. G., Jacobsen, F. M., & Wehr, T. A. (1988). Phototherapy for seasonal affective disorder. *Journal of Biological Rhythms, 3,* 101–120.

Rosenthal, T. L., Akiskal, H. S., Scott-Strauss, A., Rosenthal, R. H., & David, M. (1981). Familial and developmental factors in characterological depression. *Journal of Affective Disorders, 3,* 183–192.

Rounsaville, B. J., Sholomskas, D., & Prusoff, B. A. (1980). Chronic mood disorders in depressed outpatients. *Journal of Affective Disorders, 2,* 73–88.

Rounsaville, B., Klerman, G. L., &Weissman, M. M. (1981). Do psychotherapy and pharmacotherapy for depression conflict? *Archives of General Psychiatry, 38,* 24–28.

Rush, A. J. (1986). Diagnosis of affective disorders. In A. J. Rush & K. Z. Altshuler (Eds.), *Depression: Basic mechanism, diagnosis, and treatment.* New York: Guilford Press.

Rush, A. J., Beck, A. T., Kovacs, M., & Hollon, S. D. (1977). Comparative efficacy of cognitive therapy and pharmacotherapy in the treatment of depressed outpatients. *Cognitive Therapy and Research, 1,* 17–37.

Rush, A. J., Erman, M. K., Schlesser, M. A., Roffwarg, H. P., Vasavada, N., Khatami, M., Fairchild, C., & Giles, D. E. (1985). Alprazolam versus amitriptyline in depressions with reduced REM latency. *Archives of General Psychiatry, 42,* 1154–1159.

Scheier, M. F., & Carver, C. S. (1987). Dispositional optimism and physical well-being: The influence of generalized outcome expectancies on health. *Journal of Personality, 55,* 169–210.

Schildkraut, J. J. (1965). The catecholamine hypothesis of affective disorders: A review of supporting evidence. *American Journal of Psychiatry, 139,* 471–475.

Schoonover, S. (1984). Bipolar affective disorder and recurrent unipolar depression. In E. Bassuk, S. Schoonover, & A. Gelenberg (Eds.), *The practitioner's guide to psychoactive drugs* (2nd ed.). New York: Plenum Press.

Schuckit, M. A. (1983a). Alcoholism and other psychiatric disorders. *Hospital and Community Psychiatry, 34,* 1022–1027.

Schuckit, M. A. (1983b). Alcoholic patients with secondary depression. *American Journal of Psychiatry, 140,* 711–714.

Scovern, A. W., & Kilmann, P. R. (1980). Status of electroconvulsive therapy: Review of the outcome literature. *Psychological Bulletin, 87,* 260–303.

Segal, Z. V. (1988). Appraisal of the self-schema construct in cognitive models of depression. *Psychological Bulletin, 103*(2), 147–162.

Segal, Z. V., & Shaw, B. F. (1986a). Cognition in depression: A reappraisal of Coyne and Gotlib's critique. *Cognitive Therapy and Research, 10,* 671–684.

Segal, Z. V., & Shaw, B. F. (1986b). When cul-de-sacs are more mentality than reality: A rejoinder to Coyne and Gotlib. *Cognitive Therapy and Research, 10,* 707–714.

Shea, T., Glass, D., & Pilkonis, P. A. (1987). Frequency and implications of personality disorders in a sample of depressed outpatients. *Journal of Personality Disorders, 1,* 27–42.

Shou, M. (1968). Lithium in psychiatric therapy and prophylaxis. *Journal of Psychiatric Research, 6,* 67–95.

Sifneos, P. (1972). *Short-term psychotherapy and emotional crisis.* Cambridge: Harvard University Press.

Simons, A. D., Lustman, P. J., Murphy, G. E., & Wetzel, R. E. (1985). Predicting response to cognitive therapy of depression: The role of learned resourcefulness. *Cognitive Therapy and Research, 9,* 79–89.

Simons, A. D., Murphy, G. E., Levine, J. L., & Wetzel, R. D. (1986). Cognitive therapy and pharmacotherapy of depression: Sustained improvement over one year. *Archives of General Psychiatry, 43,* 43–50.

Simpson, G. M., & Pi, E. H. (1987). Issues in pharmacological treatment. In R. L. Morrison & A. S. Bellack (Eds.), *Medical factors and psychological disorders.* New York: Plenum Press.

Singer, J. A., & Salovey, P. (1988). Mood and memory: Evaluating the network theory of affect. *Clinical Psychology Review, 8,* 211–251.

Skinner, B. F. (1953). *Science and human behavior.* New York: Free Press.

Sklar, L. S., & Anisman, H. (1979). Stress and coping factors influence tumor growth. *Science, 205,* 513–515.

Spiker, D. G., Weiss, J. C., Dealy, R. S., Griffin, S. J., Hanin, I., Neil, J. F., Perel, J. M., Rossi, A. J., & Soloff, P. H. (1985). The pharmacological treatment of delusional depression. *American Journal of Psychiatry, 142,* 430–436.

Spitzer, R., Endicott, J., & Robins, E. (1978). Research diagnostic criteria. *Archives of General Psychiatry, 34,* 773–782.

Stewart, J. W., Quitkin, F. M., Liebowitz, M. R., McGrath, P. J., Harrison, W. M., & Klein, D. F. (1983). Efficacy of desipramine in depressed outpatients. *Archives of General Psychiatry, 40,* 202–207.

Strober, M., Salkin, B., Burroughs, J., & Morrell, W. (1982). Validity of the bulimia-restrictor distinction in anorexia nervosa. *Journal of Nervous and Mental Disease, 170,* 345–351.

Sulser, F. (1983). Mode of action of antidepressant drugs. *Journal of Clinical Psychiatry, 44,* 14–20.

Taylor, M. A., & Abrams, R. (1975). Acute mania—Clinical and genetic study of responders and nonresponders to treatments. *Archives of General Psychiatry, 32,* 863–865.

Teasdale, J. D. (1983). Negative thinking in depression: Cause, effect, or reciprocal relationship? *Advances in Behavior Research and Therapy, 5,* 3–25.

Teasdale, J. D., Fennell, M. J. V., Hibber, G. A., & Amies, P. L. (1984). Cognitive therapy for major depressive disorder in primary care. *British Journal of Psychiatry, 144,* 400–406.

Terman, M. (1988). On the question of mechanism in phototherapy for seasonal affective disorder: Considerations of clinical efficacy and epidemiology. *Journal of Biological Rhythms, 3,* 155–172.

Thase, M. E. (1987). Affective disorders. In R. L. Morrison & A. S. Bellack (Eds.), *Medical factors and psychological disorders.* New York: Plenum Press.

Thase, M. (1989). Comparison between patients with seasonal affective disorder and other recurrent forms of depression. In N. E. Rosenthal & M. Blehar (Eds.), *Seasonal affective disorders and phototherapy* (pp. 64–78). New York: Guilford Press.

Thase, M. E., & Kupfer, D. J. (1987). Characteristics of treatment resistant depressions. In J. Zohar & R. H. Belmaker (Eds.), *Treating resistant depression* (pp. 23–45). New York: PMA Publishing.

Thase, M. E., & Kupfer, D. J. (1988). MAOI treatment of imipramine-resistant depression. *American Psychiatric Association 1988 New Research Program and Abstracts,* p. 68.

Thase, M. E., & Simons, A. D. (1989). Psychobiology of recovery in depression. *World Congress of Cognitive Therapy Final Programme,* pp. 76–77.

Thase, M. E., Frank, E., & Kupfer, D. J. (1985). Biological processes in major depression. In E. E. Beckham & W. R. Leber (Eds.), *Handbook of depression: Treatment, assessment, research.* Homewood, IL: Dorsey Press.

Thase, M. E., Himmelhoch, J. M., & Mallinger, A. G. (1988). *Tranylcypromine vs. imipramine in anergic bipolar depression.* Society of Biological Psychiatry Forty-Third Annual Convention and Scientific Program, p. 300.

Thase, M. E., Himmelhoch, J. M., Mallinger, A. G., Safer, F., & McKnight, D. (1988, October 7). *Tranylcypromine in imipramine-resistant bipolar depression.* Paper presented at the First International Conference on Refractory Depression, Philadelphia.

van Praag, H. M. (1982). A transatlantic view of the diagnosis of depressions according to the DSM-III: Did the DSM-III solve the problem of depression diagnosis? *Comprehensive Psychiatry, 23,* 330–338.

Visintaine, M. A., Volpicelli, J. R., & Selyman, M. E. P. (1982). Tumor rejection in rats after inescapable and escapable shock. *Science, 216,* 437–439.

Walsh, B. T., Stewart, J. W., Roose, S. P., Gladis, M., & Glassman, A. H. (1984). Treatment of bulimia with phenelzine. *Archives of General Psychiatry, 41,* 1105–1109.

Walsh, B. T., Lo, E. S., Cooper, T., Lindy, D. C., Roose, S. P., Gladis, M., & Glassman, A. H. (1987). Dexamethasone suppression test and plasma dexamethasone levels in bulimia. *Archives of General Psychiatry, 44,* 797–803.

Wehr, T. A., & Goodwin, F. K. (1987). Can antidepressants cause mania and worsen the course of affective illness. *American Journal of Psychiatry, 144,* 1403–1411.

Wehr, T. A., Sack, D. A., Rosenthal, N. E., & Goodwin, F. K. (1987). Sleep and biological rhythms in bipolar illness. In R. E. Hales and S. J. Frances (Eds.), *Review of psychiatry* (Vol. 6, pp. 61–80). Washington, DC: American Psychiatric Press.

Weissman, M. M., & Akiskal, H. S. (1984). The role of psychotherapy in chronic depressions: A proposal. *Comprehensive Psychiatry, 25,* 23–31.

Weissman, M. M., & Klerman, G. L. (1977). The chronic depressive in the community: Underrecognized and poorly treated. *Comprehensive Psychiatry, 18,* 523–531.

Weissman, M. M., Prusoff, B. A., & DiMascio, A. (1979). The efficacy of drugs and psychotherapy in the treatment of acute depressive episodes. *American Journal of Psychiatry, 136,* 555–558.

Whybrow, P., Akiskal, H., & McKinney, W. (1984). *Mood disorders: Toward a new psychobiology.* New York: Plenum Press.

Worrall, E. P., Moody, J. P., Peet, M., Dick, P., Smith, A., Chambers, C., Adams, M., & Naylor, G. J. (1979). Controlled studies of the acute antidepressant effects of lithium. *British Journal of Psychiatry, 135,* 255–262.

Zohar, J., & Belmaker, R. H. (Eds.). (1987). *Treating resistant depression.* New York: PMA Publishing.

7

Chronic Depressive Disorders

MARTIN B. KELLER, FRANCES M. SESSA, AND LAUREN P. JONES

INTRODUCTION

Chronic depression represents a relatively new focus for psychiatry, and there have been few systematic studies on the subject. The term *dysthymic disorder* was introduced into the psychiatric nomenclature in the third edition of the American Psychiatric Association's *Diagnostic and Statistical Manual of Mental Disorders* (DSM-III; APA, 1980) to categorize chronic depressions that are of a long duration but less severe than major depressive episodes. It was used to replace the concept of *neurotic depression* in the second edition of the manual (DSM-II; APA, 1968). This revision arose as a result of studies (Akiskal, Bitar, Puzantian, Rosenthal, & Walker, 1978; Kendell, 1976; Kiloh, Andrews, Nielson, & Bianchi, 1972; Klein, 1974; Klerman, Endicott, Spitzer, & Hirschfeld, 1979; Paykel, 1971) showing substantial heterogeneity in neurotic depressions and as the result of a decision to create a diagnostic category based purely on phenomenology (Spitzer, Williams, & Skodol, 1980). An important aspect of this change is that, in the DSM-III, dysthymic disorder is included in Axis I as an affective disorder, and there is no category for chronic depression in the personality disorder section of the DSM-III. This basic structure has been maintained in the revised DSM-III (DSM-III-R; APA, 1986), although there have been several important modifications from the DSM-III criteria.

Throughout most of this chapter, the term *dysthymic disorder* is used as an inclusive label for chronic low-grade depression, so that we maintain consistency with the official American Psychiatric Association's nomenclature. However, a major thrust of the chapter

MARTIN B. KELLER and FRANCES M. SESSA • Massachusetts General Hospital, Boston, Massachusetts 02114. LAUREN P. JONES • University of California at Berkeley, Berkeley, California 94720.

is to examine the history of, the empirical data on, and the utility of conceptualizations and classifications of chronic depression, including a discussion of the utility of the term *dysthymic disorder* and its boundaries with other diagnostic groupings.

In the DSM-III-R (APA, 1986), dysthymic disorder is defined as the presence of a persistent depressed mood that lasts most of the day or is present more often than it is absent over a 2-year period. In addition to the depressed mood, the patient must report at least two of the following symptoms: poor appetite or overeating, insomnia or hypersomnia, low energy or fatigue, low self-esteem, poor concentration or difficulty making decisions, and pessimism. During the 2-year period, the patient must never have been without these symptoms for more than 2 months at a time. The exclusion criteria for dysthymia include the presence of a major depressive episode during the first 2 years of the disturbance, a manic or hypomanic episode at any time in the patient's life, psychotic symptoms or the residual phase of schizophrenia, and/or the mood's being sustained by a specific organic factor or substance.

The DSM-III-R (APA, 1986) also requires the specification of primary or secondary type and early or late onset. The primary type indicates that the dysthymia did not occur exclusively during the course of another chronic, nonmood Axis I or Axis III disorder; the secondary specification implies the converse. Early onset describes an onset before age 21, and late onset describes an onset age of 21 years or older. The age-of-onset specification is proposed in the DSM-III-R because of evidence suggesting that early onset characterizes a more homogeneous group.

The nosological precursors of dysthymic disorder include depressive temperament (Kraepelin, 1921; Kretschmer, 1936; Schneider, 1958), neurotic depression (DSM-II, 1968), depressive personality (Chodoff, 1972; Kahn, 1975), chronic minor depression (Spitzer, Endicott, Woodruff, 1977), hysteroid dysphoria (Liebowitz & Klein, 1979), characterological depression (Akiskal, Rosenthal, Haykal, Lemmi, Rosenthal, & Scott-Strauss, 1980; Yerevanian & Akiskal, 1979), and the research-diagnostic-criteria (RDC) categories of chronic and intermittent depressive disorders and minor depressive disorder of at least 2 years' duration (Spitzer, Endicott, Robins, 1985). Although not synonymous, most of these terms collectively emphasize the temperamental traits of dysphoria, a repetitive neurotic tendency toward gloomy despair, and a nebulous distinction between depression (state) and personality (trait) in the chronic course of these low-grade depressions (Akiskal, 1983; Yerevanian & Akiskal, 1979).

This chapter begins with an overview of some historical and theoretical perspectives on dysthymia, provides a description of the terminologies and classifications of chronic depression other than the definition put forward in the DSM-III-R, and then discusses the controversy about the relationship between personality disorders, dysthymia, and the major affective syndromes. Dysthymic disorder is then compared with the other chronic mood disorders (cyclothymia and labile personality). There is a section on course and outcome and a section on what is known about the psychosocial and somatic treatment of dysthymia.

It will be evident as this chapter progresses that there is a paucity of empirical data on dysthymic disorder and an abundance of diverse opinions on (1) its definition; (2) its differentiation from acute or chronic major depressive episodes; and (3) the nature of its relationship to personality. Moreover, the small number of research studies on chronic depression leaves us with an incomplete foundation of knowledge on its epidemiology, on familial aggregation, on its biology, and on its course and treatment. Nonetheless, enough studies of chronic depression have been conducted since the late 1970s to allow us to present some substantive data in each of these areas.

HISTORICAL AND THEORETICAL PERSPECTIVE

In his description of the four "fundamental" states of manic-depressive illness (the depressive, manic, irritable, and cyclothymic temperaments), Kraepelin (1921) proposed different forms of the illness. Furthermore, observing that the relatives of manic-depressives were sometimes found to have a depressive temperament without progressing to affective episodes, he hypothesized the depressive temperament as an attenuated form of a genetically determined disorder (Akiskal *et al.,* 1980).

Schneider (1958) described the "dysthymic psychopath." Rather than focusing on depressive illness, he emphasized how such individuals brought suffering to themselves or others. Schneider's "psychopaths" were not antisocial but represented a more statistically deviant personality:

> Dysthymic psychopaths were said to display the following traits: (1) quiet, passive, and nonassertive; (2) gloomy, pessimistic, and incapable of fun; (3) self-critical, self-reproaching, and self-derogatory; (4) skeptical, hypercritical, and complaining; (5) conscientious and self-disciplining; (6) brooding and given to worry; and (7) preoccupied with inadequacy, failure, and negative events to the point of morbid enjoyment of one's failures. (Akiskal *et al.*, 1980, p. 778)

Since Freud's (1946) and Abraham's (1948) references to neurotic depressives, the psychoanalytic tradition has focused little attention on neurotic depression. Although most advocates of the psychoanalytic tradition have accepted the distinction between neurotic and psychotic varieties of depression, they have tended to deemphasize the neurotic manifestations, describing them as epiphenomenal to severe character pathology of developmental origin (Akiskal, 1983; Chodoff, 1972). In contrast, proponents of the biological tradition have supported the position that the personality attributes in these low-grade depressions are the expression of an underlying affective disorder.

The DSM and the "Journey" from Neurotic Depression to Dysthymic Disorder

The most commonly diagnosed affective disorder in the DSM-III (APA, 1968) was neurotic depression (Klerman *et al.,* 1979). The use of this term was broad, and the term had multiple meanings; and it often referred to the repetitive tendency of individuals to descend into states of gloomy despair (Akiskal *et al.,* 1978). Neurotic depression was hypothesized by psychoanalytic teaching to be the result of an "excessive reaction of depression due to an internal conflict or to an identifiable event such as the loss of a love object or cherished possession" (APA, 1968, p. 40).

Growing dissatisfaction with the use of the term *neurotic depression* led to the introduction of a number of alternative diagnostic categories into the literature, and finally, the DSM-II category of neurotic depression was replaced by the DSM-III classification of dysthymia. The main reason was the belief that it was primarily the chronic "characterological" tendency toward dysphoria that was the most meaningful dimension in neurotic depressions that were otherwise nosologically heterogeneous (Akiskal *et al.,* 1978). Furthermore, the goal of having a more atheoretical and phenomenologically based definition led to classifying dysthymia under the affective disorders and also recognizing that the affective components may be secondary to an underlying personality disorder (Akiskal, 1983).

The substitution of dysthymia, a concept with strong affective connotations, for a psychological condition that was in the domain of neurotic pathology was met with much disapproval (Cooper & Michels, 1981; Frances, 1980). Similarly, criticism has been raised about the specific definition of dysthymia. It is likely that these disagreements will continue until there are more empirical data on pathogenesis, course, and the other variables associated with chronic depressive disorders. The theme of uncertainty, disagreement, and controversy about how to understand and classify the chronic depressive disorders is strongly evident throughout this chapter.

EPIDEMIOLOGY

Incidence of Dysthymia in the General Population

There are few epidemiological studies of the incidence of dysthymia in the general population (Klerman, Keller, Fawcett, Andreasen, Hirschfeld, & Endicott, 1987). However, a number of studies have indicated that it is a relatively common condition (Klerman, 1980) that may be more prevalent than formerly thought (Weissman & Klerman, 1977).

Hornstra and Klassen (1977) reported a 1-year prevalence of 47 to 105 cases per 1,000 from a community survey in Kansas City, Missouri; Barrett, Hurst, DiSalla, and Rose (1978) reported a 1-year prevalence of 60 cases per 1,000; and Weissman and Myers (1978) found a 4.7% lifetime prevalence rate of dysthymia in a New Haven, Connecticut, sample.

Weissman and Myers (1978) also found a current point-prevalence rate of 2.5% for current rates of probable and definite chronic minor depression among a same sample of 511 subjects. Robert and Vernon (1982) observed a lower current point-prevalence rate of 1.3% for minor depression in an Alameda County, California and a New Haven sample. Their finding of an annual prevalence rate of probable and definite minor depression was 4.5%.

More recently, the Epidemiologic Catchment Area (ECA) program randomly surveyed residents of three U.S. cities to assess the lifetime prevalence of psychiatric disorders and found that 3.3% of its subjects had suffered from dysthymic disorder on at least one occasion (Robins, Helzer, Weissman, Orvaschel, Gruenberg, Burke, & Regier, 1984).

Klerman and colleagues (1987) asserted that dysthymia is more prevalent in females, and that it most commonly has its onset in childhood or adolescence, or in older adulthood. In women between the ages of 45 and 65 who were surveyed for the ECA program, dysthymia was the second most common disorder, preceded only by phobic disorder (Myers, Weissman, Tischler, Holzer, Leaf, Orvaschel, Anthony, Boyd, Burke, Kramer, & Stoltzman, 1984).

Frequency of Affective Disorders among Relatives of Dysthymic Patients

Of much interest is the frequency of affective disorders among relatives of patients with dysthymia. However, little is known about the familial aggregation and the genetic transmission of dysthymia (Klerman *et al.,* 1987). In view of the heterogeneity of onset, symptom profile, and course, substantially more work is needed to define homogeneous groups of patients with dysthymia before it will be possible to establish familial patterns and to detect possible genetic factors (Winokur, Behar, Vanvalkenburg, & Lowry, 1978).

According to Weissman, Gershon, Kidd, Prusoff, Leckman, Dibble, Hamovit, Thompson, Pauls, and Guroff (1984), minor depression (not necessarily of 2 years' duration) and depressive personality aggregate in the relatives of the probands with major depression. Rates of depressive personality were slightly higher in relatives of probands with major depression (from 5.2% to 6.9%) than in relatives of probands with a bipolar I disorder (4.5%) or in relatives of never-ill normal control probands (2.1%). Minor depression was higher in the relatives of probands with major depression (from 8.6% to 13.7%) than in relatives of probands with bipolar I disorder (5.3%) or in relatives of never-ill normal control probands (6.0%).

In summary, although several studies have tried to compare the rates of the familial associations of the different depressive disorders among patients with dysthymic disorder, in comparison to patients with bipolar I or bipolar II disorder data are not yet sufficient to support specific associations of dysthymia in relatives of dysthymic patients. Although larger studies are warranted, it must be understood from the outset that the ambiguous and somewhat arbitrary distinction between major depression and dysthymia and the broad heterogeneity of the clinical characteristics of subjects diagnosed as having dysthymia make it very difficult at present to draw definitive conclusions from studies of familial aggregation and genetics.

CONTROVERSY IN THE CLASSIFICATION OF DYSTHYMIC DISORDER

As should already be evident from the preceding sections, a prevailing question is whether dysthymic disorder represents an underlying character (or personality) disorder with depressive features or is best thought of as a subsyndromal form of a major depressive disorder. It is also possible that dysthymia is a combination of a personality disturbance and a subsyndromal affective disorder.

Subsyndromal Depressions

Subaffective dysthymia refers to an intermittent, subsyndromal depression that is a symptomatically milder yet lifelong version of primary affective disorder (Akiskal, King, Rosenthal, Robinson, & Scott-Strauss, 1981). The depressive personality characteristics observed in these patients are best considered expressions of primary depressive disorder (Akiskal, 1983).

The following phenomenological criteria have been suggested for their heuristic value in future research on affective-disorder-based dysthymias. They may also help the clinician in identifying a core group of thymoleptic-responsive dysthymias:

1. Indeterminate onset, cardinal manifestations usually obvious before 25 years.
2. Fluctuating course over many years, but typically not free of affective manifestations for more than a few weeks at a time.
3. Habitually sub-syndromal in symptom profile, although the full range of depressive symptoms (which may even crystallize into superimposed syndromal episodes) occur at various times.
4. At least two of the following melancholic manifestations: a) psychomotor inertia, b) hypersomnia, c) anhedonia, and d) diurnal variation (worse in the morning).
5. Habitual introversion, with brief periods of extraversion sometimes seen during relatively "well" periods.

6. Presence of at least 5 of the 7 Schneiderian depressive personality traits (Schneider, 1958). (Akiskal, 1983, p. 18).

A later section on alternative systems for subclassifying chronic low-grade depression discusses the proposed category of a "subsyndromal depression" in more depth.

Characterological Personality Disturbance in Chronic Low-Grade Depression

By definition, characterological depression is chronic and implies a developmental origin (Akiskal *et al.*, 1980). In characterological depressions, depression and character are so enmeshed that the depression becomes an integral and prominent part of the personality (Bonime, 1966). These patients show poor premorbid adjustment, but the term *premorbid* has little meaning for this group, as these patients have been observed to present lifelong symptoms such as unhappiness, dissatisfaction, helplessness, dependency, demandingness, a sense of entitlement, irritability, anger, emotional lability, and histrionic behavior (Schildkraut, 1970). Furthermore, they tend to be poor responders to somatic and psychotherapeutic treatment (Klein, 1974, 1975; Schildkraut, 1970; Schildkraut & Klein, 1975). An alternative theory of the etiology of characterological depressions stems from their resistance to treatment, which could conceivably contribute to the maintenance of their depression. Over the course of many years, the patient may incorporate these depressive features into his or her character structure (Akiskal *et al.*, 1980).

Akiskal and colleagues (1980) contended that some characterological depressions constitute a heterogeneous group of nonaffective personality disorders: "Character spectrum disorders consist of a broad array of personality disorders with secondary dysphoria" (p. 783). Furthermore, Akiskal's character spectrum group overlaps phenomenologically with borderline personality disorders. Beeber and Pies (1983) noted that character spectrum patients typically lead lives of instability, impulsivity, interpersonal manipulativeness, chronic dysphoria, and low self-esteem.

In conclusion, there is a body of opinion that most chronic, early-onset, low-grade depressions should be thought of as personality or character disorders, but an equally strong opinion exists that such conditions are "subsyndromal" primary affective disorders. Empirical data do not support this dichotomy. At present, the evidence suggests viewing these patients from the flexible vantage point that a certain proportion have conditions that are primarily characterological in nature; that others have primarily subsyndromal variances of major depressive disorders; and that still others have an underlying disturbance in character in combination with a somewhat lifelong course of recurrent bouts of major depressive episodes *and* subsyndromal depressive conditions. There is good evidence to support this recommendation based on the phenomenology and course of chronic low-grade depression. However, the causal relationship of underlying depressive character disturbances and primary affective conditions is currently unknown. There is a more in-depth theoretical and diagnostic discussion of this issue in the section on the differential diagnosis of dysthymic disorder.

DIFFERENT APPROACHES TO SUBCLASSIFYING THE CHRONIC DEPRESSIVE DISORDERS

Believing that the categories of neurotic depression and dysthymic disorders were far too inclusive in lumping together a broad array of chronic depressive disorders, several research groups, most notably those of Akiskal (1983) and Klein (1975), have proposed more detailed nosological frameworks for subdividing "low-grade chronic depressions" into separate entities. Their categories have used the available knowledge on internal and external validators such as age of onset, concomitant personality attributes, family history, physiological correlates (including dexamethasone suppression and REM latency), and responsiveness to pharmacologic treatment (Akiskal, 1983; Akiskal *et al.*, 1980, 1981; Yerevanian & Akiskal, 1979). The details of these sub-groupings are described below.

Akiskal's System

Akiskal's subclassification of dysthymic disorder (1983) consists of the following four groups: (1) primary depression with residual chronicity; (2) chronic secondary dysphoria; (3) character spectrum disorder; and (4) subaffective dysthymia. The hallmark of the latter two categories is that they must have had an early age of onset.

Primary Depression with Residual Chronicity

Primary depression with residual chronicity is usually of late onset and occurs as a sequelae to one or more syndromal episodes of primary major depression. A history of a chronic low-grade depressive pattern preceding this episode is typically absent (Akiskal, 1983). The family history of patients with residual chronicity is positive for unipolar depression, whereas the developmental history is unremarkable. Neurotic and dependent personality features develop because of depressive episodes. These patients typically have short rapid-eye-movement (REM) latency and a positive response to antidepressants.

Chronic Secondary Dysphoria

Chronic secondary dysphoria has a variable onset age and occurs in the setting of a preexisting and incapacitating nonaffective disorder. Chronic dysphoria can be secondary to a debilitating medical illness, a psychiatric disorder, or both (Akiskal, 1983).

The dysphoric mood is typically intermittent and tends to parallel the vicissitudes of the underlying illness (Akiskal, Rosenthal, Rosenthal, Kashgarian, Khani, & Puzantian, 1979). The developmental and family histories are variable, the latter depending on the preexisting nonaffective disorder. The personality factors related to chronic secondary dysphorias also vary. Normal REM latency is found in this group, and some patients within the group may improve in response to monoamine oxidase inhibitors. Patients with preexisting anxiety disorders are most apt to respond positively to antidepressant medication (Akiskal, 1983; Klein, Gittelman, Quitkin, & Rifkin, 1980; Tyrer, 1979).

Secondary dysphoria is distinguished from primary depression with residual chronicity in that its onset is not associated with major depressive episodes of melancholic form and the family history is usually negative for affective disorder (Akiskal, 1983). The most frequent preexisting conditions found by Akiskal were neurological and rheumatological diseases, often of childhood onset, and somatization, obsessive-compulsive, panic, and phobic disorders (Akiskal *et al.*, 1981).

Character Spectrum Disorder

The designation *character spectrum* reflects the predominance of a mélange of "unstable" characterological traits, with dependent, histrionic, antisocial, or schizoid features that have an early age of onset. The character-spectrum dysphoric pattern appears as formes frustes or alternative expressions of alcoholism, sociopathy, and somatization disorders (Rosenthal, Akiskal, Scott-Strauss, Rosenthal, & David, 1981). Childhood parental loss and broken homes seem to provide the developmental roots of the characterological disturbance (Akiskal, 1983).

Familial loading of alcoholism and both maternal and paternal nonaffective illness (personality disorder and/or alcoholism) are common among patients with character spectrum disorders. Character spectrum disorders occur more often in women. Unlike subaffective dysthymia, the REM latency for character spectrum disorders is in the normal range. The most significant distinguishing feature of character spectrum disorders is that they fail to show appreciable response to clinical trials with tricyclic antidepressants, monoamine oxidase inhibitors, and lithium carbonate (Akiskal, 1983).

Subaffective Dysthymia

Subaffective dysthymia is a subsyndromal depressive disorder with mild symptomatology closely related to full-fledged episodes of major depression and begins with an early age of onset. Although the developmental history is unremarkable, the family history of these patients is positive for unipolar and/or bipolar disorder. The long-standing personality of subaffective dysthymics is characterized by passivity, pessimism, self-reproach, and conscientiousness (Akiskal, 1983).

As in primary depression with residual chronicity, the REM latency is short for subaffective dysthymic disorder. A distinguishing feature of subaffective dysthymia is that its pharmacological response to thymoleptic drugs, such as lithium carbonate and tricyclic antidepressants, is positive (Akiskal, 1983). For some patients in this group, tricyclic antidepressants can induce hypomania.

The challenge still exists of demonstrating that there are sufficient external variables to make these distinctions valid subcategories of affective disorders. Given the comprehensive schema proposed by Akiskal and the face validity of the constructs, efforts to replicate his research with larger samples and other populations appear warranted and timely.

Other Proposed Categories for Low-Grade Chronic Depressions

Subbipolar Dysthymia

Based on findings that tricyclics trigger hypomania in a subgroup of patients with characterological depressions, Rosenthal and colleagues (1981) also proposed categorizing a proportion of patients with subaffective dysthymia as subbipolar dysthymics.

Chronic Dysphoria

The category of chronic dysphoria proposed by Klein and colleagues (Stewart, Quitkin, & McGrath, 1981) is a frequently used definition for chronic low-grade depression. It includes the following six criteria:

1. A dysphoric mood for the majority of the adult life
2. Onset prior to age 25
3. Mood reactivity

4. Must also meet criteria for RDC major or minor depressive disorder or intermittent depressive disorder
5. Does not meet criteria for endogenomorphic depression
6. Did not have a period of well-being lasting at least 6 months (Keller & Lavori, 1984, p. 420)

Demoralization

Klein and associates (1980) have used the term *demoralization* to describe those patients who functioned well in life until a series of crises (usually marital or career) led to the development of a chronic dysphoria. The full dysthymic syndrome is not present; however, vegetative signs may be present. (Klein *et al.*, 1980). Demoralization also applies to those patients who are classified as chronic secondary dysphoria in Akiskal's 1983 system (Sinaikin, 1985).

DIFFERENTIAL DIAGNOSIS OF DYSTHYMIC DISORDER

An earlier section focused on the different views held on the extent to which chronic depressive disorders should be placed in the domain of personality disorders or affective disorders, or both. Although this section is entitled "Differential Diagnosis of Dysthymic Disorder," much of the material concentrates on a similar exploration of the unresolved boundary issues that exist in psychiatry's current state of knowledge about the relationship of dysthymia to major depression, double depression, other chronic mood disorders, and the coexistence of "nonaffective" personality disorders.

The Relationship of Dysthymia to Major Depression

The symptom criteria for dysthymia are similar to those for major depression, except that, by definition, the presence of delusions and hallucinations precludes the diagnosis of dysthymic disorder and the duration of dysthymia requires a duration of at least 2 years. Whether minor depression of less than 2 years' duration or whether the chronic low-grade depressions are qualitatively or quantitatively distinct from major depression has yet to bc established.

Dysthymia as Prodromal to Major Depression

There are only a few published studies that report on dysthymic patients and that are also explicit in specifying whether or not they develop a concomitant major depression before recovering from the dysthymia.

Akiskal and colleagues (1981) reported that approximately 90% of outpatients who met the DSM-III criteria for dysthymic disorder had had a course that was complicated by major affective episodes. This finding was based on a sample of 137 patients who had initially been diagnosed as having a dysthymic disorder.

In a prospective study of 19 children with a diagnosis of dysthymia, Kovacs, Feinberg, Crouse-Novak, Paulauskas, and Finkelstein (1984) found that over 70% developed a major depression during the first 5 years of follow-up. All subjects were recruited from referrals to university-affiliated outpatient child-psychiatric and pediatric clinics.

In summary, there are no psychopathological data published on a clinically identified population who had a dysthymic disorder in which more than a very small proportion of patients did not go on to develop a major depression.

Dysthymia as a Residual Syndrome

Some authors believe that most chronic depressions represent the inadequately recognized and poorly treated residual of unresolved or partially remitted acute depressions (Klerman, 1980). Clarification is needed of the diagnostic status of patients with acute episodes of major depressive disorder who do not remit. These patients could be considered either "major depressive disorder, chronic or unremitted" or "dysthymic," or both (Klerman *et al.,* 1987).

In studies reviewed by Klerman (1980), and in research by Keller, Klerman, Lavori, Coryell, Endicott, and Taylor (1984), Akiskal (1982), and Rounsaville and associates (1980), at least 15%–20% of patients experiencing acute depressions did not make a complete recovery but showed some intermittent, fluctuating, and chronic symptoms, often persisting for years. Furthermore, Keller, Lavori, Rice, Coryell, and Hirschfeld (1986) found that, following recovery from any given episode of depression, successive cohorts of prospectively observed episodes of major depressive disorder in previously recovered patients still had a 15%–20% rate of chronicity, producing "silting" in the population that undoubtedly contributed to the proportion of patients who had been diagnosed as dysthymic (Keller *et al.,* 1986).

Double Depression

The guidelines for differential diagnosis in the DSM-III-R encourage recording a diagnosis of both dysthymic disorder and major depression when a major depressive episode is superimposed on a preexisting dysthymic disorder.

The coexistence of acute episodes of major depression superimposed on dysthymia has led to the concept of *double depression* (Keller & Shapiro, 1982). Patients with a double depression are found to have an extremely pernicious long-term outcome for the dysthymic disorder and a high likelihood of recurrent episodes of major depression (Keller, 1985).

Recovery

Data from the National Institute of Mental Health's Collaborative Study of the Psychobiology of Depression indicate that the distinction between patients with and without so-called double depression may be extremely important in terms of outcome assessment (Keller & Shapiro, 1982). If recovery for such patients is defined in terms of recovery from the major depression alone, then the recovery rate at 2 years was quite high (97%). However, if recovery is defined in terms of recovery from both the acute and the chronic depression, the recovery rate was much lower (39%) (Keller & Lavori, 1984). This observation supports the validity of the DSM-III guidelines advocating diagnosing both disorders.

Relapse

Keller, Lavori, Endicott, Coryell, and Klerman (1983) found that patients with a double depression who recovered from the major depression had a significantly higher rate of relapse by 2 years than patients with major depression alone (58% to 39%). Life-table analyses demonstrate that the longer the patient remains ill with the underlying dysthymia after recovering from the major depression, the greater the likelihood that relapse into an episode of major depressive will preempt recovery from the dysthymic disorder.

Prevalence

Although prevalence or incidence rates for double depression are not available, Keller and Shapiro (1982) found that 26% of the patients who entered the NIMH Collaborative Study of the Psychobiology of Depression with a current episode of major depression also had a chronic underlying depression (dysthymic disorder) that had preceded the onset of the major depression by at least 2 years.

Conclusion

Double depression is best understood as a cross-sectional state that is likely to occur in most patients clinically identified as having a dysthymic disorder and in a significant proportion of patients identified as having a major depression. Double depression should not be thought of as a distinct disease entity that has a unique pattern of familial aggregation (Keller & Lavori, 1984).

The important issue concerning double depression is whether there is any utility in recognizing the coexistence of a dysthymia and a major depression. If so, the subtypes of chronic depression proposed by Akiskal (1983) and Klein (1975) could and should be applied to the dysthymias in patients with double depression (Keller & Lavori, 1984).

Dysthymic Disorder and Other Chronic Mood Disorders

Cyclothymia

In almost all diagnostic nomenclatures before the DSM-III-R, cyclothymia was grouped with the personality disorders. *Cyclothymic personality* referred to individuals who had long-standing patterns, sometimes cyclical and periodic, of fluctuations between depressive and hypomanic states, but not severe enough to reach the criteria for major affective disorder (Klerman *et al.*, 1987). Because of the similarities in symptom patterns to other affective disorders, particularly bipolar disorder, cyclothymia was included as an Axis I affective disorder in the DSM-III-R.

Currently, there is some consensus among researchers in psychiatry that cyclothymia is an attenuated form of bipolar disorder, based on familial and genetic data (Akiskal, Djenderedjian, Rosenthal, & Khani, 1977) and observations that a significant proportion of cyclothymics show similarities to bipolar patients in their response to treatment (Klerman, 1980).

There are empirical data to suggest that, although dysthymic patients pursue a ''unipolar'' course, they also display distinct bipolar tendencies (i.e., brief hypomanic switches activated by tricyclic challenge). It therefore seems that a proportion of dysthymic patients have affinities to patients with cyclothymic and bipolar II disorders (Akiskal, 1981, 1983; Akiskal *et al.*, 1980; Rosenthal *et al.*, 1981).

Dysthymic disorder is distinguished from cyclothymia by whether the return to normal is experienced as a relief from depression or whether there are signs of euphoria, increased activity, and poor judgment; in the latter case, the patient would be considered cyclothymic (DSM-III-R). In cyclothymia (Akiskal *et al.*, 1977), behaviorally manifested hypomania is a clinical marker distinguishing cyclothymia from nonaffective personalities. There is as yet no such clinical marker available for characterological depressions (Akiskal *et al.*, 1980).

Labile Personality Disorder

Labile personality disorder, defined in the RDC (Spitzer *et al.*, 1985) as a chronic mood disorder characterized by sudden changes from normal to irritable, angry, anxious, and depressed moods, should be distinguished from dysthymic disorder. Unlike for chronic and intermittent depression, an effort was made to establish criteria for labile personality that were not based on symptoms similar to those that define the major depressive disorder. Rather, the diagnosis was to be based more strictly on personality features.

In addition to clinical features, there are some data to suggest that response to treatment and outcome differentiate the two disorders. Rounsaville, Sholomskas, and Prusoff (1980) found that, following pharmacotherapy, labile patients had continuing greater impairment than patients with chronic depressive disorders and had tendencies toward chronic low self-esteem, envy, and pessimism after recovery from acute symptoms. Rounsaville *et al.* viewed these proclivities as attitudes and approaches to life, rather than responses to a depressive episode.

It should be noted that considerable controversy surrounds the utility and validity of the diagnostic category of labile personality. The RDC classification of labile personality most closely matches "mixed personality disorder" in the DSM-III, which does not include the diagnosis "labile personality." As the DSM-III-R also does not include the labile personality category, it is possible that this term may not be used in the coming years.

Coexistence of Dysthymia and "Nonaffective" Personality Disorders

Various theories of the etiology of depression have emphasized the importance of personality characteristics (Becker, 1979), even though disagreement exists with regard to terminology and the etiology of the characteristics themselves (Millon, 1981). From these theories, two depressive personality types have emerged (Arieti & Bemporad, 1980):

> One is characterized by low self-esteem (Becker, 1979) and high levels of obsessionality (Hirschfeld & Klerman, 1979; Kendell & Discipio, 1979), and the second by low frustration tolerance and increased dependence on others for support and approval (Brown & Harris, 1978; Hirschfeld & Klerman, 1979). (Malt, 1983, p. 19)

Because of the duration of the problems encountered by patients with dysthymia and the enduring quality of their problems with self-esteem, guilt, and poor interpersonal relations, they are often simultaneously diagnosed with Axis II personality disorders.

In Roy, Sutton, and Pickar's study (1985), 9 of the 11 dysthymic patients were clinically assessed as having an associated personality disorder that met DSM-III criteria: 4 borderline, 2 schizoid, 1 histrionic, 1 compulsive, and 1 dependent. None of the normal controls was assessed as having a personality disorder. The significantly lower self-esteem score and higher neuroticism and hostility scores of these dysthymic patients, compared with those of the controls, identified considerable personality pathology and suggested an underlying cause of their maladjustment.

Perry (1985) found that all of his subjects with borderline personality disorder who did not have antisocial personality disorder and 79% of his patients with antisocial personality disorder reported having felt depressed most of the time for 2 or more years at some point in their lives.

A number of researchers, including Stone (1979) and Akiskal (1981), have suggested that the depression of the borderline patient may be physiologically and psychologically indistinguishable from dysthymia. This suggestion raises the question of whether this lack of distinction represents the coexistence of two different disorders or whether many patients with a borderline personality disorder, as currently defined, show an alternative expression of an affective illness.

In conclusion, it is necessary to emphasize that there has been a long-standing tendency in psychiatry to minimize the intensity and the seriousness of depressive symptoms in patients with severe personality disorders (Keller & Lavori, 1984). Hence, it is important for the clinician to recognize that dysthymia that either is secondary to nonaffective character pathology or coexists with nonaffective character pathology is a serious disorder that often has a chronic course with superimposed episodes of major depression and multiple recurrences for patients who do recover.

BIOLOGICAL ASPECTS OF DYSTHYMIA

A recently conducted unpublished review by Thase (1986) indicates that insufficient data are available to draw conclusions about biological abnormalities associated with dysthymic disorder. The data that are available are speculative and require replication, and more research is needed in this domain. The major conceptual problems confronted by efforts to do biological research are that there is no consensus about what constitutes the biology of the major affective disorders and that the boundary between major depression and dysthymia is so unclear. In addition, the state-versus-trait nature of psychiatric disturbances and the heterogeneity within the dysthymic disorder category contribute to the difficulty in elucidating biological substrates. A very brief summary of some of the research on biological correlates follows.

There are speculative data describing the biological factors associated with dysthymia using neuroendocrine strategies and neurophysiological hypotheses. In Thase's review (1986) of studies published before 1985, a Dexamethasone Suppression Test (DST) found a nonsuppression rate of 9% in patients with minor depression or dysthymic disorder. This rate was not different from that of normal controls but was significantly lower than that in major depression (29%). Roy and colleagues (1985) reported an 18% DST nonsuppression rate specifically in dysthymic disorder. Neurophysiological correlates of dysthymic disorder include shortened REM sleep and diminished electrodermal activity in subgroups of affective disorder that include dysthymic disorder (Thase, 1986; Ward & Doerr, 1985). At the present time, other studies relating biological changes to dysthymia are too speculative to report.

NATURAL COURSE OF DYSTHYMIA

This section reviews the data on the course of dysthymia in settings in which treatment was not controlled by the investigators. A chronic subsyndromal depressive course may be the sequel of a major depressive episode or may arise insidiously and pursue a lifelong subsyndromal course. As described earlier, a "pure" subsyndromal depressive course that is not complicated by major affective episodes is uncommon in clinical practice and has not yet been reported in the literature.

It appears that an increasing number of patients are presenting to both outpatient and, to a smaller extent, inpatient psychiatric services with mild depressions that lack the full syndromal criteria for major depressive disorder; that are more often intermittent than sustained; and that are frequently expressions of lifelong dysphoria (Akiskal *et al.*, 1978; Kielholz, 1973; Rosenthal, 1966). Moreover, dysthymic patients may have frequent hospitalizations or visits to emergency rooms because of suicide attempts or the aggravation of somatic complaints (Klerman, 1980).

Akiskal (1983) reported that an unspecified but substantial percentage of dysthymic patients with onset in young adulthood and adolescence have a "switch in polarity" to bipolar illness. This switch has been reported by other investigators only in situations where a tricyclic antidepressant had been used (Rosenthal *et al.*, 1981).

Recovery

According to Keller and Shapiro (1982), it is difficult to assess improvement in the course of dysthmia because it is hard to know whether "improvement" in dysthymic patients means relief from an acute exacerbation of the depression or from the baseline dysthymia (Stewart, McGrath, Liebowitz, Harrison, Quitkin, & Rabkin, 1985). Nevertheless, Barrett (1984) found a 37% rate of improvement among chronic depressives based on self-reports at 2 years. Gonzales, Lewinsohn, and Clarke (1985) found a 1-year recovery rate for intermittent depressives of 43%, substantially lower than the 75% rate of recovery for major depressives. Their finding of significant differences in recovery rates for patients with intermittent versus major depressive disorder lends some support to the importance of the RDC distinction between major and chronic intermittent depression, as well as the similar DSM-III-R distinction between major depression and dysthymic disorder.

Relapse

In the same follow-up study of unipolar depressives, Gonzales and associates (1985) found a 1-year 33% relapse rate for chronically and intermittently depressed patients.

Duration of Episodes

Rounsaville and colleagues (1980) found that the average duration of intermittent depression was 5.5 years, with a range of from 2 to 20 years among chronically depressed outpatients. This finding is consistent with findings by Keller and Shapiro (1982), who reported a median duration of 5 years for dysthymia before the first superimposition of an episode of major depression.

Dysthymia as a Chronic Illness

Among the multiple pathways to a chronic low-grade depression are the two that occur most commonly. One characterizes patients with an early onset whose dysthymic symptoms have been present since adolescence and persist for many years. The other characterizes patients who become chronic because of a failure to resolve acute episodes of major depressive disorders (Keller & Shapiro, 1982; Klerman, 1980). Among the chronic depressives in Barrett's naturalistic study (1984), 63% showed no improvement or had a more severe illness at 2 years; and 61% of the patients with a double depression had not yet recovered from the underlying dysthymic disorder after 2 years (Keller *et al.*, 1983), although they may have recovered from the major depressive disorder.

TREATMENT OF DYSTHYMIC DISORDER

Low-grade chronic depressions are difficult to treat, and in most cases, the optimal treatment is a combination of psychotropic medication and psychotherapy. The specificity of which modality to use has not been studied extensively, but there is evidence to suggest that monoamine oxidase inhibitors may be effective in patients who do not respond to trials of a tricyclic antidepressant.

In terms of psychosocial treatment, most research studies have used psychodynamically oriented psychotherapy. Reports (Blackburn, Bishop, Glen, Whally, & Christie, 1981; Kovacs, Rush, Beck, & Hollon, 1981; Weissman, Klerman, Prusoff, Sholomskas, & Padian, 1981) on the success of cognitive therapy and interpersonal psychotherapy in treating major depression suggest that these treatments be tried for chronic low-grade depression.

This section examines what is known about the efficacy of psychosocial and somatic therapies in treating dysthymic disorder, and it presents data on the treatment of the different categories of low-grade chronic depression described by Akiskal and colleagues.

Psychosocial Treatment

Among the most widely used psychosocial treatments for dysthymia "are those derived from psychoanalytic and psychodynamic theories of personality (Arieti & Bemporad, 1978) . . . relating the development and the maintenance of depressive symptoms and maladaptive personality features to unresolved conflicts from early childhood" (Klerman, 1980, p. 1335). Therapy centers on an analysis of both the patient's depressive symptoms and the patient's character structure (Klerman, 1980).

Modifications of classic psychoanalytic techniques have been described by Adolf Meyer (Lief, 1948) and Harry Stack Sullivan (1953), who developed general theories of adaptation and interpersonal relations. Cohen, Baker, Cohen, Fromm-Reichmann, and Weigent (1954) described specific applications to the long-term psychotherapy of personality features related to affective disorders:

> The basic thesis is that the adult personality features predisposing to dysthymic disorder develop from a specific familial constellation related to the marginality of the family because of their religious, economic, or cultural membership and associated with excess dependency, sibling rivalry and envy, and high motivation for achievement transmitted to the child destined to become depressive. (Klerman, 1980, p. 1335).

To date, there are no controlled trials to support the efficacy of such long-term psychotherapeutic techniques; however, practitioners using these modalities have written positive anecdotal reports on their efficacy, and these procedures are often taught to trainees in the mental health profession by senior teachers and supervisors.

In addition, a variety of short-term therapies have been developed that have received systematic clinical evaluation. These include cognitive techniques (Beck, 1972; Rush, Beck, Kovacs, & Hollon, 1977), interpersonal therapy (Klerman, DiMascio, Weissman, Prusoff, & Paykel, 1974), group therapy developed by the Hopkins group (Covi, Lipman, Derogatis, Smith, & Pattison, 1974), marital therapy as reported by Friedman (1975), and psychoeducational programs developed by Lewinsohn (1974). Replication of the success of each of these therapeutic modalities is needed with other populations, different investigators, and larger samples before conclusions can be reached about their efficacy. A long-term controlled trial using social skills training is currently being conducted by Becker and Heimberg (1985), but the results are not yet available.

Somatic Treatment

Among the somatic therapies, particular attention should be given to the tricyclic antidepressants and the monoamine oxidase inhibitors, as these drugs remain the standard form of pharmacotherapy with demonstrated efficacy for depression (Klerman & Hirschfeld, 1978).

Ward, Bloom, and Friedel (1979) found that 80% of their patients diagnosed with RDC major depression, lasting over 1 year, showed marked or moderate improvement after a 4-week trial of doxepin (Kocsis, 1986). In a double-blind comparison of amitriptyline, perphenazine, and a combination of the two for treating depression, Rounsaville and colleagues (1980) studied patients with RDC major depression and some who also had the additional diagnosis of chronic and intermittent depression. Although no figures were given for responses to the three treatments separately, the overall response for patients with major depression plus the chronic and intermittent depression was comparable to the response of those with major depression alone (Kocsis, 1986).

As in the treatment of major depression, a patient with dysthymia should not be considered treatment-resistant until the equivalent of 200–300 mg of imipramine has been administered for at least 6 weeks (Klerman, 1980). Similarly, blood-level assessments are of potential value in identifying patients who are not able to absorb or metabolize antidepressant medications. The clinician should also be aware of the potential for mild elated mood swings in dysthymic patients treated with antidepressants, a finding reported by Akiskal (1981) and Rosenthal and colleagues (1981), although not yet found by other investigators.

Some reports indicate that monoamine oxidase inhibitors may have specific therapeutic efficacy for depressed patients with atypical features marked by symptoms of anxiety, hysteria, and depersonalization (Klerman, 1980; Nies, Robinson, Bartlett, & Lanborn, 1977).

Based on the results of an intensive clinical trial of desipramine in a small sample of dysthymic patients, Stewart and colleagues (1985) suggested that the drug may be ineffective in the treatment of dysthymia without panic attacks.

Amphetamines, barbiturates, and benzodiazepines are not effective in the long-term treatment of dysthymia. Clinical experience and research indicate that they are not significantly better than placebo and are at times worse (Klerman, 1980).

Combination of Psychotherapy and Somatotherapy for Treatment of Dysthymia

Several studies have reported on the combination of psychotherapy and somatotherapy in treating dysthymic patients. Lesse (1977) found that the efficacy of psychotherapy was enhanced when combined with tricyclic drug therapy. Akiskal (1981) found that 45% of 137 dysthymic probands had a positive therapeutic response to a systematic but open trial of at least two tricyclic antidepressants when given in the context of practical psychotherapeutic approaches.

Treatment of Specific Proposed Categories of Low-Grade Chronic Depression

In a series of studies, Akiskal and colleagues have examined the treatment response of dysthymia according to the categories they had developed for subclassifying chronic low-grade depression. A summary of these findings is as follows.

Primary Depression with Residual Chronicity

In a study of primary chronic depressives, Akiskal (1982) noted a significant, though only partial, treatment response in 66% of the patients when administered tricyclic antidepressants. Vegetative and psychomotor symptoms were the most responsive to this treatment (Akiskal, 1983; Sinaikin, 1985).

Chronic Secondary Dysphoric

Akiskal and associates (1981) observed symptomatic and social improvement in 35% of their chronic secondarily depressed patients treated with tricyclics and psychotherapy (Sinaikin, 1985). This percentage is compared to the 30% of the patients who received similar treatment and did not show a positive treatment response.

Characterological Depressions

In a 1980 study, Akiskal and associates found that only 33% of the patients with characterological depressions showed a positive treatment response after 1–4 years of follow-up. Desipramine and nortriptyline were generally more effective in treatment-responsive patients. Patients not responding to somatotherapy did not tolerate secondary amine tricyclics and preferred doxepin or amitriptyline. Lithium carbonate was not effective in treating the tricyclic-nonresponding patients (Akiskal *et al.*, 1980).

In another study, 40% of characterological depressives showed a positive treatment response to a combination of psychotherapy and somatotherapy (Akiskal, 1981).

Subaffective Dysthymia

Yerevanian and Akiskal (1979) noted that patients with subaffective dysthymia may respond to a combination of behavioral, psychodynamic, and individual psychotherapy, whereas their response to tricyclic antidepressants is only fair (Beeber & Pies, 1983).

Character Spectrum Disorder

Character spectrum patients are said to show poor response to both tricyclics and psychotherapy (Yerevanian & Akiskal, 1979). Beeber and Pies (1983) suggested that these patients may be responsive to psychotherapy focusing on characterological defenses, maladaptive cognitive styles, and transference.

Comments on the Treatment of Dysthymia

Clinical experience and findings from the treatment studies that have been done are in agreement that dysthymia is often an extremely difficult condition to treat, particularly when characterological features are prominent and when the condition is of long duration. Patience and perseverance are required of the clinician and the patient, especially when alleviation of the depressive symptoms reveals substantial underlying character pathology. Patients and clinicians often become demoralized by the length of time needed to show meaningful changes in the patient's mood, character, and psychosocial functioning. However, given the duration of the disorder in most patients, it would be unusual to see a marked response to relatively short-term therapies, as the long-standing depression has usually already caused disruption in many areas of the patient's functioning by the time the patient enters treatment.

SUMMARY

Psychiatry's renewed interest in chronic depression since the late 1970s is timely, given the results of recent clinical and epidemiological studies, which show that a substantial number of patients with a major depression go on to have a chronic unremitting course and that there is a relatively high incidence of chronic depression in the general population. Moreover, the high rates of relapse, the associated psychopathological and psychosocial morbidity, and the limited efficacy of the available psychotherapeutic and somatic treatments give added importance to the study of chronic depression.

The introduction of the term *dysthymic disorder* in the DSM-III was in large part a result of dissatisfaction with the vague meaning attached to *neurotic depression* and a desire for a more atheoretical and phenomenological way of defining and classifying chronic depressive disorders. The "newness" of the term to most psychiatrists' ears sparked interest in this category of disorders, as did placing these conditions with the affective disorders instead of including them with personality disorders. This shift in classification further helped to stimulate lively debate in the field of psychiatry about whether chronic low-grade depressions are best conceptualized as personality disorders or subsyndromal affective disorders.

As described in this chapter, although these issues have now been well articulated, with proponents often espousing competing viewpoints, we are far from resolving this fundamental question. The work by Akiskal and others in delineating more detailed subdivisions for defining chronic depression should continue. An awareness of the rationale for these divergent opinions and diagnostic systems and the reality that answers do not yet exist should strengthen differential diagnosis and clinical practice and should enhance research.

Furthermore, family data, course and outcome data, and information on biological markers are not yet at the point where we are able to decide whether major depression, dysthymia, and double depression are best viewed as separate affective disease entities, a continuum on the spectrum of depressive disorders, or a combination of both. Although this uncertainty does not diminish the value of the substantial number of data on the natural course of these disorders that are now available, the current boundaries defining major depression, dysthymia, and double depression should still be viewed as arbitrary.

Specifically, the knowledge that almost all children and adults identified in clinical populations as having dysthymia are at very high risk of developing a major depression, are very likely to relapse subsequently into another major affective episode if they do recover, and have a high rate of chronicity for the underlying dysthymic disorder should guide clinicians in making a prognosis and in treatment planning. The expected continued chronicity, the associated exacerbations in the severity of depression once a depression becomes chronic, and the comorbidity with other psychiatric syndromes and "nonaffective" personality disorders highlight the ubiquity of this condition. Some of the efforts currently under way to conduct controlled studies on psychosocial and somatic treatments appear promising and require further investigation. Additionally, new treatment initiatives must be undertaken so that clinicians may improve their ability to treat depression, which appears to be self-perpetuating and highly debilitating once its chronicity is established.

Hopefully, treatment research will also shed some light on whether adequate efforts at early intervention and secondary prevention will reduce the incidence, and improve the course, of "chronic depression," or whether there is an inherent underlying morbidity in these conditions that will prove to be treatment-resistant.

REFERENCES

Abraham, K. (1948). Notes on the psychoanalytic investigation and treatment of manic-depressive insanity and allied conditions. In *Selected papers on psychoanalysis* (pp. 152–172). London: Hogarth Press.

Akiskal, H. S. (1981). Subaffective disorders: Dysthymic, cyclothymic and bipolar II disorders in the "borderline" realm. *Journal of Affective Disorders, 3,* 297–315.

Akiskal, H. S. (1982). Factors associated with incomplete recovery in primary depressive illness. *Journal of Clinical Psychology, 43,* 266–271.

Akiskal, H. S. (1983). Dysthymic disorder: Psychopathology of proposed chronic depressive subtypes. *American Journal of Psychiatry, 140,* 11–21.

Akiskal, H. S., Djenderedjian, A. H., Rosenthal, R. H., & Khani, M. K. (1977). Cyclothymic disorder: Validating criteria for inclusion in the bipolar affective group. *American Journal of Psychiatry, 134,* 1227–1233.

Akiskal, H. S., Bitar, A. H., Puzantian, M. D., Rosenthal, T. L., & Walker, P. W. (1978). The nosological status of neurotic depression: A prospective three-to-four year follow-up examination in light of the primary-secondary distinction and unipolar-bipolar dichotomies. *Archives of General Psychiatry, 35,* 756–766.

Akiskal, H. S., Rosenthal, R. H., Rosenthal, T. L., Kashgarian, M., Khani, M. K., & Puzantian, V. R. (1979). Differentiation of primary affective illness from situational, symptomatic and secondary depressions. *Archives of General Psychiatry, 36,* 635–643.

Akiskal, H. S., Rosenthal, T. L., Haykal, R. F., Lemmi, H., Rosenthal, R. H., & Scott-Strauss, A. (1980). Characterological depressions: Clinical and sleep EEG findings separating 'subaffective dysthymias' from "character-spectrum disorders." *Archives of General Psychiatry, 37,* 777–783.

Akiskal, H. S., King, D., Rosenthal, T. L., Robinson, D., & Scott-Strauss, A. (1981). Chronic depression: Part 1. Clinical and familial characteristics in 137 probands. *Journal of Affective Disorders, 3,* 297–315.

American Psychiatric Association. (1968). *Diagnostic and statistical manual of mental disorders* (2nd ed.; DSM-II). Washington, DC: Author.

American Psychiatric Association. (1980). *Diagnostic and statistical manual of mental disorders* (3rd ed.; DSM-III). Washington, DC: Author.

American Psychiatric Association. (1986). *DSM-III-R in development: Work group to revise DSM-III.* Washington, DC: Author.

Arieti, S., & Bemporad, J. R. (1978). *Severe and mild depression: The psychotherapeutic approach.* New York: Basic Books.

Arieti, S., & Bemporad, J. R. (1980). The psychological organization of depression. *American Journal of Psychiatry, 137,* 1360–1365.

Barrett, J. E. (1984). Naturalistic change after 2 years in neurotic depressive disorders (RDC Categories). *Comprehensive Psychiatry, 25,* 404–418.

Barrett, J., Hurst, M. W., DiSalla, C., & Rose, R. M. (1978). Prevalence of depression over a 12 month period in a nonpatient population. *Archives of General Psychiatry, 35,* 741–744.

Beck, A. T. (1972). *Depression: Causes and treatment.* Philadelphia: University of Pennsylvania Press.

Becker, J. (1979). Vulnerable self-esteem as a predisposing factor in a depressive disorder. In R. A. Depue (Ed.), *The psychobiology of depressive disorders* (pp. 317–334). New York: Academic Press.

Becker, R. E., & Heimberg, R. G. (1985). Social skills training approaches. In M. Hersen & A. S. Bellack (Eds.), *Handbook of clinical behavior therapy with adults.* New York: Plenum Press.

Beeber, A. R., & Pies, R. W. (1983). The nonmelancholic depressive syndromes: An alternate approach to classification. *Journal of Nervous and Mental Disease, 171,* 3–9.

Bonime, W. (1966). The psychodynamics of neurotic depression. In S. Arieti (Ed.), *American handbook of psychiatry* (1st ed., pp. 239–255). New York: Basic Books.

Brown, G. W., & Harris, T. (1978). *Social origins of depression.* New York: Free Press.

Chodoff, P. (1972). The depressive personality: A critical review. *Archives of General Psychiatry, 27,* 665–673.

Cohen, M. B., Baker, G., Cohen, R. A., Fromm-Reichmann, I., & Weigent, E. V. (1954). An intensive study of twelve cases of manic-depressive psychosis. *Psychiatry, 17,* 103–110.

Cooper, A. M., & Michels, R. (1981). Book review of the American Psychiatric Association: *Diagnostic and Statistical Manual of Mental Disorders,* 3rd edition. *American Journal of Psychiatry, 138,* 128–129.

Covi, L., Lipman, R. S., Derogatis, L. R., Smith, J., & Pattison, J. (1974). Drugs and group psychotherapy in neurotic depression. *American Journal of Psychiatry, 131,* 191–196.

Frances, A. (1980). The DSM-III personality disorders section: A commentary. *American Journal of Psychiatry, 137,* 1050–1054.

Freud, S. (1946). *Mourning and melancholia: Collected papers* (Vol. 4). London: Hogarth Press.

Friedman, A. S. (1975). Interaction of drug therapy with marital therapy in depressed patients. *Archives of General Psychiatry, 32,* 619–623.

Gonzales, L. R., Lewinsohn, P. M., & Clarke, G. M. (1985). Longitudinal follow-up of unipolar depressives: An investigation of predictors of relapse. *Journal of Consulting and Clinical Psychology, 53,* 461–469.

Hirschfeld, R. M. A., & Klerman, G. L. (1979). Personality attributes and affective disorders. *American Journal of Psychiatry, 136,* 67–70.

Hornstra, R. K., & Klassen, D. (1977). The course of depression. *Comprehensive Psychiatry, 18,* 119–124.

Kahn, E. (1975). The depressive character. *Folia Psychiatrica et Neurologica Japonica, 29,* 290–303.

Keller, M. B. (1985). Chronic and recurrent affective disorders: Incidence, course and influencing factors. In D. Kemali & G. Racagni (Eds.), *Chronic treatments in neuropsychiatry* (pp. 111–120). New York: Raven Press.

Keller, M. B., & Lavori, P. W. (1984). Double depression, major depression, and dysthymia: Distinct entities or different phases of the same disorder? *Psychopharmacology Bulletin, 20,* 399–402.

Keller, M. B., & Shapiro, R. W. (1982). "Double-depression": Superimposition of acute depressive episodes on chronic depressive disorders. *American Journal of Psychiatry, 139,* 438–442.

Keller, M. B., Lavori, P. W., Endicott, J., Coryell, W., & Klerman, G. L. (1983). "Double depression": Two year follow-up. *American Journal of Psychiatry, 140,* 993–998.

Keller, M. B., Klerman, G. L., Lavori, P. W., Coryell, W., Endicott, J., & Taylor, J. (1984). Long-term outcome of episodes of major depression in clinical and public health significance. *Journal of the American Medical Association, 252,* 788–792.

Keller, M. B., Lavori, P. W., Rice, J., Coryell, W., & Hirschfeld, R. M. A. (1986). The persistent risk of chronicity in recurrent episodes of non-bipolar major depressive disorder: A prospective follow-up. *American Journal of Psychiatry, 143,* 24–28.

Kendell, R. E. (1976). The classification of depression: A review of contemporary confusion. *British Journal of Psychiatry, 129,* 15–28.

Kendell, R. E., & Discipio, W. J. (1979). Obsessional symptoms and obsessional personality traits in patients with depressive illness. *Psychological Medicine, 1,* 65–72.

Kielholz, P. (1973). *Depression in everyday practice.* Berne: Hans Huber.

Kiloh, L. G., Andrews, G., Nielsen, M., & Bianchi, G. N. (1972). The relationship of the syndromes called endogenous and neurotic depression. *British Journal of Psychiatry, 121,* 183–196.

Klein, D. F. (1974). Endogenomorphic depression: A conceptual and terminological revision. *Archives of General Psychiatry, 31,* 447–454.

Klein, D. F. (1975). Merrel Psychiatric Research Interview: A new classification of depressive disorders, *Depression notes 16.* Cincinnati: Merrell-National Laboratories.

Klein, D. F., Gittelman, R., Quitkin, F., & Rifkin, A. (1980). *Diagnosis and drug treatment of psychiatric disorders* (2nd ed.). Baltimore: Williams & Wilkins.

Klerman, G. L. (1980). Other specific affective disorders. In H. I. Kaplan & B. J. Sadock (Eds.), *Comprehensive Textbook of Psychiatry/III* (Vol. 1, 3rd ed., pp. 1332–1338). Baltimore: Williams & Wilkins.

Klerman, G. L., & Hirschfeld, R. M. A. (1978). The use of antidepressants in clinical practice. *Journal of the American Medical Association, 240,* 1403–1409.

Klerman, G. L., DiMascio, A., Weissman, M. M., Prusoff, B., & Paykel, E. S. (1974). Treatment of depression by drugs and psychotherapy. *American Journal of Psychiatry, 131,* 186–190.

Klerman, G. L., Endicott, J., Spitzer, R., & Hirschfeld, R. M. A. (1979). Neurotic depressions: A systematic analysis of multiple criteria and meanings. *American Journal of Psychiatry, 136,* 57–61.

Klerman, G. L., Keller, M. B., Fawcett, J. A., Andreasen, N. C., Hirschfeld, R. M. A., & Endicott, J. (1987). Major depression and related affective disorders. In G. L. Tischler (Ed.), *Diagnosis and classification in psychiatry: A critical appraisal of DSM-III.* New York: Cambridge University Press.

Kocsis, J. (1986). *Pharmacological treatment of dysthymic disorder.* Presented at the National Institute of Mental Health Workshop on Dysthymic Disorder, Washington, DC.

Kovacs, M., Rush, A. J., Beck, A. T., & Hollon, S. D. (1981). Depressed outpatients treated with cognitive therapy or pharmacotherapy: A one-year follow-up. *Archives of General Psychiatry, 38,* 33–39.

Kovacs, M., Feinberg, T. L., Crouse-Novak, M. A., Paulauskas, S. L., & Finkelstein, R. (1984). Depressive disorders in childhood: 1. A longitudinal prospective study of characteristics and recovery. *Archives of General Psychiatry, 41,* 229–237.

Kraepelin, E. (1921). *Manic-depressive illness and paranoia.* Edinburgh: E. & S. Livingstone.

Kretschmer, E. (1936). *Physique and character* (trans. E. Miller). London: Kegan Paul, Trench, Trubner.

Lesse, S. (1977). Psychotherapy in combination with antidepressant drugs in patients with severe masked depressions. *American Journal of Psychiatry, 31,* 185–191.

Lewinsohn, P. (1974). A behavioral approach to depression. In R. Friedman & M. Katz (Eds.), *The psychology of depression: Contemporary theory and research.* New York: Wiley.

Liebowitz, M. R., & Klein, D. F. (1979). Hysteroid dysphoria. *Psychiatric Clinics of North America, 2,* 555–575.

Lief, A. (1948). *The commonsense psychiatry of Adolph Meyer.* New York: McGraw-Hill.

Malt, U. (1983). Classification and diagnosis of depression. *Acta Psychiatrica Scandinavica, 67*(Suppl. 302), 7–35.

Millon, T. (1981). *Disorders of personality. DSM-III: Axis II.* New York: Wiley.

Myers, J. K., Weissman, M. M., Tischler, G. L., Holzer, C. E., Leaf, P. J., Orvaschel, H., Anthony, J. C., Boyd, J. H., Burke, J. D., Kramer, J., & Stoltzman, R. (1984). Six-month prevalence of psychiatric disorders in three communities. *Archives of General Psychiatry, 41,* 959–967.

Nies, A., Robinson, D. S., Bartlett, D., & Lanborn, K. R. (1977). MAO inhibitors in clinical practice: Principles based on recent research. *Psychopharmacology Bulletin, 13,* 54–59.

Paykel, E. S. (1971). Classification of depressed patients: A cluster analysis derived grouping. *British Journal of Psychiatry, 118,* 275–288.

Perry, J. C. (1985). Depression in borderline personality disorder: Lifetime prevalence at interview and longitudinal course of symptoms. *American Journal of Psychiatry, 142,* 15–21.

Robert, R. E., & Vernon, S. W. (1982). Depression in the community: Prevalence and treatment. *Archives of General Psychiatry, 39,* 1407–1409.

Rosenthal, S. H. (1966). Changes in a population of hospitalized patients with affective disorders. *Archives of General Psychiatry, 6,* 671–681.

Rosenthal, T. L., Akiskal, H. S., Scott-Strauss, A., Rosenthal, R. H., & David, M. (1981). Familial and developmental factors in characterological depressions. *Journal of Affective Disorders, 3,* 183–192.

Rounsaville, B. J., Sholomskas, D., & Prusoff, B. (1980). Chronic mood disorders in depressed outpatients: Diagnosis and response to pharmacotherapy. *Journal of Affective Disorders, 2,* 73–88.

Roy, A., Sutton, M., & Pickar, D. (1985). Neuroendocrine and personality variables in dysthymic disorder. *American Journal of Psychiatry, 142,* 94–97.

Rush, A. J., Beck, A. T., Kovacs, M., & Hollon, S. (1977). Comparative efficacy of cognitive therapy and pharmacotherapy in the treatment of depressed outpatients. *Cognitive Therapy Research, 1,* 17–26.

Schildkraut, H. (1970). Differential diagnosis and treatment of depressive disorders, In *Neuropharmacology and the affective disorders* (pp. 49–57). Boston: Little, Brown.

Schildkraut, J. J., & Klein, D. F. (1975). The classification and treatment of depressive disorders. In R. I. Shader (Ed.), *Manual of psychiatric therapeutics* (pp. 39–61). Boston: Little, Brown.

Schneider, K. (1958). *Psychopathic personalities* (trans. M. W. Hamilton). London: Cassell.

Sinaikin, P. M. (1985). A clinically relevant guide to the differential diagnosis of depression. *Journal of Nervous and Mental Disease, 173,* 199–211.

Spitzer, R. L., Endicott, J., & Woodruff, R. A. (1977). Classification of mood disorders. In E. Usdin (Ed.), *Depression: Clinical, biological and psychological perspectives.* New York: Brunner/Mazel.

Spitzer, R. L., Williams, J. B. W., & Skodol, A. E. (1980). DSM-III: The major achievements and an overview. *American Journal of Psychiatry, 137,* 151–164.

Spitzer, R. L., Endicott, J., & Robins, E. (1985). *Research diagnostic criteria (RDC) for a selected group of functional disorders* (updated 3rd ed.). New York: New York State Psychiatric Institute.

Stewart, J. W., Quitkin, F. M., & McGrath, P. J. (1981). *Efficacy of desipramine in mildly depressed patients: 1. A test of predictions of treatment response.* Unpublished manuscript.

Stewart, J. W., McGrath, P. J., Liebowitz, M. R., Harrison, W., Quitkin, F., & Rabkin, J. G. (1985). Treatment outcome validation of DSM-III depressive subtypes: Clinical usefulness in outpatients with mild to moderate depression. *Archives of General Psychiatry, 42,* 1148–1153.

Stone, M. H. (1979). Contemporary shift of the borderline concept from a subschizophrenic disorder to a subaffective disorder. *Psychiatric Clinics of North America, 2,* 577–594.

Sullivan, H. S. (1953). *The interpersonal theory of psychiatry.* New York: W. W. Norton.

Thase, M. (1986). *Biological factors related to dysthymic disorder.* Presented at the National Institute of Mental Health Workshop on Dysthymic Disorder, Washington, DC.

Tyrer, P. (1979). Clinical use of monoamine oxidase inhibitors. In E. S. Paykel & A. Coppen (Eds.), *Psychopharmacology of affective disorders* (pp. 76–89). New York: Oxford University Press.

Ward, N. G., & Doerr, O. O. (1985). *Is skin conductance a sensitive and specific marker for depression?* Paper presented at the 40th Annual Meeting of the Society of Biological Psychiatry, Dallas.

Ward, N. G., Bloom, V. L., & Friedel, R. O. (1979). The effectiveness of tricyclic antidepressants in chronic depression. *Journal of Clinical Psychiatry, 40,* 49–52.

Weissman, M. M., & Klerman, G. L. (1977). The chronic depressive in the community: Unrecognized and poorly treated. *Comprehensive Psychiatry, 43,* 523–532.

Weissman, M. M., & Myers, J. K. (1978). Affective disorders in a U.S. urban community: The use of research diagnostic criteria in an epidemiological survey. *Archives of General Psychiatry, 35,* 1304–1311.

Weissman, M. M., Klerman, G. L., Prusoff, B. A., Sholomskas, D., & Padian, N. (1981). Depressed outpatients: Results one year after treatment with drugs and/or interpersonal psychotherapy. *Archives of General Psychiatry, 38,* 51–55.

Weissman, M. M., Gershon, E. S., Kidd, K., Prusoff, B. A., Leckman, J. F., Dibble, E., Hamovit, J., Thompson, D., Pauls, D. L., & Guroff, J. J. (1984). Psychiatric disorders in the relatives of probands with affective disorders. *Archives of General Psychiatry, 41,* 13–21.

Winokur, G., Behar, D., Vanvalkenburg, C., & Lowry, M. (1978). Is a familial definition of depression both feasible and valid? *Journal of Nervous and Mental Disease, 166,* 764–768.

Yerevanian, B. I., & Akiskal, H. S. (1979). "Neurotic," characterological, and dysthymic depressions. *Psychiatric Clinics of North America, 2,* 595–617.

8

Phobia

MINNA R. FYER

INTRODUCTION

Phobias were first included as a distinct diagnostic category in the first edition of the American Psychiatric Association's *Diagnostic and Statistical Manual of Mental Disorders* (DSM-I; APA, 1952) under the heading of *phobic reaction*. This category was retained but renamed in the second edition (DSM-II; APA, 1968) as *phobic neurosis*. Subtypes of phobic disorders did not appear until the third edition (DSM-III; APA, 1980), with simple phobia and social phobia each listed as separate categories. These have been retained in the revised third edition (DSM-III-R; APA, 1987).

This chapter covers the topics of simple phobia (also sometimes referred to as specific phobia) and social phobia. The intent is to provide an overview of etiological, diagnostic, and treatment issues for the clinician.

Although simple phobias are generally well recognized, the same is not true of social phobia. This disorder has received little attention in the United States, and awareness lags behind that of the other anxiety disorders. Social phobia is often overlooked and left untreated. For this reason, somewhat more extensive clinical description, differential diagnostic, and treatment sections are provided.

EPIDEMIOLOGY

The limited available information on the epidemiology of phobic disorders comes from two sources: studies of the general population and studies of clinical populations. Results of the five year, multicenter National Institute of Mental Health's epidemiological catchment-area study (Myers, Weissman, Tischler, Holzer, Leaf, Orvaschel, Anthony,

MINNA R. FYER • Department of Psychiatry, Cornell University Medical College, New York, New York 10021.

Boyd, Burke, Kramer, & Stoltzman, 1984) indicate a 6-month prevalence of simple phobias as high as 4.3% for males and 7.0% for females. For social phobia, the 6-month prevalence was 1.3% for males and 1.7% for females. Reich (1986), in a recent literature review, suggested that a reasonable estimate of the prevalence of social phobia is 1.5% and 2.5% for simple phobias, and that the ratio of females to males is at least 2 : 1.

In the reported clinical samples of phobic disorders, social phobia appears to be less common than panic disorder and agoraphobia, but to be as frequent as or more frequent than other specific phobias. Thus, in Marks's series (1970) 8% of the monosymptomatic phobics were social phobics, 60% were agoraphobics, 3% animal phobics, and 15% illness phobics; 14% had miscellaneous phobias. Other clinics have reported higher percentages of social phobia. Liebowitz, Gorman, Fyer, and Klein (1985) found social phobia to be the third most common disorder in their anxiety clinic (panic disorder and agoraphobia were the most common). Solyom, Ledwidge, and Solyom (1986) found that 25% of their phobic population suffered from social phobia. DiNardo, O'Brien, Barlow, Waddell, and Blanchard (1983) reported that 13.3% of phobic patients were social phobics, 13.3% had panic disorder, and 38.3% were agoraphobics.

Age of Onset

Both social and simple phobias appear to have an earlier age of onset than panic disorder and agoraphobia. The mean age of onset, as estimated by Reich (1986), for both simple and social phobias, is 17 years. In contrast, the mean age is 26 years for panic disorder and agoraphobia. Others (Amies, Gelder, & Shaw, 1983; Marks & Gelder, 1966; Öst, 1987; Shafar, 1976; Sheehan, Sheehan, & Minichiello, 1981; Thyer, 1985) have reported an age of onset between 15 and 21 years for social phobia and between 4 and 23 years for simple phobias (Lidell & Lyons, 1978; Marks & Gelder, 1966; Sheehan *et al.*, 1981; Thyer, Parrish, Curtis, Nesse, & Cameron, 1985) Öst (1987) recently studied the age of onset of a variety of simple phobias in a sample of 370 phobic patients: animal phobia had the earliest onset at 7 years, followed by blood phobia at 9 years, dental phobia at 12 years, social phobia at 16 years, claustrophobia at 20 years, and agoraphobia at 28 years. The DSM-III-R (APA, 1987) states that social phobia "often begins in late childhood or early adolescence," and that simple phobias vary in age of onset: "animal phobias nearly always begin in childhood; blood-injury in adolescence or early adulthood, while circumscribed phobias of heights, driving, claustrophia and air travel appear to begin most frequently in the fourth decade of life."

In summary, simple phobias appear at a variety of ages, most of which have not been well established. Social phobia clearly tends to appear during adolescence.

Gender

In his review, Reich (1986) suggested that a reasonable estimate is that phobic disorders are at least twice as frequent among women as among men. Marks (1987) reported that, in a series of clinical samples, the proportion of female social phobics was between 52% and 60%. Others (APA, 1987; Gorman & Gorman, 1987; Leibowitz, Campeas, Levin, Sandberg, Hollander, and Papp, 1987) have stated that, in clinical samples, social phobia is more common in men.

Social Phobia

As defined in the DSM-III-R (APA, 1987), the central feature of social phobia is "a persistent fear of one or more situations . . . in which the person is exposed to possible scrutiny by others and fears that he or she may do something or act in a way that will be humiliating or embarrassing." A variety of situations may be feared—some very specific and others more general. For instance, specific fears include those of public speaking, writing or eating in front of others, or urinating in public restrooms. More generalized fears apply to a variety of social and performance situations and include meeting strangers, going to parties, going on dates, and speaking to people in authority.

When confronting the phobic situation, the social phobic consistently suffers the immediate onset of physiological anxiety symptoms, most of which involve autonomic nervous system activity. These include palpitations, sweating, flushing, shortness of breath, tremor, and faintness. A feeling of panic and a desire to flee are also common. These symptoms usually persist until the individual is able to leave the phobic situation. Often, social phobics fear that the signs of their anxiety (e.g., flushing or tremor) will be noticed by others and will thus add to their embarrassment. Nevertheless, the person with social phobia is aware that his or her fears are excessive and unreasonable.

Individuals suffering from social phobia also experience profound anticipatory anxiety before entering a phobic situation. The usual response is avoidance, although a minority force themselves to endure phobic situations with intense anxiety. The DSM-III-R diagnosis is not given unless the avoidant behavior interferes with social or occupational functioning or causes "marked distress."

Functional impairment in social phobia varies widely, but it is important to note that this can be a severe and disabling disorder. In milder forms, an individual may have one specific fear that does not interfere much with his or her lifestyle. For instance, a successful engineer with an isolated fear of public speaking was generally asymptomatic. However, for 10 days before making a presentation to a potential client, he experienced insomnia, generalized anxiety, and intermittent palpitations.

On the other end of the spectrum is the individual with multiple, severe phobias, resulting in almost total social isolation and occupational dysfunction. For example, a computer programmer worked the night shift on a job well below his capabilities because it required minimal interaction with supervisors or co-workers. He feared any conversation, as he was certain he would say the wrong things and feel humiliated. Traveling to work at night—which reduced contact with others in the street—was endured with dread. He lived with his elderly parents and had virtually no other social interactions. In the DSM-III-R, the engineer would receive a diagnosis of social phobia, and the computer programmer would be social phobia–generalized type.

Alcohol and drug abuse are frequently associated with social phobia, with reports in a clinical series of rates of 20%–50% (Liebowitz *et al.*, 1985; Marks, 1987). Others (Gorman & Gorman, 1987; Heimbert & Barlow, 1988; Mullaney & Trippett, 1979; Smail, Stockwell, Canter, & Hodgson, 1984) have pointed out the high rate of social phobia and social anxiety among alcoholics, raising the possibility that alcohol is used as self-medication.

Depression is frequently found in patients with social phobia; the reported rates vary from 30% to 50% (Amies *et al.*, 1983; Liebowitz *et al.*, 1985; Munjack & Moss, 1981). One study (Amies *et al.*, 1983) reported a 14% incidence of "parasuicidal acts," but there are no other available data on suicidal behavior among social phobics.

There is very little information about the course of social phobia. The consensus at present is that social phobia has an early onset and that it is chronic and unremitting (Leibowitz *et al.*, 1985; Turner, Beidel, Dancu, & Keys, 1986).

SIMPLE PHOBIA

The DSM-III-R describes simple phobia as "A persistent fear of a circumscribed stimulus (object or situation) other than fear of having a panic attack (as in Panic Disorder) or of humiliation or embarrassment in certain social situations (as in Social Phobia)." Fears that are considered part of agoraphobia with or without a history of panic are also exluded from the definition. Examples of some common phobias include fear of animals, insects, heights (acrophobia), closed spaces (claustrophobia), blood/injury, air travel, water, sharp objects, and driving.

As in social phobia, exposure to the phobic stimulus is reliably accompanied by an immediate, intense anxiety response. Physiological symptoms of sweating, flushing, tremor, shortness of breath, faintness, and palpitations are common. The fear response has an automatic quality, with feelings of terror, apprehension, panic, and a desire to flee. The fear is nonetheless recognized as excessive or unreasonable, and the phobic individual often says, "I know there's nothing to be afraid of but . . ." Usually, the phobic stimulus is avoided; in some cases, it is endured with intense anxiety. To receive a DSM-III-R diagnosis of simple phobia, the anxiety or avoidant behavior must interfere significantly with earlier social or occupational functioning or must cause marked distress.

Because simple phobia involves the fear of a specific object, situation, or activity, individuals are generally asymptomatic unless confronted with the phobic stimulus or anticipating the possibility of this confrontation. The degree of disability is variable and depends on how much the phobia interferes with the individual's lifestyle. A person with a fear of air travel may not be able to accept a job promotion that requires such travel but may otherwise be asymptomatic. On the other hand, a city dweller with a fear of crowds may suffer from a great deal of anticipatory anxiety, as well as many episodes of phobic anxiety. His or her lifestyle may be severely restricted by a need to avoid crowds. Individuals whose phobias involve unpredictable stimuli (e.g., thunderstorms or birds) may also suffer from more anticipatory anxiety (Fyer & Klein, 1986).

DIFFERENTIAL DIAGNOSIS

Social Phobia

Social phobia can be distinguished from "normal" social or performance anxiety by the presence of acute, intense physiological symptoms (e.g., palpitations and sweating) that persist until the person leaves the situation. A person with "normal" anxiety about public speaking may experience physiological anxiety symptoms before and at the beginning of a speech, but these usually fade quickly. In contrast, the social phobic's anxiety symptoms continue unabated, or they escalate as the speech continues. A shy person may be uncomfortable meeting new people or going to a party, but unlike the social phobic, she or he will not actively avoid these situations.

In the DSM-III-R, the diagnosis of social phobia can be made in the presence of Axis I or Axis III diagnoses as long as the social fear is not related to the other diagnoses. This distinction may be important in trying to differentiate panic disorder with agoraphobia from social phobia. Panic-disordered patients often complain of social fears, demonstrate significant avoidance, and experience physiological anxiety symptoms. Although panic-disordered patients may fear appearing foolish while having a panic attack or may express a fear that panic will make it impossible for them to act in a socially appropriate way, they do not suffer from a generalized fear of humiliation. In addition, social phobics, unlike panic-disordered patients, do not experience unexpected, unprovoked panic attacks. In social phobia, anxieties are always related to the phobic social situation and the fear of scrutiny, embarrassment, or humiliation. It is, however, possible for the two disorders to coexist, in which case both diagnoses should be assigned.

Sometimes, it is difficult to distinguish social phobia from a simple phobia. A simple phobic and a social phobic may both fear traveling on buses. For the simple phobic, this fear may be related, for instance, to concerns about safety. For the social phobic, the fear relates to a concern that he or she will be subject to scrutiny by the other passengers and will embarrass or humiliate himself or herself.

Persons with paranoid disorders or paranoid personality disorder often avoid social interactions. However, this avoidance is based on suspicion and fear of harm from others. Most social phobics do not mistrust or fear harm from others; rather, they fear that they will humiliate themselves in front of others.

Patients with schizoid personality disorder are also socially avoidant. However, the schizoid person does not crave or miss social interaction. The social phobic, on the other hand, feels the need for social interaction but avoids it because of fear.

The distinction between avoidant personality disorder and social phobia is not entirely clear and is the subject of controversy (Greenberg & Stravynski, 1983; Heimberg & Barlow, 1988; Turner *et al.*, 1986). In the DSM-III-R, avoidant personality disorder is defined as "a pervasive pattern of social discomfort, fear of negative evaluation and timidity beginning in early adulthood," which must be accompanied by four out of seven other characteristics. One of these is "fears of being embarrassed by blushing, crying, or showing signs of anxiety in front of other people." Clearly, there is room for diagnostic overlap. The DSM-III-R states that social phobia may be a complication of avoidant personality disorder and that the two may coexist. The distinction between an isolated social phobia and avoidant personality disorder is fairly straightforward, but it may be harder to determine in a patient with severe, multiple social phobias (i.e., leading to the DSM-III-R diagnosis of social phobia–generalized type). Turner *et al.* (1986) found that subjects with the DSM-III avoidant personality disorder had poorer social skills and were more interpersonally sensitive than social phobic subjects. Heimberg, Hope, and Dodge (1987) reported physiological differences between generalized and specific social phobics. Deltito and Perugi (1986) described a case of social phobia and avoidant personality disorder in which both responded to treatment with a monoamine oxidase inhibitor. The distinction between social phobia and avoidant personality disorder and the distinctions between individuals with different degrees of social phobia (i.e., generalized vs. specific) clear require further investigation.

Simple Phobia

Simple phobia is essentially a diagnosis given to any individual suffering from a specific phobia that is not a social phobia or that is not related to panic disorder and agoraphobia. Thus, it is a residual category. In differentiating simple phobias from panic-disorder-related phobias, it is essential to remember that simple phobics do not experience unexpected, unprovoked panic attacks. By definition, anxiety in simple phobia is stimulus-bound. However, simple phobia and panic disorder with or without agoraphobia do coexist. Fears and avoidance related to a trauma resulting in posttraumatic stress disorder are not considered simple phobias. Similarly, patients with obsessive-compulsive disorder may be phobic of and may avoid certain situations related to their obsessional beliefs and behaviors. Again, these are considered not simple phobias, but part of the obsessive-compulsive disorder.

ETIOLOGY

Although there are a number of hypotheses, the etiology of phobic disorders remains unexplained. At present, all of the theories have significant problems. A brief presentation of some of the major theories follows.

Conditioning and Learning Theory

According to this theory, a phobia develops when the phobic object or situation (the neutral conditioned stimulus) becomes paired with an aversive object or situation (the unconditioned stimulus). Subsequently, because of this pairing, the phobic object (conditioned stimulus) evokes a negative reaction (conditioned response) even in the absence of the aversive situation (unconditioned stimulus). Thus, if cats become associated with illness, the individual may subsequently fear cats, even though, in actuality, there is no possibility of illness resulting from a contact with cats.

The major criticisms of the learning-theory approach have been well reviewed and summarized (Fyer & Klein, 1986; Sturgis & Scott, 1984). In good part, these criticisms stem from the fact that conditioning theory does not explain several clinical observations about phobias. First, this theory cannot account for the fact that most phobias do not develop out of traumatic experiences, that is, a pairing of the conditioned and the unconditioned stimulus. Furthermore, in laboratory work (Kamen, 1969; Seligman, 1968), six to eight pairings of the conditioned and unconditioned stimuli are needed for a conditioned response. This theory also fails to explain why certain phobias are more common than others and the fact that there are many situations in which people are repeatedly exposed to traumatic and dangerous events without becoming phobic. Finally, whereas clinical phobias are not easily extinguished, laboratory-induced phobic responses (conditioned avoidance), by contrast, are easily distinguished.

Genetic Theory

There are no family studies of social or simple phobias. Torgerson (1979) looked at socially phobic features in 95 pairs of monozygotic and dizygotic twins and found that the monozygotes were significantly more concordant. Carey and Gottesman (1981) studied 21 mono- and dizygotic twin pairs in which the index twin had a diagnosis of "phobic neurosis." The concordance for phobic symptoms or features was 88% in the monozygotes and 38% in the dizygotes. Both of these studies are consistent with a familial contribution to phobic disorders; however, much more study is needed to assess this issue. In particular, studies using current diagnostic practices and adoption studies would both be useful (Fyer & Klein, 1986).

Preparedness Theory

The preparedness theory holds that there is a continuum of stimuli (objects and situations) from "most conditionable" to "least conditionable," based on natural selection (Seligman, 1971). Those stimuli that are very conditionable would correspond to situations or objects that were dangerous in an earlier, pretechnological setting (Seligman & Hager, 1972). For these situations or objects, associations are "prepared" and therefore are quickly acquired and difficult to extinguish. A phobia develops when a "prepared" stimulus becomes paired with a negative outcome. Supporting this theory are data from both animal and human analogue studies (Sturgis & Scott, 1984). However, the theory fails to explain certain clinical observations. For instance, it does not explain the fact that even phobias to "unprepared" stimuli are difficult to extinguish. In a study of clinical outcome, DeSilva, Rachman, and Seligman (1977) failed to reveal any differences between individuals with phobias to more-or-less prepared stimuli.

Cognitive Theory

In cognitive theory, a phobia is postulated to occur after an individual is informed or taught that a particular situation or object is dangerous. The person then reiterates this thought of anger to herself or himself each time she or he either contemplates or confronts the phobic object or situation. The very few studies of cognitive factors in phobias do suggest that there may be a cognitive component in phobic anxiety (Heimberg & Barlow, 1988; Sturgis & Scott, 1984).

Psychoanalytic Theory

In his early work, Freud explained phobias as being physiologically induced and as being a result of undischarged libidinal tension (see Strachey, 1961). Later on, based on his work with Little Hans (Strachey, 1961), Freud proposed a psychological theory of phobic symptoms. In this formulation, the individual is faced with libidinal and/or aggressive impulses whose gratification evokes intrapsychic conflict and/or external danger. These are displaced onto an external object which becomes the phobic stimulus, which is feared and avoided. As an example in Freud's famous case of Little Hans, the boy allegedly was sexually attracted to his mother but was jealous of his father and feared his father's anger (fear of castration). He also felt torn between his desire for his mother and his love and respect for his father. Such strong feelings—sexual, angry, and fearful—were displaced onto horses, which he feared but which he could avoid.

Social Phobia

Although the data on treatment efficacy in social phobia are sparse, there are a number of promising recent developments. Pharmacotherapy is discussed first, and then the psychosocial therapy of social phobia.

Pharmacotherapy

Most attempts to treat social phobia with medications are very recent. The lack of previous interest was explained by Liebowitz *et al.* (1987) as being due to the fact that social anxiety is often viewed as normal, and that severe social anxiety has been viewed as a personality disorder for which pharmacotherapy often is considered futile. Currently, there is interest in a possible role for beta-blockers, monoamine oxidase inhibitors, benzodiazepines, triazolobenzodiazepines, and tricyclic antidepressants in the treatment of social phobia. We discuss each of these separately.

Beta-Blockers. Interest in the use of beta-blockers in social phobia was generated by reports of their success in treating performance anxiety in normals. Leibowitz *et al.* (1985) and Gorman and Gorman (1987) have reviewed these studies and have concluded that acute beta-blocker treatment appears to decrease anxiety symptoms and to enhance performance. Furthermore, beta-blockers seem to be most effective in those individuals who experience the greatest degree of anxiety (Gorman & Gorman, 1987).

There are only two reported clinical trials of beta-blockers in patients with social phobia. Falloon, Lloyd, and Harpin (1981) studied 16 social phobics. Half received propanolol and half received placebo. All received social skills training. However, all patients improved, and there were no differences between the propanalol and placebo groups. This study was limited by small sample size and the confounding presence of unstandardized social-skills training.

Gorman, Liebowitz, Fyer, Campeas, and Klein (1985) conducted an open trial of atenolol in 10 patients with DSM-III–diagnosed social phobia. Atenolol was started at 50 mg per day, with a maximum dose of 100 mg per day. The subjects had social phobias of varying severity. None was depressed at the time of the study, although half had a history of depression and half reported alcohol abuse. Five of the ten patients were markedly improved and another four were moderately improved at the end of the 6-week trial. One patient experienced no improvement. In general, the medication was well tolerated, and the side effects were minimal.

The contradictory results of these studies and the absence of larger, more systematic trials leave the efficacy of beta-blockers in social phobia an open question. However, larger scale, controlled clinical trials are currently under way.

Monoamine Oxidase Inhibitors. Studies conducted in the 1970s using monoamine oxidase inhibitors (MAOIs) to treat groups of mixed phobics suggested their possible efficacy in the treatment of social phobia. These studies have been reviewed elsewhere (Gorman & Gorman, 1987; Leibowitz *et al.*, 1985). Unfortunately, none of these studies reported separate results for subjects with social phobia.

Further interest in the use of MAOIs for social phobia was generated by observations of their effects on depressives. Liebowitz *et al.* (1985) cited three studies (Liebowitz & Klein, 1979; Leibowitz, Quitkin, Steward, McGrath, Harrison, Rabkin, Tricamo, Markowitz, & Klein, 1984; Nies, Howard, & Robinson, 1982) in which phenelzine was useful in decreasing "interpersonal sensitivity" in patients with depressive syndromes. In two of these studies, phenelzine was superior to tricyclic antidepressants in this regard.

Liebowitz, Fyer, Gorman, Campeas, and Levin (1986) conducted the only available study—an open trial—of phenelzine in subjects with DSM-III–diagnosed social phobia. Eleven subjects received phenelzine (up to 90 mg per day) for 8 weeks. Seven experienced marked improvement and four moderate improvement.

Although the MAOIs appear to be promising for the treatment of social phobia, controlled studies are needed to establish their efficacy. One such study is under way, and the preliminary results suggest that phenelzine may be helpful in up to 70% of cases (M. Liebowitz, personal communication, 1987, as cited by Roy-Byrne & Katon, 1987).

Benzodiazepines and Triazolobenzodiazepines. We are aware of only two reports of the use of benzodiazepines and triazolobenzodiazepines in social phobics. McNair, Frankenthaler, Czerlinsky, White, Sasson, and Fisher (1982) reported that acute administration of diazepam reduced anxiety experienced during a simulated public-speaking challenge. Lydiard, Laraia, Howell, and Ballenger (1988) reported on four cases of socially phobic patients treated with alprazolam (2–8 mg po qd). All patients experienced moderate to marked improvement.

Tricyclic Antidepressants. There are only a few studies of tricyclic antidepressant treatment in social phobia. All used clomipramine, which is available in the United States only as an investigational drug. All three studies (Beaumont, 1977; Gungras, 1977; Pecknold, McClure, Appeltauer, Slan, & Wrzesinski 1982) also used mixed populations of agoraphobics, social phobics, and those with other phobic disorders. All reported improvement. However, the results with social phobics were not reported separately, so that interpretation of these data is limited. There is one recent case report (Benca, Matuzas, & Al-Sadir, 1986) of two patients with social phobia who improved markedly on imipramine. To date, there is little evidence to suggest a role for tricyclic antidepressants in the treatment of social phobia, but this area requires further investigation.

Psychosocial Treatments

Psychosocial treatments of social phobia are numerous and have been reviewed extensively (Emmelkemp, 1982; Heimberg & Barlow, 1988; Liebowitz *et al.*, 1985; Marks, 1981; Ost, Jerremalm, & Johansson, 1980; Stravynski & Shahar, 1983). Many of the studies in this area have been conducted either on heterogeneous populations of "socially anxious" individuals or on nonclinical populations. Methodological limitations, such as lack of operationalized treatments, reliable outcome measures, and control treatments, make it difficult to interpret the results and their implications for the treatment of social phobia. Although a handful of studies have involved clearly defined social phobics, no one treatment or combination of treatments has received adequate study to support its definitive efficacy (Fyer & Klein, 1986; Heimberg & Barlow, 1988). The most frequently studied treatments are described below, along with what, if anything, is known about the efficacy of their use for rigorously defined social phobia.

Graded Exposure Treatments. In graded exposure treatments, the therapist and the patient work first to establish a hierarchy (from least to most anxiety-provoking) of situations related to the specific phobic stimulus. The patient is then helped to confront these situations one at a time. When one level of the hierarchy is mastered (when the patient does not experience anxiety on exposure to the situation), the patient moves on to the next level. Exposure can either be imaginal or *in vivo*. In imaginal exposure treatment, the patient imagines the situation, which may be enhanced when the therapist also describes the feared situation. *In vivo* treatments involve the patient in actually entering the feared situations. *In vivo* exposure treatments may also involve participant modeling.

One widely used form of graded imaginal exposure is systematic desensitization. After a hierarchy of feared situations has been constructed, the patient is taught the method of deep muscle relaxation. The patient enters deep relaxation and then imagines the first situation in the hierarchy, stopping the image on experiencing any anxiety; she or he then relaxes until again in a state of deep relaxation and then imagines the situation again. When the stimulus has been imagined twice without anxiety, the patient moves on to the next item in the hierarchy. This procedure is continued until the complete hierarchy has been mastered.

Social skills training combines a number of techniques in a supportive, educational approach aimed at changing behavior and decreasing social anxiety. This treatment is often conducted in a group setting. The therapist models the behavior and the patient rehearses. The patient is also given positively framed feedback and social support.

In cognitive restructuring, the treatment goal is to alter the maladaptive thinking that underlies social phobia or anxiety. This is accomplished by teaching the patient to directly examine her or his cognitions and to challenge the assumptions on which they are based. This process is often aided by the use of a diary in which the patient records dysfunctional thoughts. After identifying and examining these cognitions, the patient is taught to use more accurate and adaptive cognitions.

Research Findings. As mentioned above, data to support the treatment efficacy in clinical populations of social phobics are sparse, and interpretation of the results is difficult. We briefly present here some of the clinically relevant data, although none of the studies is conclusive.

Emmelkamp (1982) reviewed work with systematic desensitization and concluded that it was helpful to nonclinical populations but not as effective for clinical subjects. Biran (1981) treated patients who were afraid of writing in front of others with exposure or exposure plus cognitive restructuring and found that both resulted in improvement in behavior and subjective fear. On follow-up, the behavioral gains had been maintained, but there was a recurrence of some subjective anxiety. Butler, Cullington, Munby, Amies, and Gelder (1984) studied 45 social phobics. Of these, 30 received exposure-based treatments (15 exposure and 15 exposure plus anxiety-management training), and 15 were in a waiting-list control group. Both exposure-based treatments resulted in significant improvement; the controls experienced no change. Exposure, however, had no significant, lasting effect on the fear of negative evaluation (Butler, 1985).

Studies of ill-defined populations of "socially anxious" individuals have yielded contradictory data about the relative value of social skills training and systematic desensitization. These treatment studies have been well reviewed elsewhere (Heimberg & Barlow, 1988). There are also a few comparison studies of patients with social phobia. Shaw

(1979) compared the treatment of social phobics with systematic desensitization, social skills training, and flooding. All were helpful, but there were no differences in the three treatment groups. Stravynski and Shaher, (1983) compared social skills training with social skills training plus cognitive restructuring. Again, both treatments were helpful. Some have suggested that social skills training may be more helpful to those patients who have the greatest social-skill deficits, whereas it may be less helpful to those subjects whose skills are adequate but who become immobilized by anxiety. However, convincing data are lacking.

There are very few studies of the cognitive treatment of clinical populations of social phobics. Based on their reviews, both Biran (1982) and Stravynski and Shaher (1983) suggested that cognitive restructuring does not increase the effectiveness of exposure or social skills training. In the few studies using cognitive restructuring alone, positive results have been obtained (Emmelkamp, 1982; Jerrelmalm, 1986; Meichenbaum 1977). Heimberg and Barlow (1988) recently reported work on a 12-week cognitive-behavioral group-treatment of social phobia that combined cognitive restructuring and graded exposure. In a case series, they found that all seven social phobics showed significant decreases in anxiety (subjective and behavioral). In a comparison with a control condition using education and support in a group setting, 75% of patients treated with cognitive-behavioral treatment were improved, compared with 45% of control subjects.

In summary, a number of psychosocial treatments appear to be of some benefit to ''socially anxious,'' nonclinical populations. The few available studies suggest that this may also be the case for clinical populations of social phobics. However, treatment efficacy has not been established, and systematic studies are needed. These promising treatments obviously deserve further investigation.

Simple Phobia

There is wide-ranging agreement that exposure-based behavioral treatment is most effective for simple phobias. There are many forms of exposure treatment, but none has been clearly demonstrated to be superior. The more commonly studied exposure-based treatments are described here; a discussion of some of the current clinically relevant research issues follows.

Systematic desensitization has been described above under the treatment of social phobia. The method is the same for simple phobia.

Flooding (prolonged *in vivo* exposure) is an ungraded exposure treatment in which the patient is continuously exposed to his or her most anxiety-provoking stimulus until the anxiety level begins to decline. The rationale is that such exposure causes habituation of the phobic anxiety. Flooding can be either imaginal or *in vivo*. In imaginal flooding, the patient imagines the phobic situation, and in *in vivo* flooding, the patient is actually exposed to the phobic situation. In either case, unlike in graded exposure, the initial anxiety experienced is quite intense. Marks (1987) found that anxiety began to decrease after 1 hour of exposure, and they therefore recommended this as the minimum time for a flooding session. In their review, Sturgis and Scott (1984) suggested that the therapist allow 2–5 hours for a flooding session. Clearly, flooding is appropriate only for certain patients who are well motivated and understand the treatment rationale. Patients with medical conditions that might be exacerbated by anxiety should not undergo this form of treatment.

Reinforced practice is a graded *in vivo* exposure treatment in which the aim is to reshape behavior through a series of successive approximations (O'Brien, 1981). First, a hierarchy of anxiety-provoking situations related to the phobic stimulus is constructed. The patient is then instructed to approach the phobic stimulus and to stop and/or withdraw whenever his or her anxiety level becomes too uncomfortable. After resting, the patient again approaches the stimulus. The therapist provides positive reinforcement and accurate feedback about the level of improvement. This treatment combines graded repeated practice, therapeutic support and instructions, feedback, and reinforcement (Leitenberg & Callahan, 1973).

Participant modeling is also a graded-exposure technique. The first step is the construction of a hierarchy of situations related to the phobic stimulus, from least to most anxiety-provoking. In an individual setting, the therapist approaches the phobic stimulus, and then the patient approaches the stimulus herself or himself. In a group setting, other group members may also participate in modeling. In some cases, films of modeled behavior are used. Throughout the treatment, the subject's anxiety level is maintained at moderate to low levels. The process is continued until the patient has come in contact with the phobic stimulus without anxiety. In a variant of this method, referred to as *covert modeling,* the patient imagines the model (often the therapist) progressively approaching the phobic stimulus.

These and other exposure techniques result in significant improvement in most simple phobias. However, a number of issues remain unresolved. There is controversy about whether *in vivo* exposure is more effective than imaginal exposure (Sturgis & Scott, 1984). Clearly, a times, imaginal exposure is more practical than *in vivo* exposure. Many issues concerning exposure treatment remain unknown: the optimal length of exposure, the optimal interval between exposures, and the long-term outcome of exposure treatment. Probably, long exposures are better than short ones (Stein & Marks, 1973), but again, clear-cut evidence is lacking. There are no data to indicate whether particular treatments are more effective for particular phobias or patients with specific clinical characteristics. Further research is needed to address these questions.

SUMMARY

In this chapter, the outpatient treatment of phobia (social and simple) has been described. First to be considered were the epidemiological findings, deriving from studies of the general population and clinical populations. This consideration was followed by a discussion of the clinical description of social phobia and simple phobia, focusing on DSM-III-R criteria. Next, the differential diagnosis of social phobia from normal "social anxiety" and of simple phobia from social phobia, panic disorder, and agoraphobia was outlined. Etiological hypotheses for both types of phobic disorders were examined in terms of conditioning and learning theory, genetic theory, preparedness-of-prepotency theory, cognitive theory, and psychoanalytic theory. Finally, treatments (pharmacotherapy and psychosocial treatments for social phobia) were considered, with the conclusion that those strategies showing promise require long-term, controlled evaluations. With respect to the treatment of simple phobia, variants of exposure treatment appear to be quite effective. However, data indicating which particular treatments are most effective for which particular phobias must be gathered.

American Psychiatric Association. (1952). *Diagnostic and statistical manual of mental disorders* (1st ed.; DSM-I). Washington, DC: Author.

American Psychiatric Association. (1968). *Diagnostic and statistical manual of mental disorders* (2nd ed.; DSM-II). Washington, DC: Author.

American Psychiatric Association. (1980). *Diagnostic and statistical manual of mental disorders* (3rd ed.; DSM-III). Washington, DC: Author.

American Psychiatric Association. (1987). *Diagnostic and statistical manual of mental disorders* (3rd ed., Rev.). Washington, DC: Author.

Amies, P. L., Gelder, M. G., & Shaw, P. M. (1983). Social phobia: A comparative clinical study. *British Journal of Psychiatry, 142,* 174–179.

Beaumont, G. (1977). A large open multicentre trial of clomipramine (Anafranil) in the management of phobic disorders. *Journal of Internal Medicine Research, 5,* 116–123.

Benca, R., Matuzas, W., & Al-Sadir, J. (1986). Social phobia, MVP, and response to imipramine. *Journal of Clinical Psychopharmacology, 6,* 50–51.

Butler, G. (1985). Exposure as a treatment for social phobia: Some instructive difficulties. *Behavior Research and Therapy, 23,* 651–657.

Butler, G., Cullington, A., Munby, M., Amies, P., & Gelder, M. (1984). Exposure and anxiety management in the treatment of social phobia. *Journal of Consulting and Clinical Psychology, 4,* 642–650.

Carey, G., & Gottesman, I. (1981). Twin and family studies of anxiety, phobic and obsessive disorders. In D. F. Klein & J. G. Rabkin (Eds.), *Anxiety: New research and changing concepts* (pp. 117–136). New York: Raven Press.

Deltito, J. A., & Perugi, C. (1986). A case of social phobia with avoidant personality disorder treated with monoamine oxidase inhibitors. *Comprehensive Psychiatry, 27,* 255–256.

DeSilva, P., Rachman, S., & Seligman, M. E. P. (1977). Prepared phobias and obsessions: Therapeutic outcome. *Behavior Research and Therapy, 15,* 65–77.

DiNardo, P. A., O'Brien, G. T., Barlow, D. H., Waddell, M. T., & Blanchard, E. B. (1983). Reliability of DSM-III anxiety disorder categories using a new structured interview. *Archives of General Psychiatry, 40,* 1070–1074.

Emmelkamp, P. M. G. (1982). *Phobic and obsessive-compulsive disorder: Theory research and practice.* New York: Plenum Press.

Falloon, I. R. H., Lloyd, G. G., & Harpin, R. E. (1981). Real life rehearsal with nonprofessional therapists. *Journal of Nervous and Mental Disease, 169,* 387–398.

Freud, S. (1961a). The analysis of a phobia in a 5-year-old boy. In J. Strachey (Ed.), *The standard edition of the complete works of Sigmund Freud* (Vol. 10). Longon: Hogarth Press.

Freud, S. (1961b). Obsessions and phobias. In J. Strachey (Ed.), *The standard edition of the complete works of Sigmund Freud* (Vol. 3). London: Hogarth Press.

Fyer, A. J., & Klein, D. F. (1986). Agoraphobia, social phobia, and simple phobia.

Gorman, J. M., & Gorman, L. K. (1987). Drug treatment of social phobia. *Journal of Affective Disorders, 13,* 183–192.

Gorman, J. M., Liebowitz, M. R., Fyer, A. J., Campeas, R., & Klein, D. F. (1985). Treatment of social phobia with atenolol. *Journal of Clinical Psychopharmacology, 5,* 298–301.

Greenberg, G., & Stravynski, A. (1983). Social phobia. *British Journal of Psychiatry, 143,* 526.

Gungras, M. (1977). An uncontrolled trial of clomipramine (Anafranil) in the treatment of phobic and obsessional states in general practice. *Journal of Internal Medicine Research, 5,* 111–115.

Heimberg, R. G., & Barlow, D. H. (1988). Psychosocial treatments for social phobia. *Psychosomatics, 29,* 27–37.

Heimberg, R. G., Hope, D. A., Dodge, C. S. (1987). *DSM-III-R subtypes of social phobia: Comparison of generalized social phobics and public speaking phobics.* Unpublished manuscript.

Jerremalm, A., Jansson, L., & Ost, L. G. (1986). Cognitive and physiological reactivity and the effects of different behavioral methods in the treatment of social phobia. *Behavior Research and Therapy, 24,* 171–180.

Kamen, L. J. (1969). Predictability, surprise, attention and conditioning. In B. A. Campbell & R. M. Church (Eds.), *Punishment and aversive behavior.* New York: Appleton-Century-Crofts.

Leitenberg, H., & Callahan, E. J. (1973). Reinforced practice and reduction of different kinds of fear in adults and children. *Behavior Research and Therapy, 11,* 19–30.

Lidell, A., & Lyons, M. (1978). Thunderstorm phobias. *Behaviour Research and Therapy, 16,* 306–308.
Liebowitz, M. R., & Klein, D. F. (1979). Hysteroid dysphoria. *The Psychiatric Clinics of North America, 2,* 555–575.
Liebowitz, M. R., Quitkin, F. M., Steward, J. W., McGrath, P. J., Harrison, W., Rabkin, J., Tricamo, E., Markowitz, J. S., & Klein, D. F. (1984). Phenelzine versus imipramine in atypical depression: A preliminary report. *Archives of General Psychiatry, 41,* 669–677.
Liebowitz, M. R., Gorman, J. M., Fyer, A. J., & Klein, D. F. (1985). Social phobia: Review of a neglected anxiety disorder. *Archives of General Psychiatry, 42,* 729–736.
Liebowitz, M. R., Fyer, A. J., Gorman, J. M., Campeas, R. C., & Levin, A. (1986). Phenelzine in social phobia. *Journal of Clinical Psychopharmacology, 6,* 93–98.
Liebowitz, M. R., Campeas, R., Levin, A., Sandberg, D., Hollander, E., & Papp, L. (1987). Pharmacotherapy of social phobia: A condition distinct from panic attacks. *Psychosomatics, 28,* 305–308.
Lydiard, R. B., Laraia, M. T., Howell, E. F., & Ballenger, J. C. (1988). Alprazolam in the treatment of social phobia. *Journal of Clinical Psychiatry, 49,* 17–19.
Marks, I. M. (1969). *Fears and phobias.* London: Academic Press.
Marks, I. M. (1970). The classification of phobic disorders. *British Journal of Psychiatry, 116,* 377–386.
Marks, I. M. (1978). Behavioral psychotherapy of adult neuroses. In A. E. Bergen & S. Garfield (Eds.), *Handbook of psychotherapy and behavior change.* New York: Wiley.
Marks, I. M. (1981). *Cure and care of neuroses.* New York: Wiley.
Marks, I. M., & Gelder, M. G. (1966). Different ages of onset in varieties of phobias. *American Journal of Psychiatry, 123,* 218–221.
McNair, D. M., Frankenthaler, L. M., Czerlinsky, T., White, T. W., Sasson, S., & Fisher, S. (1982). Simulated public speaking as a model of clinical anxiety. *Psychopharmacology, 77,* 7–10.
Meichenbaum, D. (1977). *Cognitive behavior modification.* New York: Plenum Press.
Mullaney, J. A., & Trippett, C. J. (1979). Alcohol dependence and phobias: Clinical description and relevance. *British Journal of Psychiatry, 135,* 563–573.
Munjack, D. J., & Moss, H. B. (1981). Affective disorder and alcoholism in families of agoraphobics. *Archives of General Psychiatry, 38,* 869–871.
Myers, J. K., Weissman, M. M., Tischler, G. L., Holzer, C. E., Leaf, P. J., Orvaschel, H., Anthony, J. C., Boyd, J. H., Burke, J. D., Kramer, M., & Stoltzman, R. (1984). Six-month prevalence of psychiatric disorders in three communities: 1980 to 1982. *Archives of General Psychiatry, 41,* 959–967.
Nies, A., Howard, D., & Robinson, D. S. (1982). Antianxiety effects of MAO inhibitors. In R. J. Mathew (Ed.), *The biology of anxiety* (pp. 123–133). New York: Brunner/Mazel.
O'Brien, G. T. (1981). Clinical treatment of specific phobias. In M. Mavissakalian & D. H. Barlow (Eds.), *Phobia: Psychological and pharmacological treatment* (pp. 63–102). New York: Guilford Press.
Ost, L. G. (1987). Age of onset in different phobias. *Journal of Abnormal Psychology, 96,* 223–239.
Ost, L. G., Jerremalm, A., & Johansson, J. (1980). Individual response patterns and the effects of different behavioral methods in the treatment of social phobia. *Behaviour Research and Therapy, 19,* 1–16.
Pecknold, J. C., McClure, D. J., Appeltauer, L., Slan, T., & Wrzesinski, L. (1982). Does tryptophan potenitate clomipramine in the treatment of agoraphobic and social phobic patients. *British Journal of Psychiatry, 140,* 484–490.
Regier, D. A., & Burke, J. D. Psychiatric disorders in the community: The epidemiologic catchment area study. In R. Hales & A. Frances (Eds.), *Annual review* (Vol. 6, pp. 610–624). Washington, DC: APA Press.
Reich, J. (1986). The epidemiology of anxiety. *Journal of Nervous and Mental Disease, 174,* 129–136.
Roy-Byrne, R., & Katon, W. (1987). An update on treatment of the anxiety disorders. *Hospital and Community Psychiatry, 38,* 835–841.
Seligman, M. E. P. (1968). Chronic fear produced by unpredictable shock. *Journal of Comparative Physiological Psychology, 66,* 402–411.
Seligman, M. E. P. (1971). Phobias and preparedness. *Behavior Therapy, 2,* 307–320.
Seligman, M. E. P., & Hager, J. (1972). *The biological boundaries of learning.* New York: Appleton-Century-Crofts.
Shafar, S. (1976). Aspects of phobic illness: A study of 90 personal cases. *British Journal of Medical Psychology, 49,* 221–236.
Shaw, P. (1979). A comparison of three behaviour therapies in the treatment of social phobia. *British Journal of Psychiatry, 134,* 620–623.
Sheehan, D. V., Sheehan, K. E., & Minichiello, W. E. (1981). Age of onset of phobic disorders: A reevaluation. *Comprehensive Psychiatry, 22,* 544–553.

Smail, P., Stockwell, T., Canter, S., & Hodgson, R. (1984). Alcohol dependence and phobic anxiety states: I.A. prevalence study. *British Journal of Psychiatry, 155,* 53–57.

Solyom, L., Ledwidge, B., & Solyom, C. (1986). Delineating social phobia. *British Journal of Psychiatry, 149,* 464–470.

Stein, R., & Marks, I. (1973). Brief and prolonged flooding: A comparison trial in agoraphobic patients. *Archives of General Psychiatry, 28,* 270–276.

Stravynski, A., & Shaher, A. (1983). The treatment of social dysfunction in nonpsychotic outpatients: A review. *Journal of Nervous and Mental Disease, 171,* 721–728.

Sturgis, E. T., & Scott, R. (1984). Simple phobia. In S. M. Turner (Ed.), *Behavioral theories and treatment of anxiety* (pp. 91–141). New York: Plenum Press.

Thyer, B. A., Parrish, R. T., Curtis, G. C., Nesse, R. M., & Cameron, O. G. (1985). Ages of onset of DSM-III anxiety disorders. *Comprehensive Psychiatry, 26,* 113–121.

Torgersen, S. (1979). The nature and origin of common phobic fears. *British Journal of Psychiatry, 134,* 343–351.

Turner, S. M., Beidel, D. C., Dancu, C. V., & Keys, D. J. (1986). Psychopathology of social phobia and comparison to avoidant personality disorder. *Journal of Abnormal Psychology, 95,* 389–394.

9

Panic Disorder

DAVID V. SHEEHAN AND B. ASHOK RAJ

INTRODUCTION

Panic disorder was first defined by Spitzer, Endicott, and Robbins (1975) in the early editions of their research diagnostic criteria (RDC). It was later included in the *Diagnostic and Statistical Manual,* third edition (DSM-III), of the American Psychiatric Association (APA, 1980). Whereas the early definition of panic disorder required at least six panic attacks within a 6-week period for a definite diagnosis to be made, the DSM-III modified these criteria to require only three panic attacks within any 3-week period. Each of these attacks was required to have at least 4 of 12 characteristic symptoms. Though the condition itself had existed long before the DSM-III, it was given separate status as a diagnostic entity based on the research findings of Donald Klein (1964, 1967). Klein's central observation in these papers was that there was a type of anxiety disorder that was particularly sensitive to imipramine, a tricyclic antidepressant. This tricyclic-sensitive anxiety disorder was characterized by spontaneous panic attacks and often failed to respond to minor tranquilizers. Such observations led the DSM-III committee to make a distinction between panic disorder and generalized anxiety disorder. The underlying assumption in making this distinction was that panic disorder is responsive to tricyclic antidepressants and not to minor tranquilizers, whereas generalized anxiety disorder is sensitive to minor tranquilizers but not to tricyclics. This observation was reinforced by a study by McNair and Kahn (1981), which found that imipramine tended to be more effective than chlordiazepoxide in the treatment of agoraphobia. Subsequently, Sheehan (1982a) and Chouinard, Annable, and Fontaine (1982) independently reported that alprazolam, a triazolobenzodiazepine, was effective in the treatment of panic disorder. This finding suggested that benzodiazepines as a class might be effective in the treatment of

DAVID V. SHEEHAN and B. ASHOK RAJ • Department of Psychiatry and Behavioral Medicine, University of South Florida College of Medicine, Tampa, Florida 33613.

panic disorder and at the same time offered a treatment for this condition that was quicker, safer, and easier to tolerate than the earlier recommended treatments with tricyclic antidepressants and monoamine oxidase inhibitors. The finding of a quicker and safer treatment for this condition proved to be a significant stimulus to research on this disorder over the following several years and gave rise to the World Wide Panic Project sponsored by the Upjohn Company, from which many new findings and more precise descriptions of panic disorder emerged. Further, Sheehan (1982b) articulated the emerging idea in the panic disorder literature that we should revise our view of panic disorder as a psychological problem in favor of a medical-illness model for this disorder. He suggested that, in contrast to stress-related situational anxiety, panic disorder appears to be associated with biological abnormalities in the central nervous system to which there is a genetic vulnerability. This new view (which was a logical outcome of the earlier work of Klein) had important implications for treatment and research. Attempts to test the strengths and weaknesses of this hypothesis guided much of the research effort in panic disorder in the 1980s.

EPIDEMIOLOGY

Anxiety and phobic disorders are the most prevalent disabling psychiatric disorders in the United States. In 1978, the President's Commission on Mental Health identified gaps in our knowledge on the prevalence of psychiatric disorders. To bridge these gaps, a large-scale, multicentered 5-year study was carried out by the National Institute of Mental Health. This study, called the ECA (Epidemiological Catchment Area) study, identified anxiety and phobic disorders as the nation's most prevalent disabling psychiatric disorders. Even with the use of conservative and precise diagnostic criteria, it identified the lifetime prevalence of anxiety and phobic disorders at 8.3% of the general adult population (Robbins, Helzer, & Weisman, 1984). Seven percent of the adult population over 18 suffers from a phobic disorder alone. Thus, these disorders are more common than depressive disorders, alcohol and drug abuse, and schizophrenia. Among women phobia ranked as the number one psychiatric disorder in all age groups (see Table 1).

Within the heterogeneous group of anxiety disorders, panic disorder has a lifetime

Table 1. Lifetime Prevalence of Anxiety Disorders[a]

Disorders	Number affected[b] (millions)	Percentage of population	Percentage receiving treatment
Anxiety/phobic	14.4	8.3	23.0
Phobic	12.2	7.0	
Alcohol/drug abuse	11.1	6.4	18.0
Affective disorders	10.4	6.0	32.0
Schizophrenia	1.7	1.0	53.0
Antisocial	1.6	0.9	39.0

[a]Adapted from Robbins *et al.* (1984).
[b]Based on 1984 census statistics: 173.99 million aged 18 and over.

Table 2. Lifetime Prevalence of DSM-III Anxiety Diagnoses by Education[a]

	New Haven (%)		Baltimore (%)		St. Louis (%)	
	College graduate (N = 839)	Other (N = 2,218)	College graduate (N = 303)	Other (N = 3,174)	College graduate (N = 416)	Other (N = 2,498)
Simple phobia	3.8	7.2***	12.8	21.4**	5.1	7.2
Agoraphobia	2.2	4.1*	4.4	9.6***	2.1	4.5*
Panic disorder	1.6	1.4	1.1	1.5	0.5	1.7*

[a]Adapted from Robbins *et al.* (1984).
*$p < .05$.
**$p < .001$.
***$p < .01$.

prevalence of approximately 1.5% of the general population (see Table 2). The sex-specific rates are approximately 2.1% for females and 0.6% for males (Robbins *et al.*, 1984). This study utilized the Diagnostic Interview Schedule (DIS), which yielded diagnoses for panic disorder according to the RDC [i.e., criteria that were harder to meet that those of DSM-III-R (APA, 1987)]. Consequently, the prevalence of uncomplicated panic disorder as assessed by the more liberal DSM-III-R criteria is undoubtedly higher than that found by the methods used in the ECA study. Further, the DSM-III-R acknowledges that many cases of agoraphobia are symptom complications of panic disorder. As a result, many of those identified as agoraphobic in the ECA would now be counted among those having the panic disorder. Overall, this could raise the lifetime prevalence of panic disorder as defined in DSM-III-R to approximately 3% or 4%.

The current adult population of the United States is approximately 174 million. Using the ECA study findings, we estimate that 14.4 million people in this country suffer from an anxiety or phobic disorder during their lifetime. Using the conservative ECA findings, we can estimate that approximately 2.6 million people in the United States have panic disorder at some point in their life. With the broader definition of panic disorder in DSM-III-R, we might expect approximately 6 million people to be affected.

THE PERCENTAGE USING THE HEALTH-CARE SYSTEM

Within any 6-month period, approximately 77% of those with anxiety and phobic disorders visit a health or mental-health-care facility to seek medical or psychiatric evaluations; approximately 23% seek care from a mental health professional (Shappiro, Skinner, Kessler, 1984). The rates for panic disorder are probably higher, as individuals suffering frequent panic attacks are more symptomatic and more driven to help-seeking behavior. In one study, we found that all of 57 consecutive panic-disorder patients had seen a physician for an evaluation of their anxiety-disorder symptoms and that 70% had seen more than 10 physicians for these symptoms (Sheehan, Ballenger, & Jacobson, 1980). The peak prevalence of the disorder is in the 20–40 age group, an age group that is otherwise generally healthy. Many have costly medical evaluations that, in the end, yield nothing positive. The cost to the health-care system is extremely high.

Table 3. *Lifetime Prevalence of DSM-III Anxiety Disorders by Age Group*[a]

	New Haven (%)				Baltimore (%)				St. Louis (%)			
	1[b]	2	3	4	1	2	3	4	1	2	3	4
Simple phobia	5.0	7.4	6.4	4.6	21.0	21.1	21.5	18.1	5.8	8.7	6.7	3.5
Agoraphobia	3.5	4.5	3.4	1.6	7.9	9.8	10.3	7.5	4.3	4.5	5.0	1.2
Panic disorder	0.7	2.4	1.2	0.2	1.2	2.1	1.5	0.1	0.9	2.2	1.8	0.1

[a]Adapted from Robbins *et al.* (1984).
[b]Age codes: 1 = 18–24 years; 2 = 25–44 years; 3 = 45–64 years; 4 = 65+ years.

AGE OF ONSET

Phobias uncomplicated by unexpected anxiety attacks can start at any age (Sheehan, Sheehan, & Minichiello, 1981). Phobias associated with spontaneous panic attacks have a uniform, unimodal age-of-onset distribution, with the peak in the 20s. It Only very infrequently does it first start before the age of 15 or after the age of 40. The lifetime prevalence data from the ECA study (see Table 3, Robbins *et al.*, 1984) reveals that the disorder becomes less common after the mid-40s. It is almost half as frequent in the 45–64 age group as in the 25–44 age group, and it drops to approximately 1⁄12th this prevalence after age 65. This age distribution is difficult to explain in psychological terms unless we posit that stress more adversely affects people in their 20s, sparing the very young and the old. This is difficult to believe. Such a distribution is consistent with a genetically inherited metabolic model of panic disorder, according to which the illness is apt to afflict a certain age group preferentially, most notably women in their child-bearing years.

GENDER DISTRIBUTION

Approximately 75%–80% of panic disorder patients are women in most studies (Marks & Lader, 1973; Sheehan *et al.*, 1981; Weissman, 1985).

FAMILIAL PATTERNS

Weissman (1985) summarized the findings of the Yale Family-Genetic Study reports that probands with panic disorder and major depression "show markedly increased rates of major depression, anxiety disorders (phobia, panic disorder and GAD), and alcoholism compared with the first degree relatives of normal controls and depressed probands without an anxiety disorder."

The majority of those affected by panic disorder have a chronic, fluctuating course for the better part of their adult lives. As many as 50% have some level of disability, and 73%–92% are symptomatic when reevaluated up to 20 years after initial diagnosis (Greer, 1969; Marks & Lader, 1973; Wheeler, White, Reed & Cohen, 1950).

Compared with controls matched for age and sex, patients with panic disorder have higher mortality rates from suicide and, among males, from cardiovascular disease (Coryell, Noyes, & Clancy, 1982).

CLINICAL DESCRIPTION

Anxiety neurosis is the historical "parent" of panic disorder. From 1895, anxiety neurosis was the diagnostic label most frequently used for patients now classified as having panic disorder. In the DSM-III, anxiety neurosis was subdivided into two major subtypes, the milder form being called *generalized anxiety disorder* and the severe form being called *panic disorder*. The assumption underlying this subdivision was that generalized anxiety disorder and panic disorder were distinct entities. However, the evidence in support of this distinction is no longer very convincing. One of the better earlier descriptions (circa 1895) of anxiety neuroses was by Sigmund Freud (1962):

> But anxiousness—which, though mostly latent as regards consciousness, is constantly lurking in the background—has other means of finding expression besides this. It can suddenly break through into consciousness without being aroused by a train of ideas, and thus provoke an anxiety attack. An anxiety attack of this sort may consist of the feeling of anxiety, alone, without any associated idea, or accompanied by the interpretation that is nearest to hand, such as ideas of the extinction of life, or of a stroke, or of a threat of madness; or else some kind of paraesthesia (similar to the hysterical aura) may be combined with the feeling of anxiety, or, finally, the feeling of anxiety may have linked to it a disturbance of one or more of the bodily functions—such as respiration, heart action, vasomotor innervation or glandular activity. From this combination the patient picks out in particular now one, now another, factor. He complains of "spasms of the heart," "difficulty in breathing," "outbreaks of sweating," "ravenous hunger," and such like; and, in his description, the feeling of anxiety often recedes into the background or is referred to quite unrecognizably as "being unwell," "feeling uncomfortable," and so on. (p. 93)

The DSM-III-R has further refined the diagnosis of panic disorder since the original publication of these criteria in the DSM-III. The central characteristic of panic disorder is the occurrence of one or more episodes of unexpected panic attacks during some stage of the patient's history. Two points need clarification here. The focus is on the central importance of the *unexpected, unprovoked* attacks rather than on the word *panic*. A panic attack is defined as any attack with at least 4 of a possible 13 symptoms (see Table 4). It is not always necessary that a patient have an intense mental feeling of panic for a panic attack to be so defined. The central point of the definition of a panic attack is the presence of four or more of the symptoms in Criterion C. For example, patients may experience shortness of breath, paresthesias, dizziness, and a sense of things around them being strange, unreal, detached, or unfamiliar. These symptoms may be accompanied by some degree of perceived anxiety, although it may not be of mental-panic-intensity proportions. Such an attack is labeled a panic attack because these four symptoms occur suddenly and unexpectedly within a 10-minute period. In contrast, patients may have sudden acceleration of the heart (and no other symptoms listed in Criterion C) and an intense feeling of mental panic. They may label such an attack a panic attack, but by definition, it does not qualify as a panic attack. Such an attack would be labeled a limited-symptom attack. Consequently, distinctions between panic attacks and limited-symptom attacks should be made not on the basis of a patient's subjective report of the intensity of the attack but on the basis of a distinction in the count of the number of symptoms occurring within 10 minutes of the sudden onset.

To be diagnosed as having a panic disorder, a patient must further have had at least four such attacks within a 1-week period at any point in his or her history or one or more attacks with four or more symptoms followed by a period of at least a month of persistent fear of having another attack. It should be emphasized that these revised criteria do not require that such attacks all have occurred in the weeks immediately before evaluation. These four attacks within a 4-week period may have occurred as long before as several months or years. If a patient has ever met the criteria for panic disorder at any stage in the natural history of the illness, thereafter he or she must be regarded as having panic disorder. The clinician who focuses on whether any of the attacks are unexpected and on counting the number of symptoms in each of the patient's attacks, rather than focusing on the intensity of each attack, will have less difficulty in making an accurate diagnosis in the majority of cases.

The typical patient with panic disorder has two to four unexpected, unprovoked anxiety attacks per week. The attacks can last from a few minutes up to 1 hour. The anxiety attacks vary considerably in the number of symptoms per attack. The classic case of panic disorder may have a great number of symptoms all occurring within the same time frame and associated with cognitive anxiety.

Table 4. Diagnostic Criteria for Panic Disorder[a]

A. At some time during the disturbance, one or more panic attacks (discrete periods of intense fear or discomfort) have occurred that were (1) unexpected, i.e., did not occur immediately before or on exposure to a situation that almost always caused anxiety, and (2) not triggered by situations in which the person was the focus of others' attention.

B. Either four attacks, as defined in criterion A, have occurred within a four-week period, or one or more attacks have been followed by a period of at least a month of persistent fear of having another attack.

C. At least four of the following symptoms developed during at least one of the attacks:

1. Shortness of breath (dyspnea) or smothering sensations
2. Dizziness, unsteady feelings, or faintness
3. Palpitations or accelerated heart rate (tachycardia)
4. Trembling or shaking
5. Sweating
6. Choking
7. Nausea or abdominal distress
8. Depersonalization or derealization
9. Numbness or tingling sensations (paresthesias)
10. Flushes (hot flashes) or chills
11. Chest pain or discomfort
12. Fear of dying
13. Fear of going crazy or of doing something uncontrolled

D. During at least some of the attacks, at least four of the C symptoms developed suddenly and increased in intensity within ten minutes of the beginning of the first C symptom noticed in the attack.

E. It cannot be established that an organic factor initiated and maintained the disturbance, e.g., Amphetamine or Caffeine Intoxication, hyperthyroidism.

[a]From American Psychiatric Association, *Diagnostic and Statistical Manual of Mental Disorders* (3rd ed. rev.), pp. 237–238. Copyright 1987 by author, Washington, DC. Reprinted with permission.
[b]Note: Attacks involving four or more symptoms are panic attacks; attacks involving fewer than four symptoms are limited symptom attacks (see Agoraphobia with History of Panic Disorder, p. 241).
Note: Mitral valve prolapse may be an associated condition, but does not preclude a diagnosis of Panic Disorder.

Many of the attacks, however, occur with three symptoms or fewer. These attacks limited to three symptoms or fewer are now referred to as *limited-symptom attacks* (Sheehan & Sheehan, 1982–1983). The 13 symptoms listed in Criterion C of the diagnostic criteria for panic disorder can occur in almost limitless permutations and combinations, and in any one patient, the clustering of these symptoms may vary from day to day and throughout the natural history of the illness.

Some patients may complain of some of these symptoms more than others. For example, some patients may be more concerned about and may experience more tachycardia and palpitations, whereas another patient may suffer predominantly from abdominal distress and attacks of diarrhea. However, the majority of the patients, if they continue to have the disorder long enough, suffer attacks with a large number of combinations of these symptoms, in varying numbers with the different attacks.

Not all of the attacks are associated with subjective anxiety. For example, the patient may have paresthesias, shortness of breath, derealization, and some lightheadedness without feeling particularly anxious. Subjective anxiety is particularly likely to be absent with some of these symptoms more than with others. For example, the chest pain and discomfort and the lightheadedness, if they occur as isolated attacks of one or two symptoms, are particularly likely not to be associated with a great deal of anxiety. The clinician should not be misled into thinking that this is a different problem or that such attacks are not a manifestation of the same syndrome. Limited-symptom attacks, or unexpected attacks limited to three symptoms or fewer in the absence of anxiety, are the lowest common denominator clinically and are the central feature of the disorder, rather than the panic attacks with four or more symptoms. This realization serves as a valuable guide not only in diagnosing the condition, but in monitoring response to treatment over time. These limited-symptom attacks, if described in isolation, may have the appearance of a conversion hysteria. Approximately half of all cases of panic disorder, in the early weeks of the condition, first present with limited-symptom attacks without yet having had the experience of a full-blown panic attack with four or more symptoms. The remaining half of patients have a panic attack with four or more symptoms as the first manifestation of their illness, usually followed by days or weeks of limited-symptom attacks.

Clinically, the limited-symptom attacks and the panic attacks seem to be manifestations of the same core phenomenon. In tracking a patient's progress during treatment, the goal is not just to eliminate the panic attacks with four or more symptoms. That is usually not difficult even with weaker and less effective treatments. Rather, the goal of treatment is to control these unexpected, unprovoked limited-symptom attacks as completely as possible. As long as such attacks continue, they will reinforce phobic avoidance behavior, will undermine the patient's progress, and will lead to incomplete therapeutic results.

Moving the limited-symptom attacks or subpanic symptom attacks to a position of central importance has significant implications for the accurate diagnosis, classification, and treatment of this disorder.

NATURAL HISTORY

Patients with this illness frequently describe several stages in the natural progression of their illness over time:

Stage 1. Limited-symptom attacks
Stage 2. Panic attacks

Stage 3. Hypochondriasis
Stage 4. Limited phobias
Stage 5. Social phobias
Stage 6. Extensive phobic avoidance or agoraphobia
Stage 7. Depression

Approximately half of all cases start with unexpected subpanic symptom attacks or limited-symptom attacks. Patients may one day be walking down the street when, for no apparent reason, they feel acutely short of breath. They are at a loss to explain why, as nothing unusual happened immediately before the attack. Several days later, they may feel a sudden burst of tachycardia and skipping of the heart. Several days later, they may experience paresthesias and numbness. Several days later, they may feel a sense of unreality, as if things are disconnected from them. If these limited-symptom attacks persist over time, eventually the majority of cases experience an attack in which several of these symptoms occur during the same time frame. The patient who feels several parts of his or her body racing out of control for no apparent reason becomes greatly alarmed and thinks that he she is going to die, lose control, or go insane. Such panic attacks are often accompanied by a flight response or immobilization (a freeze response).

Because many patients at this stage are at a loss to explain the severity and nature of their symptoms, many of which have been apparently unexpected, unprovoked, they may interpret their attacks as being a manifestation of some serious medical illness. This fear impels the patient to seek a medical evaluation. Often, they go to a specialist who is expert on the one or two symptoms that distress them most. For example, if they are particularly troubled by tachycardia and palpitations, they often first consult a cardiologist. If they are concerned about headaches, dizziness, and numbness, they may first consult a neurologist. When the specialist evaluates them and can find no serious medical illness to justify the presence of these symptoms, reassurance is usually provided that there is no cause for serious concern and that the disorder appears to be an anxiety disorder. The specialist may interpret this disorder to the patient as being a response to stress or conflict in the patient's life and may recommend a less stressful regimen or a more conflict-free environment.

When the patient thinks about this interpretation and realizes that the doctor is using a stress model to conceptualize anxiety, and that he or she is not under any unusual stress, the patient decides that it must not be an anxiety disorder. By exclusion, the patient must have some exotic medical illness and therefore seeks a specialist who has the diagnostic ability or the appropriate technology to make an accurate diagnosis. This belief leads to recurrent help-seeking behavior and an excessive health preoccupation. Although the clinician may reassure the patient that there is nothing medically wrong, and although the patient may accept this reassurance during the consultation and may even believe it, all of this reassurance will quickly vanish during the next panic attack. There is something so terrifying about the experience of a panic attack that it seems to drive away all reassurances and convinces the patient that something serious has to be wrong to justify such intense feelings. At this stage, patients are often labeled hypochondriacs and certainly often see themselves in that light. These patients often feel embarrassed about having to trouble their physicians recurrently with minor complaints for which no organic basis can be found.

If the panic attacks persist, the patients begin to have the attacks unexpectedly in a variety of situations. For example, the patient may be driving on the highway and suddenly feels acutely short of breath, experiences palpitations, and feels faint, disconnected from the ground, and so numb that the brake and the accelerator of the car cannot be felt. At that point, the patient fears that he or she will totally lose control and crash the car. It is no surprise that, after such an experience, people become frightened of driving cars on the highway. Thus, patients begin to fear and avoid the situations they associate with their bad attacks. (Editor's note: In certain locales, such a fear may generalize to tunnels and bridges.)

At this stage in the natural history of their condition, patients often describe at least two different kinds of anxiety attacks (see Figure 1). The first is the unexpected, unprovoked attack that has a sudden onset and a rapid surge of symptoms to peak intensity within the first several minutes. Then it seems to have an autonomous course and is self-driven until eventually it burns out over the next 5–60 minutes. These attacks appear to be reflections of the biological core of the illness. Over time, as patients connect these unexpected panic attacks with more situations, they develop anticipatory anxiety about entering the situations they associate with their bad attacks. Anticipatory anxiety has a profile different from that of the expected anxiety attack (see Figure 1). As patients get closer to the situation that they fear and avoid, their anxiety increases. They begin thinking, "What if I have a panic attack when I get into this frightening situation?" They know that, at any point, they can turn around and retreat, and that the intensity of the anxiety will lessen. Alternatively, if they continue in the phobic situation, they will also experience relief of this anticipatory anxiety as soon as they leave it. This type of anxiety appears to be much more within cognitive control. When the clinician sees patients several years into their condition, they usually have a combination of two to four of the unexpected anxiety attacks per week and a substantial amount of anticipatory anxiety.

How can an unexpected anxiety attack lead to avoidance behavior? Many models can be used to explain this phenomenon. As in the illustration above, in which the patient began to phobically avoid driving on highways after having a panic attack in a car, the model that leads most easily to an understanding of the phenomenon is Pavlovian or classical conditioning. Pavlov presented meat to his dogs, and in response, they salivated. The salivation was a physiological response to the presentation of the meat. At the same time, the local church bells were ringing. Over many repetitions of this pairing, the ringing of the local church bells became inextricably associated with the presentation of the meat and the onset of salivation. In time, the ringing of the local church bells elicited the salivation response even in the absence of the presentation of meat.

Precisely the same phenomenon appears to occur in panic attacks complicated by

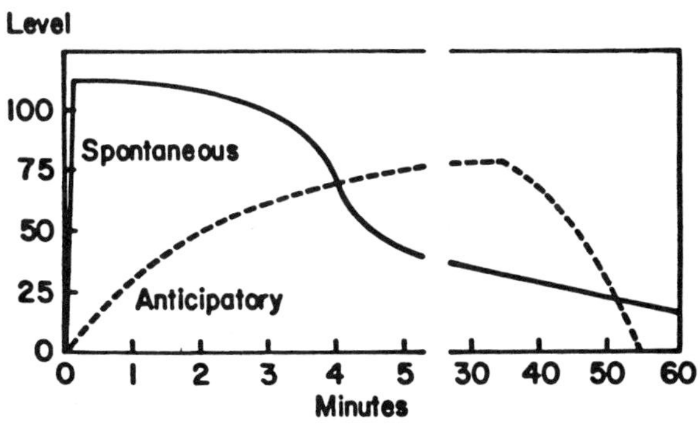

Figure 1. A graphic representation of the rise and fall of spontaneous anxiety (or panic versus anticipatory anxiety or anticipatory panic). Spontaneous anxiety comes on unpredictably, "out of the blue"; peaks almost immediately; and then gradually fades. Anticipatory anxiety builds up gradually to the time of an encounter with something that is feared and then drops sharply. (Reproduced with permission from D. V. Sheehan. Copyright 1982.)

phobic avoidance. Imagine that the spontaneous panic attack is like the presentation of the meat. It elicits a cognitive and somatic anxiety response. At the same time, other events may be occurring in the patient's life, as in the example above concerning driving a car. So the driving of the car on the highway, after a number of exposures (occasionally after only one), begins to elicit an anxiety response even in the absence of the original spontaneous panic attack. In this model of classical conditioning, then, the patient begins to fear and avoid the situations associated with bad anxiety attacks. With time, there is frequently some stimulus generalization from this core, so that the phobias begin to spread into adjacent areas in the patient's life. The phobias may be further reinforced by interoceptive conditioning and by operant conditioning (Sheehan & Sheehan, 1982–1983). It is quite possible that unexpected anxiety attacks may neurochemically facilitate conditioning or the acquisition of phobic avoidance behavior. They may put the patient into an altered mode of learning for a very short period of time, so that the imprinting of the phobic anxiety is neurochemically intensified. Subsequently, such imprinting may be reinforced by the unexpected anxiety attacks two to four times per week and by the phobic avoidance behavior that ensues. This view is reinforced by the finding that patients with this disorder, when compared to matched normal controls, have increased spontaneous fluctuations in their skin conductance and a slow habituation response to novel stimuli (Marks, 1969). When patients are treated successfully with mediation, they can more easily reenter phobic situations and more rapidly overcome their chronic phobic avoidance behavior.

If the unexpected anxiety attacks continue, the existing phobic avoidance behavior continues to generalize, and patients may become socially phobic (Stage 5). They then become more isolated and avoid mixing with friends, going to parties, or being in any situation where they might be the focus of attention. Self-consciousness may increase, and patients may, for example, become very tremulous and anxious when writing a check in a store or when going into a restaurant where there are many other people. If the panic attacks persist further, patients usually progress to a stage of extensive phobic avoidance behavior and become housebound because of agoraphobia. Literally, *agoraphobia* means a fear of the marketplace or of places where crowds assemble. It is derived from the Greek word *agora,* the marketplace at the foot of the Acropolis. The number and choice of phobias appear to be a function of the chronicity and the frequency of the unexpected anxiety attacks, as well as the situations in which they occurred. The particular choice of agoraphobia, social phobia, illness phobias, and separation anxiety, among the many possible phobic choices in severe cases, can be explained as a manifestation of high arousal regression (Sheehan, 1983). Other factors, including psychosocial stressors, may contribute to the perpetuation and even to the genesis of these phobias, and they may be further reinforced in a variety of ways. As patients become progressively more restricted by the phobic avoidance and increasingly disabled by the symptoms, and as the anxiety spreads into every sector of their life, it is not surprising that the majority of patients—at least 50%–60%—become depressed (Stage 7). The initial reaction to danger or loss is anxiety and fear. This reaction subsides when the danger lessens. When the danger is beyond control, anxiety is replaced by depression. This age-old observation was articulated elegantly by Darwin (1872) when he wrote, "If we expect to suffer, we are anxious. If we have no hope of relief, we despair."

What seems to drive the condition through its natural history is the frequency and the intensity of the attacks. If the unexpected attacks are very frequent and intense, the patient may progress through the stages very rapidly to the late chronic form of the illness. In some patients, the unexpected anxiety attacks lessen, and the patient does not progress to the late stages of the illness unless the frequency and the intensity of the attacks again increase. In approximately 15% of patients, the unexpected anxiety attacks remit completely. Such patients may move back through all of the stages to get a complete spontaneous remission. Patients who have remissions and relapses may move up and down through these stages over time. However, the majority of cases show a pattern of progression from unexpected attacks to progressive phobic avoidance behavior and increasing depression over the course of time.

Some of the stages are more stable in the way they occur in this natural sequence. Others, particularly Stage 3 (hypochondriasis) and Stage 7 (depression), sometimes occur out of the order of the natural sequence or may be bypassed entirely. The clinician who uses a cross-sectional evaluation may assign different diagnostic labels, depending on the stage at which the patient is seen. The clinician may elevate the different symptom clusters within each of these stages into discrete diagnostic entities. In contrast, by adopting a longitudinal perspective and an integrated view of the disorder, the clinician avoids much confusing diagnostic fragmentation.

PSYCHIATRIC DIFFERENTIAL DIAGNOSIS

If panic disorder is a metabolic disease to which there is a genetic vulnerability, it is likely that the current criteria in DSM-III-R do not define the boundaries of the condition accurately. It is likely that some of the victims of this illness are currently assigned to other diagnostic categories, like hypochondriasis, somatization disorder, and sometimes simple and social phobia. Most cases of agoraphobia should actually be labeled panic disorder. The debate on the optimal classification system for anxiety disorders will undoubtedly continue until laboratory techniques for diagnosing this disease are developed, such as special blood and urine tests, psychophysiological and brain-imaging measurements, genetic marking, and pharmacological dissection. Ancillary diagnostic aids will undoubtedly lend validity to one or the other of the existing classification systems and may suggest refinements that will be clinically meaningful. In the meantime, the practicing clinician can expect some diagnostic confusion when faced with many such cases and some puzzlement because patients meet the criteria for several categories simultaneously.

If a patient meets the criteria for somatization disorder or hypochondriasis in addition to meeting the criteria for panic disorder, both diagnoses should be given. In the case of agoraphobia without panic attacks, it is particularly important to rule out any past history of panic disorder even if the patient does not currently meet the criteria for this condition. It is also important in all cases of simple and social phobia to ensure that at no stage during the natural history of the phobic disorder did the patient ever meet the criteria for panic disorder. The original panic symptoms may have long subsided, and the simple or social phobia may be left as a residual symptom. In the early stages of the natural history of panic disorder, many patients pass through a phase in which they have just one or two phobias, for example, claustrophobia. A clinician who focuses on that phobia instead of taking a more complete past history of the anxiety disorder, they may be misled into diagnosing a simple phobia rather than a phobia occurring in the context of a panic disorder. It is best to restrict the diagnosis of simple phobia to the patient who develops a crescendo anxiety on exposure to a specific phobic stimulus, and who does not now have and has never had any unexpected, unprovoked attacks of anxiety. Similarly, the diagnosis of social phobia is reserved for those who develop crescendo anxiety when they are the focus of others' attention, and who do not now have and have never had any unexpected attacks.

It is not unusual for patients with chronic panic disorder to show some increase in obsessional and compulsive symptoms. They may, for example, have recurrent intrusive thoughts of loss of control or of doing something that would otherwise be ego alien, and they may engage in some minor ritualizing, for example, checking the door lock three or four times before leaving the house each morning, which they never did before the onset of the panic disorder. Clinicians who focus on these obsessional and compulsive symptoms to the exclusion of the other symptoms in the cluster could be misled into thinking that the disorder is an obsessive-compulsive disorder rather than obsessions and compulsions occurring in the context of a panic disorder.

Approximately 15% of patients with a primary major depressive episode may have recurrent panic attacks, and approximately 50%–60% of patients with panic disorder may also have a secondary depression. If a patient meets the criteria for both major depressive episode and panic disorder, both diagnoses should be given. For practical purposes, one can give primacy to whichever diagnosis came first in the natural history of the disorder or to whichever is now more prominent in the presenting symptom cluster. For example, consider the patient who had a major depressive episode at the age of 18 and subsequently developed recurrent, unexpected panic attacks. Although both diagnoses should be made, the depressive disorder is considered primary.

With the expansion of the criteria for panic disorder in the DSM-III-R to include more cases, it appears that many patients given the diagnosis of generalized anxiety disorder in the past would now be diagnosed as having panic disorder. Therefore, when the clinician feels inclined to assign a diagnosis of generalized anxiety disorder, he or she must carefully evaluate the patient's past history of anxiety to be sure that at no time did the patient ever have unexpected surges of four or more symptoms from the cluster that characterizes panic disorder.

It is often difficult to diagnose panic disorder when it occurs in a patient who is also abusing psychoactive substances. Intoxication by such drugs as marijuana, caffeine, amphetamines, or cocaine may be associated with panic attacks. Panic disorder should not be diagnosed when the panic attacks are due to the ingestion of a psychoactive substance. Panic attacks may also occur on the withdrawal of some substances, like alcohol, barbiturates, and benzodiazepines. It is often difficult to tell in the early days following withdrawal whether panic attacks are a transient rebound effect typical of the withdrawal syndrome or a manifestation of a more chronic, underlying panic disorder. The passage of time often helps clarify this issue. Typically, in most withdrawal syndromes, a peak intensity occurs between the 2nd and 7th days, and the withdrawal syndrome largely subsides within 10–12 days. If the panic attacks recur during this time, it is often not possible to tell if they are related to panic disorder. However, if the panic attacks persist beyond the normal time frame for the withdrawal syndrome (more than 2 weeks from the last ingestion of the substance), the clinician should suspect that there may be an underlying panic disorder that may require separate treatment. Indeed, approximately 10%–20% of agoraphobic and anxious neurotic outpatients are alcoholic on various criteria (Bibb & Chamless, 1986; Woodruff, Guze, & Clayton, 1972); 35% of the fathers of agoraphobics were alcoholic, compared to 10% of the fathers of nonpsychiatric patients (Harris, Noyes, & Crowe, 1983). Alcohol is remarkably effective as an antipanic drug in the first several hours after its ingestion. However, on the following day, there may be rebound reactivation of the anxiety disorder.

Many patients with panic disorder experience depersonalization or derealization. The presence of recurrent depersonalization or derealization symptoms should raise high suspicion about the presence of recurrent or past panic disorder.

Most clinicians would not find difficulty in distinguishing between panic disorder and the other major psychiatric syndromes. Although classic cases of bipolar I and bipolar II illness are quite different from panic disorder, the authors have seen some cases referred because the "panic disorder" was not responding to conventional panic disorder treatments and bipolar illness had not been suspected. A full history revealed the presence of a cyclical pattern of episodic agitation, restlessness, hyperactivity, and "anxiety" alternating with phases of depression. Several patients had a rapidly cycling bipolar illness and responded to carbamazepine. It is wise, therefore, to consider a bipolar illness (especially of the rapidly cycling or bipolar II type) in the psychiatric differential diagnosis of panic disorder.

ETIOLOGY

Historically, three major etiological models have been proposed to explain anxiety neurosis and panic disorder:

1. The psychological or psychosocial model
2. The behavioral model
3. The biological model

All the models are attempts to bring order and lucidity to many disparate observations. A good model attempts to reflect reality accurately by describing the events precisely, especially their interplay. All the models are important steps toward better understanding and prediction and frequently direct our research and clinical efforts.

The psychological model proposes that anxiety results from an interplay of environmental stressors and internal psychological conflicts (from the past and the present). The anxiety response is considered an attempt to immobilize and ward off overwhelming threat.

The behavioral model proposes that anxiety can occur even in the absence of conflict. Following the laws of learning theory, the anxiety response is believed to be acquired. It may be a classically conditioned response to trauma or stress, or an emitted behavior that has been reinforced by operant conditioning, or both.

The biological model views panic disorder as a genetically inherited and/or metabolic disease similar to other metabolic diseases such as diabetes mellitus or hyperthyroidism.

Each of these models identifies one important dimension in our overall understanding of panic disorder. Each appears to be only a partial explanation. They are not mutually exclusive. An integrated model accommodating all three of these historical models paints a richer picture for our understanding of panic disorder, while readjusting the relative importance of each and redefining their interplay.

The medical model is the most parsimonious model, because it hypothesizes that it is necessary to have genetic vulnerability for the condition to express itself. The condition may be activated by some stress, or it may switch on genetically at a certain age. As the biological core of the condition increases and attaches itself to various events and stimuli in the patient's environment, it conditions the patient to phobically avoid many situations. As mentioned previously, it is possible that a panic attack neurochemically facilitates the acquisition of this phobic avoidance behavior. Once these phobias are acquired, they may be reinforced in a variety of ways (e.g., by operant conditioning or by interoceptive conditioning). As the biological core persists and the phobic avoidance behavior worsens, new stress is added to the patient's life. If in addition there is an independent environmental stress in the patient's life, it will magnify the biological core and further amplify the conditioning. All three factors interact over time. In any one individual, these factors may operate to varying degrees. The prevailing view at this time is that the biological force is the largest contributor and that environmental stress may even be absent. Environmental stress alone is neither necessary nor sufficient to cause panic disorder. This model proposes that the lower the genetic loading for the disorder, the greater the psychosocial stress required to activate and perpetuate it. Conversely, those with a greater genetic vulnerability to the disorder require little or no stress to activate and maintain it, and the condition may appear to be quite autonomous.

Panic disorder is characterized by vertical transmission from generation to generation; approximately two thirds of affected individuals have affected relatives. The lifetime morbidity risk among first-degree relatives is 15%–25% (Crowe, Noyes, Pauls, & Slymen, 1983; Crowe, Noyes, Wilson, Elston, & Ward, 1987). Concordance rates in twins support genetic origin, and the transmission pattern within families is consistent with single-locus genetics (Crowe *et al.*, 1987; Pauls, Bocher, Crowe, & Noyes, 1980; Torgersen, 1983). Preliminary evidence suggests that panic disorder may be caused by a gene on chromosome 16q22 (Crowe *et al.*, 1987).

Several biological models of the disorder have been suggested. Four models (not necessarily mutually exclusive) have some explanatory value. Each is backed by a body of scientific data, and each probably represents a different part of the total (and still incomplete) picture:

1. *Locus coeruleus model.* In this model, panic attacks are seen to originate from central nervous system arousal that secondarily provokes peripheral events (Redmond, 1977). Speculation favors the locus coeruleus (LC) as the site of arousal. It is a small nucleus in the pons of vertebrate brain stems and contains at least 50% of all neurons in the CNS using norepinephrine as neurotransmitters. It sends numerous projections to wide areas of the brain. Stimulation of LC firing by electricity or drugs (yohimbine) tends to produce anxiety attacks and a fear response. Anxiety and fearlike responses are blocked by locus coeruleus lesions or ablation. Evidence against the involvement of the locus coeruleus in anxiety was reviewed by Insel, Ninan, & Aloy (1984).

2. *GABA–benzodiazepine receptor model.* The neurotransmitter gamma-aminobutyric acid (GABA) and chloride anions increase benzodiazepine receptor binding (Paul & Skolnick, 1981). This complex is said to open up the ion channel in the cell membrane faster and for longer periods, thus causing hyperpolarization of the cell and decreased anxiety. Compounds like beta carbolines, which also bind to benzodiazepine receptor with an opposite "inverse agonist" effect, cause anxiety. Research is under way to identify compounds that may occur naturally in the brain, that bind to the benzodiazepine receptors, and that cause or relieve anxiety.

3. *Septohippocampal hypothesis.* The septohippocampal region of the brain regulates many vital physiological functions, such as body temperature, respiration, and the fear

response. It receives significant input from the benzodiazepine receptor sites. Lesions in the septohippocampal region blunt the fear response, whereas stimulation of this region elicits anxiety. This region of the old brain acts as a comparator. It matches information from the environment, from the body, and from previous stored memories. If it detects a mismatch, it intervenes by inhibiting ongoing behavior. A panic disorder patient may have a hypersensitivity in this brain region (Gray, 1982). This is supported by the recent findings of Reiman, Raichle, and Butler (1984) in their studies of positron emission tomography (PET) scans. PET scans of panic patients during lactate infusions noted an asymmetry in the blood flow between the right and the left parahippocampal gyrus. This right–left shift in the blood flow in the parahippocampal region did not occur during lactate infusions of normal controls, nor in panic disorder patients who did not panic. It was panic-attack-specific.

4. *Redox hypothesis*. Lactate does not cross the blood–brain barrier to any significant degree. Yet, panic attacks appear to be a central phenomenon and coincide in time with the peak concentrations of lactate in the blood during a standard lactate infusion. How can lactate produce such a central response? Carr and Sheehan (1984) proposed a model that attempts to answer this question and to integrate a variety of observations. One of the few parts of the brain without a significant blood–brain barrier is the ventromedullary center. Carr and Sheehan hypothesized that panic disorder may result from a pathological hypersensitivity to carbon dioxide, pH changes, and the lactate levels of the central chemoreceptors in this region or lability in the first steps of the ventilation arousal cascade activated by these chemoreceptors. Lactic acid is the end product of the anaerobic metabolism of carbohydrates and is derived solely by the reduction of pyruvate to lactate. This process requires oxidation of the cofactor (NADH). The ratio of NADH to NAD defines the "redox" (reduction–oxidation) state of the site where the reaction is taking place, usually within the mitochondria. Carr and Sheehan hypothesized that rises in the lactate/pyruvate ratio with concomitant falls in chemoreceptor intraneuronal pH are the trigger. Experimentally, either lactate infusion or breathing of 5% carbon dioxide leads to a prompt fall in intracellular pH in these chemoreceptors. It is proposed that such changes cause the production of an "alarm" signal and then a panic attack in susceptible individuals.

Although the central defect of panic disorder appears to be a neurochemical one, it has not yet been identified precisely. Ultimately, this neurochemical abnormality is a more distal manifestation of a defect in one or more genes. It seems logical to propose that there is an alteration in a base pair of at least one gene. This results in an altered neucleotide, which in turn results in an altered sequence of amino acids in a polypeptide chain, which could result in structural and/or enzymatic alterations in the central nervous system and elsewhere. This, in turn, leads to the neurochemical defect that permits the symptom expression of the disorder.

MEDICAL DIFFERENTIAL DIAGNOSIS

A first step in the diagnosis of anxiety disorder is eliciting the presence of anxiety or panic attacks. The second step is to rule out a possible medical cause (see Figure 2). Many illnesses that have anxiety or panic attacks as part of their clinical picture are listed in Table 5. We will review a few of the conditions that are more likely to produce anxiety or that have often been listed in the differential diagnosis of anxiety-producing disorders. It is not necessary to do extensive laboratory investigations on all cases of panic disorder. Suspicions of disease elicited at each level of evaluation should suggest pursuing evaluations at the next level (see Table 6).

1. *Endocrine disorders*. Endocrine disorders can produce affective changes, including anxiety. Hyperthyroidism is usually accompanied by anxiety, restlessness, and/or nervousness. Goiter and exophthalmos may be absent in the earlier stages of the illness with diagnosis relying on abnormal T_3, T_4, or TSH levels. A case report (Katerndahl & Vandercreek, 1983) and retrospective study (Lindeman, Zitrin & Klein, 1984) have

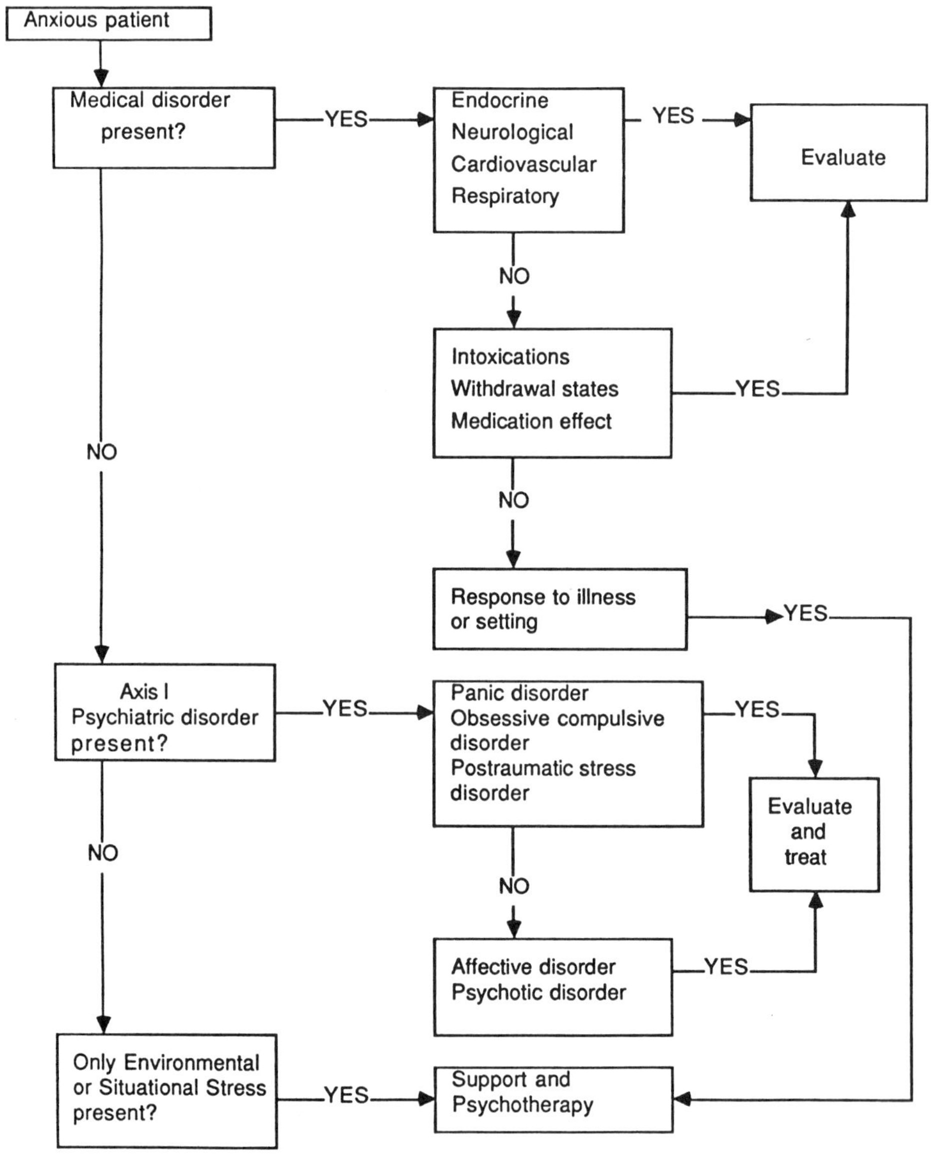

Figure 2. Evaluation strategy for the anxious patient. Copyright B. A. Raj and D. V. Sheehan, 1987. Reproduced with permission.

Table 5. Medical Disorders Associated with Anxiety[a]

A. Cardiovascular and respiratory
- Asthma
- Cardiac arrhythmias
- Chronic obstructive pulmonary disease
- Congestive heart failure
- Coronary insufficiency
- Hypertension
- Hyperventilation syndrome
- Hyperdynamic beta-adrenergic state
- Hypoxia, embolus, infections

B. Endocrine
- Carcinoid
- Cushing's syndrome
- Hyperthyroidism
- Hypothyroidism
- Hypoparathyroidism
- Hypoglycemia
- Menopause
- Pheochromocytoma
- Premenstrual syndrome
- Pregnancy

C. Neurological
- Collagen vascular disease
- Epilepsy
- Huntington's disease
- Multiple sclerosis
- Organic brain syndrome: delirium, dementia
- Parkinson's disease
- Vestibular dysfunction
- Wilson's disease

D. Substance-related
- Intoxications:
  - Anticholinergic drugs
  - Aspirin
  - Caffeine
  - Cocaine
  - Hallucinogens, including phencyclidine (''angel dust'')
  - Steroids
  - Sympathomimetics
  - THC
- Withdrawal syndromes:
  - Alcohol
  - Narcotics
  - Sedative hypnotics

[a]Reproduced with permission. Copyright B.A. Raj and D.V. Sheehan, 1987.

suggested that thyroid disorder can cause anxiety of panic proportions. Several prospective studies (Fishman, Sheehan, & Carr, 1985; Lesser, Rubin, Lydiard, *et al.*, 1987; Pariser, Jones, Pinta, *et al.*, 1979) have *not* found thyroid disease to be associated with panic disorder.

Anxiety with or without fear of impending death has been reported to be the fourth most common symptom in pheochromocytoma (Manger & Gifford, 1982). However, the condition is rare, being responsible for only 0.1% of all cases of hypertension. It occurs most often in women between the ages of 20 and 40. In addition to elevated blood pressure (sustained or paroxysmal), clues to the presence of pheochromocytoma are neurofibromata, café au lait spots, or a family history of pheochromocytoma.

The paroxysmal attacks of pheochromocytoma differ from panic attacks of primary anxiety disorder in that they are not as intense or frequent, the somatic components dominate over the cognitive symptoms, and phobic avoidance behavior is unlikely (Starrman, Zelnik, Nesse, *et al.*, 1985). When this disorder is suspected, it may be looked for by repeated determinations of 24-hour urinary catecholamines and metabolites, plasma catecholamine levels, and CAT scan of the abdomen. In some centers, scintigraphic imaging after injection of metaiodobenzyl guanidine labeled with iodine[131] may be available to detect pheochromocytomas.

Table 6. Evaluations in Anxious Patients[a]

Level 1
History
Mental status exam
Physical examination
Level 2
Urine analysis
Complete blood count
Serum electrolytes, blood urea, uric acid, calcium, phosphorus, alkaline phosphatase, total bilirubin, SGOT, SGPT
Electrocardiogram
Level 3
Urine for drug screen
Echocardiogram
Thyroid function tests
24-hour urine catecholamines
Sleep-deprived EEG
Chest X ray
Level 4
24-hour holter monitor
CAT scan of the head
CAT scan of the abdomen
Serum catecholamines
MIBGI 131 scan[b]

[a]Reproduced with permission. Copyright B.A. Raj and D.V. Sheehan, 1987.
[b]Scintigraphic imaging after injection of metaiodobenzyl guanidine labeled with iodine[131].

Anxiety is part of the clinical picture of a hypoglycemic reaction and is accompanied by tachycardia, sweating, tremors, lightheadedness, and hunger. Popkin, Callies, Lentz, *et al.* (1988) found increased prevalence of simple phobias in their female diabetic subjects. Higher rates of generalized anxiety disorder in diabetics have been suggested in several studies (Lustman, Griffith, Clouse, *et al.*, 1986; Popkin *et al.*, 1988). Anxiety and anxiety disorders may be seen as part of the reactive or psychological response to the course and prognosis of diabetic illness but may also represent a combination of organic and reactive features. Several studies suggest that hypoglycemia itself is unlikely to cause panic attacks (Gorman & Martinez, 1984; Uhde, Vittone, & Post, 1984). Hypoglycemia-induced anxiety should be suspected if the person has diabetes and is on insulin or gives a history of gastric surgery or postprandial anxiety attacks. Insulinomas should be suspected if fasting blood glucose levels are below 40 mg/dl; an insulin assay will establish the diagnosis.

2. *Cardiovascular disorders.* Paroxysmal atrial-tachycardia (PAT) is the most common paroxysmal tachycardia. It may be mistaken for a panic attack as it has a rapid onset and is frightening and exhausting. Unlike panic attacks, PAT may be triggered by postural changes of neck and head and can usually be terminated by massage of the carotid sinus. Episodes of PAT terminate abruptly (unlike panic attacks, which tend to fade gradually), and during such episodes the heart rate is usually between 140 and 220 beats per minute, whereas in panic states it is usually below 140 (Lader, 1972). Hyperdynamic beta-adrenegic circulatory state (Frohlich, Terazi, & Dustan, 1969) is a condition characterized by complaints of cardiac awareness and tachycardia at rest, as well as circulatory hyperkinesis. The symptoms may be reproduced by administering isoproterenol and may be relieved by propranolol. Palpitations, tachycardia, dizziness, lightheadedness, dyspnea, fatigue, and chest pain atypical of angina occur in panic disorder and mitral valve prolapse (MVP); both disorders have a 5% occurrence rate in the general population. MVP is diagnosed if there is a mid-systolic click or murmur on auscultation or significant mitral value leaflet prolapse on two-dimensional echocardiography. The presence of MVP in an anxious patient or a patient presenting with panic attacks does not automatically rule out primary panic disorder, as the two conditions often coexist. One study of 131 panic disorder patients found 44 (34%) with definite mitral valve prolapse (Liberthson, Sheehan, King, *et al.*, 1986). MVP is generally a benign condition, with further workup and treatment being indicated only if there is a history of transient ischemic episodes, arrhythmia, or chest pain in a person over age 45.

3. *Neurological disorders.* A complex partial seizure may resemble panic anxiety in several ways. Both may occur without a precipitating event, may be paroxysmal, and may be accompanied by feelings of fear, terror, and unreality. Autonomic symptoms such as diaphoresis, flushing, hyperventilation, and tachycardia may occur in both. Complex partial seizures should be suspected if the anxiety attack is accompanied by hallucinations or an altered state of consciousness, or by progress into other seizure types. Ictal episodes characterized by pronounced fear may occur with left- or right-temporal-lobe lesions (Strauss, Risser, & Jones, 1982). In one study, 10 patients with refractory anxiety and abnormal sleep-deprived EEG were treated with anticonvulsants, with improvement in their symptoms (Brodsky, Zuniger, Casenas, *et al.*, 1983). Panic anxiety has been reported with mass lesions of the right temporal lobe (Ghadirian, Gauthier, & Bertrand, 1986; Wall, Tuchman, & Mielke, 1985) and after right-temporal lobectomy (Wall, Mielke, & Luther, 1986).

4. *Substance-related disorders.* Sedative hypnotics, anxiolytics, anticonvulsants, over-the-counter drugs, illicit drugs, and alcohol use may lead to a withdrawal syndrome

that presents with anxiety in the early stages and severe anxiety and delirium in the latter stages. Many of these patients may be admitted to the hospital for other reasons than substance abuse or dependence and may develop anxiety later in their stay. Patients being admitted for esophagitis, gastritis, pancreatitis, liver disease, and hypertension should be viewed with suspicion. Several medications may produce anxiety as a side effect, including ephedrine derivatives, phenylproponolamine, theophylline, reserpine, and levodopa. Caffeine has been described as the most widely used psychotropic agent in the world and it may produce anxiety when consumed in large quantities (Eaton & McLeod, 1984). Anxiety may be an adverse response to the use of marijuana or hashish (Smith, 1968). Cocaine use may produce depression (83%), anxiety (83%), and panic attacks (50%) (Watson & Gold, 1984). Clues to cocaine use may be insomnia, fatigue, runny nose, nasal bleeding, tachycardia, and mydriasis.

5. *Vestibular disease.* In 125 patients referred for otological evaluation for dizziness, Drachman and Hart (1972) diagnosed vestibular problems in 38%, hyperventilation in 23%, and other psychiatric problems in 9%. These findings suggest that a large proportion of cases were psychogenic. The most common vestibular abnormality was benign paroxysmal positional vertigo. In this condition, sudden onset of vertigo is triggered by head rotation or linear acceleration when speeding up or slowing down in a car. Jacob, Moller, Turner, *et al.* (1985) found that 14 of 21 cases with panic disorder and dizziness had vestibular dysfunction.

TREATMENT

A first essential step in treating panic disorder is achieving pharmacological control of the biological core of the disorder. This step is followed by an *in vivo* exposure behavior therapy program to extinguish any remaining phobias, avoidance behaviors, and anticipatory anxiety. Finally, psychotherapy may be needed to repair strained relationships, to improve self-esteem, and to prevent relapse (see Figure 3).

Pharmacological Control

Success is most likely with the use of antipanic drugs like the triazolobenzodiazepine alprazolam (Chouinard *et al.*, 1982), the tricyclic antidepressant imipramine hydrochloride (Klein, 1964, 1967; Sheehan *et al.*, 1980; Sheehan, Claycomb, Surman, *et al.* 1984), or the monoamine oxidase inhibitor phenelzine sulphate (Sheehan, Claycomb, Surman, *et al.*, 1984). However, clinical experience suggests that all tricyclic antidepressants are equally effective in treating this disorder. Trazodone hydrochloride, a triazolopyridine antidepressant, has often been clinically effective in our experience, but Charney, Woods, Goodman, *et al.* (1986) reported otherwise. Antidepressants such as bupropion hydrochloride (Sheehan, Davidson, Manschneck, *et al.*, 1983) and amoxapine hydrochloride have not been effective. Clonazepam (Fontaine & Chouinard, 1984), a high-potency benzodiazepine, has been shown to be effective in treating panic attacks.

General Principles

These drugs are fairly equal in the treatment of early and mild cases. Their relative powers become more apparent in the severe chronic cases. Alprazolam is the least toxic and the most rapidly effective, with minimal antidepressant properties. The MAO phenelzine sulfate is probably the single most effective drug overall. Treatment failures are usually due to subtherapeutic doses of these medicines, inadequate length of treatment, or premature discontinuation of the medication. These problems can be avoided if time is spent in reviewing with the patient the dosage schedule and timing, and in monitoring the complications. Educating the patient to see the onset of mild side effects as indicating the optimal therapeutic dose encourages compliance.

Alprazolam

Alprazolam is a triazolo analogue of the 1,4 benzodiazepine class of CNS-active compounds. Following oral administration, it is readily absorbed; peak plasma concentra-

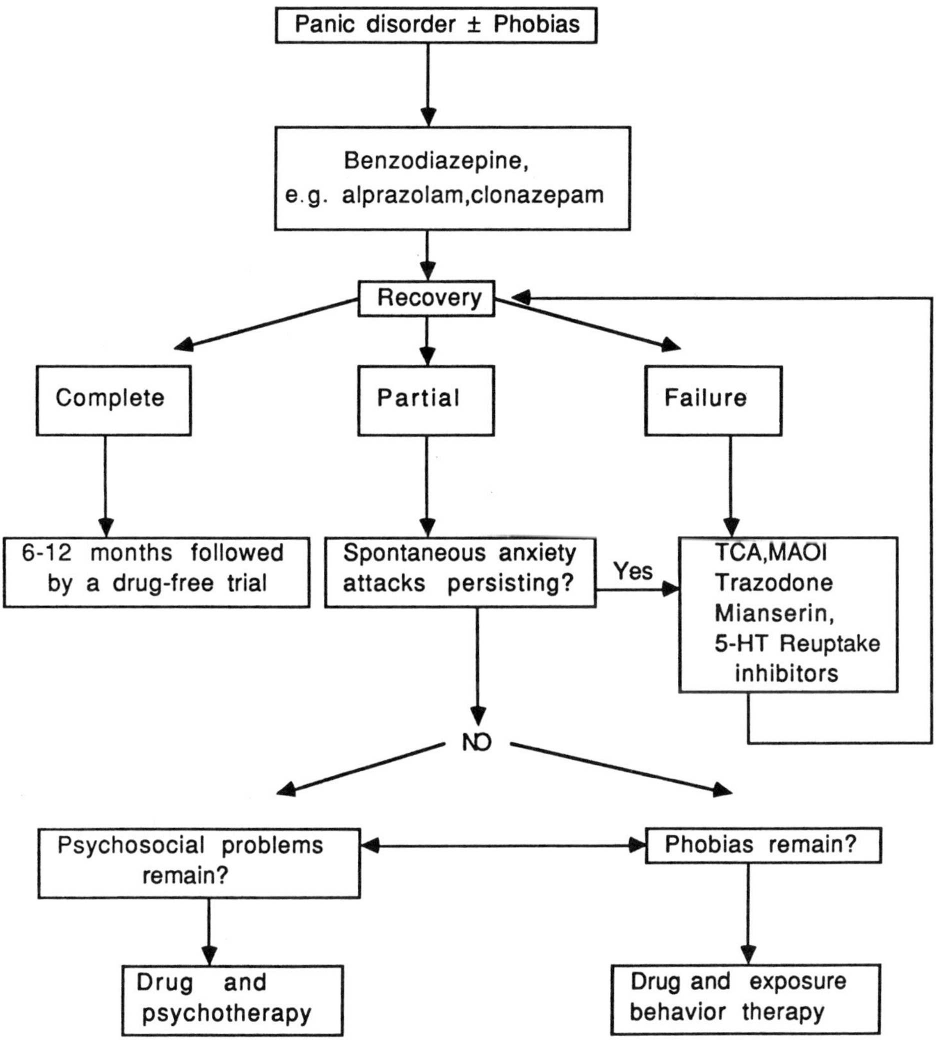

Figure 3. Treatment strategy for panic disorder. Copyright D. V. Sheehan, 1987. Reproduced with permission.

tions occur 1–2 hours later. The elimination half-life is 12–15 hours, but the drug's duration of effective therapeutic action is 4–6 hours. The starting dose is 0.5 mg three times daily, and it may be increased by 0.5 mg every 2 days until either side effects or significant benefit occurs (see Table 7). Tolerance may occur, and loss of sedation or benefit requires an increase in dosage to recapture benefit. The antipanic dosage ranges from 3 to 10 mg per day, with an average of 6 mg. Drowsiness, ataxia, and slurring of speech are the most apparent side effects of high doses. Forgetfulness, increased assertiveness, irritability, and headaches are not uncommon at first, and some patients may experience a depressed amotivational syndrome after several weeks. Alprazolam is an anticonvulsant and should not be rapidly withdrawn even when not effective, as rapid withdrawal may lead to withdrawal seizure. Withdrawal is accomplished by decreasing the total daily dose by 0.5 to 1 mg every week. After 4 weeks on alprazolam up to 10 mg a day, a change of drug should be considered if anxiety symptoms persist.

Clonazepam

Clonazepam is structurally related to chlordiazepoxide and diazepam and is indicated for the treatment of minor motor epilepsy. Its half-life and duration of action are longer than those of alprazolam, and its affinity for central benzodiazepine receptors is greater. Theoretically, clonazepam should be effective in blocking panic anxiety and should do so without the symptom rebound experienced by some patients on alprazolam at the end of typical dosing intervals (4–6 hours). Spier, Teser, Rosenbaum, & Woods (1986), in an open study of 50 patients, obtained improvement in 39 (78%). Their average dosage was 1.9 mg per day. Chouinard's group (Chouinard *et al.*, 1982) used doses of 6–9 mg/day. The side effects reported were mild depression, initial nausea, transient irritability and sedation.

Table 7. Directions for Taking Benzodiazepines[a,b]

Breakfast (tablets)	Lunch	Evening meal	Bedtime	Day
½	½	½	0	1–2
1	½	½	0	3–4
1	½	1	0	5–6
1	1	1	0	7–8
1 ½	1	1	0	9–10
1 ½	1	1 ½	0	11–12
1 ½	1 ½	1 ½	0	13–14
2	1 ½	1 ½	0	15–16
2	1 ½	2	0	17–18
2	2	2	0	19–20
2	2	2	1	21–22
2	2	2	2	23–24

[a]Reproduced with permission. Copyright D. V. Sheehan, 1985.
[b]If no side effects (drowsiness) or benefit occurs with medication, increase dose to next level every 2 days. When coming off the medicine, do not reduce dose for any reason at a rate faster than ½ tablet every 4 days. There are no food or drug restrictions with benzodiazepines as there are with MAO inhibitors. Caution when driving and operating high-speed equipment is necessary. Avoid alcohol consumption.

Among the antidepressants, there is a wide choice, differing mainly in terms of sedation and anticholinergic side effects. Patients with panic disorder tend to be sensitive to the anticholinergic effects of antidepressants (Zitrin, Klein, Woener, & Rose, 1983), so we usually start them on a drug at the less active side-effect end of the spectrum, usually desipramine or imipramine. Only when these are ineffective do we move to drugs that have greater anticholinergic side effects. Once the choice of drug is made, we start with a low dosage and then push the dose up. Imipramine is started in doses of 25 mg and then increased by 25 mg every third day (see Table 8). The final dosage is usually determined by the achievement of symptom relief or experience intolerable side effects. Dosages as high as 300 mg of imipramine a day may be needed to get relief. The clinician needs to keep in mind that there is a time lag before the tricyclic begins to work, as long as 5–10 weeks. During this latency period, the only advice one can give the patient is to try to hang on and to see that experiencing side effects is desirable as it indicates clinically that the patient is at therapeutic dosage. During the initial months of treatment, tolerance may occur, and the patient may experience a resurgence of symptoms and a decrease in side effects. All that is required at this point is an increase in dosage until some side effects are experienced again; benefit occurs 5–7 days later. Common side effects experienced are dry mouth, constipation, postural hypotension, urinary hesitancy, retrograde ejaculation, and sweating.

Monoamine Oxidase Inhibitors

There is now strong evidence from double-blind placebo-controlled studies that MAO inhibitors are effective in the treatment of panic disorder (Sheehan, Ballenger, & Jacobson, 1980; Sheehan *et al.*, 1984). The MAO inhibitors are now more widely pre-

Table 8. Directions for Taking Tricyclic Antidepressants[a,b,c]

Breakfast (tablets)	Lunch	Evening meal	Bedtime	Day
0	0	0	1	1–2
1	0	0	1	3–4
1	0	0	2	5–6
1	0	1	2	7–9
1	1	1	2	10–12
2	1	1	2	13–15
2	1	2	2	16–19
2	2	2	2	20–23
2	2	2	3	24–27
3	2	2	3	28–31
3	2	3	3	32–35
3	3	3	3	36–39

[a]Reproduced with permission. Copyright D. V. Sheehan, 1985.
[b]25-mg imipramine tablets or equivalent.
[c]If no side effects (drowsiness) or benefit occurs with medication, increase dose to next level. When coming off the medicine, do not reduce dose at a rate faster than one tablet every 3 days. There are no food or drug restrictions with tricyclics as with MAO inhibitors. Caution when driving and operating high-speed equipment is necessary. Avoid alcohol consumption.

Table 9. *Directions for Taking MAO Inhibitors*[a,b,c]

Breakfast (tablets)	Lunch	Evening meal	Bedtime	Day
0	0	1	0	1–3
1	0	1	0	4–7
1	1	1	0	8–12
1	1	2	0	13–19
2	1	2	0	20–26
2	2	2	0	27–33
2[d]	2	3	0	34–40
3[d]	2	3	0	41–47

[a]Reproduced with permission. Copyright D. V. Sheehan, 1985.
[b]10-mg tablets of Parnate or Marplan or 15-mg tablets of Nardil.
[c]If no side effects (drowsiness) or benefit occurs with medication, increase dose to next level. When coming off MAO inhibitors do not reduce dose suddenly at a rate faster than one tablet every 3 days, ideally one tablet every 2 weeks. There are food and drug restrictions with MAO inhibitors. Caution when driving and operating high-speed equipment is necessary. Avoid alcohol consumption.
[d]For Parnate and Marplan only, not Nardil.

scribed for this condition than they were 10 years ago. There is growing acceptance and awareness that, with proper dietary precautions, they are well tolerated. Blackwell, Marley, Price, *et al.* (1967) found that patients ingesting high-risk food products rarely experienced adverse hypertensive effects.

The MAO inhibitors are related chemically to isoniazid and iproniazid, which were introduced in the 1950s for their antitubercular activity. The MAO inhibitors can be divided into two classes: the hydrazines and the nonhydrazines. Phenelzine sulphate (Nardil) and isocarboxazid (Marplan) are the hydrazine compounds available, and tranylcypromine (Parnate) is the nonhydrazine most commonly prescribed. Phenelzine sulphate is the most potent and efficacious of the available drugs. Although hypertensive reactions are more likely with tranylcypromine, subjective side effects are less likely. Although more potent than the nonhydrazines, phenelzine is more hepatotoxic. Reversal of MAO inhibition may take as long as 2 weeks after stopping phenelzine; with tranylcypromine, the inhibition is largely reversed when the blood level drops to zero.

Table 10. *Dietary Restrictions on MAOI Users*[a,b]

	Danger of blood pressure rise[c]
A. Food	
1. All cheese	3
All foods containing cheese (pizza, fondue, many Italian dishes, and salad dressings).	3
Fresh cottage cheese and cream cheese are safe in moderate amounts.	Safe
Sour cream.	2
2. All fermented or aged foods, especially aged meats or aged fish (aged corned beef, salami, fermented sausage, pepperoni, summer sausage, pickled herring).	2
3. Liver (chicken, beef, or pork liver).	2
Liverwurst.	2

Table 10. (Continued)

	Danger of blood pressure rise[c]
4. Broad bean pods (English bean pods, Chinese pea pods).	3
5. Meat extracts or yeast extracts.	2
Baked products raised with yeast (bread) are safe.	Safe
Yeast is safe.	Safe
6. Spoiled fruit (spoiled bananas, pineapple, avocados).	2
Fresh fruits are safe.	Safe
B. Drinks	
1. Red wine, sherry, vermouth, and cognac.	2
2. Beer and ale.	2
3. Other alcoholic drinks are permitted in moderation. (gin, vodka, whiskey)	Safe
C. Drugs	
1. Cold medications (Dristan, Contac).	3
2. Nasal decongestants and sinus medicine.	3
3. Asthma inhalants.	3
Pure steroid asthma inhalants (e.g., Vanceril) are safe.	Safe
4. Allergy and hay fever medication.	2
5. Narcotics (e.g., Demerol).	3
Codeine is safe.	Safe
6. Amphetamines.	3
Antiappetite (diet) medicine.	2
7. Sympathomimetic amines.	
a. Direct-acting (epinephrine, isoproterenol, methoxamine, levarterenol, norepinephrine).	2
b. Indirect-acting (amphetamines, methylphenidate, phenylpropanolamine, ephedrine, cyclopatamine, pseudephedrine, tyramine).	3
c. Direct- and indirect-acting (vetaraminol, phenylephrine).	3
8. a. Local anesthetics with epinephrine.	3
b. Local anesthetics without epinephrine (Carbocaine).	Safe
9. Levodopa for Parkinsonism.	2
Dopamine.	2
10. Diabetes on insulin may have increased hypoglycemia requiring a decreased dose of insulin (otherwise safe).	Blood sugar ↓
11. Patients on hypotensive agents for high blood pressure may have more hypotension requiring a decrease in their use of hypotensive agent (otherwise safe).	Blood sugar ↓
12. Antihistamines	2
D. "Safe" Foods and Drinks[d]	
Chocolate, anchovies, caviar, coffee, colas, figs, raisins, dates, sauerkraut, mushrooms, beet root (beers), rhubarb, curry powder, junket, worcestershire sauce, soy sauce, licorice, snails, yogurt	1

[a]From D. V. Sheehan and J. B. Claycomb (1983). The Use of MAO Inhibitors in Clinical Practice. In T. C. Manschreck (Ed.), *Psychiatric Medicine Update: Massachusetts General Hospital Review for Physicians,* New York: Elsevier. With permission.
[b]Avoid for 2 days before starting and for 2 weeks after stopping drugs.
[c]Minimal danger, 1; moderate danger, 2; very dangerous, 3.
[d]These foods have been rarely reported to cause hypertensive reactions with MAOIs. The evidence supporting these claims is weak and often based on a single isolated case. Warnings based on such evidence have been uncritically perpetuated especially in view of the large numbers of patients on MAOIs who eat these foods with no problem. In practice, a blanket prohibition of these foods in small quantities seems unjustified unless they are clearly spoiled or decayed and except for specific patients in whom they have already caused symptoms.

However, it is wise to maintain the dietary restrictions for at least 1 week after tranylcypromine therapy and 2–3 weeks after phenelzine therapy.

With phenelzine, the starting dose is 15 mg/day, increasing by 15 mg every 4 days to an average dosage of 45–60 mg a day. Beyond this, increments of 15 mg every week can be made, up to doses of 90 mg/day (see Table 9). The therapeutic dosage is indicated by mild postural hypotension as measured by the sphygmomanometer. Beyond this point, the margin between benefit and side effects is narrow, so increments have to be made in very small doses with careful monitoring.

Side effects such as dry mouth, constipation, excessive sweating over the upper torso and head, delayed urination, retarded ejaculation or orgasmic delay, craving for sweets, and weight gain are common but less troublesome than at an equipotent dose of a tricyclic antidepressant. Postural hypotension is the main effect on blood pressure and is more likely in the later weeks as MAO inhibition progresses. Postural hypotension is best monitored by blood pressure checks in the sitting and standing position and may be minimized by paying attention to hydration, taking salt tablets, and taking the MAO inhibitor with coffee, cola, food, or tea, as small doses of tyramine in these foods will counteract the drug's hypotensive effect. Vitamin B_6 in doses of 200–300 mg a day and magnesium will decrease electric shock effects and carpal tunnel syndrome, as deficits of this vitamin frequently occur after 4–6 months of treatment.

Hypertensive crisis is a potentially dangerous effect of therapy with MAO inhibitors. MAO inhibitors remove the enzyme MAO from the gut wall and thus allow tyramine, a pressor amine, to enter freely and cause an acute increase in blood pressure. To minimize this problem, patients have to be instructed regarding the dietary and concomitant medication restrictions involved. In general, foods that are aged, fermented, or spoiled and over-the-counter cough and cold preparations are likely to cause a reaction (see Table 10). The hypertensive reaction, when it develops, is unmistakable even to patients who have many anxiety symptoms. It begins suddenly, within 5 minutes to 1½ hours after ingesting the pressor agent. Heart rate increases, with heavy pounding of blood vessels in the neck, face, and head. This is followed by a headache, confined initially to the occipital or temporal regions and later spreading all over the head. Patients may describe their heads as feeling "full" or ready to explode. They may be flushed, may sweat profusely, and may have nausea, vomiting, and elevated temperature. Neck stiffness, photophobia, and pulse irregularities occur less frequently. The attack may last minutes to several hours, with the patient becoming symptomatic at systolic blood pressures of 200 mmHG. Headaches may persist for several days after the blood pressure has returned to normal. Treatment consists of giving phentolamine mesylate (5 mg) slowly intravenously. Doses may have to be repeated until the blood pressure normalizes. Nifedipine is especially suited for use in the management of hypertensive crisis (Haft & Litterer, 1984) for several reasons:

1. Blood pressure is lowered in direct relation to the magnitude of the pretreatment blood pressure. Severe hypotensive responses are rarely observed, and invasive blood pressure monitoring is not required.
2. Cardiac output is maintained or increased. This reaction protects against the development of neurological deficit or oliguria that may occur when cardiac output falls considerably.
3. It has a coronary vasodilator action that protects against reflex cardiac stimulation that would precipitate angina or myocardial infarction.

4. As left ventricular afterload is reduced, the drug does not worsen any congestive failure that may accompany hypertensive crisis.
5. Finally nifedipine may be given orally or sublingually. Sublingually it has a more rapid onset of action (1–5 minutes compared to <20 minutes with the oral route). The fall in blood pressure tends to be more rapid when the drug is given sublingually, and this rapid fall may at times be undesirable. The initial dose is 10–20 mg and may be repeated at 30 minutes if necessary.

Nonbenzodiazepine Anxiolytics

Benzodiazepines, tricyclic antidepressants, and monoamine oxidase inhibitors are not single-effect drugs. The ideal anxiolytic drug should be anxioselective, should be unaccompanied by skeletal muscle relaxant or anticonvulsant activity, should not interact significantly and additionally with alcohol or other CNS-depressant compounds, and should not cause sedation or cardiovascular or autonomic effects or have effects that lead to physical or psychological dependence or abuse. Buspirone is one of a series of azaspirodecanedione psychotropic agents prepared by Wu and Rayburn in the early 1970s. Tompkins, Clemento, Taylor, and Pernach (1980) showed that this drug exerts a calming effect in aggressive rhesus monkeys. Hartman and Geller (1981) tested buspirone in a procedure highly predictive of anxiolytic activity in which rats demonstrated attenuation of shock-induced suppression in drinking behavior. On the basis of these animal studies, the potential for antianxiety activity was postulated. Goldberg and Finnerty (1982) confirmed the antianxiety effect of buspirone in a double-blind placebo-controlled study of outpatients with a diagnosis of anxiety neurosis. Richels, Weisman, Norstad, Singer, Stoltz, Brown, and Danton (1982) compared buspirone (21-mg average) to diazepam (20-mg average) and placebo in patients with generalized anxiety disorder. The results suggest that buspirone possesses anxiolytic properties similar to those of diazepam. Buspirone favored symptoms indicative of cognitive and interpersonal problems, including anger and hostility, and diazepam seemed more effective with the somatic symptoms of anxiety. Both drugs were superior to placebo. The main difference between the two drugs was in their side effect profile: diazepam produced more sedation, and buspirone produced more faintness, dizziness, headache, or nausea. Buspirone responders were more likely to be female and not previously treated. Two other studies (Feighner, 1982; Wheatley, 1982) found buspirone to be an effective anxiolytic in patients with generalized anxiety disorder.

Sheehan, Raj, Soto, *et al.* (1987, unpublished study) compared buspirone to imipramine and placebo in patients with panic disorder. Overall buspirone was less efficacious than imipramine, but only marginally, and was not significantly better than placebo. Buspirone responders tended to be older females with a late onset of their illness. The responders had less severe panic disorder, and they had minimal somatization on the SCID-P. Buspirone is effective in doses of 30–60 mg and takes 2 weeks to exert its effects. Those who have used benzodiazepines in the 2 months before starting buspirone are less likely to get a good response. Buspirone is very well tolerated, the major complaints being dizziness and lightheadedness. Buspirone can be stopped abruptly even at doses as high as 60 mg a day with no observable withdrawal syndrome. Other advantages of buspirone are in its lack of sedative hypnotic effects (Riblet, Eison, Eison, Taylor, Temple, & VanderMaelen, 1984) and its lack of potential for dependence or abuse in humans (Griffith, Jasinski, Casten, & McKinney, 1986); also, it does not interact significantly with CNS depressants like alcohol (Moskowitz & Smiley, 1982), and it does not show significant impairment of psychomotor or cognitive skills (Mattilla, Aranko, & Seppala, 1982). Overall its effect in panic disorder patients is unpredictable, but its side-effect and nonabuse profile suggest that it is worth trying in geriatric patients and those with a high risk for substance dependence and abuse.

Treatment of Phobic Behavior

Once pharmacological control of the panic attacks has been achieved, the next step is to deal with the phobic avoidance behaviors, which are a consequence of those attacks. Behavior therapy is very helpful in reducing these avoidance behaviors. The type of behavior therapy recommended has changed over the last 15 years. Initially, treatment was with systematic desensitization in fantasy. This was replaced by live exposure sessions with a therapist present, and it is now increasingly clear that most sufferers can complete live self-exposure successfully without a therapist being present (Frame, Turner, & Jacob, 1986; Ghosh & Marks, 1987). It has been suggested that imipramine in combination with exposure is more effective than either therapies alone (Mavissakalian, Michelson, & Dealy, 1983; Telch, Agras, Taylor, Roth, & Gallen, 1985).

We begin by generating a phobia profile of the patient. Each phobia identified is rated for its fearfulness and for the extent of the avoidance behavior with regard to that phobia. We next educate the patient in the principles of *in vivo* exposure. He or she is instructed to begin with the less fearful phobias. Success in eliminating these promotes confidence and risk-taking behavior. If possible, the feared situation should be entered into three or more times a week. Each exposure session should last at least 90 minutes and ideally 2–3 hours. On first entering the phobic situation, anticipatory anxiety and surges of panic may provoke a flight response. The patient should be instructed to stay in the phobic situation until the turmoil subsides before progressing further. In this manner, all the phobias can be systematically dealt with and eliminated. In treatment-resistant patients, ''megadoses'' of exposure treatment may be effective (Rapp, Thomas, & Reyes, 1983).

Long-Term Management and Relapse Prevention

Once the panic attacks are under control with the use of medications and an exposure therapy program is in place, it may be necessary to attend to several psychosocial issues. A long-standing anxiety disorder may have caused low self-esteem and a defeatist attitude; it may have strained the marital or family situation, and it may have forced compromises and limitations that the patient is no longer willing to accept. Despite benefit from the medication, patients feel conflict about their reliance on it. This conflict may lead them to prematurely and inappropriately discontinue the medication. This dependence–independence conflict is best dealt with by educating patients and their families regarding the biological nature of the illness and by outlining a long-term course of action. We recommend being on the medication for a period of 6–12 months and then gradually tapering off. The relapse rates are so high (Sheehan, 1986) that we need to consider the possibility of ongoing pharmacotherapy for a majority of patients with panic disorder. It has been suggested that relapse rates tend to be lower if drugs have been combined with behavioral treatment (Mavissakalian & Michelson, 1986).

FUTURE DIRECTIONS

The past decade has seen a great proliferation of knowledge about panic disorder. Indeed, the information about and the conceptualization and treatment of panic disorder have changed more in the past decade than perhaps for any other disorder in psychiatry. This does not now appear to be a passing fashion. It has been a high-yield trend that is likely to continue to be a potent stimulus to new research directions and treatment approaches.

It appears likely that we will identify very precisely the exact genetic locus—or base-pair alteration—at the root of the disorder. This will help us identify those at risk of developing the condition before they begin to have symptoms. This may permit us to intervene earlier to block the symptomatic expression of the disorder.

Better laboratory diagnostic tests will emerge to support the physician's clinical impression of the diagnosis. The neurochemical basis for the disorder will be more fully elucidated. This in turn will permit more accurate classification studies and a precise delineation of the boundaries of the disorder.

There is an acute need to develop good animal models for this disorder. Perhaps a genetic strain that is lactate-infusion-sensitive would be a logical place to begin searching for such a model. Animal models usually result in a much greater acceleration in the knowledge about any disease and permit more high-yield and precisely controlled studies.

All of these developments should provide the groundwork for safer, more rapid, and more precise treatments.

REFERENCES

American Psychiatric Association. (1980). *Diagnostic and statistical manual of mental disorders* (3rd ed.; DSM-III). Washington, DC: Author.

American Psychiatric Association. (1987). *Diagnostic and statistical manual of mental disorders* (3rd ed. rev.; DSM-III-R). Washington, DC: Author.

Bibb, J. L., & Chambless, D. L. (1986). *Behavior Research and Therapy, 24,* 49–58.

Blackwell, B., Marley, E., Price, J., & Taylor, D. (1967). Hypertensive interaction between monoamine oxidase inhibitors and food stuffs. *British Journal of Psychiatry, 113,* 349–365.

Brodsky, L., Zuniger, J. S., Casenas, E. R. *et al.* (1983). Refractory anxiety: A mashed epileptiform disorder. *Psychiatric Journal of the University of Ottawa, 8,* 42–45.

Carr, D. B., & Sheehan, D. V. (1984). Panic anxiety: A new biological model. *Journal of Clinical Psychiatry, 45,* 323–330.

Charney, D. S., Woods, S. W., Goodman, W. K., *et al.* (1986). Drug treatment of panic disorder: The comparative efficacy of imipramine, alprazolam and trazodone. *Journal of Clinical Psychiatry, 47,* 580–586.

Chouinard, G. Annable, L., Fontaine, R., *et al.* (1982). Alprazolam in the treatment of generalized anxiety and panic disorders: A double blind placebo controlled study. *Psychopharmacology, 77,* 229–233.

Coryell, W., Noyes, R., & Clancy, J. (1982). Excess mortality in panic disorder. *Archives of General Psychiatry, 39,* 701–703.

Crowe, R. R., Noyes, R., Pauls, D. L., & Slymen, D. (1983). A family study of panic disorder. *Archives of General Psychiatry, 40,* 1065–1069.

Crowe, R. R., Noyes, R., Wilson, A. F., Elston, R. C., & Ward, L. J. (1987). A linkage study of panic disorder. *Archives of General Psychiatry, 44,* 933–937.

Darwin, C. (1872). *The expressions of the emotions in man and animals.* London: J. Murray.

Drachman, D. A., & Hart, C. W. (1972). An approach to the dizzy patient. *Neurology, 22,* 323–334.

Eaton, W. W., & McLeod, J. (1984). Consumption of coffee or tea and symptoms of anxiety. *American Journal of Public Health, 74,* 66–68.

Feighner, J. P. (1982). A double blind comparison of buspirone and diazepam in outpatients with generalized anxiety disorder. *Journal of Clinical Psychiatry, 43,* 103–107.
Fishman, S. M., Sheehan, D. V., & Carr, D. B. (1985). Thyroid indices in panic disorder. *Journal of Clinical Psychiatry, 46,* 422–423.
Fontaine, R., & Chouinard, G. (1948). Antipanic effect of clonazepam (letter to the editor). *American Journal of Psychiatry, 141,* 149.
frame, C. L., Turner, S. M., & Jacob, R. G. (1986). Self-exposure treatment of agoraphobia. *Behavior Modification, 8,* 115–122.
Freud, S. (1962). On the grounds for detaching a particular syndrome from neurasthenia under the description "Anxiety neurosis." In J. Strachey (Ed. and Trans.), *The standard edition of the complete psychological works of Sigmund Freud (Vol. 3).* London: Hogarth Press. (Original work published 1895.)
Frohlich, E. D., Terazi, R. C., & Dustan, H. P. (1969). Hyperdynamic beta-adrenergic circulatory state. *Archives of Internal Medicine, 123,* 1–7.
Ghadirian, A. M., Gauthier, S., & Bertrand, S. (1986). Anxiety attacks in a patient with a right temporal meningioma. *Journal of Clinical Psychiatry, 47,* 270–271.
Ghosh, A., & Marks, I. M. (1987). Self-treatment of agoraphobia by exposure. *Behavior Therapy, 18,* 3–16.
Goldberg, H. L., & Finnerty, R. (1982). Comparison of buspirone in two separate studies. *Journal of Clinical Psychiatry, 43,* 87–91.
Gorman, J. M., & Martinez, J. M. (1984). Hypoglycemia and panic attacks. *American Journal of Psychiatry, 141,* 101–102.
Gray, J. A. (1982). *The neuropsychology of anxiety: An enquiry into the functions of the septo-hippocampal system.* Oxford: University Press.
Greer, S. (1969). The prognosis of anxiety states. In M. H. Leder (Ed.), *Studies of anxiety* (pp. 161–157). London: Royal Medical Psychological Association.
Griffith, J. D., Jasinski, D. R., Casten, G. P., & McKinney, G. R. (1986). Investigation of the abuse liability of buspirone in alcohol dependent patients. *American Journal of Medicine, 80,* 30–35.
Haft, J. L., & Litterer, W. E., III. (1984). Chewing nifedipine to rapidly treat hypertension. *Archives of Internal Medicine, 144,* 2357–2359.
Harris, E. L., Noyes, R., & Crowe, R. R. (1983). A family study of agoraphobia: A pilot study. *Archives of General Psychology, 40,* 1061–1064.
Hartman, R. J., & Geller, J. (1981). Effects of buspirone on conflict behavior of laboratory rats and monkeys. *Proceedings of the Western Pharmacological Society, 24,* 179–181.
Insel, T. R., Ninan, P. T., & Aloy, J. (1984). A benzodiazepine receptor meditated model of anxiety: Studies in nonhuman primates and clinical implications. *Archives of General Psychiatry, 41,* 741–750.
Jacob, R. G., Moller, M. B., Turner, S. M., *et al.* (1985, December). *Otoneurological dysfunction in patients with panic disorder or agoraphobia with panic attacks.* Paper presented at the 17th Annual Convention of the World Congress on Behavior Therapy, Washington, DC.
Katerndahl, D. H., & Vandercreek, L. (1983). Hyperthyroidism and panic attacks. *Psychosomatic, 24,* 491–496.
Klein, D. F. (1964). Delineation of two drug responsive anxiety syndromes. *Psychopharmacologia, 5,* 397–408.
Klein, D. F. (1967). Importance of psychiatric diagnosis and prediction of clinical drug effects. *Archives of General Psychiatry, 16,* 118–126.
Lader, M. H. (1972). The nature of anxiety. *British Journal of Psychiatry, 121,* 481.
Lesser, I. M., Rubin, R. T., Lydiard, R. B., *et al.* (1987). Past and current thyroid function in subjects with panic disorder. *Journal of Clinical Psychiatry, 48,* 473–476.
Liberthson, R., Sheehan, D. V., King, M. E., & Weyman, A. E. (1986). The prevalence of mitral valve prolapse in patients with panic disorder. *American Journal of Psychiatry, 143,* 511–515.
Lindeman, C. G., Zitrin, C. M., & Klein, D. F. (1984). Thyroid dysfunction in phobic patients. *Psychosomatics, 26,* 603–606.
Lustman, P. J., Griffith, L. S., Clouse, E. R., *et al.* (1986). Psychiatric illness in diabetes mellitus: Relationship to symptoms and glucose control. *Journal of Nervous and Mental Disease, 174,* 736–742.
Manger, W. M., & Gifford, R. W. (1982). Hypertension secondary to pheochromoaton. *Bulletin of the New York Academy of Medicine, 58,* 139–158.
Marks, I. S. (1969). *Fears and phobias.* New York: Academic Press.
Marks, I. S., & Lader, M. (1973). Anxiety states (anxiety neurosis: A review). *Journal of Nervous and Mental Disease, 156,* 3–18.

Mattilla, M. J., Aranko, K., & Seppala, T. (1982). Acute effects of buspirone and alcohol on psychomotor skills. *Journal of Clinical Psychiatry, 43,* 56–60.

Mavissakalian, M., & Michelson, L. (1986). Two year follow-up of exposure and imipramine treatment of agoraphobia. *American Journal of Psychiatry, 143,* 1106–1112.

Mavissakalian, M., Michelson, L., & Dealy, R. S. (1983). Pharmacological treatment of agoraphobia: Imipramine versus imipramine with programmed practice. *British Journal of Psychiatry, 143,* 348–355.

McNair, D., & Kahn, R. J. (1981). Imipramine compared with the benzodiazepine for agoraphobia. In D. F. Klein & J. G. Rabkin (Eds.), *Anxiety: New research and current concepts* (pp. 60–79). New York: Raven Press.

Moskowitz, H., & Smiley, A. (1982). Effects of chronically administered buspirone and diazepam in driving related skills performance. *Journal of Clinical Psychiatry, 34,* 45–55.

Pariser, S. F., Jones, B. A., Pinta, E. R. *et al.* (1979). Panic attacks: Diagnostic evaluations of 17 patients. *American Journal of Psychiatry 136,* 105–106.

Paul, S. M., & Skolnick, P. (1981). Benzodiazepine receptors and psychopathological states: towards the neurobiology of anxiety. In D. F. Kline & J. Rabkin (Eds.), *Anxiety; New research and changing concepts.* New York: Raven Press.

Pauls, D. L., Bocher, K. D., Crowe, R. R., & Noyes, R. (1980). A genetic study of panic disorder pedigrees. *American Journal of Human Genetics, 32,* 639–644.

Popkin, M. K., Callies, H. L., Lentz, R. D., *et al.* (1988). Prevalence of major depression, simple phobia and other psychiatric disorders in patients with long standing Type 1 diabetes mellitus. *Archives of General Psychiatry, 45,* 64–68.

Rapp, M. S., Thomas, M. R., & Reyes, E. C. (1983). Mega doses of behavior therapy for treatment resistant agoraphobics. *Canadian Journal of Psychiatry, 28,* 105–109.

Redmond, D. E. (1977). Alterations in the functions of the nucleus locus coeruleus: A possible model for studies of anxiety. In I. Hanin & E. Usdin (Eds.), *Animal models in psychiatry and neurology.* New York: Pergamon Press.

Reiman, E. M., Raichle, M. E., & Butler, F. K. (1984). PET focal brain abnormality in panic disorder. *Nature, 310,* 683–685.

Riblet, L. A., Eison, A. S., Eison, M. S., Taylor, D. P., Temple, D. L., & VanderMaelen, C. P. (1984). Neuropharmacology of busiprone. *Psychopathology, 17,* 69–78.

Richels, K., Weisman, K., Norstad, N., Singer, M. Stoltz, D., Brown, A., & Danton, J. (1984). Busiprone and diazepam in anxiety. A controlled study. *Journal of Clinical Psychiatry, 43,* 81–86.

Robins, L. N., Helzer, J. E., & Weissman, M. M. (1984). Lifetime prevalence of specific psychiatric disorders in three sites. *Archives of General Psychiatry, 41,* 949–958.

Shappiro, S., Skinner, E. A., & Kessler, L. G. (1984). Utilization of health and mental health services. *Archives of General Psychiatry, 41,* 977.

Sheehan, D. V. (1982). Panic attacks and phobias. *New England Journal of Medicine, 307,* 156–158.

Sheehan, D. V. (1983). *The anxiety disease.* New York: Scribner's.

Sheehan, D. V. (1986). Tricyclic antidepressants in the treatment of panic and anxiety disorders. *Psychosomatics, 27,* 10–16.

Sheehan, D. V., & Claycomb, J. B. (1983). The use of MAO inhibitors in clinical practice. In T. C. Manschreck (Ed.), *Psychiatric medicine update: Massachusetts General Hospital review for physicians.* New York: Elsevier.

Sheehan, D. V., & Sheehan, K. E. (1982–1983). The classification of phobic disorders. *International Journal of Psychiatric Medicine, 12,* 243–264.

Sheehan, D. V., Ballenger, J., & Jacobson, G. (1980). Treatment of endogenous anxiety with phobic, hysterical, and hypochondrical symptoms. *Archives of General Psychiatry, 31,* 51–59.

Sheehan, D. V., Sheehan, K. E., & Minichiello, W. E. (1981). Age of onset of phobic disorders: A reevaluation. *Comprehensive Psychiatry, 22,* 544–553.

Sheehan, D. V., Davidson, J., Manschneck, T. C., *et al.* (1983). Lack of efficacy of a new antidepressant (bupropion) in the treatment of panic disorder with phobias. *Journal of Clinical Psychopharmacology, 3,* 28–31.

Sheehan, D. V., Claycomb, J. B., Surman, O. S., *et al.* (1984). *The relative efficacy of alprazolam, phenelzine, and imipramine in treating panic attacks and phobias.* Annual meeting of the American Psychiatric Association, Los Angeles, May 8.

Sheehan, D. V., Raj, B. A., Soto, S., *et al.* (1987, May). Is buspirone effective for panic disorders? A double blind placebo controlled study. Paper presented at NCDEU Annual Meeting, Bay Biscayne, FL.

Smith, D. E. (1968). Acute and chronic toxicity of marijuana. *Journal of Psychoactive Drugs, 2,* 37–47.

Spier, S. A., Teser, G. E., Rosenbaum, J. F., & Woods, S. W. (1986). Treatment of panic disorder with clonazepam. *Journal of Clinical Psychiatry, 47,* 238–242.

Spitzer, R. L., Endicott, J., & Robbins, E. (1975). *Research diagnostic criteria.* New York: New York State Psychiatric Institute, Division of Biometric Research.

Starrman, M. N., Zelnik, T. C., Nesse, R. M., *et al.* (1958). Anxiety in patients with pheochromocytoma. *Archives of Internal Medicine, 145,* 248–252.

Strauss, E., Risser, A., & Jones, M. W. (1982). Fear responses in patients with epilepsy. *Archives of Neurology, 39,* 626–630.

Telch, M. J., Agras, W. S., Taylor, C. B., Roth, W. T., & Gallen, C. C. (1958). Combined pharmacological and behavioral treatment for agoraphobia. *Behavior Research and Therapy, 23,* 325–355.

Tompkins, E. C., Clemento, A. J., Taylor, D. P., & Pernach, J. L. (1980). Inhibition of aggressive behavior in rhesus monkeys by buspirone. *Research Communications in Psychology, Psychiatry and Behavior, 5,* 337–352.

Torgersen, S. (1983). Genetic factors in anxiety disorders. *Archives of General Psychiatry, 40,* 1085–1089.

Uhde, T. W., Vittone, B. J., & Post, R. M. (1984). Glucose tolerance testing in panic disorder. *American Journal of Psychiatry, 141,* 1461–1463.

Wall, M., Tuchman, M., & Mielke, D. (1958). Panic attacks and temporal lobe seizures associated with a right temporal lobe arteriovenous malformation: Case report. *Journal of Clinical Psychiatry, 46,* 145.

Wall, M., Mielke, D., & Luther, J. S. (1986). Panic attacks and psychomotor seizures following right temporal lobectomy. *Journal of Clinical Psychiatry, 47,* 219.

Watson, A. M., & Gold, M. S. (1948). Chronic cocaine abuse: Evidence for adverse effects on health and functioning. *Psychological Annals, 14,* 733–745.

Weissman, M. M. (1985). Rates, risks, and familial patterns. In A. H. Tuma & J. D. Maser (Eds.), *Anxiety and the anxiety disorders.* Hillsdale, NJ: Erlbaum.

Wheatley, D. (1982). Buspirone: Multicenter efficacy study. *Journal of Clinical Psychiatry, 43,* 92–94.

Wheeler, E. O., White, P. D., Reed, E. W., & Cohen, M. E. (1950). Neurocirculatory asthenia (anxiety neurosis, effort syndrome, neurasthenia): a 20 year follow up study of 173 patients. *Journal of the American Medical Association, 142,* 878–889.

Woodruff, R. H., Guze, S. B., & Clayton, P. J. (1972). Anxiety neurosis among psychiatric outpatients. *Comprehensive Psychiatry, 13,* 165–170.

Zitrin, C. M., Klein, D. F., Woener, M. G., & Rose, D. C. (1983). Treatment of phobias: 1. Comparison of imipramine and placebo. *Archives of General Psychiatry, 40,* 125–138.

10

Obsessive-Compulsive Disorder

P. R. McCARTHY AND E. B. FOA

INTRODUCTION

In the third edition of the *Diagnostic and Statistical Manual of Mental Disorders* (DSM-III; APA, 1980), the official diagnostic manual of the American Psychiatric Association, obsessive-compulsive disorder (OCD) is listed among the anxiety disorders. Requisite for the diagnosis of this disorder are the presence of obsessions and/or compulsions. Obsessions are recurrent and persistent thoughts or images experienced as intrusive, unwanted, and senseless. They are recognized by the person as a product of the mind, and as not being imposed externally on him or her. Typically, the individual attempts to ignore or suppress them. The most common obsessions include repetitive thoughts of violence, contamination, and doubt.

Compulsions are repetitive and purposeful behavior performed according to certain rules or in a rigid, stereotyped fashion. The compulsive act is not an end in itself; rather, it is an attempt to neutralize or prevent discomfort arising from an event or situation that is feared unrealistically. Usually, the individual is able to recognize and acknowledge the excessive and irrational nature of the compulsion. Obsessions and compulsions produce marked distress, are time-consuming, and can interfere markedly with the social and occupational functioning of the individual. Among the most common compulsions seen clinically are repetitive hand-washing, counting, checking, and touching (APA, 1986).

Historical Overview

Accounts of obsessive-compulsive behaviors have been present in popular and technical literature for well over 100 years. Obsessive thought patterns were briefly discussed by Esquirol in 1838. Labeling them as a form of intellectual monomania in his rudemen-

---

P. R. McCARTHY • Biobehavioral Research Institute, Chester Springs, Pennsylvania 19425. E. B. FOA • Medical College of Pennsylvania, Philadelphia, Pennsylvania 19129.

tary classificatory schema, he characterized these thought patterns as an intense concentration on a single object and the formation of false principles from which pseudological reasonings and consequents were derived. These thought patterns, Esquirol suggested, modified affect, behavior, and willpower.

It was the French philosopher Janet who in 1903 provided the first significant treatise on obsessions and anxiety, describing obsessional individuals as *scrupuleux*. Like Esquirol, he viewed obsessionals as suffering primarily from problems of willpower and of controlling mentation. For Janet, obsessions, rather than compulsions, were the core of this mental disorder; consequently, the treatment he proposed focused primarily on obsessions. According to his classification schema, obsessions were divided by content into five categories: crime, sacrilege, shame, physical inadequacy, and hypochondriasis. Further, Janet distinguished four components common to all types of obsessive thinking. First, obsessional thoughts are focused not on external objects, but on a patient's behavior. For example, a fear of knives may, in reality, be a fear of committing murder. Second, obsessional thoughts involve only "bad" or unacceptable acts. The degree of "badness" or unacceptability of these acts is not always dictated by common morality. Instead, it is influenced by their disparity from the individual's desires and will. An example is an individual who is obsessed by the thought that his prayers must be perfect in form. Third, obsessions typically focus on extreme negative behaviors such as sacrilegious or dangerous acts. Fourth, obsessions emanate from within but are also influenced by external events, which do not cause them but do shape their content.

Freud used his now well-known case of the ratman (1909) to conceptualize obsessional neurosis. For Freud, obsessionals have been fixated at the anal stage of psychosexual development as a result of conflicts between parents and the child over early toilet training. During toilet training, conflict arises between the child's desire to eliminate at will and the parents' request that anal activities be regulated to meet the cultural standards of cleanliness and impulse control. When parents are too punishing, when training is too early or too late, or when training is experienced by the child as too frustrating, the parent–child conflict intensifies. Such conflict results in anal fixation and, consequently, in the development of a predominantly anal (obsessive-compulsive) character structure in the child. According to Freud, stress in later life produces a regression to the anal stage, which is the basis of obsessional phenomena.

According to the psychoanalytic view, a number of defense mechanisms play a role in obsessive-compulsive disorder; the three that predominate are undoing, emotional isolation, and reaction formation. Perhaps the most readily apparent is "undoing," which can be recognized directly in the individual who feels compelled to engage in a thought or an action in order to nullify a negative event. As a defense, emotional isolation is the mechanism by which affective thoughts and images are repressed into the unconscious. When effective, this defense filters the access to awareness so that only affectless mentation is available, thereby *dissassociating existing negative feelings*. A third mechanism, reaction formation, is the emission of behaviors directly opposed to unconscious impulses. It is thought that the aggressive impulses underlying obsessive-compulsive disorder are suppressed, so that the patient is enabled to appear caring, cooperative, and devoid of anger.

Classification

In contrast to the focus of Janet on obsessions, modern attempts at classifying the phenomenology of obsessive-compulsive disorder have focused primarily on compulsions, organizing the disorder on the basis of ritualistic activity (e.g., washers, checkers, and orderers). Many patients manifest more than one type of ritualistic behavior. However, in most cases, one specific type prevails, the most common compulsions being washing and cleaning, followed by checking (Stern & Cobb, 1978). A subgroup of checking is the repeating of actions multiple times. Like checkers, repeaters ritualize in order to circumvent disaster. They differ from checkers in that their rituals are *not logically* related to the feared consequences. If one is afraid of burglary, checking windows and doors is a logical action; dressing and redressing to prevent one's husband's death lacks obvious logic. A third type of ritual consists of ordering objects in a precise manner to create a state of symmetry or balance. Disturbance of this order causes extreme discomfort. An additional category, obsessional slowness, was suggested by Rachman and Hodgson (1980). These patients do not appear to have distinct obsessions followed by ritualistic behavior designed to reduce anxiety. Rather, they carry out daily activities, particularly toileting, with extreme care and many hours of effort. Other authors have attempted to provide a classification based on the form of the obsessions (e.g., Akhtar, Wig, Verma, Pershad, & Verma, 1975; Capstick & Seldrup, 1973; Dowson, 1977).

A shortcoming inherent in the above classifications is their absence of bearing on treatment strategies. Foa, Steketee, and Ozarow (1985) offered a classification resting on the class of cues that evokes anxiety and the type of activity (cognitive or overt) that reduces it. In this manner, they related typology to treatment. All obsessive-compulsives, they proposed, suffer from intrusive thoughts, images, or impulses. This mentation may be triggered by external stimuli, such as a perceived contaminant, or may arise without clear external cues. A further distinction is the presence or absence of feared disasters. For example, the thought "Was I driving carefully?" may be associated with the fear of injuring a pedestrian and leaving him or her to die. On the other hand, an intrusive thought such as "Are my hands dirty?" may elicit discomfort in the absence of a fear that dirt may be harmful.

Accordingly, Foa *et al.* (1985) divided obsessions into different types: (1) the presence of intrusive cognitive material, external cues, and fears of disasters; (2) the presence of intrusive material and external cues (in the absence of disasters); and (3) the presence of intrusive material and a fear of disasters (in the absence of external cues). An additional type of intrusive cognitive material with neither external cues nor a fear of disasters is possible according to this framework but has not been observed clinically. Rachman's division (1976b) of "restorative" and "preventive" compulsions provides an explanation for the absence of this pattern. It is difficult to imagine repetitive thoughts without the urge either to restore a state of relative calm or to prevent a future disaster that would evoke anxiety sufficient to constitute an obsession. Thus, the development of obsessions requires fear of external cues.

The present conceptualization posits that all rituals are anxiety-reducing. The type of ritual (e.g., washing or checking) is irrelevant, because it does not lead to differential treatment. A more useful approach categorizes compulsions according to their mode of action (i.e., cognitive or behavioral). These two classes do not differ in their functional relationship to anxiety; yet they carry different treatment implications.

The combination of the four classes of obsessions and the two classes of compulsions described above yields eight types of obsessive compulsives (see Figure 1). Only six of the eight possible types have been observed clinically. It should be stressed that these types are not mutually exclusive. A patient may experience obsessions of several different types. Similarly, a given obsession may give rise to both covert and overt rituals. As depicted in Figure 1, three obsessive-compulsive types are distinguished by the absence of

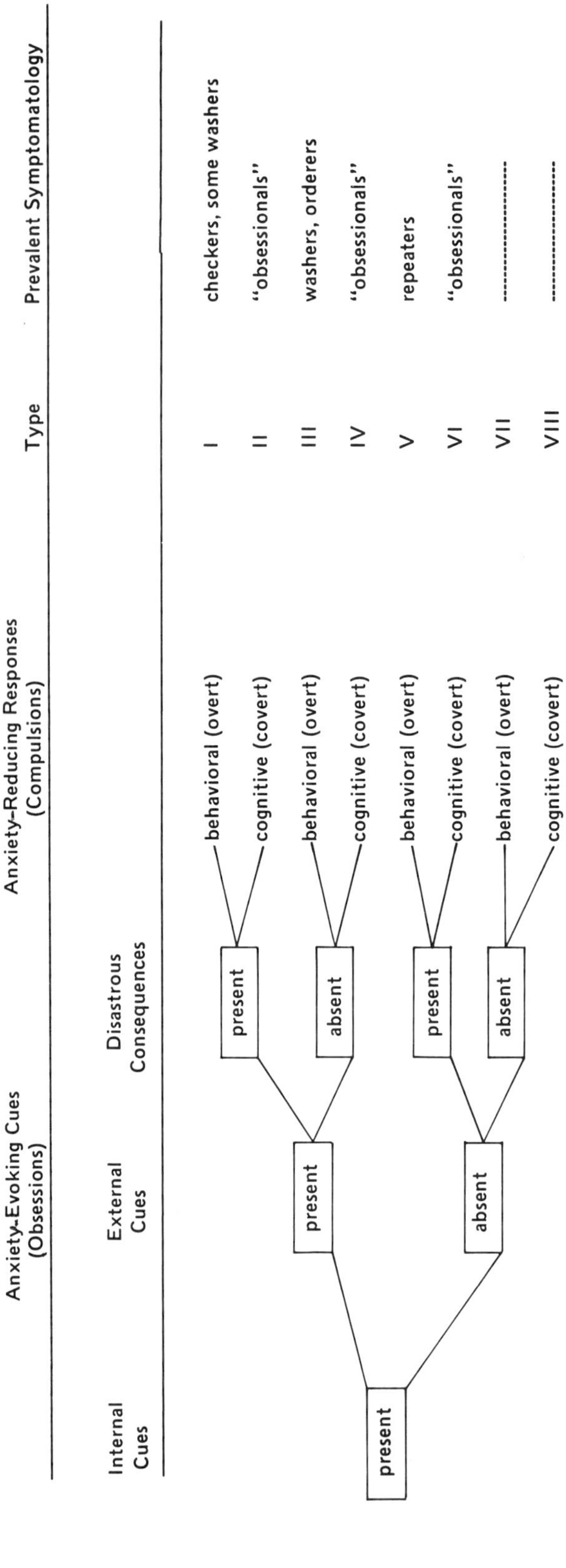

Figure 1. Typology of obsessive-compulsive manifestations.

overt rituals. Patients manifesting this pattern have been labeled *obsessional;* they may vary, however, with respect to whether or not their obsessions include external cues and/or anticipated disasters. Overt compulsions triggered by external cues and by anticipated disasters (Type 1) are found in nearly all checkers and in many washers and cleaners. Externally triggered obsessions without feared consequences (Type 3) occur in orderers and also exist in washers. Obsessions triggered by internal cues and by anticipated disaster (Type 5) are most often observed in repeaters.

This classification reflects the view that the patterns of obsessive-compulsive symptomatology include both obsessions and compulsions. Hence, Foa *et al.* (1985) suggested that individuals who have been referred to in the literature as pure obsessionals, if carefully evaluated, will be found to manifest cognitive compulsions.

Frequent Clinical Problems

Depression

A strong association between depression and obsessive-compulsive symptoms has been noted by numerous authors (Beech, 1971; Cammer, 1973; Mellett, 1974; Rachman, 1976a; Walker & Beech, 1969). Kendell and DiScipio (1970) and Vaughn (1976) have studied the incidence of obsessional symptoms in large samples of depressed patients and have found a joint occurrence of the two symptomatologies in a range of 17%–35%. When the incidence of depression was studied in an obsessive-compulsive population, a somewhat similar picture emerged. Solyom, Zamanzadeh, Ledwidge, and Kenney (1971) found that two thirds of a sample of 15 obsessionals showed mild to moderate depression; only two were severely depressed. In observing 20 obsessive-compulsives, Mellett (1974) reported that 95% were "unusually prone to depressive reactions." In a study of 21 obsessive-compulsives, mild to moderate depression was evident, with a mean depression rating of 4.8 on a scale ranging from 0 to 8 (Foa & Goldstein, 1978). Only 3 of this sample were classified as severely depressed. In a more recent study of 38 obsessive-compulsives, the mean score on the Beck Depression Inventory was 23, indicating a moderate to high level of depression (Foa, Steketee, Kozak, & Dugger, 1987).

Whereas the existence of a relationship between obsessive-compulsive symptoms and depression is unquestionable, its nature remains unclear. Does depression produce obsessive symptoms? Do patients become depressed as a result of the discomfort and limitations imposed by obsessive-compulsive symptoms, or are the two related through a third unidentified variable? The first hypothesis has been investigated in studies on antidepressants, primarily with clomipramine. If depression causes obsessive-compulsive symptoms, antidepressants would reduce obsessive-compulsive symptoms only if they first reduce depression. If, on the other hand, depression is caused by the discomfort arising from obsessive-compulsive symptoms, then improvement in these symptoms following any treatment will result in a reduction in depression.

The joint occurrence of obsessive-compulsive symptomatology and depression may be due to a common factor of hyperreactivity. Lewinsohn, Lobitz, and Wilson (1973) demonstrated that depressives show more sensitivity to aversive events than normals. Periods of depression, with a concomitant increase in obsessions and compulsions, have been observed in obsessional patients (Marks, 1965).

Overvalued Ideation

A subpopulation of obsessive-compulsives maintain a strong belief that their fears are realistic and that their ritualistic behaviors actually prevent the occurrence of disaster.

When asked how likely their feared consequences are in the absence of preventive rituals, these patients estimate a high likelihood. This belief is uncharacteristic of the majority of obsessive-compulsives, who recognize the senselessness of their fears and therefore assign a low probability to their occurrence, despite their compulsion to behave as if actual danger does exist. Foa (1979) presented the example of a patient who feared contact with "leukemia germs," which she believed would kill her husband and children. Despite repeated assurances from professionals that no such germs exist, the patient found ways to devalue outside information, holding to her belief that such germs did exist and could be spread interpersonally. When asked to estimate the likelihood that her loved ones would die if she did not perform preventive washing rituals, she responded, "100 percent."

The problem of the differential diagnosis of obsessive-compulsive disorder and schizophrenic process is still an unresolved issue (Insel & Akiskal, 1986). As indicated in the latest revision of the DSM (DSM-III-R; APA, 1986), "the individual with an overvalued idea can usually, after considerable discussion, acknowledge that his/her belief may be unfounded in contrast with a true delusion that cannot be shaped" (p. 246). Although good measures do not yet exist for assessing overvalued ideation, the study of this concept may throw light on what factors differentiate psychotic delusion from neurotic conviction.

THEORETICAL MODELS

Behavioral Theory

Mowrer's two-stage theory (1939) for the acquisition and maintenance of fear and avoidance behavior has commonly been adopted to explain phobic and obsessive-compulsive disorders. Following further elaboration by Dollard and Miller in 1950 and again by Mowrer in 1960, this theory postulates that, first, a neutral event becomes associated with fear by being paired with a stimulus, which, by its nature, provokes discomfort or anxiety. Through an associative process, concrete objects, as well as thoughts and images, acquire the ability to produce discomfort. In the second stage of the course of symptoms, escape or avoidance responses develop to reduce the anxiety or discomfort evoked by the various conditioned stimuli and are maintained by their success in doing so. Because of extensive generalization, many of the fear-provoking situations of obsessive-compulsives cannot be readily avoided. Passive avoidance behaviors, such as those used by phobics, are rendered ineffective in controlling anxiety. Active avoidance patterns, in the form of ritualistic behaviors, are then developed.

Support for the fear acquisition stage of this model is inadequate (e.g., Rachman & Wilson, 1980). The majority of patients cannot recall conditioning events associated with symptom onset. Onset does, however, often follow stressful life events, which, as suggested by Watts (1971), may serve to sensitize the individual to cues that have an innate tendency to elicit fear. Teasdale (1974) proposed that anxiety responses learned during early experiences may be enhanced by stress. In the same vein, Rachman (1971) posited that, for obsessive-compulsives, a state of heightened arousal may lead to sensitization of thoughts that have special significance to the individual. Related to these notions is Eysenck's theory (1979) that brief exposure to events that upset the individual above his or her tolerance threshold produces sensitization; fear may then be acquired. Accordingly, individuals who are highly arousable physiologically may be prone to developing anxiety disorders. Indeed, there is evidence to suggest that obsessive-compulsives are more physiologically reactive to threat anticipation than normals (Boulougouris, 1977). However, these data were obtained after symptom onset, and arousability may have been the effect rather than the cause of the obsessive-compulsive disorder. Nonetheless, it is not unreasonable to presume that heightened physiological arousal combined with a general stressor and with specific fear cues may produce such symptoms.

Whereas the factors related to the acquisition of obsessive-compulsive disorder are still largely unclear, there is evidence to suggest that obsessions give rise to anxiety-discomfort and that compulsions reduce it. Ruminative thoughts were found to increase heart-rate and skin conductance responding more than neutral thoughts (Boulougouris, Rabavilas, & Stefanis, 1977; Rabavilas & Boulougouris, 1974). Likewise, contact with contaminated objects resulted in increased heart rate and subjective anxiety (Hodgson & Rachman, 1972), as well as skin conductance level (Hornsveld, Kraaimaat, & van Dam-Baggen, 1979). A series of experiments with washers and checkers revealed that, in most instances, their anxiety decreased following the performance of a ritual after the deliberate provocation of an urge to ritualize (Hodgson & Rachman, 1972; Hornsveld *et al.*, 1979; Roper & Rachman, 1976; Roper, Rachman, & Hodgson, 1973).

Cognitive Theories

In an attempt to explain obsessive-compulsive symptoms, Carr (1974) proposed that obsessive-compulsives have abnormally high expectations of unpleasant outcomes; that is, they overestimate the risk of negative consequences for a variety of actions. He noted that obsessional content typically includes exaggerations of the normal concerns of most individuals: health, death, others' welfare, sex, religious matters, performance at work, and the like. Similarly, McFall and Wollersheim (1979) stressed the erroneous beliefs of obsessive-compulsives. These include the idea that one must be perfectly competent in all endeavors to be worthwhile, the belief that a failure to live up to perfectionistic ideals should be punished, and the belief that certain magical rituals can prevent catastrophes. Such mistaken beliefs, the authors suggested, lead to erroneous perceptions of threat, which in turn provoke anxiety. The obsessive-compulsive's tendency to devalue his or her ability to deal adequately with such threats compounds the dysfunctional process. The resulting feelings of uncertainty, discomfort, and helplessness are reduced through magical rituals, which are viewed by the patient as the only available method for coping with the perceived threat, as he or she lacks other, more appropriate coping resources.

Experimental findings lend some support to the above assertions. Obsessive-compulsives were observed to catalog events discretely without being able to link concepts integratively, thus creating "islands of certainty" amidst confusion in an effort to control and predict events (Makhlouf-Norris, Jones, & Norris, 1970; Makhlouf-Norris & Norris, 1972). Reed (1969) found that obsessive-compulsive thinking was characterized by the underinclusion or the overspecification of concepts. He attributed the doubt and indecision of obsessive-compulsives to a distrust of their own conclusions (Reed, 1968). Consistent with these findings, Persons and Foa (1984) observed that ritualizers used overly specific concepts in their thought patterns with respect to both obsessional and neutral cues. An analogue study of college students scoring high on the Maudsley Obsessive-Compulsive Inventory (MOCI) checking subscale indicated that these individuals had poorer recall of prior actions and greater difficulty in distinguishing real from imagined events than did subjects who had low scores (Sher, Frost, & Otto, 1983). These findings suggest that memory deficits in checkers may motivate repetitious checking behavior. The greater tendency of obsessive-compulsives than of other psychiatric patients, to request a repetition of information before rendering a decision was observed by Milner, Beech, and Walker (1971). Volans (1976) found similar trends, although the differences in experiments failed to reach significance.

The above findings suggest that obsessive-compulsives are more rigid, perfectionistic, and doubting, requiring excessive amounts of information to make a decision, only to distrust their choice. These observations must be interpreted with some caution, however, as several of the studies included individuals deemed to have a compulsive personality style rather than an obsessive-compulsive disorder.

Foa and Kozak (1984) conceptualized ''anxiety disorders'' as specific impairments in affective memory networks. They viewed ''fear'' within Lang's bioinformational theory of emotions (1979), as an affective memory that includes information about feared ''stimuli,'' fear ''responses,'' and their ''meanings.'' Foa and Kozak proposed that neurotic fears differ structurally from normal fears: The former are characterized by the presence of erroneous estimates of threat, an unusually high negative valence for the threatening event, and excessive response elements (e.g., physiological and avoidance). Additionally, neurotic fear structures are resistant to modification. This persistence may reflect a failure to access the fear structure, either because of active avoidance or because the content of the fear network precludes spontaneous encounters with situations that evoke anxiety in everyday life. Anxiety may also persist because of some impairment in the mechanism of change. Cognitive defenses, excessive arousal with failure to habituate, faulty premises, and erroneous rules of inference are all impairments that would hinder the processing of information necessary to change the fear structure of the obsessive-compulsive.

Biological Theories

There is no clear evidence to indicate the presence of structural organic neural impairment in obsessive-compulsive disorder. Several psychosurgical procedures, frontal leukotomy and capsulotomy, have been used somewhat successfully with treatment-intractible obsessive-compulsives. However, there is no rationale to guide the specific choice of the procedure or the location for surgical intervention. Therefore, it is impossible to determine the mechanisms involved in the improvement observed in obsessive-compulsive patients following such a procedure, or to use this work for an understanding of the etiology of this disorder.

In contrast, studies examining electrocortical function in obsessive-compulsives have provided support for the presence of a CNS-based pathophysiology. Two major recording techniques, the electroencephelogram (EEG) and sensory evoked potentials, were used to study cortical activity. The results are summarized below.

EEG Studies

Early studies examining the role of neurological factors in obsessive-compulsive disorder suggested a possible connection between early traumatic or infectious processes (e.g., epidemic encephalitis) and the development of this disorder (e.g., Grimshaw, 1964; Ingram & McAdam, 1960; Pacella, Polatin, & Nagler, 1964). Neurological examinations and clinical EEG recordings were used in these studies. In this early work, the reported size of the subpopulation of obsessive-compulsives showing abnormal EEGs varied widely from study to study (e.g., 10% in Ingram & McAdam, 1960; 65% in Pacella *et al.*, 1964). Because of considerable variation in the criteria used for the diagnosis of obsessive-compulsive disorder and to the relatively large variance of the electrocortical recording techniques of that time, interpretation of these early clinical reports is difficult.

Since the late 1970s, only a few studies have examined the EEGs of obsessive-compulsives. In one such study, Flor-Henry, Yendall, Koles, and Howarth (1979) examined both the neuropsychological profile and the EEG of 11 obsessive-compulsive patients and compared them with those of 23 controls. Based on the pattern of difference on neuropsychological tests between the patients and the normal controls, the authors inferred an anterior, dominant-hemisphere dysfunction in obsessive-compulsives. Further, lower score impairments on the WAIS subtests of digit span and digit symbol, which were observed in obsessive-compulsives when compared with normals, were interpreted as implicating the frontal lobe as the specific site of this dysfunction. This apparent frontal-lobe dysfunction with greater left-hemisphere involvement was found in 10 of the 11 obsessive-compulsive patients examined. Flor-Henry *et al.* also recorded electrocortical activity during mental rest and during verbal and spatial tasks and analyzed it spectrally, using a Fourier analysis algorithm. Obsessive-compulsives' EEGs differed significantly from those of normals on two dimensions: they showed less left-temporal-lobe variability in the beta (13–50 Hz) range during eyes-closed conditions and more right-parietal variability in the beta 1 (13–20 Hz) range. The authors interpreted this finding as indicating frontal-lobe dysfunction in obsessive-compulsives, particularly in the dominant hemisphere. This dysfunction, they suggested, may result in a loss of the normal inhibitory processes in that region, accounting for the inability of obsessive-compulsives to inhibit verbal representations.

In an attempt to replicate the above findings, Insel, Donnelly, Lalakee, Alterman, and Murphy (1983) collected EEG data from OCD patients using a more clinical method of analysis (EEG tracings were visually inspected during conditions of hyperventilation and photic stimulation). These researchers reported no clear indication of dysfunction. The differences in the findings of the two studies may be due to methodological differences. Visual analysis of the EEG is useful in detecting gross manifestations of biological-organic dysfunction; however, it is not sufficiently sensitive for the study of cognitive processes. In the Insel *et al.* (1983) study, the EEG was recorded during experimental conditions which would be expected to physically activate the subject. Although this method is useful in evoking EEG anomalies with biological bases, it does not directly access the effects of various states of cognitive activation. If OCD is manifested at a cognitive processing level, Insel *et al.*'s methods might not have detected electrocortical differences due to this disorder. In contrast, the methodology used by Flor-Henry *et al.* on EEG recordings taken during the manipulation of cognitive activation increased the likelihood of detecting differences between obsessive-compulsive patients and normals.

More recently, McCarthy (1986) studied obsessive-compulsives, anxious controls, and normals via spectral analysis of EEGs recorded during various attentional tasks. At rest, obsessive-compulsives showed EEG patterns different from normals, but similar to those of anxious controls. During cognitive task performance, however, excessive bilateral frontal slow-wave activity distinguished obsessives from both control groups. These results are compatible with those of Flor-Henry *et al.*'s and seem to indicate some frontal-lobe dysfunction during information processing.

Evoked-Potential Studies

As in EEG research, very few studies have used the electrophysiological technique of evoked potentials to study the electrocortical activity of obsessive-compulsives. Like EEG recording, this technique purports that its object of measure is the electrical activity of the brain.

One of the first studies to use sensory evoked potentials with obsessive-compulsives versus control subjects found no differences between groups for simple flash-induced visual evoked potentials for the major component, P130 (Ceiseilski, Beech, & Gordon, 1981). However, in obsessive-compulsives, Ceiseilski *et al.* (1981) found a significant decrease in the amplitude of the P130 when a patterned flash stimulus was presented. Further, obsessive-compulsives demonstrated decreases in both latency and amplitude for the N220 component when engaged in cognitive activity (same vs. different figure matching).

In a follow-up study, Beech, Ceiseilski, and Gordon (1983) reported a decreased latency for N220 and P350 components for obsessive-compulsives versus normal subjects. This was found with the two-shape figure-matching task used previously by Ceiseilski *et al.* (1981). The amplitudes of these components were approximately equivalent across groups. To increase further the complexity of the cognitive task, a three-shape version of the figure-matching task was used. Reduced latency and amplitude were found for N220 and P350 components in obsessive-compulsives versus normal subjects on this more complex task. The authors noted that, whereas the control subjects showed increased amplitude for N220 and P350 components for the three-shape matching tasks as compared to the two-shape version of the task, both components showed a markedly decreased amplitude in obsessive-compulsives as the task complexity increased.

The above studies suggest that differences may exist between the evoked-potential components (i.e., N220 and P350) in obsessive-compulsives and those in control subjects. However, these differences become most evident when greater demands are placed on the information-processing capacity of obsessive-compulsives.

Using stimulation in several sensory modalities (visual, auditory, and shock-stimulated), Shagass, Roemer, Straumanis, and Josiassen (1984) found that evoked-potential components with peak latencies under 100 msec distinguished obsessive-compulsives from other groups. For auditory evoked potentials, decreased amplitude of the P50 component was seen in obsessive-compulsives. Visually evoked potentials showed decreased amplitude and latency of the N75 component. Electrical shock increased the amplitude of the N60 component for both the right and the left sides.

Although these results appear to be in conflict with the findings of Beech and coworkers, the differences noted by Shagass *et al.* occurred while the subjects receive sensory stimulation. No demands on informational capacity were made. The differences in later evoked-potential components reported by Beech *et al.* became more pronounced as the demand on processing capacity was increased. Consequently, the findings of Shagass *et al.* are of interest in that some suggestion of baseline sensory evoked-potential differences between groups was found. The data initially reported by Ceiseilski *et al.* (1981) and replicated and extended by Beech *et al.* (1983) indicated that differences in the latency and the amplitude of later evoked-potential components (N220 and P350) occurred with reliability, distinguishing obsessive-compulsives from normals.

In sum, electrocortical data suggest that a centrally based pathophysiological component exists for OCD and that the frontal-lobe region is the site of the dysfunction. These atypical neural response patterns are found primarily during cognitive processing.

Psychopharmacological Studies

It has been hypothesized that neural serotonergic deficiency underlies OCD. This hypothesis has been derived primarily from treatment studies using antidepressant medication with obsessive-compulsive patients. Clomipramine has emerged as the most effective tricyclic in controlling symptoms of this disorder. In comparison with other tricyclic antidepressants, clomipramine is a strong inhibitor of serotonin uptake (Asberg, Ringberger, Sjoqvist, Thoren, Traskman, & Tuck, 1977). Hence, reports of the efficacy of this drug have led to a serotonergic hypothesis of the disorder. Several recent studies have examined the effects of two new antidepressant medications, fluoxetine and fluvoxamine (Perse, Greist, Jefferson, Rosenfeld, & Dar, 1987; Price, Goodman, Charney, & Heninger, 1987; Turner, Jacob, Beidel, & Himmelhoch, 1985). These drugs have demonstrated even greater specificity than clomipramine in enhancing neural serotonergic transmission by blocking serotonin uptake. Whereas the results of this work are still preliminary, they are clinically promising and potentially support the presence of a serotonergic dysfunction in this disorder.

Further support for a serotonergic abnormality in the brains of obsessive-compulsive patients is derived from examining the levels of 5-hydroxyindoleacetic acid (5-HIAA), a metabolite of serotonin, in the cerebrospinal fluid (CSF) of these patients. The administration of a monoamine-reuptake inhibitor, such as clomipramine, alters the turnover of the specific amine, reducing its metabolite in the spinal fluid. Thoren, Asberg, Bertilsson, Mellstrom, Sjoqvist, and Traskman (1980) compared 5-HIAA levels obtained before and after a 3-week period of clomipramine administration. As expected, reductions in obsessive-compulsive symptoms were found to be significantly correlated with decreases in cerebral spinal fluid concentrations of 5-HIAA. Although this finding supports the serotonergic hypothesis, somewhat contradictory results have been reported by Insel, Mueller, Alterman, Linnoila, and Murphy (1985). These authors compared the effects of clomipramine and zimelidine (a potent serotonin-uptake blocker) on obsessive-compulsive symptoms and on spinal fluid 5-HIAA levels of eight obsessive-compulsive patients. Interestingly, before drug administration, an elevated 5-HIAA level was found in a small cohort of obsessionals, as compared to normals, possibly reflecting increased serotonin turnover. Significant elevations in 5-HIAA occurred in obsessive-compulsives following the administrations of both clomipramine and zimelidine. However, no significant improvement was found on any measure of obsessive-compulsive symptoms for the zimelidine group, whereas clomipramine patients were found to improve on several measures. The authors concluded that the pharmacological blockade of serotonergic uptake alone may not be sufficient for a reduction of obsessive-compulsive symptoms.

TREATMENT: BEHAVIOR THERAPY

Traditional psychotherapy has not proved effective in ameliorating obsessive-compulsive symptoms (Black, 1974). In a sample of 90 inpatients, Kringlen (1965) found that only 20% had improved in 13–20 years posttreatment. Somewhat more favorable results were reported by Grimshaw (1965): 40% of an outpatient sample had improved at a 1- to 14-year follow-up. Considerable prognostic improvement emerged from the introduction of behavioral techniques derived from the learning theories described earlier. The learning model proposed that obsessions evoke anxiety or discomfort, which is reduced by compulsions. It follows that treatment should include anxiety-reducing procedures as well as ways to block the reinforcement embedded in the emission of rituals.

Although the treatment of obsessionals has often differed from that of overt ritualizers, variants of exposure and blocking procedures have been used for both populations. Exposure techniques such as systematic desensitization, paradoxical intention, flooding, and satiation consist of deliberately confronting the patient with anxiety-evoking material, either *in vivo* or in imagination. Blocking, on the other hand, cuts short the patient's ruminations or ritualistic behaviors via such procedures as response prevention, thought stopping, aversion, and distraction. We first review the use of exposure procedures in the treatment of obsessive-compulsive ritualizers and in the treatment of obsessionals. Blocking techniques are discussed next, followed by an overview of the literature on the effects of *in vivo* exposure combined with response prevention—the current treatment of choice for ritualizers.

Early Behavioral Procedures

The implementation of procedures directed at the anxiety associated with obsessions is based on the rationale that, once the obsessional cues cease to evoke anxiety, compulsive behavior will extinguish because it will no longer be reinforced by its anxiety-reducing properties. To this end, "systematic desensitization" (Wolpe, 1958) has often been used. This procedure consists of the induction of a relaxed state and the concomitant presentation of anxiety-evoking items arranged in a hierarchical order. It is hypothesized that the pairing of relaxation with the disturbing stimuli will eventually result in deconditioning of the associated anxiety. Usually, no direct effort to treat the ritualistic behavior has been attempted when systematic desensitization is used.

The largest series of patients treated by this technique was reported by Cooper, Gelder, and Marks (1965). Of 10 obsessive-compulsives, only 3 improved; a comparison group treated with supportive psychotherapy and drugs showed greater gains. The results of single-case reports are less bleak but still ambiguous (e.g., Furst & Cooper, 1970; Haslam, 1965; Marks, Crowe, Drewe, Young, & Dewhurst, 1969; Tanner, 1971; Worsley, 1970). In reviewing 21 cases treated by 5–100 sessions of systematic desensitization, Beech and Vaughn (1978) reported that 4 out of 10 patients treated with imaginal desensitization were improved, in contrast to 7 of the 11 who received this procedure *in vivo*. Although this difference is not striking, the latter technique seems to have fared better.

Walton and Mathers (1963) examined the differential effects of systematic desensitization on chronic versus recently acquired symptoms. The factors responsible for the elicitation and maintenance of compulsive behavior, they felt, varied with symptom duration. Recently acquired symptoms were presumed to be elicited by conditioned anxiety, whereas long-standing symptoms were hypothesized to be functionally autonomous and independent of anxiety. In accordance with this hypothesis, the authors predicted that only patients whose symptoms were of recent onset would benefit from systematic desensitization. As expected, compulsions were extinguished in two of three patients with recently acquired symptoms. Conversely, in two of the three patients with chronic symptoms, desensitization reduced anxiety, but the compulsions remained unchanged. Interestingly, Marks *et al.* (1969) also found that the elimination of anxiety had no effect on avoidance behavior and rituals.

Desensitization has also been used in the treatment of obsessionals who do not manifest overt rituals. Bevan (1960) treated a patient who ruminated about war and illness by combining 6 weeks of desensitization *in vivo* (reading anxiety-provoking material) with chlorpromazine. Some reduction in the treated obsessions was evident, but new ones emerged. Better results were reported by Agras, Leitenberg, Barlow, Curtis, Edwards, and Wright (1971), who used systematic desensitization with and without relaxation in treating patients who ruminated about harming others. Both procedures markedly reduced the frequency of the obsessions, the improvement being greater with the addition of relaxation.

Overall, the reported effectiveness of systematic desensitization in the treatment of both ritualizers and obsessionals leaves much to be desired. Nevertheless, there is some justification for its use with patients with a recent onset of symptoms; *in vivo* administration seems to improve the outcome.

Procedures using prolonged exposure have also been employed with ritualizers. Noonan (1971) used a procedure he labeled "induced anxiety." Although conceptualized within a traditional insight framework, this procedure resembled implosive therapy (Stampfl & Levis, 1967). The patient was instructed to experience intense anxiety and to describe the images that arose spontaneously. After seven sessions, he was symptom-free. A related approach, "paradoxical intention," has also been used with obsessive-compulsives (Frankl, 1960). This procedure typically involves deliberate attempts to increase the frequency or the intensity of problem thoughts or behaviors. An obsessive-compulsive individual may be asked to imagine in an exaggerated fashion that feared consequences ensuing from a failure to perform a ritual have actually occurred. A patient with checking rituals who feared making mistakes might be asked to think that he was the "greatest mistake-maker in the world." This procedure resembles implosion or flooding in imagination; the difference is that, in paradoxical intention, the patient is usually asked to carry out the procedure on his or her own, whereas in implosion or flooding, the stimulus input for the images is provided by the therapist. Additionally, deliberate attempts to evoke humor are included in the former but not in the latter. Using paradoxical intention with six obsessive-compulsives, Gertz (1966) reported that four recovered and two improved. Paradoxical intention has also been used with obsessionals who do not exhibit overt rituals. Solyom, Garza-Perez, Ledwidge, and Solyom (1972) treated 10 such patients with this technique and reported that 5 markedly improved, 3 remained unchanged, and 2 failed to follow the instructions.

Two studies compared the effect of exposure with that of thought stopping, a blocking procedure that will be discussed in the next section. In the first study, Emmelkamp and Kwee (1977) examined the difference in effectiveness of five sessions of thought stopping and five sessions of imaginal exposure. Three of the five obsessional patients improved equally with either procedure, and the remaining two failed to improve regardless of treatment. In the second investigation, Stern (1978) compared the efficacy of yet another exposure technique, "satiation," with thought stopping. Seven patients with obsessive ruminations were given four sessions of satiation treatment followed by four sessions of thought stopping. A 1-month interval separated the two treatments. Each satiation session lasted 1 hour and consisted of having the patient verbalize his or her rumination in the presence of the therapist, who encouraged him or her in this regard by using verbal prompts. Daily practice of writing thoughts repeatedly was assigned, and the patients were further instructed to expose themselves to external cues that elicited the obsession. The results of this study were disappointing: only two of the seven patients improved with satiation.

"Exposure" combined with "aversive relief" was used by Solyom and his colleagues. Four patients suffering from ruminations and horrific temptations were treated by the following procedure: A previously taped narrative of the obsessional thought sequence was played for the patient and was periodically interrupted by a 20-second silence that was followed by a mild electric shock. When the shock was terminated by the patient, the taped obsessional material resumed. In effect, relief from shock (negative reinforcement) was associated with the anxiety-arousing stimuli. All four patients were improved and maintained gains at follow-up (Solyom *et al.*, 1971). In a later study, the same technique was successfully used to treat sexual and aggressive ruminations (Solyom & Kingstone, 1973). The authors viewed this aversion-relief procedure as a form of reciprocal inhibition rather than as negative reinforcement. They posited that, because horrific temptations are anxiety-augmenting stimuli, they would be most affected by this procedure, whereas ruminations might be more successfully treated with other behavioral techniques.

In summary, variations of prolonged exposure do not seem to affect ritualistic behavior, nor do they appear to improve obsessions. Positive results have been obtained with the aversion-relief procedure used by Solyom and his associates. However, this technique has been used in one center only and requires replication.

Treatment by Exposure and Response Prevention

In 1966, Victor Meyer introduced a treatment for OCD called *apotrepic therapy,* which consisted of a combination of exposure with response prevention. The success of this treatment generated much interest and instigated studies, both controlled and uncontrolled, that have provided information on the procedures and the processes involved. In a series of studies in which procedural variants of exposure were examined, the effects of exposure and response prevention were compared with a control condition of treatment by relaxation for a determination of whether the improvement observed was not merely a function of time spent in therapy (Hodgson, Rachman, & Marks, 1972; Marks, Hodgson, & Rachman, 1975; Rachman, Marks, & Hodgson, 1973). Fifteen daily sessions of variants of exposure *in vivo* were used along with response prevention for obsessive-compulsive inpatients. Although five patients showed no improvement, eight patients were much improved and seven were improved. In contrast, no effect was found in patients receiving relaxation training. Fourteen patients remained much improved, one was improved, and five were unchanged at 2-year follow-up. Similar results were reported in a study using 10 washers (Roper, Rachman, & Marks, 1975). For 5 patients, the treatment included 15 weeks of therapist-modeled exposure to disturbing objects (passive modeling). The 5 control patients received an equivalent period of relaxation training. Following this, both groups were given an additional 15 sessions of *in vivo* exposure and response prevention. Three patients were much improved, five were improved, and two were unchanged at posttreatment. At follow-up, similar results (4 much improved, 4 improved, and 2 unchanged) were found.

Three studies were conducted with outpatients in Holland by Emmelkamp and colleagues. In the first of these studies, 13 obsessive-compulsive patients were treated at home with 15 two-hour sessions of exposure and response prevention (Boersma, Den Hengst, Dekker, & Emmelkamp, 1976). At posttreatment, 7 of these patients were found to be symptom-free, 3 showed some improvement, and 3 remained unchanged. The findings were similar at follow-up. Comparing therapist-aided and self-controlled exposures, Emmelkamp and Kraanen (1977) provided 13 patients with 10 two-hour sessions of exposure to anxiety-evoking cues. At both posttreatment and follow-up, data indicated a significant overall reduction in both anxiety and ritualistic behavior. However, most of the patients required additional therapy sessions, and two patients failed to benefit from treatment. In a third study, Emmelkamp, van der Helm, van Zanten, and Plochy (1980) treated 15 obsessive-compulsive patients with 10 sessions of exposure and response prevention. Although only group means were reported, evidence of improvement was found at posttreatment and at 1- and 6-month follow-ups. A slight relapse occurred at 1-month follow-up, and the patients were given an average of an additional 15 sessions. These authors suggested that 10 sessions of exposure and response prevention may not generally be adequate to protect patients against future relapse. Foa and Goldstein (1978) provided more detailed information about the effects of exposure and response prevention. Continuous exposure and complete response prevention were used with 21 ritualizers (14 outpatients and 7 inpatients). These patients received 10 daily 2-hour sessions of imaginal and *in vivo* exposures and were supervised in response prevention. At posttreatment, 18 patients were symptom-free on measures of rituals, 2 were improved, and 1 was unchanged. Three patients were found to have relapsed at follow-up. For obsessions, 12 patients were asymptomatic at posttreatment, 8 were mildly to moderately symptomatic, and 1 showed no improvement. Two patients had relapsed at follow-up.

In a later study investigating the effects of using both imaginal exposure to feared consequences and *in vivo* exposure to external cues, Foa, Steketee, Turner, and Fischer (1980) compared seven checkers from the Foa and Goldstein (1978) study with eight checkers treated with 10 daily 2-hour sessions of exposure and response prevention. The average overall improvement in the 15 patients was comparable to that reported in the earlier study and in other research centers. Half of the patients receiving exposure *in vivo* were found to have relapsed to various degrees at 9-month follow-up, whereas patients receiving both imaginal and *in vivo* exposure had maintained their gains.

Foa and colleagues analyzed data collected from 50 patients who had participated in various experiments in which treatment using exposure and response prevention was applied (Foa, Grayson, Steketee, Doppelt, Turner, & Latimer, 1983). As a measure of improvement, 9-point Likert-type ratings of obsessions and compulsions by independent assessors were transformed by subject into scores of percentage change from pretreatment baseline. These scores were then averaged, and comparisons were made of pretreatment, posttreatment, and follow-up evaluations. These patients were divided into three groups on the basis of their percentage-change scores: patients with gains of 70% or more were categorized as much improved; those with gains of 31% 69% were classified as improved; and failures demonstrated 30% or less symptom reduction. At posttreatment, 58% (29) were much improved, 38% (19) were improved, and 4% (2) were treatment failures. At follow-up, which ranged from 3 months to 3 years, with a mean of 1 year, 59% of the 50 patients treated (27) were much improved, 17% (8) were improved, and 24% (11) were treatment failures. The authors noted that much improved patients tended to maintain their gains, and that those patients who failed posttreatment did not improve by follow-up. Further, partial gains that were evident immediately posttreatment were generally unstable, often resulting in relapse.

The results of a number of treatment studies (e.g., Catts & McConaghy, 1975; Julien, Rivere, & Note, 1980) and case reports (e.g., Farkas & Beck, 1981; Haynes, 1978; Lipper & Feignbaum, 1976; Meyer, Robertson, & Tatlow, 1975; Rainey, 1972) have been closely congruent with the findings cited previously and have been reported in other centers regarding high treatment efficacy and low relapse rates. Three well-designed single-case studies (Mills, Agras, Barlow, & Mills, 1973; Turner, Hersen, Bellack, & Wells, 1979; Turner, Hersen, Bellack, Andrasik, & Capparell, 1980) are of particular interest in that behavioral observations of the time spent ritualizing was their primary measure of outcome. The results reported in these designs provide further corroboration of the findings reported in earlier studies that instead used global measures of symptomatology.

At this time, well over 200 obsessive-compulsive ritualizers have been treated by means of prolonged exposure and response prevention. Contrasting with the information available for obsessionals (without overt rituals), the majority of outcome data for ritualizers have come from studies using group designs rather than single-case reports, so that they add confidence to the interpretation of the findings. Although these studies were conducted in many centers with numerous therapists, a remarkable convergence in their findings is apparent, attesting to the strength and generalizability of the treatment effects. In a summary of some 20 studies using exposure and response prevention with obsessive-compulsive ritualizers, Foa *et al.* (1985) observe that 51% of patients treated by this method were either symptom-free or much improved at post-treatment and that an additional 39% were moderately improved. Only 10% of obsessive-compulsive ritualizers failed to benefit from this treatment. Although at follow-up the number of failures increased to 24%, the high efficacy of this treatment is evident, and it may be viewed as the treatment of choice for the obsessive-compulsive ritualizer.

The treatment in most of these studies was conducted most often on a daily basis and in a hospital setting. Was the intensity of the treatment sufficient to account for its demonstrated efficacy? This does not appear to be the case. In each of the previously cited studies by Marks and his colleagues at the Maudsley Hospital, treatment with exposure and response prevention was compared with an equivalent amount of relaxation training. The latter treatment was found to be entirely ineffective in producing symptom reductions. However, it could be argued that extraneous variables such as patient expectancy contributed to the outcome of the Maudsley studies in that no measure of expectancy was obtained. Steketee, Foa, and Grayson (1982) examined the separate and combined effects of exposure and response prevention while controlling for expectancy and the frequency and duration of treatment. Comparisons of each treatment alone, as well as a treatment combining exposure and response prevention, were conducted. Although the treatment outcome was superior for the combined-treatment group, expectancy was equivalent across groups. Hence, expectancy could not be concluded to be a significant explanatory factor in these results.

TREATMENT: DRUG ADMINISTRATION

A variety of drugs have been used in the treatment of obsessive-compulsive disorder. Although some degree of symptom reduction has been reported in clinical case studies using antipsychotic and anxiolytic agents as well as lithium, antidepressants (primarily tricyclic compounds) are most commonly used in clinical practice. Perhaps because of the strong concurrence of depression and obsessive-compulsive disorder (e.g., Foa, Grayson, & Steketee, 1982).

Numerous case studies have attested to the efficacy of tricyclics with obsessive-compulsives (for review see Ananth, 1985), and 11 controlled studies have been conducted. Of these 11 studies, 7 used clomipramine, a tricyclic that has gained a reputation as an antiobsessional agent (e.g., Wyndowe, Solyom, & Ananth, 1975). These studies are summarized in Table 1.

Using a crossover design, Montgomery (1980) compared 4 weeks of clomipramine to placebo. Even with a low dosage (75 mg), clomipramine was superior to placebo for

Table 1. Antidepressant Trials in Obsessive-Compulsive Disorders

Study	*N*	Drug	Mean daily dosage (mg, p.o.)	Length of trial (wks)	Improvement in depression	Improvement in OCD
Cammer (1973)	20	Desipramine	Not reported	24+	70%	0%
Wyndowe *et al.* (1975)	15	Clomipramine	225	4	44%	26%–55% of cases
Thoren *et al.* (1980)	24	Clomipramine Nortriptyline Placebo	150 150	5	Not reported	CMI > PBO CMI = NOR NOR = PBO
Montgomery (1980)	14	Clomipramine	75	4	CMI = PBO No improvement	CMI > PBO
Ananth *et al.* (1981)	20	Clomipramine Amitriptyline	133 197	4	CMI > AMI	CMI = AMI only CMI produced improvement pre-post
Marks *et al.* (1980)	40	Clomipramine Placebo	183	7	CMI > PBO	CMI > PBO (2 of 8 measures)
Insel *et al.* (1982)	12	Clominpramine Clorgyline Placebo	200 30	6	CMI > CGL = PBO	CMI > CGL = PBO
Mavissakalian *et al.* (1985)	12	Clomipramine Placebo	229	12	CMI = PBO	CMI > PBO
Mavissakalian & Michelson (1983)	20	Clomipramine Imipramine	167 250	12	CMI = IMI	CMI = IMI both produced
Volavka *et al.* (1985)		Clomipramine Imipramine	275 265	12	CMI > IMI	CMI = IMI except for obsessive thoughts; both produced improvement pre-post
Turner *et al.* (1985)	8	Fluoxetine Placebo	80	10	FLU > PBO	FLU > PBO
Foa *et al.* (1987)	37	Imipramine Placebo	225	6	IMI > PBO	IMI = PBO minimal improvement for both
Perse *et al.* (1987)	16	Fluvoxamine Placebo	300	8	FLV > PBO	FLV > PBO
Price *et al.* (1987)	10	Fluvoxamine Placebo	300	4	FLV > PBO	FLV > PBO

obsessions and general anxiety although it did not affect ritualistic behaviors. Because clomipramine reduced obsessions but not depression, the study supports the view that this drug has direct antiobsessional properties. A 4-week comparison of clomipramine and placebo was conducted with a larger sample (Marks, Stern, Mawson, Cobb, & McDonald, 1980). Clomipramine was superior in reducing depression. Effects of the active drug were observed on only three of eight measures of obsessive-compulsive (OC) symptoms. When the 10 most and 10 least depressed patients were compared, only the former showed drug effects on OC and on depressive symptoms. The authors suggested that clomipramine's effects on OC symptoms were mediated by reduction in depression. A longer comparison (12 weeks) of clomipramine with placebo indicated a stronger effect of the active drug on OC symptoms (Mavissakalian, Turner, Michelson, & Jacob, 1985). A faster decline in depressive than in obsessive symptoms was observed and interpreted by the authors to indicate the independence of these symptoms. In all the above studies, then, clomipramine appeared to reduce both OC and depressive symptoms to a greater degree than did placebo.

Clomipramine has also been compared with other antidepressants. When compared to nortriptyline and placebo, clomipramine produced more improvement on the OC subscale of the Comprehensive Psychiatric Rating Scale (CPRS) than did nortriptyline, but the effects of both drugs were modest; only the difference between clomipramine and placebo reached statistical significance (Thoren *et al.*, 1980). Because the CPRS subscale contains items pertaining to depressive symptoms, it is unclear whether the observed improvement reflected a reduction in depression, in OC symptoms, or in both. No posttreatment data on depression were reported. The initial level of depression was not found to be related to improvement in OC symptoms. In a comparison of clomipramine and amitriptyline, Ananth, Pecknold, Van Der Steen, and Engelsmann (1981) found that clomipramine reduced depression more than amitriptyline. On OC symptoms, clomipramine produced significant improvement pre- and posttreatment but did not differ significantly from amitriptyline. Change in OC symptoms was not associated with change in depression. In a crossover design, Insel, Alterman, Donnelly, and Murphy (1982) compared clomipramine with the MAOI clorgyline and with placebo. After 6 weeks, clomipramine reduced both depressive and OC symptoms by about 30%, whereas clorgyline did not. Initial depression was not related to a reduction in OC symptoms. In summary, all of the above comparisons evidenced a tendency for clomipramine to produce more improvement than other antidepressants in both sets of symptoms, but the observed differences did not always reach statistical or clinical significance.

Two investigations compared clomipramine and imipramine (Mavissakalian *et al.*, 1985; Volavka, Neziroglu, & Yaryura-Tobias, 1985). Mavissakalian and Michelsen (1983) reported on eight patients who received either imipramine or clomipramine. A significant reduction in obsessive-compulsive symptoms and in depression were reported for the 12-week trial. Reduction in depression preceded reduction in obsessional symptoms, and greater initial depression was associated with a better response in OC symptoms. When data from this study were combined with data from the 1985 study mentioned above, no differences between clomipramine and imipramine were detected. In contrast to the findings of the 1983 study, in the combined data initial depression did not affect outcome. A controlled comparison of clomipramine with imipramine conducted by Volavka *et al.* (1985) indicated that both OC and depressive symptoms were improved with both drugs. Clomipramine reduced depression and obsessive thoughts more than imipramine, but on other measures (SRONS and Beaumont Scale), the two drugs reduced OC symptoms to the same extent. Unfortunately, the two groups showed large initial differences in the severity of the OC symptoms. Although the use of analysis of covariance corrected statistically for these initial differences, it may have influenced the measures of clinical improvement: lower initial levels of symptoms may be more easily reduced. Pretreatment depression was not found to be related to outcome on OC symptoms.

A comparison of imipramine and placebo was conducted over a 6-week period by Foa, Steketee, Kozak, and Dugger (1987) with 37 obsessive-compulsive ritualizers. They found imipramine to produce significantly greater reductions than placebo in depressive symptoms, whereas the little drug effect observed for obsessive-compulsive symptoms paralleled that seen for placebo. These findings seem to be incongruent with those of Mavissakalian *et al.* (1985) and of Volavka *et al.* (1985) described above. However, the lack of a placebo group in these two earlier studies prevents one from drawing the conclusion that the significant improvement for imipramine on five of eight measures of obsessive-compulsive symptoms by Foa *et al.* (1987) was found in the placebo group as well. Thus, the reduction in obsessive-compulsive symptoms cannot be construed as a specific action of imipramine.

As previously indicated, recent preliminary work has generated considerable interest in two highly specific seretonergic-uptake-blocking agents, fluoxetine and fluvoxamine. In a single blind crossover design, Turner *et al.* (1985) compared 10 weeks of fluoxetine with placebo in eight obsessive-compulsives. An inspection of the data indicates that the drug produced a clinically significant reduction in depression. However, for obsessive-compulsive measures, a statistically significant drug effect was found on the Hopkins Obsessive-Compulsive Scale, yet no improvement was evidenced for scores on the Maudsley Obsessional-Compulsive Inventory (MOCI). Despite the small size of the overall drug effect on obsessive-compulsive symptomatology, five of the eight patients completing this study were rated as demonstrating clinical improvement on a global rating of improvement. These ratings appear to be somewhat incongruent with the rating observed on other measures of OC symptoms, perhaps because the ratings of global improvement were affected by the sizable drug effect on depression.

A recently completed study by Perse *et al.* (1987) using a double-blind crossover methodology compared the effects of 8 weeks of fluvoxamine to 8 weeks of placebo in 16 obsessive-compulsives. Statistically significant patterns of reduction in depression and OC symptoms were reported, and moderate improvement was reported in 9 of 16 patients. However, an inspection of the means reveals a minimal reduction in OC symptoms that may not have clinical significance.

Using a double-blind procedure, Price *et al.* (1987) compared the effect of a 4-week trial of fluvoxamine and placebo in 10 OC patients. Whereas significant reductions on the Yale-Brown Obsessive-Compulsive scale and the Hamilton measures of depression and anxiety were reported, no drug effect was found for scores on the MOCI. Six of ten patients improved moderately on a global rating of improvement. As previously indicated, changes in ratings of global improvement may, at least in part, be the result of reductions in depression.

In sum, the available data suggest that the majority of OC patients experience some degree of improvement with the use of the more specific seretonin-uptake-blocking agents. However, the size of this effect is moderate at best.

The application of standard leukotomy to obsessive-compulsives has been reported since the early 1940s (e.g., Berliner, Beveridge, Meyer-Gross, & Moore, 1945). A review of variants of leukotomy indicated results ranging from 70%–90% improvement (Pippard, 1956). It is hard to evaluate these figures because the measures of improvement appeared to differ from those used in other treatments. Often, only anxiety associated with obsessions was rated, and ritualistic behavior was ignored. In reviewing the cases of 15,000 patients treated with leukotomy between 1942 and 1962, Sargent (1962) suggested that anxious ruminative patients had benefited from this procedure, but not those with long-standing compulsions.

Comparing leukotomized and nonleukotomized obsessionals, Pollitt (1956) found no substantial difference in the degree of symptomatology at follow-up. However, the two groups had not been matched on severity of symptoms; one would suspect that the leukotomized patients had more severe symptoms. Indeed, when matched on this variable in a *post hoc* analysis (Tan, Marks, & Marset, 1971), leukotomized obsessive-compulsives fared better than controls on obsessions and general anxiety. At a 5-year follow-up, 50% of the leukotomized, as opposed to 23% of the nonleukotomized patients, were much improved. Kelly and Cobb (1985) reported that, of 49 obsessive-compulsive patients who had undergone stereotactically performed limbic leukotomy, 78% showed long-term improvement. Further support for the effects of psychosurgical intervention was provided by Mindus, Bergstrom, Levander, Noren, and Nyman (1985), who examined the effects of gama-produced bilateral lesions of the anterior interior capsules in six severely obsessive-compulsive patients. These assessments indicated considerable reduction in obsessive-compulsive symptoms at 3- and 7-year follow-ups.

Comparisons of the effectiveness of stereotactic psychosurgical operations cast doubt on their specific "antiobsessional" effects. When 24 obsessive ritualizers were compared with 24 depressed patients, all treated with bilateral stereotactic tractotomy, no differences were found (Bridges, Goktepe, Maratos, Browne, & Young, 1973). Some differential effects across patient groups were obtained by Mitchell-Heggs, Kelly, and Richardson (1976), using stereotactic limbic leukotomy. Chronic anxiety was least effected (66%), and obsessive-compulsive symptoms improved most (89%). Depressed patients benefited less than obsessionals, and schizophrenics were approximately equivalent. A report on 100 patients and the use of the same technique substantiated these findings (Mitchell-Heggs, Kelly, Richardson, & McLeish, 1978). These authors observed that a good outcome was found for obsessional neurosis, while outcome for depression was poor. The small differences in outcome among groups, as well as the findings of Bridges *et al.* (1973), do not seem to warrant this conclusion.

There seems to be no doubt that leukotomy results in improvement in obsessive-compulsives. Because it is a drastic measure, however, the procedure has been reserved for those who fail to benefit from behavioral and psychopharmacological interventions.

SUMMARY

Evaluations of treatment outcome studies demonstrate that behavior therapy, specifically exposure and response prevention, produces a 60%–70% reduction in the symptomatology of obsessive-compulsive ritualizers (e.g., Foa *et al.*, 1983; Marks *et al.*,

1980). It is important to note that 25% of patients who seek help refuse this form of treatment.

What is the drug of choice for OCD? Psychopharmacological studies comparing clomipramine with placebo have consistently shown a drug effect on OC symptoms. In contrast, no significant difference from placebo was found for nortriptyline (Thoren *et al.*, 1980), amitriptyline (Ananth *et al.*, 1981), or imipramine (Foa *et al.*, 1987), whereas, in direct comparisons with other tricyclics, clomipramine has not proved superior in reducing obsessive-compulsive symptoms. Its consistent superiority to placebo suggests that it is somewhat more effective than other antidepressants. Preliminary work examining the more pure serotonin blockers, fluoxetine and fluvoxamine, does not appear to suggest that these drugs show enhanced treatment efficacy over that seen for clomipramine.

It is important to note that, when drugs produced change in obsessive-compulsive symptoms, the reduction was relatively small by comparison with the effects of behavioral treatment. Approximately 30% improvement has been reported with clomipramine (Insel *et al.*, 1982; Marks *et al.*, 1980; Volavka *et al.*, 1985). The only exception is the study by Mavissakalian *et al.* (1985), who found 50% improvement. Even if the efficacy of drug and that of behavior therapy were equal, relapse rates on drug withdrawal are a problem. Indeed, Thoren *et al.* (1980) reported that "amelioration of obsessive-compulsive disorder with clomipramine is only maintained as long as the drug treatment continues" (p. 1285); all six patients who stopped the drug relapsed. Further, the gains achieved by the drug may often be accompanied by uncomfortable side effects. It appears, then, that antidepressant agents may not be the treatment of choice for obsessive-compulsive ritualizers; exposure plus response prevention is preferable. Adding drug to behavioral treatment does not appear to improve on the effects of the latter (Foa *et al.*, 1987; Marks *et al.*, 1980).

It is clear that effective therapies exist for obsessive-compulsive disorder. However, the numbers of patients who fail to benefit from the existing treatments and who show later relapse call for further investigation and development of clinical methods. Perhaps, the limits in treatment efficacy that are currently seen reflect a lack of understanding of the etiology and maintenance of this disorder. Future studies should focus on potentially promising avenues such as the study of brain function (e.g., neural function and electrocortical activity), of deficits in information processing, and of the interrelationships between depression and obsessive-compulsive symptoms. At the same time, the processes involved in behavioral treatment should be further investigated. Such investigations may show us why subpopulations of patients benefit from this treatment and others do not and may suggest ways to improve our treatment modalities.

REFERENCES

Agras, W. S., Leitenberg, H., Barlow, D. H., Curtis, N., Edwards, J., & Wright, D. (1971). Relaxation in systematic desensitization. *Archives of General Psychiatry, 625*, 511–514.

American Psychiatric Association (1980). *Diagnostic and statistical manual of mental disorders* (3rd ed.; DSM-III). Washington, DC: Author.

American Psychiatric Association (1986). *Diagnostic and statistical manual of mental disorders,* (3rd ed. rev.; DSM-III-R). Washington, DC: Author.

Ananth, J., Pecknold, J. C., Van Der Steen, N., & Engelsmann, F. (1981). Double blind comparative study of clomipramine and amitriptyline in obsessive-neurosis. *Progress in Neuropsychopharmacology, 5*, 257–262.

Asberg, M., Ringberger, V., Sjoqvist, F., Thoren, P., Traskman, L., & Tuck, J. (1977). Monoamine metabolites in the cerebrospinal fluid and serotonin uptake inhibition during treatment with clomipramine. *Clinical Pharmacology and Therapeutics, 21,* 201–207.

Beech, H. R. (1971). Ritualistic activity in obsessional patients. *Journal of Psychosomatic Research, 15,* 417–422.

Beech, H. R., & Vaughn, M. (1978). *Behavioral treatment of obsessional states.* New York: Wiley.

Beech, H. R., Ceiseilski, K. T., & Gordon, P. K. (1983). Further observations of evoked potentials in obsessional patients. *British Journal of Psychology, 142,* 605–609.

Berliner, F., Beveridge, R. L., Meyer-Gross, W., & Moore, J. N. P. (1945). Prefrontal leucotomy: Report on 100 cases. *Lancet, 2,* 325.

Bevan, J. R. (1960). Learning theory applied to the treatment of a patient with obsessional ruminations. In H. J. Eysenck (Ed.), *Behaviour therapy and neurosis.* Oxford: Pergamon Press.

Black, A. (1974). The natural history of obsessional neurosis. In H. R. Beech (Ed.), *Obsessional states.* London: Methuen.

Boersma, K., Den Hengst, S., Dekker, J., & Emmelkamp, P. M. G. (1976). Exposure and response prevention: A comparison with obsessive-compulsive patients. *Behaviour Research and Therapy, 14,* 19–24.

Boulougouris, J. C. (1977). Variables affecting the behavior modification of obsessive-compulsive patients treated by flooding. In J. C. Boulougouris & A. D. Rabavilas (Eds.), *The treatment of phobic and obsessive-compulsive disorders.* New York: Pergamon Press.

Boulougouris, J. C., Rabivillas, A. D., & Stefanis, C. (1977). Psychophysiological responses in obsessive-compulsive patients. *Behavior Research & Therapy, 15,* 221–230.

Bridges, P. K., Goktepe, E. O., Maratos, J., Browne, A., & Young, L. A. (1973). A comparative review of patients with obsessional neurosis and with depression treated by psychosurgery. *British Journal of Psychiatry, 123,* 663–674.

Cammer, L. (1973). Antidepressants as a prophylasix against depression in the obsessive-compulsive person. *Psychosomatics, 123,* 663–674.

Capstick, N., & Seldrup, J. (1973). Phenomenological aspects of obsessional patients treated with clomipramine. *British Journal of Psychiatry, 122,* 719–720.

Carr, A. I. (1974). Compulsive neurosis: A review of the literature. *Psychological Bulletin, 8,* 311–318.

Catts, S., & McConaghy, M. (1975). Ritual prevention in the treatment of obsessive-compulsive neurosis. *Australian and New Zealand Journal of Psychiatry, 9,* 37–41.

Ceiseilski, K. T., Beech, H. R., & Gordon, P. K. (1981). Some electrophysiological observations in obsessional states. *British Journal of Psychiatry, 138,* 479–484.

Cooper, J. E., Gelder, M. G., & Marks, I. M. (1965). The results of behavior therapy in 77 psychiatric patients. *British Medical Journal, 1,* 1222–1225.

Dollard, J., & Miller, N. E. (1950). *Personality and psychotherapy: An analysis in terms of learning, thinking, and culture.* New York: McGraw-Hill.

Dowson, H. H. (1977). The phenomenology of severe obsessive-compulsive neurosis. *British Journal of Psychiatry, 131,* 75–78.

Emmelkamp, P. M. G., & Kraanen, J. (1977). Therapist-controlled exposure *in vivo:* A comparison with obsessive-compulsive patients. *Behaviour Research and Therapy, 15,* 491–495.

Emmelkamp, P. M. G., & Kwee, K. G. (1977). Obsessional ruminations: A comparison between thought-stopping and prolonged exposure in investigation. *Behaviour Research and Therapy, 15,* 441–444.

Emmelkamp, P. M. G., van der Helm, M., van Zanten, B. L., & Plochy, I. (1980). Contributions of self-instructional training to the effectiveness of exposure *in vivo:* A comparison with obsessive-compulsive patients. *Behaviour Research and Therapy, 18,* 61–66.

Esquirol, J. E. D. (1838). *Des maladies mentalis* (Vol. 2). Paris: Bailliere.

Eysenck, H. J. (1979). The conditioning model of neurosis. *The Behavioral and Brain Sciences, 2,* 155–159.

Farkas, G. M., & Beck, S. (1981). Exposure and response prevention of morbid ruminations and compulsive avoidance. *Behaviour Research and Therapy, 19,* 257–261.

Flor-Henry, P., Yendall, L. T., Koles, Z. J., & Howarth, B. G. (1979). Neuropsychological and power spectral EEG investigations of the obsessive-compulsive syndrome. *Biological Psychiatry, 14,* 119–130.

Foa, E. B. (1979). Treatment of obsessive-compulsives with prolonged exposure and strict response prevention. *Archives of Greek Association for Behavioral Modification and Research, 1,* 5–17.

Foa, E. B., & Goldstein, A. (1978). Continuous exposure and complete response prevention of obsessive-compulsive disorder. *Behaviour Therapy, 9,* 821–829.

Foa, E. B., & Kozak, M. J. (1984). Treatment of anxiety disorders: Implications for psychopathology. In A. H. Tuma & J. D. Maser (Eds.), *Anxiety and the anxiety disorders*. Hillsdale, NY: Erlbaum.

Foa, E. B., Steketee, G. S., Turner, R. M., & Fischer, S. C. (1980). Effects of imaginal exposure to feared disasters in obsessive-compulsive checkers. *Behaviour Research and Therapy, 18,* 449–455.

Foa, E. B., Grayson, J. B., & Steketee, G. (1982). Depression, habituation and treatment outcome in obsessive-compulsives. In J. C. Boulougouris (Ed.), *Practical applications of learning theories in psychiatry.* New York: Wiley.

Foa, E. B., Grayson, J. B., Steketee, G. S., Doppelt, H. G., Turner, R. M., & Latimer, P. R. (1983). Success and failure in the behavioral treatment of obsessive-compulsives. *Journal of Consulting and Clinical Psychology, 51,* 287–297.

Foa, E. B., Steketee, G. S., & Ozarow, B. J. (1985). Behavior therapy with obsessive-compulsives: From theory to treatment. In M. Mavissakalian (Ed.) *Obsessive-compulsive disorders: Psychological and pharmacological treatments.* New York: Plenum Press.

Foa, E. B., Steketee, B., Kozak, M. J., & Dugger, D. (1987). Imipramine and placebo in the treatment of obsessive-compulsives: Their effect on depression and on obsessional symptoms. *Psychopharmacology Bulletin, 23,* 8–11.

Frankl, V. E. (1960). Paradoxical intention: A logotherapeutic technique. *American Journal of Psychotherapy, 14,* 520–525.

Freud, S. (1909). Notes upon a case of obsessional neurosis. In S. Freud, *Collected Papers* (Vol. 3, pp. 291–383). London: Hogarth Press, 1957.

Furst, J. B., & Cooper, A. (1970). Failure of systematic desensitization in two cases of obsessive-compulsive neurosis marked by fears of insecticide. *Behaviour Research and Therapy, 8,* 203–206.

Grimshaw, L. (1964). Obsessional disorder and neurological illness. *Journal of Neurological and Neurosurgical Psychiatry, 27,* 229–231.

Grimshaw, L. (1965). The outcome of obsessional disorder, a follow-up study of 100 cases. *British Journal of Psychiatry, 111,* 1051–1056.

Haslam, M. T. (1965). The treatment of an obsessional patient by reciprocal inhibition. *Behaviour Research and Therapy, 2,* 213–216.

Haynes, R. (1978). Treatment of an obsessive-compulsive checker. *Behaviour Research and Therapy, 16,* 260–278.

Hodgson, R. J., & Rachman, S. (1972). The effects of contamination and washing in obsessional patients. *Behaviour Research and Therapy, 10,* 111–117.

Hodgson, R. J., Rachman, S., & Marks, I. M. (1972). The treatment of chronic obsessive-compulsive neurosis: Follow-up and further findings. *Behaviour Research and Therapy, 10,* 181–189.

Hornsveld, R. H. J., Kraaimaat, E. W., & van Dam-Baggen, R. M. J. (1979). Anxiety/discomfort and handwashing in obsessive-compulsive and psychiatric control patients. *Behaviour Research and Therapy, 17,* 223–228.

Ingram, I. M., & McAdam, W. A. (1960). The electroencephalogram, obsessional illness and obsessional personality. *Journal of Mental Science, 106,* 686–691.

Insel, T. R., & Akiskal, H. (1986). Obsessive-compulsive disorder with psychotic features: A phenomenologic analysis. *American Journal of Psychiatry, 12,* 1527–1533.

Insel, T. R., Alterman, T., Donnelly, E. F., & Murphy, D. L. (1982). Antiobsessional and antidepressant effects of clomipramine in the treatment of obsessive-compulsive disorder. *Psychopharmacology Bulletin, 18,* 115–117.

Insel, T. R., Donnelly, E. F., Lalakee, M. L., Alterman, I. S., & Murphy, D. L. (1983). Neurological and neuropsychological studies of patients with obsessive-compulsive disorder. *Biological Psychiatry, 18,* 741–751.

Insel, T. R., Mueller, E., Alterman, I., Linnoila, M., & Murphy, D. (1985). Obsessive-compulsive disorder and serotonin: Is there a connection? *Biological Psychiatry, 20,* 1174–1188.

Janet, P. (1903). *Les obsessions et al psychosthenie.* Paris: Bailliere.

Julien, R. A., Rivere, B., & Note, I. D. (1980). Traitement comportenmental et cognitif des obsessions et compulsions resultats et discussion. *Seance due Lundi 27 Octobre,* 1123–133.

Kelly, D., & Cobb, J. P. (1985). *Limbic leucotomy in the treatment of severe intractable obsessive-compulsive neurosis.* Paper presented at the Fifth World Congress of Biological Psychiatry, Philadelphia.

Kendell, R. E., & DiScipio, W. J. (1970). Obsessional symptoms and obsessional personality traits in patients with depressive illness. *Psychological Medicine, 1,* 65–72.

Kringlen, E. (1965). Obsessional neurotics, a long-term follow-up. *British Journal of Psychiatry, 111,* 709–722.

Lang, P. J. (1979). A bio-informational theory of emotional imagery. *Psychophysiology, 16,* 495–512.

Lewinsohn, P. M., Lobitzs, W. C., & Wilson, S. (1973). "Sensitivity" of depressed individuals to aversive stimuli. *Journal of Abnormal Psychology, 81,* 259–263.

Lipper, S., & Feignbaum, W. M. (1976). Obsessive-compulsive neurosis after viewing the fetus during therapeutic abortion. *American Journal of Psychotherapy, 30,* 666–674.

Makhlouf-Norris, F., & Norris, H. (1972). The obsessive-compulsive syndrome as a neurotic device for the reduction of self-uncertainty. *British Journal of Psychiatry, 121,* 277–288.

Makhlouf-Norris, F., Jones, H. G., & Norris, H. (1970). Articulation of the conceptual structure in obsessive-neurosis. *British Journal of Social and Clinical Psychology, 9,* 264–274.

Marks, I. M. (1965). *Patterns of meaning in psychiatric patients.* London: Oxford University Press.

Marks, I. M., Crowe, E., Drewe, E., Young, J., & Dewhurst, W. G. (1969). Obsessive-compulsive neurosis in identical twins. *British Journal of Psychiatry, 15,* 991–998.

Marks, I. M., Hodgson, R., & Rachman, S. (1975). Treatment of chronic obsessive-compulsive neurosis by *in vivo* exposure. *British Journal of Psychiatry, 127,* 349–364.

Marks, I. M., Stern, R. S., Mawson, D., Cobb, J., & McDonald, R. (1980). Clomipramine and exposure for obsessive-compulsive rituals: 1. *British Journal of Psychiatry, 136,* 1–25.

Mavissakalian, M., & Michelson, L. (1983). Tricyclic antidepressants in obsessive-compulsive disorder: Anti-obsessional or antidepressant agents? *Journal of Nervous and Mental Disease, 171,* 301–306.

Mavissakalian, M., Turner, S. M., Michelson, L., & Jacob, R. (1985). Tricyclic antidepressants in obsessive-compulsive disorders: Antiobsessional or antidepressant agents? *American Journal of Psychiatry, 142,* 572–576.

McCarthy, P. R. (1986). Cognitive influences on autonomic and central nervous system activity in obsessive-compulsive disorder. (Doctoral Dissertation, Pennsylvania State University, 1986). *Dissertation Abstracts International, 47,* 2378/2B.

McFall, M. E., & Wollersheim, J. P. (1979). Obsessive-compulsive neurosis: A cognitive behavioral formulation and approach to treatment. *Cognitive Therapy and Research, 3,* 333–348.

Mellett, P. G. (1974). The clinical problems. In H. R. Beech (Ed.), *Obsessional states.* London: Methuen.

Meyer, V. (1966). Modification of expectations in cases with obsessional rituals. *Behaviour Research and Therapy, 4,* 273–280.

Meyer, V., Robertson, J., & Tatlow, A. (1975). Home treatment of an obsessive-compulsive disorder by response prevention. *Journal of Behavior Therapy and Experimental Psychiatry, 6,* 37–38.

Mills, H. L., Agras, W. S., Barlow, D. H., & Mills, J. R. (1973). Compulsive rituals treated by response prevention. *Archives of General Psychiatry, 28,* 524–527.

Milner, A. D., Beech, H. R., & Walker, V. J. (1971). Decision processes and obsessional behaviour. *British Journal of Social and Clinical Psychology, 10,* 88–89.

Mindus, P., Bergstrom, M. K., Levander, S. E., Noren, G., & Nyman, H. (1985). *Stereotactic GAMA capsulotomy in anxiety and obsessive-compulsive states.* Paper presented at the Fifth World Congress of Biological Psychiatry, Philadelphia.

Mitchell-Heggs, N., Kelly, D., & Richardson, A. (1976). Stereotactic limbic leucotomy—A follow-up at 16 months. *British Journal of Psychiatry, 128,* 226–240.

Mitchell-Heggs, N., Kelly, D., Richardson, A., & McLeish, J. (1978). *Further experience of limbic leucotomy.* Unpublished manuscript.

Montgomery, S. A. (1980). Clomipramine in obsessional neurosis: A placebo controlled trial. *Pharmaceutical Medicine, 1,* 189–192.

Mowrer, O. A. (1939). Stimulus-response analysis of anxiety and its role as a reinforcing agent. *Psychological Review, 46,* 553–565.

Mowrer, O. H. (1960). *Learning theory and behavior.* New York: Wiley.

Noonan, J. R. (1971). An obsessive-compulsive reaction treated by inducing anxiety. *American Journal of Psychotherapy, 25,* 293–295.

Pacella, B. L., Polatin, P., & Nagler, S. H. (1964). Clinical and EEG studies in obsessive-compulsive states. *American Journal of Psychiatry, 100,* 830–838.

Perse, T. L., Greist, J. H., Jefferson, J. W., Rosenfeld, R., & Dar, R. (1987). Fluvoxamine treatment of obsessive-compulsive disorder. *American Journal of Psychiatry, 144,* 1543–1548.

Persons, J. B., & Foa, E. B. (1984). Processing of fearful and neutral information by obsessive-compulsives. *Behaviour Research and Therapy, 22,* 259–265.

Pippard, J. (1956). Discussion: Obsessional-compulsive states, the surgical treatment of obsessional states (abridged). *Proceedings of the Royal Society of Medicine, 49,* 846–849.

Pollitt, J. (1956). Discussion: Obsessive-compulsive states (abridged). *Proceedings of the Royal Society of Medicine, 49,* 842–845.

Price, L. H., Goodman, W. K., Charney, D. S., & Heninger, G. R. (1987). Treatment of severe obsessive-compulsive disorder with fluvoxamine. *American Journal of Psychiatry, 144,* 1059–1061.

Rabavilas, A. D., & Boulougouris, J. C. (1974). Physiological accompaniments of ruminations, flooding and thought-stopping in obsessive patients. *Behaviour Research and Therapy, 12,* 239–243.

Rachman, S. (1971). Obsessional ruminations. *Behaviour Research and Therapy, 9,* 229–235.

Rachman, S. (1976a). Obsessional-compulsive checking. *Behaviour Research and Therapy, 14,* 437–443.

Rachman, S. (1976b). Obsessional ruminations. *Behaviour Research and Therapy, 9,* 229–235.

Rachman, S., & Hodgson, R. (1980). *Obsessions and compulsions.* Englewood Cliffs, NJ: Prentice-Hall.

Rachman, S. J., & Wilson, G. T. (1980). *The effects of psychological therapy.* Oxford: Pergamon Press.

Rachman, S., Marks, I. M., & Hodgson, R. (1973). The treatment of obsessive-compulsive neurotics by modelling and flooding *in vivo. Behaviour Research and Therapy, 11,* 463–471.

Rainey, C. A. (1972). An obsessive-compulsive neurosis treated by flooding *in vivo. Journal of Behavior Therapy and Experimental Psychiatry, 3,* 117–121.

Reed, G. F. (1968). Some formal qualities of obsessional thinking. *Psychiatria Clinica, 1,* 382–392.

Reed, G. F. (1969). "Under-inclosion"—A characteristic of obsessional personality disorder: 1. *British Journal of Psychiatry, 115,* 787–790.

Roper, G., & Rachman, S. (1976). Obsessional-compulsive checking: Experimental replication and development. *Behaviour Research and Therapy, 14,* 25–32.

Roper, G., Rachman, S., & Hodgson, R. (1973). An experiment on obsessional checking. *Behaviour Research and Therapy, 11,* 271–277.

Roper, G., Rachman, S., & Marks, I. M. (1975). Passive and participant modeling in exposure treatment of obsessive-compulsive neurotics. *Behaviour Research and Therapy, 13,* 271–279.

Sargent, W. (1962). The present indication for leucotomy. *Lancet, 1,* 1197.

Shagass, C., Roemer, R. A., Straumanis, J. J., & Josiassen, R. C. (1984). Evoked potentials in obsessive-compulsive disorder. *Advances in Biological Psychiatry, 15,* 69–75.

Sher, K. K., Frost, R. O., & Otto, R. (1983). Cognitive dysfunction in compulsive checkers: An exploratory study. *Behaviour Research and Therapy, 21,* 357–364.

Solyom, L., & Kingstone, E. (1973). An obsessive neurosis following morning glory seed ingestion treated by aversion relief. *Journal of Behavior Therapy and Experimental Psychiatry, 4,* 293–295.

Solyom, L., Zamanzadeh, D., Ledwidge, B., & Kenny, K. (1971). Aversion relief treatment of obsessive-neurosis. In R. D. Rubin, J. P. Brady, & J. D. Henderson (Eds.), *Advances in behavior therapy.* New York: Academic Press.

Solyom, L., Garza-Perez, J., Ledwidge, B. L., & Solyom, C. (1972). Paradoxical intention in the treatment of obsessive-thoughts: A pilot study. *Comprehensive Psychiatry, 13,* 291–297.

Stampfl, T. G., & Levis, D. J. (1967). Essentials of implosive therapy: A learning-theory-based psychodynamic behavioral therapy. *Journal of Abnormal Psychology, 72,* 496–503.

Steketee, G. S., Foa, E. B., & Grayson, J. B. (1982). Recent advances in treatment of obsessive-compulsives. *Archives of General Psychiatry, 39,* 1365–1371.

Stern, R. S. (1978). Obsessive thoughts: The problem of therapy. *British Journal of Psychiatry, 133,* 200–205.

Stern, R. S., & Cobb, J. P. (1978). Phenomenology of obsessive-compulsive neurosis. *British Journal of Psychiatry, 132,* 233–239.

Tan, E., Marks, I. M., & Marset, P. (1971). Bimedial leucotomy in obsessive-compulsive neurosis: A controlled serial enquiry. *British Journal of Psychiatry, 118,* 155–164.

Tanner, B. A. (1971). A case report on the use of relaxation and systematic desensitization to control multiple compulsive behaviors. *Journal of Behavior Therapy and Experimental Psychiatry, 2,* 267–272.

Teasdale, Y. D. (1974). Learning models of obsessional-compulsive disorder. In H. R. Beech (Ed.), *Obsessional states.* London: Methuen.

Thoren, P., Asberg, M., Bertilsson, L., Millstrom, A., Sjoqvist, F., & Traskman, L. (1980). Clomipramine treatment of obsessive-compulsive disorder. *Archives of General Psychiatry, 37,* 1289–1294.

Turner, S. M., Hersen, M., Bellack, A. S., & Wells, K. C. (1979). Behavioral treatment of obsessive-compulsive neurosis. *Behavioural Research and Therapy, 17,* 95–106.

Turner, S. M., Hersen, M., Bellack, A. S., Andrasik, F., & Capparell, H. V. (1980). Behavioral and pharmacological treatment of obsessive-compulsive disorders. *Journal of Nervous and Mental Disorder, 168,* 651–657.

Turner, S. M., Jacob, R. G., Beidel, D. C., & Himmelhoch, J. (1985). Fluoxetine treatment of obsessive-compulsive disorder. *Journal of Clinical Psychopharmacology, 5,* 207–212.

Vaughn, M. (1976). The relationships between obsessional personality, obsessions in depression, and symptoms of depression. *British Journal of Psychiatry, 129,* 36–39.

Volans, P. J. (1976). Styles of decision making and probability appraisal in selected obsessional and phobic patients. *British Journal of Social and Clinical Psychology, 15,* 305–317.

Volavka, J., Neziroglu, E., & Yaryura-Tobias, J. A. (1985). Clomipramine and imipramine in obsessive-compulsive disorder. *Psychiatry Research, 14,* 85–93.

Walker, V. J., & Beech, H. R. (1969). Mood state and the ritualistic behavior of obsessional patients. *Journal of Behavior Therapy and Experimental Psychiatry, 1,* 257–262.

Walton, D., & Mathers, M. D. (1963). The application of learning principles to the treatment of obsessive-compulsive states in the acute and chronic phases of illness. *Behaviour Research and Therapy, 1,* 163–174.

Watts, E. N. (1971). *An investigation of imaginal desensitization as an habituation process.* Unpublished doctoral dissertation, University of London.

Wolpe, J. (1958). *Psychotherapy by reciprocal inhibition.* Stanford, CA: Stanford University Press.

Worsley, J. L. (1970). The causation and treatment of obsessionality. In L. E. Burns & J. L. Worsley (Eds.), *Behaviour therapy in the 1970s.* Bristol: Wright.

Wyndowe, J., Solyom, L., & Ananth, J. (1975). Anafranil in obsessive-compulsive neurosis. *Current Therapeutic Research, 18,* 611–617.

11

Sexual Dysfunction

KATHRYN S. K. HALL AND SANDRA R. LEIBLUM

INTRODUCTION

Browse through any bookstore today and you will see books and magazine articles devoted to the description of how to, when to, why to, who to, and what to do in relation to sex. Sexual activity is probably one of Western society's leading recreational pastimes. Consequently, there is pressure on people to become ''good'' at sex, just as one might strive to be a good golfer or tennis player. Despite the proliferation of gourmet guides to ''good sex,'' recent studies have highlighted the fact that many people are dissatisfied with their sexual functioning.

In fact, the prevalence of sexual problems in the general population is high, with incidence figures ranging anywhere from 20% to 75%. In a recent survey of 212 patients attending a family medicine practice over a 4-month period, Schein, Levine, Zyzanski, Medalie, Dichman, and Alemangno (1986) reported that 75% of patients had at least one problem involving sexual identity or function and 26% of patients described their overall sexual lives as being a problem. Bachmann and Leiblum (1987) found that nearly one fifth of 887 consecutive female patients seeking gynecological care reported at least one sexual problem.

Even ''happily married'' couples often experience less than satisfactory sex lives. As part of a larger study involving 100 married couples, Frank, Anderson, and Rubinstein (1978) found that 40% of the males and 63% of the females reported one or more sexual dysfunctions! The incidence of sexual complaints was even higher. That the couples in this study described themselves as happily married attests to the fact that sex is not the sole determinant of a successful marriage. Nevertheless, it is obvious that despite our society's enthusiastic endorsement of sexual freedom and permissiveness since the 1970s, most people have difficulty spontaneously and ''naturally'' enjoying a carefree sexual life.

KATHRYN S. K. HALL and SANDRA R. LEIBLUM • Department of Psychiatry, UMDNJ–Robert Wood Johnson Medical School, Piscataway, New Jersey 08854.

As little as 100 years ago, human sexuality was not considered a legitimate topic for discussion in scientific or medical circles but was a moral issue that belonged exclusively in the domain of religion. The importance of sexuality was understood primarily in terms of procreation, and pleasure was not considered a significant factor. Erectile dysfunction or "impotence" was the only recognized sexual dysfunction, and the treatment of this disorder has been traced back to 2000 B.C. (Rosen, 1983). In the Victorian era, the early sex researchers viewed sexuality as a dangerous force that should be contained within matrimonial bonds, and "normal" sexuality continued to be rigidly defined as intercourse. Other sexual acts were no longer labeled as sinful, but as physically and psychologically damaging to the individual who engaged in them. In 1886, for example, Richard von Krafft-Ebing published his collosal work *Psychopathis Sexualis,* in which he depicted sex in almost all of its manifestations as a collection of loathsome diseases (Brecher, 1969). He insisted that masturbation was at the root of all sexual perversions, from simple fetishism to violent lust murder (Leiblum & Pervin, 1980). One can only wonder at one of his remedies for this "problem," which involved applying a white hot iron to the clitoris of a 4-year-old girl!

Fortunately, however, the turn of the century brought with it several key figures who were responsible for questioning some of the earlier beliefs concerning sexual expressiveness. One of the most influential figures of this time was Henry Havelock Ellis. In his seven-volume *Studies in the Psychology of Sex* (1899–1928), Ellis attempted an integrated view of human sexuality, one that included biological, sociological, and anthropological perspectives. The panorama of human sexuality that emerges from Ellis's work anticipate many of the later findings of Kinsey and Masters and Johnson in its acceptance of masturbation as a common phenomenon in men and women, in its view of homosexuality and heterosexuality as relative terms, and in its understanding of the presence and complexity of the female sexual response. This broader view of sexuality paved the way for viewing sexual difficulties other than erectile dysfunction as legitimate.

Sigmund Freud must be regarded as a monumental figure in any history of sexuality. Although he was aware of the high incidence of sexual problems among his patients (indeed, his whole theory of psychosexual development revolved around the exigencies of the sexual drive and the difficulty in achieving sexual maturity), Freud's diagnostic and treatment approach to sexual problems differed radically from that currently practiced. He endorsed intercourse as the *sine qua non* of sexual exchange between couples, and viewed masturbation and oral and anal sex as immature sexual outlets. His notions concerning female orgasm are well known and widely rejected among women today. His belief that the so-called vaginal orgasm was indicative of greater psychosexual maturity than the infantile clitoral one would come to be hotly challenged both by sexual physiologists and by clinicians. "Freudian" treatment of sexual problems involved years on the proverbial couch, analyzing and understanding the source of one's sexual conflicts and inhibitions, and attempting to overcome the destructive consequences of unresolved "Oedipal and Electra complexes." Although such treatment often promoted "insight," it rarely resulted in "recovery." Indeed, a recent article by an analytic psychiatrist illustrates the limitations of psychoanalytic therapy in the treatment of sexual problems. Simpson (1985) reported seeing a man with erectile dysfunction in analytical psychotherapy for over 1,000 hours without notable improvement in his erections. Some 15 years later, after the analyst had been trained in directive sex therapy techniques, he saw the same man, who again presented with erectile problems. In 10 sessions with this man and his wife, therapy was completed with a successful outcome.

In this latter half of the 20th century, there has been a change in sexual attitudes, so that sex is seen as a potential source of pleasure for both men and women. Partly responsible are the changes inherent in a postwar society, but much is owed to the contributions of Alfred Kinsey, Virginia Johnson, and William Masters.

Alfred Kinsey, a respected biologist, was asked to teach a course on sex education and marriage at Indiana University in 1937. In preparation for the course, Kinsey discovered that information on the sexual behaviors of people was sorely lacking. Kinsey took the task upon himself, and more than 17,000 interviews later came the first published descriptions of what Americans were up to both in and out of their bedrooms (Kinsey, Pomeroy & Martin, 1948; Kinsey, Pomeroy, Martin, & Gebhard, 1953). To some, the news was shocking. For example, over 90% of the men and 62% of the women respondents reported that they masturbated, percentages too high to make masturbation seem immature and immoral. Alfred Kinsey helped set the stage for the scientific study of sex that was to come with the efforts of Masters and Johnson.

Over a span of 12 years, Masters and Johnson (1966) conducted a study of human sexual response based on laboratory observations of 694 individuals. Their results challenged many former ideas about sexuality. They concluded that, during the sexual response cycle, men and women responded more similarly than differently; they discounted the distinction between vaginal and clitoral orgasms; and they validated the experience of masturbation as a means of arousal, pleasure, and orgasm. With the publication of *Human Sexual Inadequacy* in 1970, Masters and Johnson outlined their treatment approach to sexual dysfunction and claimed a "cure" rate that was surprisingly high. In essence, Masters and Johnson challenged the traditional Freudian notion of sexual dysfunction as a symptom of deep-seated psychological problems. Rather, they insisted that successful sexual performance was a "natural" ability that is affected by various sociocultural influences and by ignorance and anxiety.

Today, sex therapy is based largely on the work of Masters and Johnson, with important contributions and modifications by the behaviorists and, perhaps most significantly, by the work of Helen Singer Kaplan. Kaplan (1974) is the leading synthesizer of behavioral and psychoanalytic approaches to the treatment and understanding of sexual dysfunction. In essence, she has a multicausal conceptualization of the etiology of sexual dysfunction that includes immediate causes such as ignorance, anxiety, and communication failures as well as more remote causes such as internal conflicts between sexual wishes and fears.

THE SEXUAL DYSFUNCTIONS

Masters and Johnson (1966) conceptualized sexual dysfunctions according to a biphasic model of sexuality in which there are disorders of sexual excitement and disorders of orgasm. Kaplan (1977) highlighted the importance of an initial phase (desire) of this model, thereby making it triphasic. Thus, she introduced a new category of sexual dysfunctions: disorders of sexual desire. Disorders of sexual excitement include erectile dysfunction in the male and lack of sexual arousal in the female. Disorders of orgasm include retarded and premature ejaculation in males and female orgasmic dysfunction. Vaginismus and dyspareunia form a distinct category of disorders that involve pain with sexual activity. (See Table 1 for a summary classification of sexual disorders.)

Disorders of Desire

Exactly what constitutes low or inhibited sexual desire (ISD) remains controversial. There is no agreed-upon definition of how often one should experience sexual desire, nor even how to measure sexual desire. One may assess sexual desire by the number of times a person engages in sexual activity, either alone or with a partner. However, many people do not have an available sexual partner and may not consider masturbation a reasonable option for religious or moral reasons. On the other hand, some individuals engage in sexual acts with a partner for the sole purpose of procreation, satisfying their partner, or avoiding conflict and may experience little desire for such activity. Even masturbation may be undertaken solely for physical tension release, rather than for sexual pleasure. The presence or absence of sexual thoughts or fantasies, as well as time spent reading or watching erotica, may provide additional diagnostic information, although again one has to tease out whether the absence of these activities is indicative of low desire or religious or moral restraints. To given the definition of low sexual desire some clinical relevance, both objective and subjective components as well as situational issues must be considered (Levine, 1984).

The DSM-III (APA, 1980), the *Diagnostic and Statistical Manual* of the American Psychiatric Association, acknowledges the subjective nature of the diagnosis and defines ISD as the "persistent and pervasive inhibition of sexual desire." Such factors as the individual's age, sex, health, and intensity and frequency of sexual desire, and the context of the individual's life must be taken into account. The revised DSM-III, the DSM-III-R (APA, 1986), differentiates desire disorders into two categories: hypoactive sexual desire and sexual aversion. The former disorder is diagnosed when there is a persistent absence or deficiency of both sexual fantasies and desire for sexual activity, and the latter diag-

Table 1. Summary Classification of Sexual Dysfunctions According to the DSM-III-R[a]

Sexual desire disorders
Hypoactive sexual desire disorder
Sexual aversion disorder
Sexual arousal disorders
Female sexual arousal disorder
Male erectile disorder
Orgasm disorders
Inhibited female orgasm
Inhibited male orgasm
Premature ejaculation
Sexual pain disorders
Functional dyspareunia
Functional vaginismus

[a]American Psychiatric Association (1986).

nosis is given when there is evidence of "extreme aversion to, and avoidance of all or almost all genital sexual contact with a sexual partner." There is little consensus on whether hyperactive sexual desire should be considered a sexual dysfunction. Quadland (1985) defined sexual compulsivity as a unique problem characterized by a lack of control over one's sexual behavior. He argued that sexual compulsives do not display more neurotic symptoms than would be expected in the general population but differ primarily in terms of the greater frequency of sexual activities and partners. Some of our clients have complained that they think about sex "all the time" or masturbate "too much." In many instances, such thoughts or behavior is symptomatic of another disorder, such as obsessive-compulsive disorder or the manic phase of bipolar disorder. The diagnosis of ISD does not include cases of desire discrepancy in which neither partner in a relationship would be viewed as having a desire disorder but seek sexual contact with markedly different frequencies (Zilbergeld & Ellison, 1980).

Etiological Considerations and Theoretical Formulations

In the Victorian era, lack of sexual desire on the part of a woman was considered perfectly normal, and before that time, a man's lack of desire was praiseworthy and a sign of high moral character. However, in 1905, in *Three Essays on the Theory of Sexuality,* Freud wrote of the existence of an innate sexual drive or libido. Low sexual desire would result only from an active repression or inhibition due to intrapsychic conflict. Since the publication of the *Three Essays,* our understanding of ISD has become increasingly complicated by an awareness of the many factors that can contribute to it.

Kaplan (1979) regarded persons with ISD as actively suppressing the desire they would otherwise normally experience. According to Kaplan (1974, 1979), all sexual dysfunctions have both immediate and remote causes. The immediate causes of ISD, as of other dysfunctions, is performance anxiety or fear of failure. The anxiety, however, is evoked earlier in the sexual response cycle, so that arousal is denied or avoided altogether. On the other hand, according to Kaplan, ISD can also be symptomatic of a repression of earlier unresolved sexual conflict that arises in childhood out of the desire to act on libidinal impulses and the fear of doing so. For these individuals, later sexual arousal or desire evokes anxiety and unconscious guilt, which is dealt with through the mechanism of repression. Although Kaplan has emphasized the importance of intrapsychic determinants of desire, she has neglected biological, hormonal, cognitive, and interpersonal factors (Rosen & Leiblum, 1987b).

Levine (1984) attempted to integrate several elements into his formulation of ISD. He identified a drive element in sexual desire, a biologically based brain mechanism for the perpetuation of the species. Levine also stressed the importance of interpersonal attraction and "voyeuristic stimulation," by which he meant the verbal, visual, and auditory representations of sexual stimulation that an individual may carry. Finally, Levine detailed the importance of the degree to which an individual wants to feel sexual—the cognitive aspiration to be sexual.

Other theorists have highlighted other aspects of low sexual desire. The emphasis on the interpersonal and social context of desire disorders comes from proponents of systemic-interactional models (Regas & Sprenkle, 1984; Verhulst & Heiman, 1979) and most recently from Apfelbaum and Apfelbaum (1985). The systems-interactional model focuses on partner interactions in the genesis and maintenance of low desire, as desire is interpreted as the experience of, or attraction to, another person as a sexual being (Verhulst & Heiman, 1979). The Apfelbaums suggested that desire disorders might best be viewed as stemming from societal pressure to be sexually active, especially in a committed relationship. They took exception to the notion that the person with a lack of desire is withholding sexual feelings, and they claimed that this is a moral judgment rather than a psychological statement. The Apfelbaums drew attention to the fact that we rarely consider the partner with "higher" desire abnormal for retaining his or her sexual interest despite lack of reciprocation by the identified patient. According to the Apfelbaums, the underlying issue is the "response anxiety" of the low-desire person, which is invoked primarily in reaction to societal or partner pressure to be sexual. "Sexual apathy," as the Apfelbaums referred to it, is conceptualized not simply as a lack of desire, but as a withdrawn state created by the pressure to feel or be sexual.

These (and other) theoretical models of sexual desire have evolved, in part, as a response to demands placed on the clinician for assistance with problems of desire. Although some theories attempt to integrate most of the existing knowledge about desire, others focus only on certain major components, such as intrapsychic or systemic determinants. There are shortcomings in each of these models, but given that sexual desire problems are so heterogeneous, it is unlikely that any one theory can account for the diversity of problems and patients encountered.

Issues in Evaluation

There is little consensus regarding the choice of format or content for the evaluation of desire problems. Indeed, it is difficult for the evaluation process to keep up with the many factors that may be associated with ISD. Nevertheless, Rosen and Leiblum (1987b) outlined one of the most comprehensive evaluations to date (see Figure 1).

The primary diagnostic issue is whether the desire problem is primary and global (lifelong and pervasive) or whether it is situational and secondary, as this distinction has important treatment implications. To make this distinction, the clinician must assess the extent and duration of the problem. A consistent absence of sexual fantasies, a history of infrequent masturbation, restricted sexual experiences with a limited number of sexual partners, and little or no pleasure in sexual or sensual activity is the typical pattern of primary ISD. These characteristics have usually persisted since early adolescence. Individuals with secondary or situational ISD usually describe an earlier period of sexual interest and involvement and may retain an interest in fantasy or masturbation, or an attraction to partners other than the primary one. Where the onset of ISD is insidious, biological factors may be implicated (e.g., chronic alcoholism). When the onset is acute and can be related to a specific event(s), the therapeutic outcome tends to be more favorable. Another important element is the degree to which a sexual performance problem antedates or coincides with the desire problem. It is not uncommon for a man who cannot get an erection, or a woman who cannot achieve an orgasm, to lose his or her desire for sexual activity. However, the reverse is also often true, and ISD may be masked by a performance difficulty (sexual dysfunction).

A complete medical history is also important in the evaluation of ISD as any major physical illness, disability, or surgical procedure (e.g., postcoronary adjustment syndrome, cancer of the reproductive organs or breasts in both men and women, and the effects of chronically administered medications such as the adrenergic-inhibiting antihypertensives) may depress sexual interest, either chronically or temporarily (Rosen & Kostis, 1985). However, health problems may also impact on sexual interest indirectly

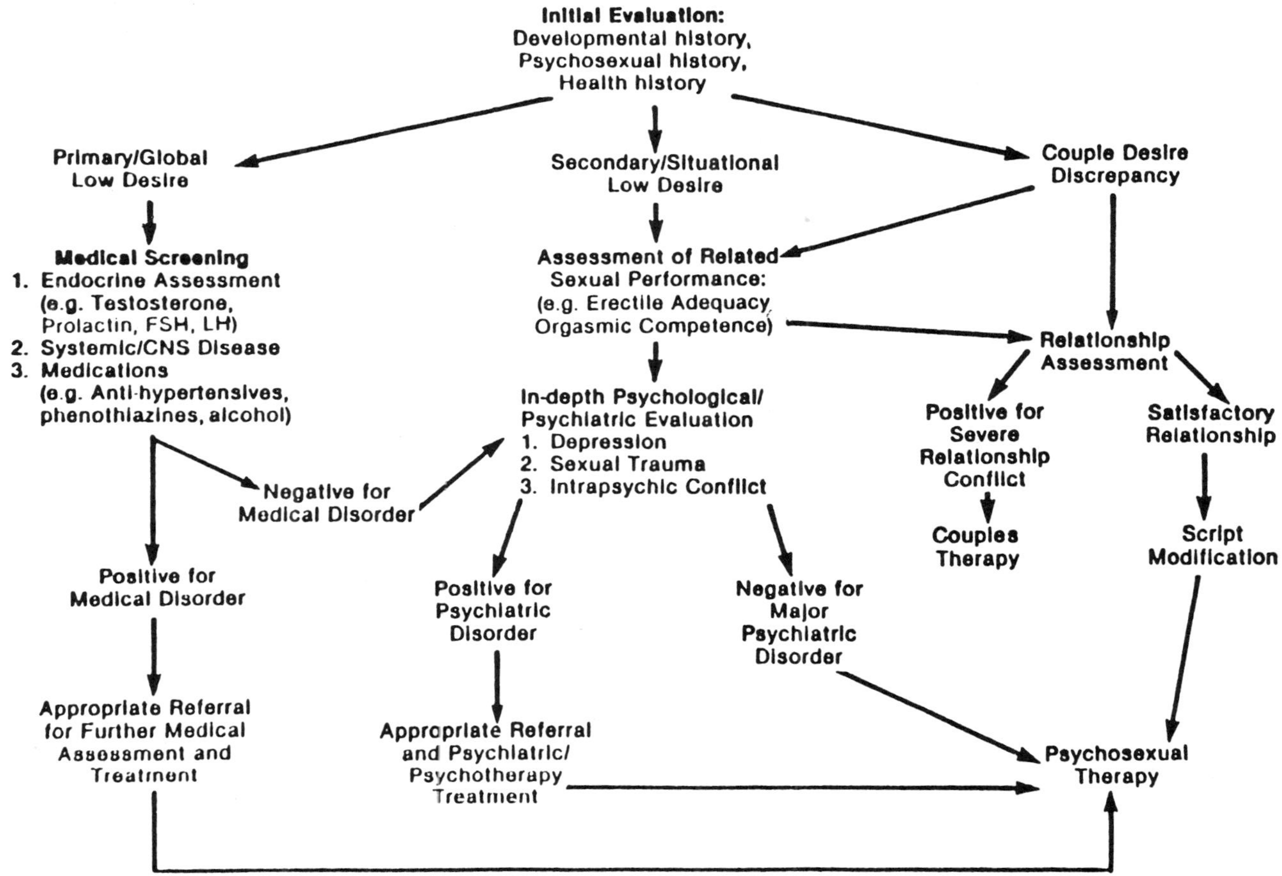

Figure 1. A flowchart model for the evaluation of sexual desire problems in individuals and couples. (From "Current Approaches to the Evaluation of Sexual Desire Disorders" by R. C. Rosen and S. R. Leiblum in *Journal of Sex and Marital Therapy*, 1987a.)

through the effects on body image and self-esteem (e.g., post-mastectomy patients and ileostomy and colostomy patients).

Endocrine screening is sometimes helpful. Bancroft (1983) found a correlation between a clear-cut deficiency in endogenous androgen levels and absent or diminished desire in both males and females. Exogenous replacement of androgens is beneficial in most of these cases (e.g., hypogonadal males and young, surgically menopausal women). However, there is no hard evidence that problems of sexual desire experienced by otherwise healthy individuals can be reversed by androgen administration. Administering high levels of testosterone to enhance desire in such a population is currently felt to be medically unsound and ethically questionable. (Rosen & Leiblum, 1987).

Also related to a decrease in sexual desire are psychiatric illnesses, such as schizophrenia, chronic alcoholism, and depression. Other psychological factors to be assessed include a past history of sexual abuse or trauma, sexual preference conflicts, and interpersonal problems.

Inhibited sexual desire often appears to be constitutional; that is, the individual displays a lifelong lack of interest in sex, although remaining capable of a degree of performance. The following case vignette describes a man who has primary, global ISD:

> Mr. and Mrs. S presented to the Sexual Counseling Service with Mrs. S complaining of her husband's lack of sexual desire. Mr. S did not perceive himself as having a desire problem. He reported a lifelong history of low sexual interest, with no fantasies or daydreams about sex. He had masturbated only infrequently since adolescence, and although he had dated before he was married, he had had limited sexual experiences. Mrs. S had assumed that the frequency of sex would improve after marriage, but such was not the case. Intercourse remained at about once per month over the course of their 6-year marriage. Mrs. S also felt that Mr. S was inattentive to her in bed and seemed concerned primarily with achieving his orgasm. Mr. S failed to see "what all the fuss is about." He indicated no desire or curiosity with regard to changing their sexual script. He claimed that he loved his wife very much and showed it to her by going to work every day and coming home every night.

The case of the Ss is quite different from one in which ISD is situational and symptomatic of underlying marital conflict. This conflict may reflect power issues or problems with intimacy as is illustrated by the following case vignette:

> Mrs. G requested therapy for her husband, who had not approached her sexually for several months. When Mr. G was seen alone, he reported no difficulty with erections and indicated that he was turned on by erotic materials. Although he did not engage in sexual activities with his wife, or anyone else, he masturbated several times monthly. He reported that he did not feel any "urge" to have sex with his wife. During the course of therapy, Mr. G expressed anger at his spouse for trying to take charge of the relationship and dominate him. He was also angry at her because, despite his efforts to please her, she continued to be critical of him. The sexual relationship with his wife was the only area in which Mr. G felt he had some control. He found that he could assert his independence and also punish his wife by withholding sex.

Treatment

The treatment of ISD depends to a large extent on one's theoretical orientation to the problem. Those who advocate a systems-interactional perspective argue that the treatment of choice should be marital or couples therapy (Fish, Fish, & Sprenkle, 1984; Regas & Sprenkle, 1984). The Apfelbaums (Apfelbaum & Apfelbaum, 1985) recommended "reframing'' as a major intervention. Reframing refers to the process of making individuals aware that their low desire is their reaction to the pressure placed on them to be or feel sexual. The Apfelbaums believe that, once response anxiety is removed, sexual interest returns rather readily. Although it is undeniably true that individuals labeled as having ISD tolerate considerable spousal and societal pressure to respond enthusiastically to sexual overtures, it is not always the case that removing the pressure to be sexual results in active sexual interest. Kaplan (1974) argued that, as intrapsychic conflicts are often at the root of ISD, we well as conflicts about intimacy, insight-oriented psychotherapy is the treatment of choice.

In cases where the issue appears to be a problem of desire discrepancy rather than inhibited desire on the part of one individual, guided compromise has been suggested as having value (Rosen & Leiblum, 1976). Where fatigue, boredom, or a deficient or unacceptable sexual repertoire appears to be a major problem, script modification has been suggested as an effective intervention (Gagnon, Rosen, & Leiblum, 1982). The following case demonstrates the use of both techniques:

Mr. and Mrs. M had been married for several years and came to the Sexual Counseling Service complaining of Mr. M's loss of sexual desire. Indeed, the frequency of their lovemaking had declined from once a day to less than once a week. Unknown to Mrs. M, however, Mr. M had continued to engage in weekly masturbation. Both Mr. and Mrs. M had been married previously and had had very unsatisfactory sexual relations with their first spouses. Following the death of her first husband, Mrs. M felt ''liberated'' sexually and began to enjoy sex for the first time in her life. On the other hand, after his divorce, Mr. M felt inadequate sexually with the many women he was encountering through a dating service. He had difficulty getting and maintaining an erection. When he met his present wife, he had found her a patient and considerate lover and was eventually able to achieve an erection with her. They developed an elaborate, but rather rigid, sexual script, from which they had not deviated. Mrs. M had become dissatisfied with the invariant nature of their lovemaking and had suggested changes. Mr. M, who was exquisitely sensitive to criticism and worried lest his erectile difficulties should return, withdrew sexually from his wife. Over the course of eight sessions, the Ms gradually widened their sexual repertoire, in both the timing and the variety of activities. They reached a compromise on sexual frequency of once weekly. Their earlier higher level of coitus reflected the need both had to feel that they were sexually desirable and to confirm that they were loved. When they found other avenues to express their mutual love and caring, they agreed that they did not need or want to have sex daily.

In conclusion, it seems that inhibited sexual desire is a complex and heterogeneous disorder. Assessment is paramount in pinpointing the biological, psychological, and interpersonal variables that may be etiologically relevant. More research on the factors contributing to inhibited sexual desire is necessary before a comprehensive theory and treatment can be formulated. At present, there is no one valid approach to either evaluation or treatment.

Disorders of Sexual Excitement

Erectile Dysfunction

Erectile dysfunction (ED) is a broad term for a difficulty in achieving or maintaining an erection. This difficulty can be total or partial, omnipresent or situational (for example, during intercourse, but not during masturbation). Furthermore, ED can be primary (lifelong), or it can be secondary. Although it is true that most men experience erectile difficulty at some time in their lives (e.g., when fatigued, ill, or depressed), ED refers to a long-standing loss of erection. What degree of erectile loss constitutes ED, however, is not clear and is often left up to the discretion of the clinician. In many cases a useful guideline is whether the penis becomes rigid and full enough for vaginal penetration. For many men, the ability to achieve a full erection is a salient index of their sexual prowess, and they are very concerned with any dimunition in erectile ability. Furthermore, it has been our experience that many men are not open to the suggestion that psychogenic rather than physical factors account for their difficulty. They are often convinced that they have a medical problem and want medical treatment for it. Some of the reason for their belief in an organogenic etiology rests with their assertion that they continue to feel sexually aroused and desire sexual contact.

The DSM-III-R diagnosis of ED is two-pronged and involves (1) persistent or recurrent failure in attaining or maintaining erection until completion of intercourse and/or (2) persistent or recurrent lack of subjective sexual excitement and pleasure during sexual activity.

The addition of the latter specification indicates that there are males who function automatically with prompt, rigid erections but who, nevertheless, derive little pleasure from these erections.

Etiological Considerations and Theoretical Formulations. Psychoanalytic theory identifies unconscious intrapsychic conflicts as the source of ED. These conflicts are said to have their roots in unresolved Oedipal problems that produce feelings of guilt and fear about sex and, most importantly, result in unconscious castration anxiety. However, Kaplan (1974) argued that ED may be better conceptualized as the physiological concomitant of anxiety rather than as the defense against it. This anxiety need not be due to castration fears or an unresolved Oedipal conflict but may be the result of sexual arousal being associated with negative contingencies (shame, fear of punishment or of physical illness) during a child's formative years.

Performance anxiety was identified by Masters and Johnson (1970) and also by Kaplan (1974) as a prime cause of ED. Some men have such a fear of failure that they are constantly monitoring their performance. These men may have unrealistically high expectations of their performance or may feel that they have (or indeed may have) a demanding sexual partner. Cognitive-behavioral theories emphasize the importance of being focused on sexual stimuli for arousal and erection to occur. When a man focuses instead on nonsexual thoughts, such as work problems or the idea that he has to succeed at sex, erection is often impaired (Ellis, 1980).

Other formulations of the etiology of ED include learning theory, which postulates the existence, in some cases, of a phobia of women's genitalia. Systems formulations focus on maladaptive patterns in the relationship as causing and maintaining ED.

Issues in Evaluation. The evaluation of ED is complex and often requires considerable collaboration with other health professionals. Until recently, erectile failure was thought to be primarily psychogenic in etiology. Then, in 1980, Spark, White, & Connolly, published a paper reporting that 37 of 105 men referred to their endocrine clinic for assessment of ED showed disorders of the hypothalamic-pituitary-gonadal axis. The press publicized this report and suggested that the role of organic factors in ED was greater than had previously been acknowledged. Some even suggested that as much as 50% of erectile failure was due to endocrine, neurological, or vascular problems (Nolen, 1981). Current assessment strategies recognize the importance of identifying both psychogenic and organogenic contributions to the erectile difficulty, as most such problems are the result of many contributory factors. Treating the organic component without acknowledging the role of psychogenic factors is often doomed to failure, as is the reverse situation.

A thorough assessment and screening process is outlined in Figure 2. A detailed sexual and medical history is taken in order to determine if the problem appears to be acute or chronic in its development and whether the problem onset may be traced to some discernible factor such as a divorce or the administration of antihypertensive medication. If the client reports that the problem occurs *only* with certain people or in certain situations, a psychogenic etiology is likely. Often, for example, the male can obtain an erection during masturbation or awakens with a strong erection but cannot achieve or sustain an erection when in bed with his wife. If the male complains that he can achieve only a partial erection despite high arousal or is unable to achieve an erection with both self and partner stimulation, a complete physical evaluation is necessary. Endocrine screening, which includes a determination of the levels of serum testosterone, prolactin,

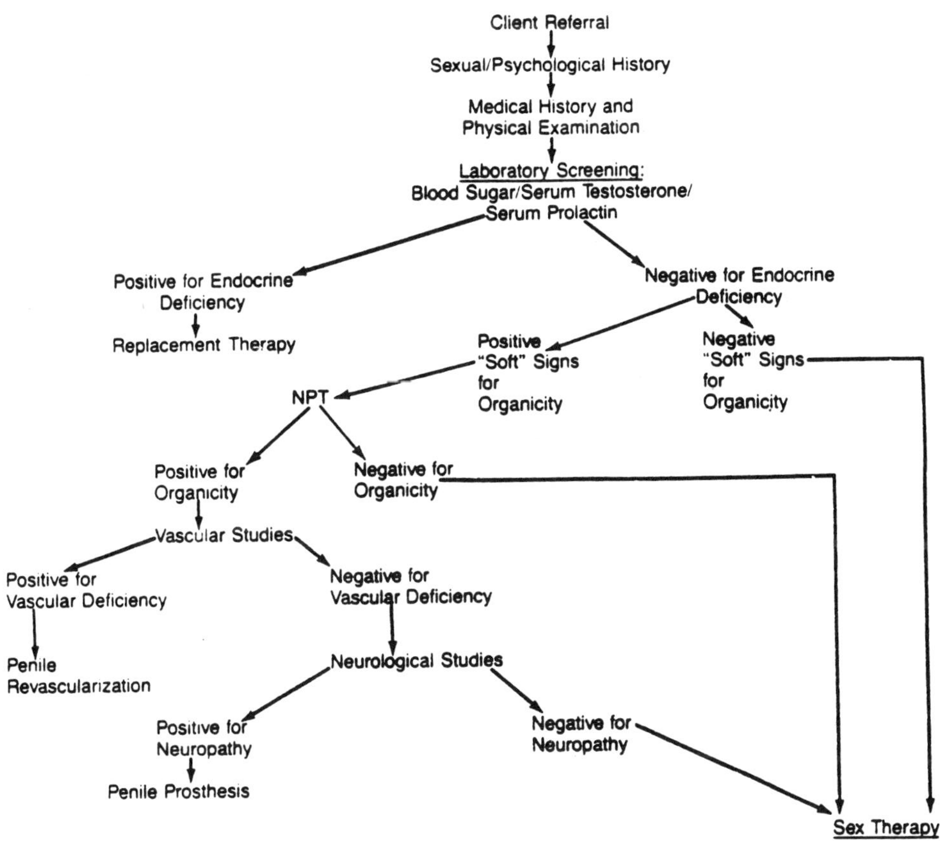

Figure 2. A flowchart model for comprehensive assessment of erectile dysfunction. (From "Clinical Issues in the Assessment and Treatment of Impotence: A New Look at an Old Problem" by R. C. Rosen in *The Behavior Therapist,* 1983.)

luteinizing hormone (LH), follicle-simulating hormone (FSH), and glucose, is part of this process. Although it is rare to find a man with abnormally low free or bound testosterone, if a case of hypogonadism is uncovered testosterone replacement is usually effective in restoring satisfactory functioning. In cases where there is an abnormal elevation of prolactin, bromocryptine treatment is indicated. Other elements of the physical evaluation are the penile Doppler test and the nocturnal penile tumescence (NPT) test. The Doppler gives an index of penile blood pressure, indicating whether there is sufficient flow of blood into the penis.

Healthy males have erections during random-eye-movement (REM) sleep. These erections have little to do with the content of dreams and are a normal physiological reaction during this phase of sleep. The presence of nocturnal erections indicates a predominantly psychogenic origin, whereas the absence usually indicates a predominantly organogenic etiology of the ED. There is recent evidence that nocturnal erections are inhibited by depression (Thase, Reynolds, Glanz, Jennings, Sewitch, Kupfer, & Frank, 1986).

The following case vignette demonstrates the multiple factors that may contribute to the experience of ED:

> Mr. C, a 63-year-old businessperson, consulted the Sexual Counseling Service at the insistence of his wife, because of his lack of sexual contact with her over the past several years. Assessment revealed that Mr. C had been experiencing erectile failure for 2 years, although before that time he had been able to obtain an erection through oral sex with a mistress. His medical history revealed several factors that may have contributed to the ED. Mr. C had a history of hypertension, which was being controlled by antihypertensive medication with occasional use of diuretics. He also overindulged in alcohol and may have been suffering from sleep apnea, which might have been instrumental in causing both the hypertension and the erectile problem. However, there were a number of psychological factors that also seemed relevant. Mr. C felt alienated from his wife, particularly as, 2 years before, she had insisted on separate bedrooms because of his noisy and sleep-disruptive snoring. Sessions with the couple together revealed a number of potentially significant and unresolved marital issues, such as questions of power and conflict about the use of leisure time.

This case, which is not atypical, illustrates the number of overlapping physical and psychological factors that may be instrumental in causing ED. It also demonstrates a situation in which lack of sexual desire was secondary to a sexual dysfunction problem.

Treatment. Medical and surgical interventions for the treatment of ED are becoming increasingly common and complex. They range from hormone replacement therapy to penile revascularization and prosthetic devices. The administration of testosterone to men who have normal baseline levels is usually ineffective and always ethically questionable. Men may experience additional hopelessness if their problem persists despite the hormone therapy (Rosen, 1983). Vascular surgery has been found to be of limited value in the treatment of ED. It is effective only if there is a specific blockage in the large-gauge artery leading to the penis or if there is a fistula in the corpora cavernosa allowing leakage of blood out of the corpora. These two types of problems are not very common. What is more often the case is diffuse small-vessel atherosclerotic disease in the pelvic region, which is not treatable by vascular surgery (LoPiccolo, 1985). Surgical implantation of prosthetic devices is also an increasingly popular treatment. Such devices come in two types: inflatable and semirigid. They permit a man to attain an erection that is sufficient for intercourse. Tactile sensitivity and ejaculation are unaffected by the procedure. Nevertheless, as Rosen (1983) noted, partner satisfaction and self-satisfaction with the device show considerable variability. Who should receive an implant is also an issue. At opposite ends of the spectrum are those who argue that all men should be given a course of sex therapy first, as some diagnosed organogenic cases respond favorably to therapy (Bullard, Mann, Caplan, & Stoklosa, 1978); others feel that an implant may be indicated in those cases of psychogenic ED where the prognosis for therapy is poor (Brooks, 1981). Schover and von Eschenbach (1985) outlined a comprehensive treatment plan relying on input from urologists and sex therapists; it includes both the evaluation and the treatment of candidates for a prosthesis pre- and postoperatively.

The most recent medical advance in the treatment of ED is the intracavernosal injection of papavarine hydrochloride and phentolamine mesylate. Injection of these substances into the corporal body of the penis results in relaxation of the smooth muscles in the corporal arterioles and in the area surrounding the corporal lacunae. The effect is an increase in arterial blood inflow and a decrease in drainage from the corporal lacunae. With this increase in intracavernosal pressure, the penis may become sufficiently erect to allow vaginal penetration. This pharmacological erection can be enhanced in duration and rigidity with sexual stimulation, and administration of these drugs does not interfere with ejaculation or orgasm. The major side effect of papavarine and phentolamine has been priapism, or prolonged erections (Goldstein, 1986).

At present, programs for the self-administration of papavarine are in the initial stages, but the early results are promising. The best success has been found in those men with neurological ED, who have normal penile tissue and blood supply, but abnormal nerve supply to the corporal erectile tissue (Goldstein, 1986). Success has even been reported for cases of ED in spinal-cord-injured men (Leyson, 1986). For men with ED of vasculogenic etiology, higher doses of papavarine are required, and the resulting erections are not as rigid or as long-lasting as for men with neurological ED (Goldstein, 1986). Finally, intracavernosal injections of papavarine have been suggested for those men with psychogenic ED who have not responded to an adequate trial of psychotherapy, but preliminary results suggest that papavarine is least effective in these instances (Althof, Turner, Levine, Risen, Hursh, Resnick, & Bodner, 1986).

The trend in recent years toward focusing on medical interventions for the treatment of ED results in part from our greater awareness of the organic causes, but it also reflects the reluctance many men display in addressing the psychological issues that may be related to their sexual difficulties.

Psychological interventions continue to be effective in the treatment of ED, although high relapse rates are also reported (Levine & Agle, 1978). Rosen (1983) provided a good overview of the behavioral approach to the treatment of ED. Cognitive restructuring (Ellis, 1980) is considered the first step in the treatment program. The aim is to encourage a more flexible and pleasure-oriented approach to sexual activities. At times, it is also necessary to conduct several sessions of marital therapy before dealing directly with the sexual problem. However, the decision to focus initially on marital or sexual issues is really up to the clinician. We have found that a successful outcome may be attained with couples and individuals typically considered poor prognostic risks (Leiblum & Kopel, 1977; Mobarak, Tamerin & Tamerin, 1986). Next, a graded series of sexual assignments is introduced:

1. Intercourse, or attempts at intercourse, is banned. The couple is then given a series of exercises that focus on sensual interaction, called "sensate focus" by Masters and Johnson (1970). These exercises typically progress from nongenital massage to more

direct genital stimulation. The ability to communicate likes and dislikes to one's partner in a positive, nonthreatening manner is also a focus of treatment at this stage. These graded exercises are often sufficient to produce an erection.

2. The next step is to deal with the fear of failure (e.g., fear of losing the erection), which becomes a self-fulfilling prophecy for many men. This extends to the fear that once lost, the erection will not return. Kaplan (1974) and Zilbergeld (1978) recommended exercises in which the man and his partner practice obtaining erections and then deliberately losing them by withdrawing the stimulation. The man often experiences new confidence in his erectile ability as he finds that, once lost, erections can indeed return with adequate stimulation and a relaxed setting.

3. Once confidence in erectile ability is achieved, the couple is ready to attempt intercourse. Initially, the male is encouraged to relax as much as possible. The female partner stimulates the male, orally or manually, to erection and then guides his penis inside her vagina, while in the female-superior position. Some therapists recommend that the man become comfortable with vaginal containment before attempting to thrust to orgasm and before attempting other positions. The goal is to eliminate as much performance pressure as possible.

This treatment program raises several issues. As is obvious, considerable attention is directed at the male partner. The clinician must recognize the female partner's needs and desires as well, if only to keep her an interested and involved ally in the treatment. A second issue is the problem of the single male, or the male without a partner. Some therapists have advocated the use of surrogates in such cases (Apfelbaum, 1980), but this option has been questioned on both ethical and psychological grounds. Zilbergeld (1978) outlined fantasy and masturbation exercises that a single male may practice and also advocated a group approach (Zilbergeld, 1975), which is not widely practiced today.

Finally, in those cases in which the behavioral approach is unsuccessful and no organogenic basis can be found, Kaplan (1974) advocated psychotherapy to deal with the remote or underlying issues responsible for the ED.

Disorders of Orgasm

Premature Ejaculation

Premature ejaculation (PE) means, simply, to ejaculate too early. The question that is left unanswered is what is too early? In the past, therapists and researchers tried to quantify the criterion for the diagnosis of PE. They focused either on the duration of intercourse (ranging from 30 seconds to 2 minutes) or the number of thrusts (fewer than 10). In their early work, Masters and Johnson (1970) proposed that PE be diagnosed in those cases where the male partner cannot control his ejaculation long enough for the female partner to reach orgasm at least 50% of the time. The problem, of course, was that this diagnosis rested on someone else's sexual ability or pleasure. By this definition, a man who can delay his ejaculation for 30 minutes would be given a diagnosis of premature ejaculation if his partner were not orgasmic in that time. However, most sex therapists now agree that the crucial factor in making a diagnosis of premature ejaculation is the absence of an ability, or a perceived ability, to control ejaculation, with only secondary consideration given to the elapsed time.

Etiological Considerations and Theoretical Formulations. The psychoanalytic understanding of PE holds that it is an expression of unconscious conflicts toward women. By ejaculating quickly, a man is assumed to be denying pleasure to his partner, while acknowledging her sexual needs. In essence, the male is expressing his hostility toward women. However, there does not appear to be a relationship between PE and psychopathology, marital disharmony, sexual conflict, or socioeconomic status (Perelman, 1980). Men who suffer from PE appear to be a diverse group that cannot be classified by an underlying hostility toward women.

Some researchers have suggested that PE is a psychophysiological disorder that is characterized by the male's inability to tolerate high levels of sexual arousal without ejaculation. It has been suggested that men with PE are more sensitive to sexual stimulation or have a lower threshold for ejaculation than other men (Speiss, 1977). Such a hypothesis, however, awaits further investigation.

Learning theory proposes that PE is acquired as a result of an early history in which rapid ejaculation was not only necessary but beneficial. Such situations would be lack of sufficient privacy for masturbation, such as hurried masturbation in the family bathroom, or early intercourse experiences in the back seat of a car, in the parental home complete with the threat of discovery, or with prostitutes, who actively encourage prompt ejaculation from their clients. Learning theorists argue that rapid ejaculation is a learned response to sexual excitement. Indeed, from a sociobiological point of view, rapid ejaculation is a superior response, given that a man can impregnate more women quickly and in potentially dangerous situations (Kinsey *et al.*, 1948). Needless to say, this "superiority" is small compensation for either partner where PE is a problem.

Today, most sex therapists regard PE as an inability to recognize the premonitory sensations of ejaculation and a consequent inability to delay it. To some men, the concept of actively delaying ejaculation is new and needs to be learned. Some men believe that sex should "just happen" and that they have no control over when they ejaculate. What is probably common to all men with PE is some degree of performance anxiety that detracts from their ability to recognize impending orgasm. A common device tried by men to control their ejaculation is distraction. Some think about what they have to do the next day; some do mathematics in their head; one man tried to recall baseball scores and statistics of previous games (one wonders what he did in the off season). Primarily, however, these men's thoughts are occupied by worries about how long they will "last." Not only do such thoughts detract from the sexual pleasure these men could be experiencing, but they are a further distraction from sensing the warning signs of ejaculation.

Issues in Evaluation. The important factors to consider when evaluating PE are the sense of control over ejaculation and when, in the sequence of sexual activity, ejaculation occurs. If ejaculation occurs before vaginal penetration (when not desired), this is readily diagnosed as PE. If ejaculation occurs during intercourse, but the timing of ejaculation is perceived as involuntary (e.g., the man experiences no control over ejaculation), then PE may be suspected. However, in this case, one must also consider how much time has elapsed during intercourse. Some men may have unrealistic expectations and are discontent with lasting "only" 10–15 minutes. For these men, the evaluation of cognitions and performance demands is important.

Premature ejaculation may also be situational. Some men may be able to control their ejaculation during masturbation, but not when they are with their partner. Often, they attribute this discrepancy to the fact that being with a partner is more stimulating than being alone. Although this may be true, it may also be the case that these men are concerned about displeasing or ''failing'' their partner.

Finally, PE may also be secondary. That is, it may develop after a period of time in which the man did have the ability to control his ejaculation. Some possible precipitating events include changes in partner or in life circumstances. Further, PE is often secondary to erectile dysfunction. A man may be so distracted by his fear of losing his erection that he does not attend to the warning signs of impending ejaculation, or he may want to ejaculate quickly when he fears he will lose his erection, and thereby, he may set up a maladaptive learning pattern.

At times, a man's partner may contribute to his experience of PE. If his partner does not enjoy sex, she may try to hurry her partner so that sex is over quickly. It is therefore important to evaluate the status of the relationship and the partner's attitude toward sex. This evaluation is especially necessary because the partner plays a key role in the treatment.

As a final note, it is always important to examine the cognitions or thoughts that occur during sexual activity. If the source of distraction is anxiety, it must be recognized and dealt with therapeutically.

Treatment of PE. There are numerous ''home remedies'' marketed for the treatment of premature ejaculation. In addition, men have used a variety of techniques to help themselves prolong their ejaculation. Usually, these are unsuccessful and may even exacerbate the problem. Some of the more commonly tried methods are distraction (thinking about something else to decrease excitement), use of condoms to reduce sensations, avoidance of foreplay, and even self-infliction of pain to physically distract oneself from excessive arousal. Finally, there are numerous anesthetizing creams marketed under a variety of brand names, such as Mr. Maintain, Stay-Hard, Stay-Awhile, and Prolong. Unfortunately, one of the side effects of these creams is that they reduce the partner's sensations of pleasure as well.

The most successful treatment for premature ejaculation is the stop–start technique, which was originally described by Semans in 1956 and has since been elaborated on. Basically, this technique involves stimulation of the penis until the premonitory sensations of ejaculation are experienced. Stimulation is interrupted until these sensations diminish. The process is then repeated until the stimulation can be tolerated for longer periods of time. Kaplan (1974) emphasized the importance of having the patient focus on the sensations of impending orgasm as the ''essential therapeutic ingredient'' (p. 303); others have emphasized the importance of a graded hierarchy of stimulation, which provides gradual mastery and diminishes performance anxiety (Masters & Johnson, 1970). In most applications of this procedure, the penis is initially stimulated extravaginally, and then the stimulation is increased in successive approximations until coitus is achieved. The following case outlines the treatment of PE:

Mr. B was a 48-year-old man who presented to the Sexual Counseling Service with his second wife, a 28-year-old woman. The Bs had been married for 9 years. In the past year, Mr. B had found that his wife was refusing sexual contact with increasing frequency, saying she experienced little pleasure from their sexual activities. She was not orgasmic with intercourse and complained that intercourse was frustrating because she would begin to get aroused just as ''it was all over.'' Both agreed that Mr. B ejaculated within 2 minutes of penetration.

Treatment

The Bs were instructed in the method and rationale of the stop-and-start method. Mrs. B was asked to manually stimulate her husband's penis. When he felt that he was going to have an orgasm, Mr. B was to signal her to stop. They were to repeat this three times, and on the fourth and final time, they were permitted to continue until Mr. B reached orgasm. They were not permitted to have intercourse but were encouraged to make the experience pleasurable for both. The Bs returned the next week to report that the exercise had gone very well. They had done it three times, and by the end of the week, Mr. B could delay his ejaculation for about 5 minutes between periods of stimulation. The subsequent exercises were essentially a repeat of the first, increasing the level of sexual stimulation by using lubricants and engaging in more sex play. Mrs. B adamantly refused to engage in oral sex, however, despite her husband's entreaties.

The next sessions introduced intercourse. With the use of the female-superior position, Mr. B was surprised to find that, even though he was concentrating on his own sensations, his wife experienced an orgasm during intercourse! Nevertheless, Mrs. B complained that, in general, her husband seemed to stop thrusting just as she was about to climax. She was frustrated and angry. After some discussion, it became evident that Mrs. B was angry because she felt that her husband was too demanding sexually. He wanted sex more often than she did, and he seemed to want it at inopportune times for her. The treatment, focused as it was on her husband, highlighted the inequality in their sexual relationship and elicited her previously unexpressed anger. With some modifications in the timing and frequency of sex, the couple attempted intercourse in the male-superior position, the most exciting position for Mr. B. At termination, Mr. B could delay his ejaculation with a few rest periods, or by slowing down the pace of his thrusting. Mrs. B was orgasmic only some of the time but indicated that this was acceptable to her.

A variant of the stop–start technique is the squeeze technique (Masters & Johnson, 1970). Instead of stopping stimulation at the point of impending orgasm, the partner places her thumb and forefinger around the penis, just below the coronal ridge, and gently squeezes. The feeling of impending orgasm subsides, and there may be some diminution of erection. However, most therapists prefer the stop–start technique, which is just as effective and less obtrusive.

Orgasmic Dysfunction

The sexual revolution has brought with it an increasing awareness by women, not only that they can enjoy sex, but that they should enjoy it, and enjoyment of sex is often equated with the ability to have orgasms: "Today, not only are women expected to have orgasms, they are expected to have multiple orgasms, through a variety of means, in a reasonable period of time, and to enjoy them with pleasure and pride" (Leiblum & Pervin, 1980, p. 107). These expectations may be partly responsible for the fact that difficulty in achieving orgasm is the most common complaint of women presenting to the Sexual Counseling Service.

There is some debate, however, about exactly what defines an orgasm. According to Kaplan (1974), an orgasm is a reflex event located in the lumbrosacral spinal cord. As such, it is subject to facilitory and inhibitory influences both from direct sensory input and from input from higher neural centers. Others conceptualize an orgasm as more of a CNS event (Cohen, Rosen, & Goldstein, 1976). In any event, what does seem to be important is that the orgasm be both physically and psychologically experienced as pleasurable. The following is a description of an orgasm by a previously nonorgasmic female client, as dictated to her therapist:

I'm pretty much at a resting state, testing areas of my body. I find a spot, and all of a sudden I know it will start to build. I lose consciousness. There is warmth. I can feel it in my toes, a tingling. It goes straight down my body to my toes. My body starts to tense from head to toe. My breathing and my heartbeat quicken. When the good, intense feeling comes, it comes suddenly. It is an intensely, intensely pleasurable feeling, a rolling feeling of pleasure, and I say to myself, "Oh my God." I experience an intense need in my genitals. In my head, I have the feeling of going up, up to the top of something. When it's over, sometimes I try again, but my brain says, "No, you can't handle this."

Just as there is debate about what constitutes an orgasm, there is also controversy over the diagnosis of orgasmic dysfunction. The DSM-III category "Inhibited Female Orgasm" is vague and broad. It covers those instances in which some difficulty is experienced in achieving an orgasm that cannot be accounted for by physical factors. Unfortunately, it does not clearly specify under what circumstances such a diagnosis is warranted. Instead, it is left up to the judgment of the clinician whether the difficulty in achieving orgasm is due to psychological inhibition. Masters and Johnson (1970) distinguished between primary, situational, and random orgasmic inadequacy. Kaplan (1974) discriminated between women who have never experienced an orgasm (primary dysfunction) and those who have at some point in their lives (secondary dysfunction), but she further distinguished between absolute and situational orgasmic dysfunction. If it is absolute, the woman is unable to achieve an orgasm in any situation, either by coital or clitoral stimulation, whereas if the dysfunction is situational, the woman can achieve an orgasm only under specific circumstances (for example, during masturbation, but not with a partner). It is important to note that the woman who has orgasmic dysfunction may still have a high desire for sexual activity and may experience high levels of arousal.

Derogatis, Fagan, Schmidt, Wise, and Gilden (1986) identified two psychological subtypes of anorgasmia that they labeled Type A and Type B. Type A anorgasmics appear to be more psychologically "healthy," are better informed about sex, possess sexually liberal attitudes, and have a high sex drive. Derogatis *et al*, postulated that these women have a higher prevalence of constitutional or interpersonal etiologies underlying their anorgasmia. On the other hand, Type B anorgasmic women display higher levels of psychological distress, lower levels of investment in sexuality, and poor body images and self-concepts. The etiology of anorgasmia in this group was labeled by these authors as "psychogenic." We would propose at least one additional subtype based on the women we have seen in our clinic. These women are generally young, single, well-educated, and sexually experienced. They have accurate information about their genital anatomy; have engaged in masturbation, perhaps even with vibrators; and may or may not have caring and attentive partners. For these women, sex triggers thoughts and feelings of shame (Lewis, 1986) or raises conflicts about intimacy and control that may be related to childhood issues. These women express present feelings of shame and distress concerning their present sexual "inadequacy."

There is some controversy about whether the inability to achieve orgasm during coitus should be considered a dysfunction, especially given the results of the Hite report (1976), which found that only 30% of the women surveyed regularly achieved orgasm from intercourse alone. Nevertheless, it is not an uncommon complaint of women, or their partners, that they are not having orgasms "the right way," by which they mean during coitus.

The issue of the "vaginal orgasm" was once again raised in the popular press with the publication of the book *The G Spot* (Ladas, Whipple, & Perry, 1982). The "G" spot, or Grafenberg spot, is purported to be an erogenous zone on the anterior wall of the vagina, which swells with stimulation. This stimulation may result in the expulsion of a fluid through the urethra, a so-called female ejaculate, a "partial, infertile homologue of male ejaculation" (Addiego, Belzer, Comolli, Moger, Perry, & Whipple, 1981, p. 17). Alzate and Hoch (1986) reviewed the research literature on the G spot. They claimed that evidence in support of a discrete anatomical structure is inconclusive, although women probably do possess a zone of tactile erotic sensitivity on the anterior vaginal wall, which in many women may extend to the entire anterior wall, and for some to the posterior wall as well. Summarizing these findings, these authors concluded "that some women emit a fluid through the urethra at orgasm, yet the fluid's true nature and anatomical origin are still unclear. . . . no advantage is obtained by calling the urethral emission a 'female ejaculation' " (p. 218).

The DSM-III and the DSM-III-R state that, in most cases, the inability to have coital orgasms should be considered a normal variation of the female sexual response, except in those instances in which the clinician judges there to be significant psychological inhibition.

Etiological Considerations and Theoretical Formulations. There is general consensus that the causes of orgasmic dysfunction are primarily psychological. Beyond this agreement, however, one will find any number of factors listed as potential causes. These may be as simple as lack of adequate stimulation to unconscious conflicts regarding sexuality. Essentially, contributing factors may be categorized into three areas: educational, interpersonal, and intrapersonal psychological determinants.

EDUCATIONAL FACTORS: The difficulty or inability to achieve orgasm may stem from a lack of information or, indeed, from misinformation. For many women, the presence of the clitoris as part of their genital anatomy has been one of the best kept secrets of all time. When they become aware of the clitoris and its potential for transmitting sexually pleasurable sensations, many women still believe that to be "normal" they should have orgasms solely from coital stimulation. As a result of prohibitions against female masturbation, as well as the fact that women often do not discuss their sexuality with other women, many women do not know what will please them sexually. In these cases, guided masturbation training and groups are the treatment of choice (see, for example, Barbach, 1975).

INTERPERSONAL FACTORS: Ambivalence about commitment to a relationship may inhibit a woman's sexual feelings in general or her orgasmic ability in particular. Indeed, one way a woman may express anger or dissatisfaction to her partner is by "denying" him her orgasm, especially if the couple perceive the man to be the one who "gives" his partner an orgasm. Often, however, a woman is committed to a relationship, but she and her partner are caught in sex roles that are so clearly and rigidly defined as to be dysfunctional. In these cases, men are assumed to be the experts on sex. As Lonnie Barbach (1980) pointed out:

> With no instruction, each man is somehow expected to understand each woman's unique sexuality. This, of course, is presumed to occur without any input from the woman herself, who, if she is decent and respectable, is expected to be innocent and have no sexual knowledge. The man cannot ask her for information, since he is supposed to know, and not knowing would make him appear less than masculine. The woman, on the other hand, cannot tell him, because she is not supposed to know or fears that if she directed him in any way she might hurt his ego. (p. 110)

It is evident from Barbach's analysis that both men and women are hurt by this rigid role-scripting.

Communication failures are often responsible for a woman's inability to achieve orgasm with her partner. Even when she does not feel constrained by her feminine role, and when she has a partner who is receptive to instruction on how to please her, a woman—and indeed the couple—may not have the language or the skills necessary to discuss a topic that is filled with such potential for hurt, embarrassment, or intimidation.

Where relationship factors appear to be the cause of the orgasmic dysfunction, the treatment of choice is conjoint therapy that focuses on sex roles, scripting, or relationship conflicts. In these cases, the woman, if she masturbates, should be able to achieve orgasm on her own.

INTRAPERSONAL PSYCHOLOGICAL FACTORS: Although the status of a woman's mental health does not appear to be related to her ability to have an orgasm (Fisher, 1973), many psychoanalysts continue to believe that deep-seated psychological problems are at the root of orgasmic dysfunction. Notions such as "penis envy" and the Electra complex have generally been dismissed as valid explanations of a woman's orgasmic difficulty. It does appear, however, that fear is one of the leading causes of orgasmic dysfunction, especially the fear of loss of control.

Kaplan (1974) asserted that, in preorgasmic women, the fear of losing control over their feelings or behavior is very prevalent and that the concomitant defense mechanisms of "holding back" and overcontrol are probably crucial to the pathogenesis of orgasmic dysfunction. Barbach (1980) similarly argued the importance of the fear of loss of control in preorgasmic women. She contended that many women are "trained" as young girls to be passive and to relinquish control over their lives to others. The resulting sense of insufficient control then leads to problems such as lack of ego differentiation and an inability to express feelings, as well as orgasmic difficulties. With no initial sense of control, relinquishing conscious control in experiencing an orgasm can be extremely anxiety-provoking for women. These fears may be consciously expressed as embarrassment and fear of appearing unattractive, of losing consciousness, or even of "dissolving" away completely. Most often, however, these women cannot verbalize their fears; instead, they recognize mounting anxiety with increasing sexual excitement or report that, with high levels of arousal, they "shut themselves off."

Issues in Evaluation. Several issues are important in the evaluation of orgasmic dysfunction. First, the clinician must determine whether the woman is experiencing any arousal or whether the problem is better conceptualized as lack of arousal. If a woman does not experience arousal, does not lubricate, or reports pain or discomfort during sex, these issues need to be addressed. If the orgasmic dysfunction still persists, it can then be treated. However, a secondary loss of desire or diminished sexual arousal can result from a chronic inability to experience an orgasm.

The clinician must also determine whether the inability to experience an orgasm is absolute or situational, as this determination has important treatment implications. In those cases where a woman has never experienced an orgasm, it is probably most efficacious to teach her to achieve orgasm on her own, and then to help her generalize this experience to a partner. On the other hand, when a woman can achieve orgasm in certain situations and not in others, it is necessary to assess what is unique about those situations that facilitate orgasm, and why the orgasm is otherwise inhibited.

The evaluation should focus on the knowledge, perceptions, and beliefs a woman holds about herself and her body. It is often the case that she lacks knowledge or, more seriously, that she has negative ideas about her body, that her genitals are "dirty" or "smelly" or that somehow it is not nice to touch them. In such cases, it is hard for a woman to receive pleasure from genital stimulation or even to permit the extended stimulation it may take to achieve orgasm.

Treatment. The most widely used and effective treatment for primary orgasmic dysfunction is a program of guided masturbation. This treatment approach assumes that what women need to become orgasmic is education, an awareness and acceptance of their body, and directed masturbation. Kaplan (1974) stated that, unlike other dysfunctions, the orgasmic dysfunction is inversely related, in its severity to the outcome of treatment. It is her experience, and one that we share, that primary, absolute orgasmic dysfunction is most amenable to treatment, whereas treatment gains for women with secondary or situational orgasmic dysfunction are less spectacular, although there is usually some improvement. What we may have is an excellent example of the law of diminishing returns. Lonnie Barbach (1980) is a proponent of group treatment for preorgasmic women and has reported high success rates. Unlike others, we do not limit inclusion in our groups to preorgasmic women; we extend involvement to any sexually inhibited or dissatisfied women. The women we are currently seeing seem to suffer less from misinformation; rather they display internal psychological conflicts related to their orgasmic inability. This group of women is more often resistant to treatment, but we, like Barbach (1980), have had good outcomes with both group and individual treatment. The following case description demonstrates the complexity that the treatment of anorgasmia often entails:

Nicole is a 27-year-old graduate student who presented with primary orgasmic dysfunction. She had a history of sexual abuse. At the age of 16, she had begun a 5-year relationship with a 20-year-old man. She reported being very aroused by sexual activity with him but felt he regarded her arousal as "inappropriate." Nicole's boyfriend was chronically unfaithful to her, and after repeated disappointments, she recalled that she "shut off" sexually. At college, Nicole dated but was not orgasmic and experienced only transitory sexual arousal. When she presented for treatment, Nicole was living with a 27-year-old man with whom she was very much in love. However, she was pessimistic about her ability to become sexually aroused and to experience orgasm. She did not feel that she was "sexually healthy" and felt irreparably scarred by her early experiences. The only time Nicole reported feeling sexual arousal was during sexually explicit dreams.

Treatment

Nicole entered one of our eight-session therapy groups. Although she faithfully carried out the homework assignments, even to the extreme of masturbating for 2½ hours on two occasions, Nicole did not reveal or share her past experiences with the group. Neither did she experience any change in her sexuality.

Individual therapy with Nicole initially focused on the issue of intimacy. Nicole revealed that she had not told her boyfriend about her anorgasmia, nor of her involvement in therapy. Her subsequent decision to inform him was the first sign that she was dealing with this issue. Nevertheless, Nicole continued to have difficulty discussing her past with her therapist. She felt ashamed and guilty about the sexual abuse, and any discussion of it overwhelmed her. Nicole was therefore instructed to write on separate index cards those incidents that had caused her shame, or that she felt had "scarred" her. In subsequent sessions, Nicole and her therapist dealt with each card or incident separately. Nicole soon began to feel that she had a right to be sad about her past, which she then described as a "holocaust of abuse." Yet, she still had to explore and deal with her feelings of guilt and her anger at her parents for not "taking care of me." During this time, Nicole began enjoying sexual activity with her boyfriend, was aware of sexual attraction to other men, and began experiencing more intense sexual dreams.

At the 20th session, the therapist brought up the issue of trying to masturbate again. Although Nicole said she had been toying with the idea of buying a vibrator, she expressed a fear that, if she tried and did not succeed, the therapist would realize that she was indeed a "hopeless case" and that therapy would end. The therapist reassured her that, regardless of whether she experienced an orgasm or not, termination of therapy would be by mutual discussion at some later date. Nicole did buy a vibrator and, to her surprise, experienced very high levels of arousal when she used it.

At the 25th session, Nicole announced that she "may have had an orgasm." In subsequent sessions, Nicole was more sure that what she was experiencing was an orgasm. At the 27th session, Nicole and her therapist went outside and burned the index cards, signalling that the incidents on them were in the past and no longer a present source of shame. Nicole reported feeling elated after the ceremony. At the time of this writing, Nicole is continuing to experience orgasms on her own, and therapy is continuing to focus on helping her to experience orgasms with a partner.

Retarded Ejaculation

Retarded ejaculation refers to a man's inability to ejaculate or having difficulty doing so, even though he has an erection, wishes to ejaculate, and is receiving sufficient stimulation to trigger his orgastic reflex. The severity of this disorder varies considerably, from cases in which only those conditions that evoke anxiety or guilt result in retarded ejaculation to cases in which a man has never experienced ejaculation in his life. In its mildest form, retarded ejaculation may be quite common; its severest manifestation is reportedly rare. The more common clinical situation is that in which the man cannot reach orgasm during coitus but can upon masturbation, or via oral or manual stimulation by his partner. Some men, however, cannot ejaculate in the presence of another and must leave the room to masturbate to orgasm.

Kaplan (1974) described a variant of retarded ejaculation, which she labeled "partial ejaculatory incompetence." A man suffering from this disorder experiences only the seepage of semen and does not experience the ejaculatory contractions of the penile urethra and perineal muscles. He may complain that his orgasm is not as intense or is only a partial climax. According to Kaplan, in this condition, the emission and ejaculatory phases of orgasm are separated. Unfortunately, the absent ejaculatory phase is what is experienced as pleasurable. The underlying causes and treatment are similar to those in retarded ejaculation, and so they will be dealt with together for the remainder of this section.

Etiological Considerations and Theoretical Formulations. Retarded ejaculation may have an organic basis. Any condition or drug that depresses androgen levels may have this result, although more often, erectile dysfunction occurs. Prostate and bladder surgery may result in retrograde ejaculation (ejaculation into the bladder), which is often confused with retarded ejaculation.

According to a psychoanalytic formulation, retarded ejaculation is the result of a reactivation of castration anxiety: the male fears that if he ejaculates in the vagina, he will be punished or castrated. This formulation, however, does not adequately address those cases in which there is a difficulty ejaculating extravaginally as well. According to Kaplan (1974), retarded ejaculation is a reactivation of the fear of losing the primary love object, now the wife or sexual partner instead of the mother. The man fears, unconsciously, that his partner will leave him should he "let go" or ejaculate. In support of her argument, Kaplan claimed that these men often have conflicts about expressing anger and use the defense of "holding back."

Systems theory stresses the importance of the couple interaction in the genesis and maintenance of retarded ejaculation. Retarded ejaculation may result from ambivalence about the relationship, power struggles, a fear of impregnation, or either partner's reaction to semen as "dirty" or "messy."

Learning theory states that the ejaculatory reflex becomes inhibited through its association with a traumatic event. An actual trauma, or painful event, may occur at the point of ejaculation, or ejaculation may be associated with guilt-laden fantasies. Sometimes, retarded ejaculation results from a history of trying to prolong intercourse by using methods that detract from or diminish the arousal normally experienced during intercourse. Dow (1981) offered a different learning-theory model. According to his model, retarded ejaculation occurs because orgasm is associated almost exclusively with masturbation, so that the contrasting conditions of sexual intercourse are less likely to produce orgasm. Shull and Sprenkle (1980) proposed simply that some men have a high ejaculatory threshold, so that intercourse and genital thrusting are not sufficient to trigger the orgasm.

Finally, Apfelbaum (1980) proposed an innovative view of the etiology of retarded ejaculation, suggesting that men who suffer from retarded ejaculation may be genitally reactive. In other words, these men are automatic responders: they develop erections even when sexual arousal is minimal or absent, if the situation appears to demand it. Indeed, these men appear to have a compulsion to satisfy their partners. They themselves do not experience an increase in sexual arousal, even though they are being stimulated. These men are inhibited by the touch or presence of their sexual partner, and were it not for their genital reactivity and their compulsion to satisfy their partner, they would suffer instead from erectile dysfunction. Apfelbaum noted that this situation is ripe with the potential for the male partner to feel used, and this may account for the fact that men with retarded ejaculation are so often described as having hostility or harboring resentment toward their partner, or toward women in general.

Issues in Evaluation. As with the other dysfunctions, medical screening is important as well as a sexual history that identifies those situations in which retarded ejaculation occurs. Not unlike premature ejaculation, no specific time period defines retarded ejaculation. Rather, the inability to control ejaculation is the key. The difference, of course, is that, for men with retarded ejaculation, the conscious desire to ejaculate precedes the ejaculation, if indeed it does occur at all. It is important to determine if the male is receiving adequate stimulation for orgasm to occur. This is difficult to determine as there are no established criteria, but usually, the stimulation is what would be considered by most to be sufficient. What is often neglected is an evaluation of the degree of *subjective* arousal that is experienced during sexual activity. Often, this is quite low.

Treatment. The goal of treatment is to desensitize the male to ejaculation in those circumstances in which he has difficulty, typically intercourse. In learning-theory terms, treatment is aimed at extinguishing the learned inhibition of ejaculation. The process varies somewhat according to the severity of the symptom. In essence, treatment begins with having the male ejaculate in whatever circumstance he can, and then, his behavior is gradually shaped until he can experience coital orgasm. For example, if a man can ejaculate only by masturbating away from his partner, he is instructed to begin masturbating in closer proximity to her (the next room, the same room, beside her) and then to experience orgasm from sexual activity that gradually involves his partner, until finally, vaginal stimulation can trigger orgasm. The man may first learn to ejaculate when his partner masturbates him, then when she orally stimulates him, and finally, he learns to ejaculate in closer proximity to her vagina, until the last phase is coital orgasm. If he experiences difficulty at any stage, the man is encouraged to use fantasy to bring himself to orgasm, as it is necessary to experience orgasm without negative consequences in those previously inhibiting conditions. We also believe it is important to ensure a high degree of subjective arousal at each phase of treatment, or the outcome may be only what Kaplan (1974) described as partial ejaculatory incompetence.

The most difficult case is the one in which the man has never experienced ejaculation, except, perhaps, through nocturnal emission. In such cases, it is usual to have the male experience an orgasm initially on his own. Erection and sexual arousal thus become associated under low-demand, minimal-anxiety conditions. Sometimes, it is necessary to deal with unconscious conflicts or guilt before proceeding to the sexual tasks.

The following vignette outlines the treatment of a man with retarded ejaculation:

> Mr. J, a 26-year-old engineer, consulted us because of his inability to ejaculate intravaginally with his fiancée. He was perfectly capable of ejaculating during self-stimulation. However, both he and his partner were distressed over his inability to ejaculate inside her vagina, particularly as they recognized that the problem would need to be resolved by the time they wanted to start a family.
>
> When we spoke with Mr. J alone, it became apparent that his inability to ejaculate was initially a rather deliberate strategy, learned in order to delay his orgasm during his early sexual experiences with prostitutes. He wanted, he said, "to make them work for their money," and he used ejaculatory delay as a way of exercising control over them. However, over time, this pattern became more invariant, and he was unable to readily ejaculate voluntarily with his fiancée. The only stimulus that could induce orgasm was viewing explicit pornographic films during intercourse with her, a strategy his fiancée vehemently objected to!
>
> Treatment involved both cognitive and behavioral elements. Mr. J was helped to recognize the hostile and controlling aspects of his behavior, and how, through conditioning, he had overlearned a "bad" habit. He and his therapist discussed how to "break the habit" by gradual steps, involving masturbation to orgasm with his fiancée in close proximity and then having his fiancée manually stimulate him to orgasm. Mr. J was able to move rather smoothly throughout each of the graduated steps toward intravaginal ejaculation. Helpful to his progress was his fiancée's love, support, and enthusiastic participation in the treatment. Arousal was not a problem for either of them, and so the therapy progressed smoothly to a successful outcome.

Disorders Involving Pain with Sexual Activity

Vaginismus

Vaginismus is the involuntary, spasmodic contraction of the pubococygeus (PC) and related muscles controlling the vaginal opening, so that intercourse is either impossible or extremely painful. The woman who suffers from vaginismus is often able to enjoy sexual activity and may even be orgasmic. However, whenever penetration of the vaginal opening is attempted, or whenever the woman feels that it may be attempted, the musculature around the vagina tightens. For these women, gynecological pelvic examinations are either impossible or extremely difficult. Often, these women cannot tolerate even digital penetration, nor do they use tampons during menstruation. For most women with vaginismus, the first contact is with their gynecologist. However, many of them are only given the advice to "keep trying" or are encouraged to "relax" by taking a drink before intercourse. These interventions are not particularly helpful and suggest to the troubled woman that, as the origin is psychological, she should be able to overcome her difficulty through sheer willpower. In fact, repeated efforts to force penetration serve only to reinforce the notion that intercourse is painful and thus heighten the woman's fear of it. Although most often vaginismus is primary, it may develop after sexual trauma, dyspareunia, or gynecological surgery. A striking fact about vaginismus is the length of time that passes before the couple seeks treatment, and then often only when they want to have children.

Etiological Considerations and Theoretical Formulations. Vaginismus is now commonly conceptualized as a conditioned response. Kaplan (1974) stated that "any adverse stimulus which is associated with intercourse or vaginal entry may be responsible for the acquisition of this response, regardless of whether this contingency is real or fantasized, and regardless of whether it does or does not lie within the patient's conscious awareness" (p. 417). There are, therefore, a great number of etiologial factors associated with vaginismus, solely by virtue of the fact that they cause pain or fear to be linked to vaginal penetration. Often, the pain has a physical source, such as pelvic inflammatory disease or endometriosis. Once this is corrected, however, the vaginismus may still remain, as intercourse has become associated with pain. Other factors that have been identified are traumatic pelvic examinations, rape or other brutal sexual experiences such as incest, a fear of men, a homosexual orientation, hostility toward one's husband, a reaction to the husband's erectile dysfunction, or a fear of childbirth. In still other women, no specific cause can be identified. Masters and Johnson (1970) argued that ignorance and misinformation are often the source of vaginismus. They blamed a strict religious upbringing for invoking guilt about sex, which leads to a fear of intercourse. What is important to remember, however, is that many of these factors are present in the backgrounds of women who do enjoy a variety of sexual experiences, including intercourse.

Ellison (1972) highlighted the importance of the partner in maintaining a woman's vaginismic response to intercourse. He claimed that the partners are usually passive men and that, in general, both members of the couple shy away from the fundamental aggressiveness of the act of vaginal penetration. It is our clinical experience that the partners of women with vaginismus are often also sexually inexperienced, at least in the role of "aggressor." If they have had previous experience with intercourse, it often has been with a woman more sexually experienced than themselves. These men also claim that they were attracted to their partner because of her sexual innocence or "purity." A woman may find it hard to reconcile being sexually active with this image of herself and so remains a "virgin bride." That other sexual activity is often enjoyed may be a result of the notion that "real sex" equals intercourse.

Psychoanalytic formulations about vaginismus are not popular, perhaps because psychoanalysis is relatively ineffective compared to behavioral treatment approaches. Briefly, the theory is that vaginismus is a result of unresolved penis envy and is the woman's attempt to frustrate the male partner, or to "castrate" him in revenge for her own, earlier "castration."

Issues in Evaluation. The accurate evaluation and diagnosis of vaginismus is essential to a good therapeutic outcome. Essential to the evaluation process is a thorough examination by a gynecologist to confirm the diagnosis and to rule out a physical basis for the pain. If there is a physical cause, it must be treated first. However, the vaginismus will not always disappear as a result. It is also important to discover if ignorance and/or misinformation is contributing to the problem so that an educational component should be emphasized during treatment. Finally, it is often important to uncover and deal with previous sexual trauma before effective treatment can begin.

Treatment. The recommended treatment for vaginismus is a cognitive-behavioral approach. First, it is important that the couple be aware that vaginismus is an involuntary response. This awareness often relieves guilt and hostility that may have been building up in the relationship. Fordney (1978) stated that demonstration of the nonvolitional contractions is essential before treatment can begin. For a gynecologist, this may be feasible, but for a therapist, it is more reasonable to ask the couple to do this on their own. The next step is to teach the woman relaxation and control over the PC muscle. The woman is taught to identify this muscle by stopping the flow of her urine midstream when she is using the toilet. She is then told to mimic that movement and to observe, in a mirror, the contraction and relaxation of this muscle. When she feels she has control over the PC muscle and is able to relax, she is ready for the next phase of the treatment process. This phase involves the insertion of Hegar dilators in graduated sizes, while the woman is relaxed and is relaxing her PC muscle, until she is able to insert a dilator the size of a penis. We have modified this treatment approach slightly and encourage the woman to insert her fingers and then her partner's fingers, starting in both cases with one finger and working up to three. The dilators, fingers, or other objects should, of course, be clean and should also be lubricated to allow for easier insertion. We feel that fingers are preferable over dilators because they encourage the woman and her partner to touch the vagina and to get used to the feel of it. Digital penetration can help to uncover issues such as aversion to one's genitalia. Intercourse is banned during these phases of treatment, but the couple is encouraged to engage in other mutually pleasurable sexual activity.

When this stage of treatment has been successfully completed, the couple is ready to attempt intercourse. It is important in this phase, as it is in the others, that the woman feel that she has control over what is going on. Vaginismus can be conceptualized as an exaggerated response to the need for control. The male partner lubricates his erect penis, and then, the female partner guides it into her vagina with her hand. He leaves his penis in the vagina without thrusting and then withdraws. When the couple is comfortable with this stage, they move on to gentle thrusting and, finally, thrusting to male orgasm.

In cases where there is a strong phobic element, this may have to be dealt with first in imagination before it is attempted in actuality. The essential therapeutic element is the repeated exposure, in imagination and reality, to the feared situation, while keeping anxiety, and therefore pain, at a minimum (Leiblum, Pervin, & Campbell, 1980).

Dyspareunia

Quite simply, dyspareunia is pain from penile-vaginal intercourse. Although there are cases in which men experience pain, this section deals only with the pain experienced by women. Like the other dysfunctions, dyspareunia may be primary, secondary, global or situational. The location of the pain may also vary from deep pain, located at the cervix or lower abdominal area, to that localized near the introitus (Fordney, 1978). However, the pain is not due to an involuntary spasm of the muscles surrounding the vagina, as in vaginismus.

Etiological Considerations and Theoretical Formulations. Dyspareunia is presumed to have a high incidence of physical disease etiology. Subacute vaginitis is the most common physical cause of superficial pain (Fordney, 1978). The characteristic pattern is the report of a burning sensation that does not disappear after penetration has ceased, and that may be exacerbated by ejaculation. The burning sensation is usually reproduced in the gynecologist's office when the speculum or a finger is inserted and is also present on insertion of a tampon. Typically, these women have had incidents of vaginitis before but do not currently report any other acute symptoms.

The presence of small scars can also cause pain on intercourse. Usually, these scars are so small that they are overlooked in a routine gynecological examination. Scarring can be the result of childbirth, introital injury, episiotomy, or gynecological surgery. When scarring is the problem, the pain is more localized and can be reproduced by the gynecologist when pressure is applied to that area. The pain typically ceases when penetration does. Other factors include endometriosis, ovarian fixation, uterine descensus, and ligament tears.

Finally, dyspareunia is somewhat more prevalent in postmenopausal women than in other age categories, perhaps because of vaginal atrophy or reduced lubrication.

Psychological factors can also be responsible for dyspareunia. In these cases, the women are more likely to have a history of prior sexual dysfunction for either themselves or their partners and are less likely to have a history of gynecological disease. They typically cannot localize or specifically describe their pain. As with vaginismus, the specific etiological factors are varied. Dyspareunia may result when the woman is anxious and tense about intercourse, perhaps because of misinformation, ignorance, lack of interest, guilt, or relationship difficulties. Repeatedly unsatisfactory sexual interactions with one's partner may lead to painful intercourse. Sexual activity that is less than satisfactory may be due to a partner's naïveté or lack of interest or to a failure of the woman to adequately communicate her needs to her partner. If a woman fails to lubricate before intercourse, penetration is bound to be painful. Finally, intrapsychic factors due to unresolved sexual conflicts may also lead to the development of dyspareunia.

Issues in Evaluation. Lazarus (1980) outlined an evaluation procedure that covers seven parameters; behavior, affect, cognition, imagery, sensation, and interpersonal and medical factors. Under the behavioral category, the couple's sexual technique must be examined to determine if there is sufficient stimulation to produce arousal and vaginal lubrication in the woman, so that she feels ready and desires penetration. A negative attitude toward sex can be determined by examining affect, cognitions, and imagery (mental pictures). Evaluation of these three parameters may also provide important clues to the presence of intrapsychic conflict or conflict arising from negative sexual experiences. The couple's interaction can also contribute to dyspareunia if it is conflicted of if there is the absence of love, desire, or sexual attraction. A detailed description of the pain is also very important, as is a complete medical history to ascertain whether there is a physical or psychological basis for the pain. However, such a diagnosis should never be made in the absence of a complete gynecological examination.

Treatment. The treatment of dyspareunia depends on its etiology. Where there is a physical cause, this must be treated first, although behavioral intervention may subsequently be required. The exception to this rule is the case of scarring, which is not effectively treated medically, except for surgically repeated episiotomies, but which responds to behavioral treatment. In the case of postmenopausal women, hormone replacement therapy is usually the treatment of choice, with the possible addition of external lubrication (saliva or jellies) (Leiblum & Bachmann, 1987).

When there is a psychological etiology, the treatment of dyspareunia closely resembles that of vaginismus. In essence, it involves progressive desensitization to intercourse, sometimes in fantasy and almost always *in vivo,* by the use of graduated vaginal dilation. In the case of scarring, there is an emphasis on putting pressure on the area of the scar and, in essence, stretching and loosening the tissue surrounding it.

THE EFFECTIVENESS OF SEX THERAPY

After the publication of *Human Sexual Inadequacy* (Masters & Johnson, 1970), sex therapy was hailed as a fast and effective treatment for sexual dysfunction. Masters and Johnson reported that only 20% of their clients failed to improve after approximately 2 weeks of intensive sex therapy. Thus, many people, both professional and lay, have assumed a ''cure'' rate of 80%. However, the Masters and Johnson approach, which involves couples in 2–3 weeks of residential treatment with a mixed-sex cotherapy team, is impracticable for many clients and therapists. The approach has therefore been modified so that it is more accessible to the general public in terms of the expenditure of time and money. A single therapist and weekly sessions spaced over the course of months are now the standard manner in which sex therapy is practiced. It has been assumed that these modifications, as well as a less motivated clientele, are the reasons behind the continued failure to replicate the astonishingly high success rates inferred from the Masters and Johnson data. However, neither cotherapy teams nor massed treatment sessions have been found to be more effective in the treatment of sexual dysfunction than a single therapist and spaced sessions (Marks, 1981).

Zilbergeld and Evans (1980) took a second, critical look at the Masters and Johnson (1970) study and concluded that ''Masters and Johnson's research is so flawed by methodological errors and slipshod reporting that it fails to meet customary standards—and their own—for evaluation research. . . . Because of this, the effectiveness of sex therapy—widely assumed to be high since the advent of Masters and Johnson—is thrown into question'' (pp. 29–30). Although this conclusion may appear to be catastrophizing, it is true that the Masters and Johnson outcome statistics have not been replicated by other clinics and investigators. As Zilbergeld and Evans pointed out, ''If their study is not as sound as most people have thought, the empirical support for sex therapy's effectiveness is greatly diminished'' (p. 33).

Zilbergeld and Evans (1980) criticized Masters and Johnson (1970) for omitting details of their study regarding definition of the subject sample, duration of the therapy process, and criteria for success, failure, and relapse. Most significant, perhaps, are the problems they identified in Masters and Johnson's outcome criteria. In order to circumvent the biases inherent in measuring outcome, Masters and Johnson chose not to measure success at all, but to measure failure. However, there is nothing more inherently objective about determining failure than there is about deciding success. Furthermore, their definition of ''failure'' is vague. As most clinicians realize, there are some instances in which therapy is unquestionably successful or unsuccessful, by both the therapist's and the client's standards. Most outcomes, however, are more ambiguous and fall into neither category. Masters and Johnson did not specify whether ''nonfailure'' meant slight, moderate, or significant improvement or complete resolution of the sexual problem. Furthermore, they had no category for *deterioration,* those cases in which treatment actually appeared to cause the sexual problem, or the relationship, to worsen.

Kolodny (1981) responded to many of the criticisms posed by Zilbergeld and Evans (1980). He stated that the "nonfailure category" included only those cases that were "unequivocal successes in the reversal of sexual symptomatology" (p. 303); the "failure" group therefore included some cases that improved. Unfortunately, this explanation is not entirely helpful in clarifying what is meant by "failure" and "nonfailure." For example, it is not clear whether a preorgasmic woman is a "nonfailure" case if she experiences orgasm by self-stimulation but cannot with her partner, or if a man with erectile dysfunction who still experiences transitory erectile failure is a "success," or if a woman with vaginismus who can have intercourse but experiences no pleasure from it is "cured." Clearly, there is definite improvement in these cases, but the gains are not sufficient to allow one to say that the sexual problem has been completely and unequivocally resolved.

Kolodny (1981) defended the shortcomings of the Masters and Johnson (1970) study by stating that their primary concern was to present the concepts of their therapeutic approach and to summarize outcome instead of providing a "definitive statement, leaving no loose ends" (p. 314). Kolodny threw the responsibility for good outcome research back at sex therapists in general, and perhaps at Zilbergeld and Evans in particular, with the following statement: "Taking pot shots at one another cannot make up for a lack of research data, and research cannot be magically conjured up" (p. 314).

What is highlighted by this controversy is not that the Masters and Johnson study is woefully inadequate, but that the field of outcome research in general is fraught with difficulties. Outcome research in sex therapy shares these problems and has its own unique difficulties as well. It is true that there are usually specific behaviors that can be examined when investigating the outcome of sex therapy, such as frequency of penetration, frequency of orgasmic attainment, and duration of intercourse. However, most clinicians realize that focusing on these discrete behaviors does an injustice both to sex therapy and to the couple's or client's sexuality. Sexual satisfaction entails more than the number of orgasms or the duration of penetration, although these are important and relevant factors. As there is no universally agreed-upon definition of "sexual adjustment," client-reported satisfaction should be included in the assessment of treatment outcome. Finally, because sex therapy often involves couples, it is important to examine the impact of therapy on the relationship. It is not always the case that the relationship and the sexual difficulty improve or deteriorate together. Often, the relationship improves, but the sexual dysfunction persists. Alternatively, the sexual difficulty may improve, but the relationship, built around the problem, may deteriorate.

In evaluating the effectiveness of therapy at our own clinic, we have devised a dual-focus, multilevel classification of outcome (Rosen, Leiblum, & Hall, 1987). We assess the effects of therapy on both the sexual dysfunction and the relationship, and we do so along a continuum ranging from deterioration to complete resolution. These ratings are based on the therapist's assessment, which includes the therapist's judgment regarding the client's satisfaction with the outcome. We are aware of the biases inherent in relying exclusively on the treating therapist's assessments and the limitations involved in the exclusion of the client's report and/or the judgments of impartial examiners. Nevertheless, our 5-year study of over 500 clients represents one of the more ambitious attempts to examine the outcome of sex therapy in an outpatient setting.

Despite the problems inherent in outcome research, some general conclusions can be reached regarding the efficacy of sex therapy for specific sexual dysfunctions. In general, vaginismus and PE have the best prognosis for success, have less risk for prolonged relapse, and entail the fewest number of therapy hours for successful treatment (Kilmann, Boland, Norton, Davidson, & Caid, 1986). It is no coincidence that these dysfunctions have a clear psychogenic etiology and that specific behavioral techniques are used in their treatment. Reported success rates for PE are often as high as 96%–100% (Kilmann & Auerbach, 1979; Kolodny, 1981), although rates as ''low'' as 64% and 62% have also been reported (Hawton & Catalan, 1986; Kilmann *et al.*, 1986). Success rates for vaginismus, treated with dilation, are also very good and tend to fall in the range of 70%–80% (Pasmore, 1967; Walker, 1977). Although success is not contingent on the involvement of the male partner in treatment sessions (Bramley, Brown, Draper, & Kilvington, 1981; Cooper, 1969), success rates for treatment directly involving both members of the couple are generally higher and have been reported to be as high as 98% (Kolodny, 1981).

Reported success rates for orgasmic dysfunction fall in the range of 65%–100% for primary manifestations and 50%–87% for secondary or situational symptomatology (Anderson, 1983). However, the tendency for treatment successes for primary orgasmic dysfunction to exceed those for secondary orgasmic dysfunction appears to be changing (Kilmann, Mills, Caid, Davidson, Bella, Milan, Drose, & Boland, Follingstad, Montgomery, Wanlasa, 1986; Spence, 1985). It may be that, because women & now have greater access to excellent self-help guides, many are achieving their first orgasm on their own. Indeed, primary orgasmic dysfunction is often amenable to self-help treatments (Morokoff & LoPiccolo, 1986). The women who do not respond to self-help programs may be the ones presenting for treatment and possibly represent a greater challenge to sex therapists. However, this possibility must remain conjecture, as there are few data regarding changing client characteristics over time.

Secondary erectile dysfunction has also been found to have good results with sex therapy. Rosen (1983) suggested that 50%–75% of men can be seen as showing some improvement in erectile functioning with behavioral sex therapy. Kilmann and Auerbach (1979) reviewed the outcome studies and concluded that 60%–90% of men show improvement posttreatment. However, a treatment study by Levine and Agle (1978) highlights the fact that treatment gains for secondary ED are often relatively unstable over time. Only 1 man out of 16 maintained treatment gains at 12-month follow-up, although 70% could still be considered ''improved.''

The dysfunctions that are the most resistent to change are retarded ejaculation, primary erectile dysfunction, and inhibited sexual desire. Success with retarded ejaculation is inversely related to the severity of the disorder. Treatment is very successful in mild cases (Dow, 1981; Shull & Sprenkle, 1980), whereas success rates fall to about 20% for the more severe manifestations (Hawton & Catalan, 1986). There are relatively few studies examining the efficacy of sex therapy for primary erectile dysfunction, perhaps because it is less common than secondary erectile dysfunction or is more often perceived to be of organic etiology and is therefore regarded as requiring medical intervention. The providers of sex therapy in the Kilmann *et al.* (1986a) study reported primary erectile dysfunction to be the most difficult sexual problem to treat. Men with primary erectile failure often display considerable psychological conflict and interpersonal problems that require attention in addition to the erectile failure. Improvement in erectile functioning has been reported for diabetic men with secondary erectile dysfunction in which there are both organic and psychogenic factors present (Jensen, 1986). At the Masters and Johnson Institute, where extensive screening for medical complications is purported to take place, success with primary ED is estimated at 67%. Finally, ISD is often considered the bane of sex therapists, being one of the most prevalent of presenting complaints and the one that requires the most therapy hours to treat (Kilmann *et al.*, 1986a). Despite the pessimistic reports of many clinicians that ISD is often not amenable to sex therapy (Kaplan, 1979), the reported rates of improvement are in the range of 49%–56% (Hawton & Catalan, 1986; Kilmann *et al.*, 1986a; Schover & LoPiccolo, 1982).

An examination of the characteristics of treatment "failures" and "successes" can lead to some interesting speculation about those cases in which sex therapy is most helpful. Reynolds (1977) concluded that a history of adequate sexual functioning, an acute versus an insidious onset of the problem, and a short duration of sexual impairment were predictive of greater success of men in sex therapy. Kaplan, Fyer, and Novick (1982) also highlighted client characteristics that may limit the effectiveness of sex therapy. They concluded that when sexual problems are the product of "complex and tenacious neurotic and characterological problems," or when the sexual difficulty exists in a relationship that is characterized by profound hostility and ambivalence, there is a poor prognosis with brief sex therapy. Finally, Kaplan *et al.* stated that treatment failures may be due to the presence of undetected medical problems.

Hawton and Catalan (1986) conducted a prospective investigation of sex therapy with 154 couples who presented with a diversity of sexual dysfunctions. Of the factors identified at the start of treatment, three emerged as powerful predictors of success: the quality of the couple's general and sexual relationship, as assessed by the therapist, and the couple's motivation as assessed by the therapist, and as rated by the husband. However, the most powerful prognostic factor was the extent to which a couple had become engaged in the therapy, in terms of carrying out the homework assignments by the third session. The outcome of therapy was not related to the presence of psychiatric symptoms, age, the duration of the problem, or the extent of religious beliefs. In general, it appears that therapist ratings of the couple's relationship and motivation are predictive of treatment success. It may be that the therapist's judgment regarding the couple functions as a self-fulfilling prophecy, in that the more hopeful a therapist is about outcome, the more hopeful the couple may be, and the more engaged both the therapist and the couple will be in treatment.

In summary, as with outcome studies, more investigations are needed into the identification of prognostic factors. Knowledge of prognostic factors would allow clinicians to be aware of who is most likely to benefit from sex therapy and who may require other forms of intervention. Such knowledge may also explain why there is often such a wide range in the reported treatment effects of sex therapy for many dysfunctions.

SUMMARY

It is less than two decades since sex therapy first appeared as a distinct clinical entity, and yet, it has made remarkable advances in that short time. Sex therapy has become increasingly sophisticated in its recognition of the complexity of sexual dysfunction and, indeed, of people in general. We no longer take a "cook book" approach to treatment, and sex therapy is far from being a "bag of tricks." As the case examples highlight, it requires good diagnostic and therapeutic skill, as well as sensitivity and versatility on the part of the clinician, to treat people with sexual dysfunction. Indeed, a review of 289 providers of sex therapy reveals that the therapeutic process involves a considerable focus on nonsexual individual and relationship issues (Kilmann *et al.*, 1986a). Sex therapy has borrowed principles and techniques from behavior therapy, psychodynamic psychotherapy, and, most recently, from family therapy (Hof & Berman, 1986). However, the inclusion of behavioral strategies and a focus on the sexual relationship are what distinguishes sex therapy from other therapeutic modalities, in which sexual dysfunction is dismissed as being symptomatic of underlying conflict. Sex therapy may best be conceptualized as a specialized form of psychotherapy for clients with sexual problems.

The treatment of sexual dysfunction is proceeding in two separate directions. On the one hand, as discussed above, sex therapy is becoming less behavioral and is incorporating psychodynamic and systems formulations and therapeutic "technique." On the other hand, there is an increased focus on technological solutions such as penile prostheses and drugs to enhance desire and/or erectile ability. Although we applaud these innovations, we believe that this technology should be reserved for cases of organic dysfunction, and we are concerned about the potential for misuse in cases of psychogenic sexual dysfunction. This potential appears to be high, given the desire, of men in particular, for quick and easy solutions to what we regard as complex problems. Medical interventions alone are often less effective, or altogether ineffective, in treating cases where there are psychogenic components in the sexual dysfunction, and these include almost all cases.

The tremendous optimism accompanying the publication of Masters and Johnson's *Human Sexual Inadequacy* (1970) is more muted today, but not gone. The sexual problems we are currently treating are becoming more complex as individuals seek to deal with their sexuality in an increasingly complicated world. The epidemic rise in sexually transmitted diseases, teenage pregnancies, infertility, and other consequences of sexual activity have all contributed to making people more cautious about how they express their sexuality. The liberalism of the 1970s has been replaced by the conservatism of the 1980s. Nevertheless, the demand for sexual therapy is increasing as the population ages and as couples seek to improve existing sexual relationships rather than trade partners when sexual satisfaction wanes. The challenge facing sex therapist is great as we attempt to modify our approaches and treatment to the ever-changing issues and problems of the coming decades.

REFERENCES

Addiego, F., Belzer, E. G., Jr., Comolli, J., Moger, W., Perry, J. D., & Whipple, B. (1981). Female ejaculation: A case study. *Journal of Sex Research, 17,* 13–21.

Althof, S. E., Turner, L. A., Levine, S. B., Risen, C. B., Kursh, E. D., Resnick, M. I., & Bodner, D. (1986). *Preliminary results of the treatment of impotence by intracavernosal injection of papavarine and phentolamine: Impact upon sexual, psychological and marital functioning.* Paper presented at the Annual Meeting of the Society for Sex Therapy and Research, Philadelphia.

Alzate, H., & Hoch, Z. (1986). The "G spot" and "female ejaculation": A current appraisal. *Journal of Sex and Marital Therapy, 12,* 211–220.

American Psychiatric Association. (1980). *Diagnostic and statistical manual of mental disorders* (3rd ed.; DSM-III). Washington, DC: Author.

American Psychiatric Association. (1986). *DSM-III-R in development* (2nd draft). Washington, DC: Author.

Anderson, B. L. (1983). Primary orgasmic dysfunction: Diagnostic considerations and review of treatment. *Psychological Bulletin, 93,* 105–136.

Apfelbaum, B. (1980). The diagnosis and treatment of retarded ejaculation. In S. R. Leiblum & L. A. Pervin (Eds.), *Principles and practices of sex therapy.* New York: Guilford Press.

Apfelbaum, B., & Apfelbaum, C. (1985). The ego-analytic approach to sexual apathy. In D. C. Goldberg (Ed.), *Contemporary marriage: Special issues in couples therapy.* Homewood, IL: Dorsey Press.

Bachmann, G., & Leiblum, S. R. (1987). *Sexual inquiry in gynecological practice: Rationale and results.* Unpublished manuscript.

Bancroft, J. (1983). *Human sexuality and its problems.* London: Churchill, Livingstone.

Barbach, L. G. (1975). *For yourself: The fulfillment of female sexuality.* New York: Doubleday.

Barbach, L. (1980). Group treatment of anorgasmic women. In S. R. Leiblum & L. A. Pervin (Eds.), *Principles and practices of sex therapy.* New York: Guilford Press.

Bramley, H. M., Brown, J., Draper, K. C., & Kilvington, J. Y. (1981). Brief psychosomatic therapy for consummation of marriage. *British Journal of Obstetrics and Gynecology, 88,* 819–824.

Brecher, E. M. (1969). *The sex researchers.* Boston: Little, Brown.

Brooks, M. B. (1981). *Lifelong sexual vigor: How to avoid and overcome impotence.* New York: Doubleday.

Bullard, D. G., Mann, J., Caplan, H., & Stoklosa, J. M. (1978). Sex counseling and the penile prosthesis. *Sexuality and Disability, 1,* 184–189.

Cohen, H. D., Rosen, R. C., & Goldstein, L. (1976). Electroencephalographic laterality changes during human sexual orgasm. *Archives of Sexual Behavior, 5,* 189–199.

Cooper, A. J. (1969). An innovation in the ''behavioral'' treatment of a case of non-consummation due to vaginismus. *British Journal of Psychiatry, 115,* 721–722.

Derogatis, L. R., Fagan, P. J., Schmidt, C. W., Wise, T. N., & Gilden, K. (1986). Psychological subtypes of anorgasmia: A marker variable approach. *Journal of Sex and Marital Therapy, 12,* 197–210.

Dow, M. G. T. (1981). Retarded ejaculation as a function of non-aversive conditioning and discrimination: A hypothesis. *Journal of Sex and Marital Therapy, 7,* 49–53.

Ellis, A. (1980). Treatment of erectile dysfunction. In S. R. Leiblum & L. A. Pervin (Eds.), *Principles and practices of sex therapy.* New York: Guilford Press.

Ellis, H. H. (1899–1928). *Studies in the psychology of sex* (Vols. 1–7). Philadelphia: Davis.

Ellison, C. (1972). Vaginismus. *Medical Aspects of Human Sexuality, 8,* 34–54.

Fish, L. S., Fish, R. C., & Sprenkle, D. H. (1984). Treating inhibited sexual desire: A marital therapy approach. *The American Journal of Family Therapy, 12,* 3–12.

Fisher, S. (1973). *The female orgasm.* New York: Basic Books.

Fordney, D. S. (1978). Dyspareunia and vaginismus. *Clinical Obstetrics and Gynecology, 21,* 205–220.

Frank, E., Anderson, C., & Rubinstein, D. (1978). Frequency of sexual dysfunction in ''normal'' couples. *New England Journal of Medicine, 299,* 111–115.

Freud, S. (1920). *Three essays on the theory of sexuality* (J. Strachey, Ed.). New York: Avon Books. (Originally published 1905).

Gagnon, J. H., Rosen, R. C., & Leiblum, S. R. (1982). Cognitive and social aspects of sexual dysfunction: Sexual scripts in sex therapy. *Journal of Sex and Marital Therapy, 8,* 44–56.

Goldstein, I. (1986). *The use of intracavernosal pharmacological agents.* Paper presented at the annual meeting of the Society for Sex Therapy and Research, Philadelphia.

Hawton, K., & Catalan, J. (1986). Prognostic factors in sex therapy. *Behaviour, Research and Therapy, 24,* 377–385.

Hite, S. (1976). *The Hite report: A nationwide study of female sexuality.* New York: Dell.

Hof, L., & Berman, E. (1986). The sexual genogram. *Journal of Marital and Family Therapy, 12,* 39–47.

Jensen, S. B. (1986). Sexual dysfunction in insulin-treated diabetics: A six year follow-up study of 101 patients. *Archives of Sexual Behavior, 15,* 271–283.

Kaplan, H. S. (1974). *The new sex therapy.* New York: Brunner/Mazel.

Kaplan, H. S. (1977). Hypoactive sexual desire. *Journal of Sex and Marital Therapy, 3,* 3–9.

Kaplan, H. S. (1979). *Disorders of sexual desire.* New York: Brunner/Mazel.

Kaplan, H. S., Fyer, A. J., & Novick, A. (1982). The treatment of sexual phobias: The combined use of antipanic medication and sex therapy. *Journal of Sex and Marital Therapy, 8,* 3–28.

Kilmann, P. R., & Auerbach, R. (1979). Treatments of premature ejaculation and psychogenic impotence: A critical review of the literature. *Archives of Sexual Behavior, 8,* 81–100.

Kilmann, P. R., Boland, J. P., Norton, S. P., Davidson, E., & Caid, C. (1986a). Perspectives of sex therapy outcome: A survey of AASECT providers. *Journal of Sex and Marital Therapy, 12,* 116–138.

Kilmann, P. R., Mills, K. H., Caid, C., Davidson, E., Bella, B., Milan, R., Drose, G., Boland, J., Follingstad, D., Montgomery, B., & Wanlasa, R. (1986b). Treatment of secondary orgasmic dysfunction: An outcome study. *Archives of Sexual Behavior, 15,* 211–229.

Kinsey, A. C., Pomeroy, W. B., & Martin, C. E. (1948). *Sexual behavior in the human male.* Philadelphia and London: W. B. Saunders.

Kinsey, A. C., Pomeroy, W. B., Martin, C. E., & Gebhard, P. H. (1953). *Sexual behavior in the human female.* Philadelphia and London: W. B. Saunders.

Kolodny, R. C. (1981). Evaluating sex therapy: Process and outcome at the Masters and Johnson Institute. *Journal of Sex Research, 17,* 301–318.

Krafft-Ebing, R. von. (1902). *Psychopathia sexualis.* Brooklyn: Physicians and Surgeons Books. (Originally published 1886.)

Ladas, A. K., Whipple, B., & Perry, J. D. (1982). *The G spot.* New York: Holt, Rinehart & Winston.

Lazarus, A. A. (1980). Psychological treatment of dyspareunia. In S. R. Leiblum & L. A. Pervin (Eds.), *Principles and practices of sex therapy,* New York: Guilford Press.

Leiblum, S. R., & Bachmann, G. (1987). The sexuality of the climacteric woman. In B. Eskin (Ed.), *The menopause: Comprehensive management. Second edition.* New York: Yearbook Publications.

Leiblum, S. R. & Kopel, S. A. (1977). Screening and prognosis in sex therapy: To treat or not to treat. *Behavior Therapy, 8,* 480–486.

Leiblum, S. R., & Pervin, L. A. (1980). The development of sex therapy from a sociocultural perspective. In S. R. Leiblum & L. A. Pervin (Eds.), *Principles and practices of sex therapy.* New York: Guilford Press.

Leiblum, S. R., Pervin, L. A., & Campbell, E. H. (1980). The treatment of vaginismus: Success and failure. In S. R. Leiblum & L. A. Pervin (Eds.), *Principles and practices of sex therapy.* New York: Guilford Press.

Levine, S. (1984). An essay on the nature of sexual desire. *Journal of Sex and Marital Therapy, 10,* 83–96.

Levine, S. B., & Agle, D. (1978). The effectiveness of sex therapy for chronic secondary psychological impotence. *Journal of Sex and Marital Therapy, 4,* 235–258.

Lewis, A. C. (1986). *Shame and its sexual implications.* Paper presented at the annual meeting of the Society for Sex Therapy and Research, Philadelphia.

Leyson, J. (1986). *Comparative study of erectiogenic drugs in the management of impotence in spinal cord injured men.* Paper presented at the annual meeting of the Society for Sex Therapy and Research, Philadelphia.

LoPiccolo, J. (1985). Diagnosis and treatment of male sexual dysfunction. *Journal of Sex and Marital Therapy, 11,* 215–232.

Marks, I. M. (1981). Review of behavioral psychotherapy, II: Sexual disorders. *American Journal of Psychiatry, 138,* 750–756.

Masters, W. H., & Johnson, V. E. (1966). *Human sexual response.* Boston: Little, Brown.

Masters, W. H., & Johnson, V. E. (1970). *Human sexual inadequacy.* Boston: Little, Brown.

Mobarak, A., Tamerin, J. S., & Tamerin, N. G. (1986). Sex therapy: An adjunct in the treatment of marital discord. *Journal of Sex and Marital Therapy, 12,* 229–238.

Morokoff, P. J., & LoPiccolo, J. (1986). A comparative evaluation of minimal therapist contact and 15-session treatment for female orgasmic dysfunction. *Journal of Consulting and Clinical Psychology, 54,* 294–300.

Nolen, W. A. (1981). Impotence. *Esquire,* (Nov) 132–141.

Pasmore, J. (1967). The treatment of non-consummation in prevention of marriage problems. *Psychotherapy and Psychosomatics, 15,* 52.

Perelman, M. A. (1980). Treatment of premature ejaculation. In S. R Leiblum & L. A. Pervin (Eds.), *Principles and practices of sex therapy.* New York: Guilford Press.

Quadland, M. C. (1985). Compulsive sexual behavior: Definition of a problem and an approach to treatment. *Journal of Sex and Marital Therapy, 11,* 121–132.

Regas, S. J., & Sprenkle, D. H. (1984). Functional family therapy and the treatment of inhibited sexual desire. *Journal of Marital and Family Therapy, 10,* 63–72.

Reynolds, B. S. (1977). Psychological treatment models and outcome results for erectile dysfunction: A critical review. *Psychological Bulletin, 84,* 1218–1238.

Rosen, R. C. (1983). Clinical issues in the assessment and treatment of impotence: A new look at an old problem. *The Behavior Therapist, 6,* 81–85.

Rosen, R. C., & Kostis, J. B. (1985). Biobehavioral sequellae associated with adrenergic-inhibiting antihypertensive therapy: A critical review. *Health Psychology, 4,* 579–604.

Rosen, R. C., & Leiblum, S. R. (1976). Unequal sex drives: Helping couples match up. *Sexology, 42,* 11–16.

Rosen, R. C., & Leiblum, S. R. (1987a). Current approaches to the evaluation of sexual desire disorders. *Journal of Sex and Marital Therapy.*

Rosen, R. C., & Leiblum, S. R. (1987b). Current approaches to the evaluation of sexual desire disorders. *Journal of Sex Research, 23,* 141–162.

Rosen, R. C., Leiblum, S. R., & Hall, K. S. (1987). *Etiological and predictive factors in sex therapy: A review of 500 cases.* Paper presented at the annual meeting of the Society for Sex Therapy and Research, New Orleans.

Schein, M., Levine, S., Zyzanski, S., Medalie, J., Dickman, R., & Alemangno, S. (1986). *Frequency of sexual problems in a family medicine practice.* Paper presented at the annual meeting of the Society for Sex Therapy and Research, Philadelphia.

Schover, L., & LoPiccolo, J. (1982). Effectiveness of treatment for dysfunctions of sexual desire. *Journal of Sex and Marital Therapy, 8,* 179–197.

Schover, L. R., & von Eschenbach, A. C. (1985). Sex therapy and the penile prosthesis: A synthesis. *Journal of Sex and Marital Therapy, 11,* 57–66.

Semans, J. H. (1956). Premature ejaculation: A new approach. *Southern Medical Journal, 49,* 353–358.

Shull, G. R., & Sprenkle, D. H. (1980). Retarded ejaculation, reconceptualization and implications for treatment. *Journal of Sex and Marital Therapy, 6,* 234–246.

Simpson, W. S. (1985). Psychoanalysis and sex therapy: A case report. *Bulletin of the Menninger Clinic, 49,* 565–582.

Spark, R., White, R., & Connolly, P. (1980). Impotence is not always psychogenic: Newer insights into hypothalamic-pituitary-gonadal dysfunction. *Journal of the American Medical Association, 243,* 750–755.

Speiss, W. (1977). *The psycho-physiology of premature ejaculation: Some factors related to ejaculatory latency.* Unpublished doctoral dissertation, State University of New York at Stony Brook.

Spence, S. H. (1985). Group versus individual treatment of primary and secondary female orgasmic dysfunction. *Behaviour, Research and Therapy, 23,* 539–548.

Thase, M. E., Reynolds, C. F., Glanz, L. M., Jennings, J. R., Sewitch, D. E., Kupfer, D. J., & Frank, E. (1986). *Noctural penile tumescence in depressed men.* Paper presented at the annual meeting of the Society for Sex Therapy and Research, Philadelphia.

Verhulst, J., & Heiman, J. (1979). An interactional approach to sexual dysfunction. *The American Journal of Family Therapy, 7,* 19–36.

Walker, B. A. (1977). Unconsummated marriages: An innovative and successful therapeutic approach. *Family Therapy, 4,* 121–128.

Zilbergeld, B. (1975). Group treatment of sexual dysfunction in men without partners. *Journal of Sex and Marital Therapy, 1,* 204–214.

Zilbergeld, B. (1978). *Male sexuality.* New York: Bantam Books.

Zilbergeld, B., & Ellison, C. R. (1980). Desire discrepancies and arousal problems in sex therapy. In S. R. Leiblum & L. A. Pervin (Eds.), *Principles and practices of sex therapy.* New York: Guilford Press.

Zilbergeld, B., & Evans, M. (1980). The inadequacy of Masters and Johnson. *Psychology Today, 14,* 29–43.

12

Male Sex Offenders

GENE G. ABEL AND JOANNE-L. ROULEAU

INTRODUCTION

Individuals who commit deviant sex acts have always posed a difficult problem for society. In many respects, their crimes are felonious, antisocial acts and clearly fall within the purview of the criminal justice system. However, their compulsive, repetitive, driven behavior, which at times has no rational, logical reward, appears to fit the criteria of an emotional or psychiatric illness.

Treatment for sex offenders on an outpatient basis is likewise the subject of considerable and ongoing controversy. Individuals opposed to such programs assert that, regardless of the treatment modality, the risk of reoffense by nonincarcerated offenders poses a significant threat to society. These individuals are convinced that the best prevention of recidivism is incarceration and/or the removal of the offender from his or her social milieu. The proponents of outpatient treatment for sex offenders cite the lack of effective treatment programs within the prison setting, the continuing problem of prison overcrowding, and the high recidivism where a strict criminal-justice model is followed.

Numerous attempts have been made to carry out psychological treatment for sex offenders within certain penal institutions. These attempts have, for the most part, been unsuccessful because such institutions do not usually have appropriately trained individuals to provide the treatment. In addition, prisons lack the necessary equipment to provide adequate psychophysiological assessment. Prisons do not provide an appropriate environment in which to practice some of the necessary components of treatment. Finally, some forms of deviant sexual behavior frequently do not lead to incarceration (i.e., exhibitionism, voyeurism, incest, and transvestitism). Zussman and Moore (1984) reported that approximately 9 out of 10 sex offenders are not known or held within the criminal justice system.

GENE G. ABEL and JOANNE-L. ROULEAU • Behavioral Medicine Institute, Atlanta, Georgia 30327–4104; and Emory University School of Medicine, Atlanta, Georgia 30302.

An additional problem relates to the treatment process itself in the prison setting. Only 20% of incarcerated sex offenders volunteer for treatment, and those who do are motivated primarily by attempts to give a favorable impression to their parole board (Christie, Marshall, & Lanthier, 1977). Therefore, among incarcerated offenders, there is the problem of working with subjects who are resistant to treatment and who are likely to be noncompliant with the treatment components. Under these circumstances, treatment can be viewed as excessively coercive, thus possibly leading to ethical conflicts.

Another limitation of treatment in prison is the social milieu in which the treatment is conducted. Heterosocial skills training, the development of sexual arousal to adult females, and appropriate assertiveness training cannot be reinforced within the prison setting, which provides the offender with minimal opportunities to practice these skills. For example, teaching a hostile, inappropriately aggressive inmate more appropriate methods of social and sexual expression may be ineffective within the prison setting, where violent confrontations and overt anger help protect the offender against other inmates. Therefore, the net effects of these treatment components rapidly deteriorate because of the lack of reinforcement.

A further problem associated with treatment conducted within the prison relates to the therapeutic alliance between therapist and offender. Effective therapy requires the offender to be able to talk openly with the therapist about his deviant arousal, including the thoughts and behaviors that precede his commission of sex crimes (Short & Nye, 1957). Offenders often fear that the appearance of such information in their records will have a profound influence on any decisions regarding probation or release. Even though the valid reporting of the offender's deviant interests may be absolutely essential to effective treatment, incarceration may be prolonged if such information is made available to probation authorities. Therefore, what often results is an accelerating game of offenders attempting to suppress their true arousal pattern as the therapist attempts to expose it. The final result is destruction of the therapeutic relationship with offenders and a marked reduction in the effectiveness of the treatment.

Finally, sex-offender treatment programs within the prison would, in optimal circumstances, reach only 15% of sex offenders because, on the average, less than 15% of sexual offenses lead to incarceration. The majority of sex offenders are not within the prison system but are "on the street." If the increasing incidence of sex crimes is to be stopped, it is essential that affordable outpatient treatment for sexual deviation be provided.

DETERMINING SPECIFIC DIAGNOSIS

In order to provide efficient treatment for individuals with sexual deviations, specific areas of deviant interest must be determined. A number of steps may be taken to increase the validity of the offender's self-reports of deviant interests.

Confidentiality of Information

As most patients are aware of the illegality of deviant sexual behavior as well as of the consequences attendant on the disclosure of such acts, a clarification regarding the confidentiality of their histories must be provided before beginning assessment.

In earlier publications (Abel, Becker, Mittelman, Cunningham-Rathner, Rouleau, & Murphy, 1987; Abel & Rouleau, 1986), we have described the steps to be taken to preserve the confidentiality of information given by nonincarcerated sex offenders. Within the framework of a research study, it was possible to obtain a Certificate of Confidentiality from the Department of Health and Human Services of the federal government. This certificate ensures that no city, county, state, or federal agency may oblige an investigator to reveal the identity of subjects participating in a research project involving sensitive data pertaining to criminal activities such as drug abuse or deviant sexual behavior.

Although the Certificate of Confidentiality does not apply to information gained from offenders undergoing treatment outside a research project, several steps may be taken to maintain the confidentiality of patient records.

First, each patient should be assigned a confidential identification number, and all recorded information should be coded only by the ID number. The code matching the patient's name with his identification number can be held outside the treatment setting, preferably outside the country. Access to the patient's chart by persons not specifically involved in the treatment program is thus inhibited. Patients should be told to be careful with the release of their ID numbers, as access to their records is possible only if the patients voluntarily provide their ID numbers to others.

Second, patients should be aware that details that are irrelevant to treatment will not be recorded in their charts. For example, a patient will be requested to describe the age range and gender of victims and the frequency of various sex crimes. Extraneous (and possibly incriminating) information not germane to the planning of the treatment will not be recorded. In other words, patients should be aware that their charts contain only material pertinent to their treatment.

Third, in order to encourage more accurate self-reports and cooperation with the therapists, patients should be aware that the goal of interviews with the therapist is to arrive at effective ways of understanding their problem and to establish efficient treatment methods to help them gain control over their deviant behavior.

Finally, to reduce the patient's fear of reports being used against them by others, all reports should be provided only to the offenders. In this way, the offenders are in a position to consider the findings and recommendations of the therapist and to make their own decision regarding the dissemination of this information.

Structured Clinical Interview

At the beginning of the interview, assurances about the protection of the patient's self-reported information should be repeated. The function of the structured interview is to target specifically the type and number of various paraphilic acts, the age of onset of these interests, the type of sexual fantasies, and the number of victims. If patients are easily able to recall and describe the variety and complexity of their paraphilic interests, the structured clinical interview may last 1 hour. If subjects experience difficulty recalling their paraphilic acts or have been involved in numerous categories of paraphilic acts, the interview may require up to 5 hours.

Numerous problems can be anticipated during the clinical interview. First, it is sometimes difficult for patients to describe the frequency of their involvement with paraphilias that developed much earlier in their lives. To assist patients with the chronology of their deviant arousal and to improve the validity of their reports, the interviewer should attempt to associate important events in the patient's lives with the onset and frequency of their paraphilias.

Second, some subjects may report several paraphilias occurring simultaneously but at different frequencies and at different times in their lives (Abel, Becker, Cunningham-Rathner, Mittelman & Rouleau, 1988). Such reports tend to indicate that, as one paraphilia rises to become the predominating deviant behavior, others become less dominant. This wave effect continues as another paraphilia rises to dominance and other deviant interests diminish. Special care should be taken under these circumstances to separate the occurrences and frequencies of the various paraphilias. If patients report a range in the frequency of their deviant behaviors (e.g., one to three times a week), we prefer to select the minimal figures to avoid exaggeration of the paraphiliac's deviant behavior (Abel *et al.*, 1987). In the very rare instances of suspected overreporting, the interview should be repeated until the data become consistent.

In addition to the traditional clinical interview, the therapist can collect further information that, in some cases, contributes considerably to an understanding of the patient's treatment needs. Such data include information gained from self-reports or attitudinal measures (paper-and-pencil testing), direct observation of the patient's motor behavior (assessments of role-played behavior), or recording of the offender's physiological responses to stimuli that are expected to provoke responses corresponding to the offender's deviant behavior (psychophysiological assessment).

Paper-and-Pencil Testing

Cognitive Scale

This questionnaire was developed by our research team to evaluate cognitive deficits, that is, misconceptions about specific crimes and their impact on the victim and society. It has been administered to over 287 sex offenders and 150 non-sex-offending adults (Abel, Mittelman, & Becker, 1983).

Sexual Interest Cardsort

This test was also developed by our team and has been administered to over 600 sex offenders; it contains 15 categories of sexual behavior. The goal of the cardsort is to determine the subject's self-reported paraphilic and nonparaphilic sexual arousal patterns (Abel *et al.*, 1983).

Sexual Knowledge Inventory

This standardized questionnaire was used in this research to evaluate the level of sexual knowledge.

Behavioral Measurement

Assessment Role-Play

Role-play social skills and assertiveness skills were videotaped and were scored to objectively assess each subject's level of social and assertive skills (Abel *et al.*, 1983).

Probably no other means of assessment has proved to be as helpful to our understanding of the treatment needs of paraphiliacs as psychophysiological assessment. This technique was discovered in the early part of this century and was developed further by Freund and others in the 1960s (Freund, 1961, 1967). The system involves recording the genital responses of offenders while presenting them with various categories of paraphilic and nonparaphilic stimuli. The male offender's erection responses to the various stimulus categories are recorded. The validity of these measures rest on a number of factors, such as the degree of confidentiality of the data, the extent to which the patient admits to deviant arousal, the category or means of presenting the stimuli (such as slide projection, audiotape recordings, and videotape presentations), and the instructional set given to the offender prior to his experience with psychophysiological measurement. Because positive erection responses to stimuli have greater validity than an absence of erection responses to the various stimuli, we have found it most helpful to confront the patient with any discrepancies between his self-reported deviant interests and the psychophysiological assessment results.

The major advantage of psychophysiological assessment is that it uncovers deviant patterns of arousal by stimuli that, for numerous reasons, the patients attempted to conceal. Because a thorough investigation of all of the offender's deviant interests is essential to the formulation of an effective treatment approach, the use of psychophysiological assessment is very valuable. The highly sensitive equipment of the psychophysiological laboratories, the start-up costs of such equipment, and the need for special technical training tend to limit psychophysiological assessment laboratories to programs in which large numbers of offenders are evaluated and treated.

The psychophysiological measurement of sexual arousal patterns includes two types of measurements: (1) the visual physiological measurement of erection, consisting of 40 slides depicting 10 categories of stimuli, and (2) the audio physiological assessment of erection, consisting of audiotaped descriptions of deviant and nondeviant sexual behaviors.

DEVELOPMENTAL CONSIDERATIONS

How Deviant Arousal Develops

A number of theories (Abel & Blanchard, 1974; Avery-Clark & Laws, 1984; Evans, 1968) indicate that the development of sexual arousal is a primary component in the etiology of sexual identification and of deviant and nondeviant sexual behaviors.

A normal part of one's sexual development is sex play with same-aged peers (Constantine & Martinson, 1982; Kinsey, Pomeroy, & Martin, 1948). It follows that if sex play occurs between two 10-year-old boys, either boy can become classically conditioned to the sight, feel, and emotional responses of a 10-year-old boy and find him and boys similar to him sexually exciting. This process occurs during the critical period of puberty and can be considered a type of "imprinting." The likelihood that this will occur is directly proportional to the degree of pleasure (reinforcement) that the developing pedophile experiences. The cues that can be classically conditioned are slightness of build, the absence of secondary sexual characteristics (pubic and facial hair, deepened voice, etc.), and a childlike attitude toward play.

McGuire, Carlisle, and Young (1965) proposed that what is important in the development of a "fixation" on an early sexual object is for the developing offender's early experience of arousal (stemming from what they called the first "real" sexual experience) to become incorporated into a fantasy that is repeated and becomes increasingly prominent in the individual's fantasy life. They further proposed that the sexual experience of being molested provides the content of future erotic fantasies (McGuire *et al.*, 1965). These fantasies become progressively more deeply incorporated into an individual's masturbatory fantasies. Because masturbation is one of the most potent reinforcers available to humans, these masturbatory fantasies become increasingly erotic as they are consistently paired with orgasm. This connection of masturbation and deviant fantasies may help to explain the initiating and maintaining of the desires for molestation behavior.

Upon examination of the masturbatory fantasies of sex offenders, several investigators (Feldman & MacCulloch, 1973; Gebhard, Gagnon, Pomeroy, & Christenson, 1965; Mohr, Turner, & Jerry, 1964) have reported a high rate of masturbation to deviant fantasies by sexual deviates. In viewing deviant fantasies as a mechanism that leads to the maintenance of deviant behavior, Tausk (1951) and Abel and Blanchard (1974) have asserted that the consistent pairing of pleasurable orgasm with a memory makes that memory arousing and pleasurable, even if the original experience was not pleasurable.

In view of the frequency with which most individuals have early sexual experiences with young peers, it could be expected that child molestation would be the most common of sexual deviations and would occur at a very high frequency. Such would undoubtedly be the case were it not for the evaluative processes that we all learn during acculturation. All individuals grow up in an environment that communicates behavior considered normative for our society. We observe the behavior of our parents, siblings, and others. Through our academic and religious institutions, we gain information about appropriate and inappropriate behavior. In the majority of cases, we are given clear messages about what is acceptable and unacceptable. We learn that physical attacks on children are unacceptable. Unfortunately, our culture, in general, feels the need to protect its children from any discussion of sexuality as well as of what constitutes appropriate sexual behavior. Children are taught that they should not talk about or discuss sexual things because sex is a private matter, not a public one, and therefore, early sexual experiences do not come under the scrutiny of parents and/or cultural institutions. As a result, the normal evaluative processes fail to give the child feedback about the appropriateness or inappropriateness of his or her sexual behavior.

If participation in deviant stimuli persists as the child grows, he will eventually realize the need to conceal his sexual interests and behaviors particularly after he realizes that his sexual involvement with young children, for example, is severely sanctioned by society. The self-statements or internal attitudes and beliefs that shape much of his nonsexual behavior in our society do not incorporate society's sexual norms. Therefore, the developing paraphiliac develops his own set of cognitive distortions or beliefs, which justify a behavior that is inconsistent with the norms of society. These internal attitudes may include such self-statements as "It's all right to involve myself sexually with a younger child as long as no force is used;" "I cannot tell if sexual involvement with a young child will harm that child when the child grows up": or "Someday, the attitudes of society will change regarding sex between adults and children, and therefore, it matters little what society believes now, as those attitudes are changing." This process of the persistent pairing of deviant fantasies with the pleasure of masturbation and/or orgasm and the concomitant development of inappropriate beliefs about what constitutes appropriate sexual behavior work together to create not only the deviant arousal pattern but the belief system that supports its maintenance into adulthood. The mechanism that explains the development of pedophilia is also applicable to other paraphilias, such as fetishism, bestiality, voyeurism, exhibitionism, and rape.

If we are to understand the development of paraphilic influence, we would do better by attempting to understand the development of the inhibitory processes that allow each individual to evaluate and appraise the appropriateness or inappropriateness of his sexual behavior.

The Coexistence of Multiple Diagnoses

Another consideration regarding the diagnosis of paraphilia is whether an arousal pattern should be considered paraphilic only if it is the patient's predominant sexual activity or interest. According to the third edition of the *Diagnostic and Statistical Manual* of the American Psychiatric Association (DSM-III, APA, 1980), the diagnosis of paraphilia is possible only when the individual fantasizes or uses images that are predominantly paraphilic. This criterion is inconsistent with the findings of our research with sex offenders (Abel *et al.*, 1988). The majority of our patients reported sexual involvement with adult partners without relying on paraphilic fantasies. Many indicated that they preferred paraphilic fantasies to nonparaphilic fantasies. We found, however, that both deviant and nondeviant behavior clearly coexisted in most patients who used both paraphilic and nonparaphilic fantasies. Our clinical experience with sex offenders also indicates that multiple paraphilias may exist concomitantly and nonconcomitantly in a single individual.

In cases of multiple, concomitant paraphilic diagnoses, one paraphilic interest initially takes dominance. As a second deviant interest develops, the initial paraphilia appears to lose some of its arousal properties and may continue at a reduced intensity. Many paraphiliacs have had significant experience with as many as 10 separate types of deviant sexual behavior (Abel, 1986). Therefore, a careful assessment of the full scope of the patient's deviant interests must be undertaken in order to facilitate effective treatment.

To illustrate the importance of such careful investigation, consider the following different views of incest cases. Many researchers who have studied the family dynamics of incest have stated that, when the normal sexual outlet (the mother) is not available to the father, he then turns to his daughter (De Young, 1982; Justice & Justice, 1979; Meiselman, 1978). What is the difference between the man who will seek sexual gratification with his daughter and the man who will seek the attentions of another adult woman when he finds that appropriate forms of sexual expression within the home are not available to him?

Our assessment of incest cases indicates that the man who chooses his daughter as a sex partner has developed a sexual attraction to young girls in general, including his daughter. The man who opts for an extramarital affair has not developed paraphilic interests. Furthermore, the results of psychophysiological evaluations of incestuous and nonincestuous pedophiles (Abel, Becker, Murphy, & Flanagan, 1981; Abel *et al.*, 1988) indicate that incest cases frequently involve individuals who participate in both incestuous and nonincestuous activities, and individuals involved with children outside the home frequently have concurrent involvement with children within the home.

COMPLICATIONS

When assessing and treating individuals with deviant sexual interests and/or behaviors, major complications can arise if alcoholism, drug abuse, or a high frequency of aggressive, deviant sexual behavior is also present in the patient's profile. Each of these problems require additional treatment planning.

Alcoholism

When alcoholism is closely associated with paraphilia, effective treatment for sexual deviation cannot ignore the patient's possible dependence on alcohol. Such consideration is especially important as the paraphiliac may be at greater risk of reoffending because alcohol frequently causes a temporary decrease in his ability to control paraphilic urges. Therefore, the treatment plan must include a strategy aimed at making the patient less likely to drink. We have found that a highly effective biological approach is the use of disulfiram (Antabuse), which, when taken orally, remains in the bloodstream for 7–14 days. Individuals who drink alcohol while disulfiram is in the bloodstream experience a profound acetaldehyde reaction, an unpleasant complex of symptoms including sweating, palpitations, shortness of breath, hypotension, nausea, and possible fainting. The advantage of this medication is the relative ease with which compliance can be assessed. If taken on Day 1, it will still be evident in the individual's bloodstream up to Day 14.

The use of disulfiram serves not as a replacement for a standard treatment package for the paraphiliac, but as an invaluable adjunct to assist him in the control of his sexually deviant urges by decreasing his use of alcohol.

Drug Abuse

In some cases, the patient's deviant arousal is associated with illicit drugs, such as amphetamines, cocaine, or tranquilizers. Therefore, effective treatment also requires some attention to the patient's drug involvement. It is recommended that random drug screens be done throughout the treatment. It is felt that positive screens should be viewed as failure of outpatient treatment and the need for incarceration. Drug screens are frequently a condition of an individual's probation, and these tests, if conducted randomly, provide the therapist with the necessary documentation.

Once a means of surveillance of drug use has been established, attention must be focused on the emotional conflicts precipitating the drug use, and steps should be taken to reduce or eliminate the stresses associated with illicit drug use.

The Need for Biological Intervention

The function of therapeutic interventions with sex offenders is to prevent the recurrence of the sex offense. Sex offenders commit sexual crimes because of an attraction to deviant sexual stimuli and not as a result of excessive sexual arousal. The treatment components described in the following section outline specific treatment interventions that selectively reduce deviant sexual arousal while maintaining or increasing nondeviant sexual arousal. However, in some patients such as highly aggressive offenders, immediate and drastic reduction of the patient's sexual drive is indicated.

A typical behavioral-treatment approach requires time for the patient to learn how to disrupt his deviant fantasies and thoughts. During the time the patient is receiving treatment, he may reoffend. When those reoffenses are nuisance crimes such as voyeurism or fetishism, the consequences for society and the offender are not extensive. However, if reoffenses during the course of treatment involve rape, child molestation, or sadomasochistic acts, such acts carry much graver ramifications for the victim and for the offender.

The various behavioral and dynamically oriented interventions also require considerable cognitive skills. When these skills are absent, particularly among patients who are highly resistant to cognitive treatment or who have limited intellectual functioning, treatment is less effective. As a result, these individuals continue to be at risk of reoffending.

Biological interventions are unique in that the effects of these treatments are immediate and the patients receiving biological treatment are at a greatly decreased risk of reoffending. Biological interventions have focused primarily on surgical castration and, more recently, on chemical castration. The latter involves the use of drugs to reduce the circulating testosterone that forms the substrate for the offender's sexual fantasies and behavior. Currently, two drugs appear to be effective. These are cyproterone acetate (currently available in Canada but not in the United States) and medroxyprogesterone acetate (available in both Canada and the United States under the trade name Provera). Expressions of sexual urges and desires necessitate an adequate quantity of testosterone. Both of these drugs act by decreasing testosterone to levels that reduce sexual functioning (Berlin & Meinecke, 1981; Money, 1970).

Medroxyprogesterone is available in two forms: an oral preparation (10 mg per tablet) and an intramuscular preparation (Depo-Provera, either 100 or 400 mg/cc). One of the advantages of oral Provera is that the half-life is minimal, so if side effects occur, the medication can be discontinued relatively rapidly. However, because it is administered by mouth, it can easily be voluntarily discontinued by the patient. Therefore compliance with this intervention must be monitored. The customary starting dosage is 200 mg per day, which is adjusted according to the impact of the medication on the patient's deviant sexual urges and drives.

Depo-Provera in the intramuscular form has advantages in that it is released slowly from the injection site and remains in the individual's system for 7–14 days (Spodak, Falck & Rappeport, 1978). However, because the half-life of the drug is approximately 80 days, side effects, if developed, are likely to persist for a considerable period of time. The usual starting dosage of Depo-Provera is 400 mg per day (given in the 100-mg/cc doses, which do not cause the pain associated with the 400 mg/cc doses). The drug is then titrated according to the patient's responses, as measured by his deviant sexual fantasies, urges, and drive. Because Depo-Provera is administered intramuscularly by the therapist, it cannot be voluntarily discontinued by the patient. Compliance is therefore ensured.

Both forms of medroxyprogesterone lead to a reduction in the patient's circulating testosterone and a consequent decrease in sexual drive and sexual fantasies and urges and to decreased ejaculate, decreased sperm production, and a decreased ability to achieve or maintain an erection. Although in some cases there are some side effects such as hot and cold flashes, weight gain, increased blood pressure, and lethargy, they appear to be infrequent and do not usually warrant discontinuation of the drug.

There have been no double-blind controlled studies of the effectiveness of either cyproterone acetate or medroxyprogesterone acetate. However, given the lengthy baseline of patients who repeatedly reoffend without drug intervention but who experience marked curtailment of their deviant sexual behavior when started on medroxyprogesterone, there is ample evidence that these drugs are effective in helping the patient gain control over his deviant urges and behavior.

The major limitation of this biological intervention is the high relapse rate when the medication is discontinued if no other form of intervention has been implemented. Therefore, chemical therapy should be viewed as a valuable adjunct to global treatment of the paraphiliac.

TREATMENT APPLICATIONS

Thirty years ago, sex offenders were treated with traditional, dynamically oriented psychotherapy. The results of this general treatment strategy were minimal. Treatments that focus on the specific excesses or deficits of the offender and use a specific treatment intervention to help the paraphiliac normalize these excesses and deficits have proved more effective. The first and most critical aspect of the treatment is decreasing the patient's deviant sexual arousal.

Since the late 1970s, we have been involved in determining which specific treatments are most effective for treating sex offenders. As described elsewhere (Abel *et al.*, 1983), we initially implemented a treatment program using six components (Abel, Becker, Cunningham-Rathner, Rouleau, Kaplan, & Reich, 1984). The goal of the treatment was to decrease deviant sexual arousal by using covert sensitization and masturbatory satiation, and to increase nondeviant sexual arousal by treating cognitive deficits, improving the subject's sexual knowledge, treating specific sexual dysfunctions that interfere with nondeviant sexual functioning, and developing appropriate sociosexual skills and appropriate assertiveness skills. Recently, an additional element, ammonia-aversion therapy, has been added to the treatment program.

Decreasing Deviant Arousal

Satiation Therapy

One of the most effective treatments currently available for eliminating deviant arousal is satiation (Abel, Rouleau, & Cunningham-Rathner, 1984; Marshall, 1973, 1975, 1979). This is a treatment in which the individual uses his most erotic (usually deviant) thoughts, fantasies, and images in such a way that they become repulsive and are no longer sexually arousing. The satiation treatment involves teaching the patient how to satiate himself with the fantasies that he finds erotic. The treatment is unusual in that the patient practices and applies it by himself in the privacy of his home. The patient is required to audiotape 20 hours of satiation and to bring the tapes to the therapy sessions so that the therapist can review them and provide comments about how the patient may improve and can also ensure compliance with the treatment regimen. The patient then continues to practice the satiation treatment at home. In this way, the patient can apply the satiation treatment at any time, and in any place. It is our goal to help the patient acquire inexpensive treatment interventions that he can initiate himself.

Covert Sensitization

A second form of treatment teaches the patient the dangers connected with any behaviors that have preceded deviant sexual behavior in the past (Abel *et al.*, 1984a). A number of nonparaphilic behaviors generally precede the actual deviant behavior. For example, among child molesters, such behaviors may include having too much unstructured time, working in a job that brings the individual in close proximity to children, spending leisure time with children, and fantasizing about prior experiences of child molestation. The patient is shown the various antecedents to his deviant behavior and then, in the treatment setting, is taught the covert sensitization methodology. This treatment teaches the patient how to fantasize the early links in the chain leading toward deviant behavior and then to imagine the worst possible consequences of participating in these early behaviors. For example, the aversive consequences may be images of being raped in prison, being humiliated in front of fellow workers as they learn of his deviant behavior, or the patient's mother or wife's committing suicide as a result of learning of his behavior. The patient is taught to practice forming these aversive images should any of the early links occur. This treatment is also audiotaped by the patient and is reviewed by the therapist to ensure that the therapy has been learned successfully.

Ammonia-Aversion Therapy

When properly applied, satiation and covert sensitization help the patient to make major strides toward controlling his deviant behavior. However, the inherent limitations of both of these components are their complexities, the time needed to complete them, the intellectual concentration required, and the privacy involved in practicing them. When patients are unable to complete satiation or sensitization successfully, ammonia-aversion therapy has proved to be a valuable treatment adjunct.

Odor aversion has been used for a number of years (Colson, 1972; Laws, Meyer, and Holmen, 1978). Because ammonia aversion therapy has not been extensively described in the literature as a means of assisting the sex offender in controlling his deviant fantasy and behavior, a detailed explanation of its use is included here. Ammonia is a volatile gas commonly used in smelling salts to provide a sharp, aversive stimulus to individuals who have fainted. Although ammonia is readily available in various forms, the ampules of ammonia used as smelling salts appear to be the preferred method of administering ammonia aversion. The ampules are relatively small and easy for the offender to carry unobtrusively. When they are crushed between the fingers and inhaled, a strong jolt of ammonia is delivered, producing lacrimation, nasal stuffiness and rhinorrhea, coughing, speech disfluency (as the patient catches his breath), and burning of the eyes and nose. If used in excess, the ammonia can cause burning of the nasal mucosa, so a periodic evaluation of the patient's nasal mucosa is advised.

Treatment begins by explaining to the patient the principles of aversive conditioning, that is, the association of stimuli with a positive valence (such as images or fantasies of young children for a child molester) with a powerful aversive stimulus (such as ammonia) to associate those images with the aversive consequence of inhaling ammonia. In the office, the patient is first taught how to do the procedure. To provide the therapist with an opportunity to monitor compliance, the offender audiotapes the treatment in 10-minute segments.

The offender begins his audiotaped ammonia-aversion-therapy sessions by describing the chain of events that led him to participate in deviant sexual behavior. He is instructed to verbalize the scenes as vividly as possible and to capture the feelings, emotions, and images surrounding the perpetration of the behavior to make the experience and the feelings associated with it as realistic as possible. Once the antecedents are clearly fixed in the patient's consciousness, he brings an ammonia capsule to his nose and crushes it. The audiotape should record the popping of the capsule as well as the patient's verbalizations. As he inhales the ammonia, the patient switches the fantasies from the antecedents of deviant behavior to his current physiological experience of smelling the ammonia. These verbalizations serve as a further check on treatment compliance. He describes the physiological consequences of the ammonia. He then makes the connection verbally between his current feeling of aversion to the ammonia and the fact that his fantasies of deviant behavior have led to the aversive experience that he is now having. Because the ammonia experience is aversive at this point, he removes the ammonia from his nose (continuous aversion is not necessary) and begins the cycle again.

Learning occurs through repeated trials. Many times, two to three capsules are necessary per 10-minute session, as some offenders report that the ammonia loses its effectiveness after four or five inhalations.

When the patient demonstrates that he has acquired the proper technique for ammonia aversion through a critique of his tapes by the therapist, he carries ammonia capsules into his natural environment for use *in vivo*. Under these circumstances, when the patient finds himself fantasizing or approaching the antecedents to child molestation, he is able to apply the aversion therapy. An added advantage of this technique is that, when it is used *in vivo*, there is reasonable assurance that the antecedents to the deviant sexual urges have actually occurred, and therefore, it is an ideal time to associate an aversive experience with these images and thoughts. Of course, the aversive experience serves as a prompt disrupter of the antecedent behavior.

To assist the patient (and the therapist) with his ammonia therapy sessions, the patient should complete a self-report form (see Figure 1) after each ammonia-aversion session. The offender reports the date and time of the session and its duration and then rates his feelings regarding the clarity and intensity of the antecedents to deviant behavior, the degree of his sexual attraction to the antecedent images, and the degree to which those same images are aversive to him. Next, the patient rates the clarity with which he experienced the ammonia sensations physiologically and the degree to which the experience was aversive to him. Finally, he tries to observe what made the session go well or poorly.

The therapist should carefully check the patient's ammonia aversion therapy audiotapes. Common errors that offenders make include (1) not breaking the ammonia capsule close enough to the audiotape recorder so that the ''pop'' of the smelling salts capsule can be heard; (2) giving long descriptions of the antecedents or of the ammonia, rather than many brief pairings per session; and (3) making pauses in the audiotape during which the patient is not describing either the antecedents or the physiological experiences of the aversive ammonia inhalations. Such pauses usually indicate noncompliance or a reduction in the number of treatment pairings.

Ammonia aversion has definite advantages over other forms of aversive conditioning. The treatment is unobtrusive and discreet; the capsules themselves are small and relatively inexpensive. Most important, the aversive technique provide immediate pairings between the antecedents to deviant behavior and an aversive stimulus. Finally, the treatment is patient-controlled and can be applied at almost any place and at any time.

As with all therapies, there may be evidences of anticipated failure. Some offenders do not find the ammonia particularly aversive, and therefore, the appropriate aversive associations do not develop. Some offenders have such limited intellectual skills that they

Name or ID # ______________________

					Rating of fantasy						
					Deviant behavior scene			Ammonia scene			
Session #	Date	Time (include AM or PM)	How long did the session take?	Instructions	Sexual arousal (10 = extremely arousing)	Clarity of image (10 = extremely clear)	Aversive or upsetting (10 = extremely aversive)	Sexual arousal (10 = extremely arousing)	Clarity of image (10 = extremely clear)	Aversive or upsetting (10 = extremely aversive)	How did the session go? Problem? What helped it go well?

Figure 1. Self-report form for ammonia-aversion therapy.

fail to grasp the principles of ammonia aversion and therefore are poor candidates for its use.

Increasing Nondeviant Arousal

Social Skills Training

Some offenders have deficits in initiating and maintaining peer relationships. This component of treatment involves teaching the offender appropriate ways of relating to adult partners. In order to improve their interpersonal skills in this regard, offenders are taught, within the treatment setting, how to begin conversations, continue conversations, maintain eye contact, and make appropriate follow-up comments.

Assertiveness Training

This technique teaches the individual how to express himself more directly to adults and to relate more effectively to them. It involves modeling, role playing, social reinforcement, and feedback to improve assertive skills with adults.

Sex Education

This is a course that teaches the individual how to be more sexually responsive to adult partners and that eliminates any false ideas about appropriate sexual behavior.

Treatment of Faulty Cognitions

This treatment examines the patient's distorted beliefs and attitudes that, in the past, have supported his deviant behavior. The treatment technique involves confrontation of these faulty ideas and an examination of how the faulty beliefs developed.

Following completion of the structured treatment program, a final component of treatment deals with surveillance of the patient's behavior outside the treatment setting.

The Establishment of Surveillance Groups

From the beginning of treatment and throughout its various components, one of the most important objectives for the patient and the therapist is the recognition of situations in the patient's environment that cause the most problems for him, that is, situations in which the patient is concerned about his ability to control his deviant urges. In order to obtain a clearer picture of the various influences found in the patient's daily environment and of his reaction to them, the therapist will find it useful to gather information in addition to the patient's self-report, the therapist's clinical impression, paper-and-pencil testing, and psychophysiological assessment. Such information is most reliably obtained from persons identified by the patient and with whom he is well acquainted (e.g., coworkers, supervisors, neighbors, and clergy). These individuals, if they agree to participate in the patient's treatment, will form a surveillance group.

Because the perpetration of a sex crime is usually preceded by a chain of antecedent events, the first step is to inform the members of the surveillance group of the behaviors that may suggest that the patient is in danger of reoffending. For example, a child molester's antecedent behaviors may include increased interest in pornography, a failure to assert himself with others, long or frequent visits to shopping malls, or increased drinking or drug use. Figure 2 is a typical surveillance form for a child molester, with a means of scaling the possible antecedent behaviors. Surveillance group members are asked to complete this form two times a month.

A meeting is held with the patient, the therapist, and the five candidates to be surveillance group members, and details of the patient's deviant behavior are described, including what factors have tended to precede commission of the deviant behavior, and how the surveillance group members may identify these antecedent behaviors. The report forms are explained in detail to the surveillance group members, and they are then asked to consider participation. Surveillance group members are told that they may withdraw from further participation at any point without negative repercussions either to the patient or to themselves. It is especially helpful to clarify to surveillance group members that they are not to act as spies and that they are not to go out of their way to put themselves in close proximity to the offender to observe his behavior.

Each surveillance group member agrees to complete the surveillance form (Figure 2) on the 1st and 15th of each month. The therapist then reviews these forms to determine if the offender is demonstrating any of the early behaviors antecedent to reoffense. Group members are instructed to contact the therapist immediately should any acute potential problems of recidivism be suspected.

The establishment of a surveillance group does not guarantee that the patient will not reoffend, nor will the implementation of any single therapeutic intervention ensure complete protection of society from possible recidivism. On the other hand, treatments like these described above that are specifically designed to normalize the patient's behavior, as well as the gathering of detailed information regarding his behavior outside the therapeutic situation, increase the likelihood that reoffense will not occur.

Sequencing of Treatment Components

In this chapter, we have described specific components of the assessment and outpatient treatment of individuals with deviant sexual interests. The first three treatment elements assist the offender in decreasing his deviant sexual arousal. Satiation reduces arousal by satiating the sex offender with his own deviant sexual fantasies. Covert sensitization and ammonia therapy teach the offender to disrupt the behaviors that precede paraphilic acts by matching them with aversive images or aversive physiological experiences.

The next three elements, social skills, assertiveness training, and sex education, are deigned to help the offender achieve improved sexual, social, and emotion relationships with his peers. Cognitive therapy, the final element, attempts to disrupt the attitudes and beliefs that the offender has used to justify his deviant sexual behavior.

An important issue in providing treatment to sex offenders has been to determine the most effective order of treatment component presentation. Our clinical experience indicates that, immediately following their initial assessment and entrance into therapy, offenders are very willing to deal with their deviant arousal pattern, admitting its presence and need for correction. If treatment to decrease deviant arousal is introduced later in the course of treatment, offenders tend to become reluctant to reopen the issue of their deviant arousal (Abel *et al.*, 1984a). Therefore, we believe that covert sensitization, masturbatory satiation, and ammonia aversion should be provided first. Within these first three treat-

1. Is he having frequent social contact with adults without young children being around?
   Never Rarely Frequently Always
2. Is he spending time with children when there is no other adult around?
   Never Rarely Frequently Always
3. Is he working any kind of job that brings him into contact with children as part of the job, i.e., working in a grocery store, working with church youth groups, etc.?
   Never Rarely Frequently Always
4. Does he have a large amount of time on his hands, that is, time in which he has nothing to do?
   Never Rarely Frequently Always
5. Does he seem unwilling to talk with you about what he is doing and how he is spending his time?
   Never Rarely Frequently Always
6. Is he socially isolating himself from others?
   Never Rarely Frequently Always
7. Does he ask you to "trust him" that he is not involving himself with children rather than letting you ask him specifically about his behavior?
   Never Rarely Frequently Always
8. Is he baby-sitting children?
   Never Rarely Frequently Always
9. Is he sad or depressed?
   Never Rarely Frequently Always

I realize that you may not wish to participate in this surveillance aspect of my treatment. If you do not wish to participate, discard this letter. If you are willing to participate, please sign your name at the bottom of the letter, provide your address and telephone number, and return it. If you agree to participate now but change your mind and wish to withdraw in the future, that will be perfectly acceptable. Please let us know your decision. Thank you in advance.

Sincerely yours,

Gene G. Abel, M.D. Joanne-L. Rouleau, Ph.D.

____________________ ____________________
(Signature) (Print name)

____________________ ____________________
(Address) (Telephone number)

____
(City, state, zip code)

____
(Date)

Figure 2. Surveillance form.

ments, there is also an important order. Offenders tend to find the logic behind covert sensitization and ammonia aversion, and their help in disrupting the behavioral chains leading to deviant sexual behavior, easily understandable. Therefore, these two elements should be introduced first and followed by masturbatory satiation once greater trust exists between the therapist and the patient.

Social skills and assertiveness training should be given next, followed by cognitive restructuring and sex education/sexual dysfunction for two reasons. The most important reason is that the completion of cognitive restructuring requires excellent rapport between therapist and offender because one is dealing with basic belief discrepancies). This component of treatment needs to be introduced into treatment when rapport between the therapist and the offender is at a maximum. Social skills and assertiveness training are applicable to almost all offenders and easily engage the offender's attention. They are relevant to his everyday routine, and when the offender sees the impact of this training on his life, his rapport with the therapist improves; thus, the stage is set for the cognitive restructuring to follow.

We prefer the order of social skills training followed by assertiveness training because social skills begin with the rudiments of interacting with others (e.g., beginning a conversation, maintaining conversational flow, and asking nonthreatening questions). Assertiveness training involves a more complex communication of the offender's wants, needs, and emotions. The need for assertiveness skills is therefore predicated on an existing relationship.

Finally, cognitive restructuring should precede the sex education/sexual dysfunction component because the offender should consider the cognitive restructuring issues before treatment ends (Rouleau, Abel, Mittelman, Becker, & Cunningham-Rathner, 1986). Concluding the total treatment package with cognitive restructuring would be a problem because this component tends to lead to an upheaval in the patient's long-standing belief system about his paraphilic behavior. As a result, considerable strain frequently develops between the offender and the therapist. Therefore, we feel that cognitive restructuring should precede the sex education/sex dysfunction component so that the intensive therapy will end with a positive relationship between the offender and the therapist.

Regarding the elimination of distorted beliefs, we have observed that covert sensitization, ammonia aversion, and masturbatory satiation are more effective than cognitive therapy in decreasing faulty cognitions. This discovery supports our clinical impression that the onset of deviant arousal occurs first and is followed by the development of faulty beliefs or distorted cognitions that maintain and justify the deviant behavior. Therefore, if deviant arousal is eliminated first, cognitive distortion is more easily treated later. The remaining distorted beliefs indicate persistent deviant arousal (Rouleau *et al.*, 1986).

Maintenance of Therapeutic Gains

Once the paraphiliac has completed each of the treatment components described above, he enters the maintenance phase of treatment. It is especially important to point out that treatment programs for sex offenders should not be presented as an approach that, on completion, represents total cure and that no further contact with the therapist will be needed. This might be possible if the patient were being treated for more benign symptoms whose recurrence would not jeopardize the safety and welfare of others. Each of the treatment components described above operates on the premise that there may be situations in the patient's near or distant future in which his deviant sexual proclivities will reappear. If the offender has not been prepared for this possible eventuality, recurrences of urges to commit paraphilic acts are viewed as treatment failure and positive proof that the patient's behavior is beyond his control. These attitudes in themselves contribute to the breakdown of the patient's control over his paraphilic urges. We prefer to present therapy as training that will teach the offender the skills necessary to meet the challenge if the deviant urges recur.

The continuation of less intense treatment and the entrance into a maintenance group provide important reinforcement of the offender's treatment gains. The frequency of contact between therapist and patient in such maintenance groups is infrequent (once a week), but this contact provides a valuable support system for the offender. The length of time that treatment should continue on the maintenance level depends in part on the degree of aggression that the offender has evidenced in his deviant behavior, the degree to which a typical victim of the paraphilic act might be able to defend himself or herself against assault, and the frequency and complexity of the paraphiliac's deviant sexual behavior(s). Behaviors involving aggressive assaults on the victim, acts against victims who are less prepared to protect themselves (the very young or the very old), and acts that in the past have occurred at high frequencies or in which multiple paraphilic behaviors are involved require prolonged contact with maintenance groups, possibly for the offender's lifetime.

SUMMARY AND CONCLUSIONS

Contrary to popular belief, successful treatment strategies that help paraphiliacs control their deviant sexual behavior have been available for a number of years. The perplexing question is why these techniques and methods have been unavailable to the perpetrators. We suspect that society is so enraged by the perpetration of such acts that it prefers to direct its therapeutic efforts to the injured victim and to incarcerate the perpetrator. The obvious problem with this mentality is that there will never be enough therapists to provide treatment services for all of the victims and potential victims of sex offenders. Furthermore, the provision of valuable treatment to victims, although certainly a worthwhile and important service, is predicated on the commission of a deviant sexual act and therefore functions after the fact. The prevention of such acts is an important and effective public-health approach to the reduction of sexual violence in our society. At the core of the prevention issue is the fact that deviant sexual acts are committed by people who are highly likely to reoffend if specific treatment is not provided to them. Treatment for deviant sexual behavior should not be promoted simply as a humanitarian service for perpetrators whose lives are disrupted by the commission of deviant sex acts. The perpetrator of unwanted sexual acts can be prevented, and potential victims can be saved from being victimized. Preventing victimization is a high ideal that should be supported by our society; to wait until acts of sexual violence are committed against others is wrong.

ACKNOWLEDGMENT. The authors gratefully acknowledge the editorial assistance of Larry Brown.

REFERENCES

Abel, G. G. (1986). *The treatment of child molesters*, Final Report. Grant R01MH36347. Rockville, MD: National Institute of Mental Health.

Abel, G. G., & Blanchard, E. B. (1974). The role of fantasy in the treatment of sexual deviation. *Archives of General Psychiatry, 30,* 467–475.

Abel, G. G., & Rouleau, J.-L. (1986). Sexual Disorders. In G. Winokur & P. Clayton (Eds.), *Medical basis of psychiatry.* Philadelphia: W. B. Saunders.

Abel, G. G., Becker, J. V., Murphy, W. D., & Flanagan, B. (1981). Identifying dangerous child molesters. In R. B. Stuart (Eds.), *Violent behavior.* New York: Brunner/Mazel.

Abel, G. G., Mittelman, M. S., & Becker, J. V. (1983, December). *Sexual offenders: Results of assessment and recommendations for treatment.* Paper presented at the World Congress of Behavior Therapy, Washington, DC.

Abel, G. G., Becker, J. V., Cunningham-Rathner, J., Rouleau, J-L., Kaplan, M., & Reich, J. (1984a). *The treatment of child molesters.* Department of Psychiatry, Emory University, Atlanta.

Abel, G. G., Rouleau, J.-L., & Cunningham-Rathner, J. (1984b). Sexually aggressive behavior. In W. Curran, A. McGarry, & S. Shah (Eds.), *Forensic psychiatry and psychology.* Philadelphia: F. A. Davis.

Abel, G. G., Becker, J. V., Cunningham-Rathner, J., Mittelman, M., & Rouleau, J-L. (1988). Multiple paraphilic diagnoses among sex offenders. *Bulletin of the American Academy of Psychiatry and the Law, 16* (1).

Abel, G. G., Becker, J. V., Mittelman, M., Cunningham-Rathner, J., Rouleau, J-L., & Murphy, W. L. (1987). Self-reported crimes of non-incarcerated paraphiliacs. *Journal of Interpersonal Violence, 2,* 3–25.

American Psychiatric Association. (1980). *Diagnostic and statistical manual of mental disorders* (3rd ed.; DSM-III). Washington, DC: Author.

Avery-Clark, C. A., & Laws, D. R. (1984). Differential erection response patterns of sexual child abusers to stimuli describing activities with children. *Behavior Therapy, 15,* 71–83.

Berlin, F. S., & Meinecke, C. (1981). Treatment of sex offenders with antiandrogenic medication: Conceptualization, review of treatment modalities, and preliminary findings. *American Journal of Psychiatry, 138,* 601–607.

Christie, M. M., Marshall, W. L., & Lanthier, R. D. (1977). *A descriptive study of incarcerated rapists and pedophiles.* Kingston, Ontario: Canadian Penitentiary Services.

Colson, C. E. (1972). Olfactory aversion therapy for homosexual behavior. *Journal of Behavior Therapy and Experimental Psychiatry, 3,* 185–187.

Constantine, L., & Martinson, F. (1982). *Children and sex: New findings and new perspectives.* Boston: Little, Brown.

De Young, M. (1982). *The sexual victimization of children.* Jefferson, NC: McFarland.

Evans, D. R. (1968). Masturbatory fantasy and sexual deviation. *Behavior Research and Therapy, 6,* 17–19.

Feldman, M. P., & MacCulloch, A. (1973). *Homosexual behavior: Therapy and assessment.* Oxford, Pergamon.

Freund, K. (1961). Laboratory differential diagnoses of homo- and heterosexuality—An experiment with faking. *Review of Czeckoslovak Medicine, 7,* 20–31.

Freund, K. (1967). Diagnosing homo- or heterosexuality and erotic age-preference by means of psychophysiological test. *Behaviour Research and Therapy, 1,* 85–93.

Gebhard, P. H., Gagnon, J. H., Pomeroy, W., & Christenson, C. V. (1965). *Sex offenders: An analysis of types.* New York: Harper & Row.

Justice, B., & Justice, R. (1979). *The broken taboo.* New York: Human Sciences.

Kinsey, A. C., Pomeroy, W., & Martin, C. (1948). *Sexual behavior in the human male.* Philadelphia: W. B. Saunders.

Laws, D. R., Meyer, J., & Holmen, M. L. (1978). Reduction of sadistic sexual arousal by olfactory aversion: A case study. *Behavior Research and Therapy, 16,* 281–285.

Marshall, W. L. (1973). The modification of sexual fantasies: A combined treatment approach to the reduction of deviant sexual arousal. *Behavior Research and Therapy, 11,* 557–564.

Marshall, W. L. (1975). *Prediction of treatment outcome with sexual deviants based on changes in erectile response to deviant and nondeviant stimuli.* Unpublished report, Queen's University, Kingston, Ontario, Canada.

Marshall, W. L. (1979). Satiation therapy: A procedure for reducing deviant sexual arousal. *Journal of Applied Behavior Analysis, 12,* 10–22.

McGuire, R. J., Carlisle, J. M., & Young, B. G. (1965). Sexual deviation as a conditioned behavior: A hypothesis. *Behaviour Research and Therapy, 2,* 185–190.

Meiselman, K. (1978). *Incest: A psychological study of causes and effects with treatment recommendations.* San Francisco: Jossey-Bass.

Mohr, J. W., Turner, R. E., & Jerry, M. B. (1964). *Pedophilia and exhibitionism: A handbook*. Toronto: University of Toronto Press.

Money, J. (1970). Use of androgen-depleting hormone in the treatment of male sex offenders. *Journal of Sex Research, 6,* 165–172.

Rouleau, J-L., Abel, G. G., Mittelman, M. S., Becker, J. V., & Cunningham-Rathner, J. (1986, February). *Effectiveness of each component of a treatment program for non-incarcerated pedophiles*. Paper presented at the NIMH Conference on Sex Offenders at the Florida Mental Health Institute. Tampa, FL.

Short, J. F., & Nye, F. I. (1957). Reported behavior as a criterion of deviant behavior. *Social Problems, 5,* 207–213.

Spodak, M. F., Falck, A. A., & Rappeport, J. R. (1978). The hormonal treatment of paraphiliacs with Depo-provera. *Criminal Justice and Behavior, 5,* 304–314.

Tausk, V. (1951). On masturbation. *Psychoanalytic study of the child, 6,* 61–79.

Zussman, J., & Moore, H. A. (1984). *Report on treatment programs: Summary and recommendations*. Tampa: Florida Mental Health Institute.

13

Somatoform Disorders

CHARLES V. FORD AND PAMELA E. PARKER

INTRODUCTION

Persons who have somatoform disorders do not seek psychiatric help on their own initiative because of the nature of these disorders. Instead, they perceive their difficulties as being physical and conceptualize their distress in terms of organic disease. Consequently, they seek help from medical doctors, stating their complaints in terms of physical symptoms. When a diagnosis of a somatoform disorder is made by a physician, somatizing patients typically resist any implication that there is a psychiatric problem. However, they may reluctantly seek treatment at a psychiatric clinic, when referred, and an occasional patient demonstrates enthusiasm about such treatment if a positive referral has been made by a physician with whom he or she has a good relationship.

One possible exception is patients who seek pain clinics. These multidisciplinary treatment facilities often appeal to patients who have chronic pain, and although they may resist any implication that their pain is "psychogenic," they will seek outpatient care for the symptom of pain and often accept ancillary psychological or psychiatric services. Pain clinics are discussed further below.

The outpatient psychotherapist should be cognizant of the various problems of somatoform disorders because they may also occur during the process of psychiatric treatment and/or psychotherapy. In diagnosis, there is a need to differentiate physical disease from somatic symptoms that may represent reactions to the therapist (transference and/or resistance) or to stressors in the patient's life.

CHARLES V. FORD and PAMELA E. PARKER • Department of Psychiatry and Behavioral Sciences, University of Arkansas for Medical Sciences, Little Rock, Arkansas 72205.

HISTORICAL OVERVIEW

Conversion disorders (hysteria) have been recognized since antiquity. Egyptian physicians were quite aware of the phenomenon and attributed the symptoms to the wandering of the uterus (Veith, 1965). Hippocratic medicine also described conversion phenomena and similarly linked the symptoms to sexual issues.

The symptom of hypochondriasis has been recognized since the time of Galen and was associated with the humoral theory of medicine. Hypochondriasis, quite literally, means below the cartilage, referring to the xiphoid process. This anatomical area contains the liver and the spleen, both previously believed to generate humors that affected both physical health and mood (Adams, 1844).

Thomas Sydenham, the great 17th-century English physician, believed that hysteria was a disease of women and that hypochondriasis was its equivalent in men. However, Paul Briquet took exception to this idea and clearly stated that the two diseases could not be more different. He contrasted the obsessive quality of hypochondriacs with the hysterical aspects of patients who had multiple conversion disorders (Mai & Merskey, 1981). To add confusion to the historical perspective, until recently conversion disorders, hysterical personality, and pain syndromes (psychalgia) were all loosely grouped together. The relationship of these three disorders to hypochondriasis was not clear.

Recent concepts in the area of "hysteria" have largely developed from the phenomenological research of Purtell, Robins, and Cohen (1951) and the later work of Guze (1983) at Washington University in St. Louis. In brief summary, conversion symptoms are common phenomena and are associated with a wide variety of psychiatric disorders. There is a subgroup of persons (mostly women) who have recurrent conversion disorders along with other somatic symptoms. The symptomatology of these women is stable, falls in the spectrum of hysteria, and has been labeled *Briquet's syndrome*. The third edition of the American Psychiatric Association's *Diagnostic and Statistical Manual of Mental Disorders* (APA, 1980) split "hysteria" into three categories: conversion disorders, psychogenic pain (formerly subsumed under conversion disorder), and "somatization disorder." The last disorder is based on the phenomenology of Briquet's syndrome, although the criteria are not quite as rigid.

Modern concepts of hypochondriasis emanated largely from Gillespie (1928), were later defined by Pilowsky (1970), and are currently specified by diagnostic criteria in the DSM-III-R (APA, 1987). These concepts have emphasized the conviction that one has a disease and the preoccupation with physical symptoms, which are interpreted as representing physical disease. These fears can be alleviated only transiently by reassurance by a physician. In general, it is the fear and the worry that characterize these patients rather than dramatic symptoms.

Some authors (Ford, 1983; Nadelson, 1979; Phillips, Ward, & Reis, 1983) have suggested that the somatoform disorders are not discrete diagnostic categories but represent differing points on a continuum of abnormal illness behavior. Ford (1983) suggested that there are actually two continua. One is characterized by the obsessive cognitive style, of which the prototype is hypochondriasis; and the other is characterized by the hysterical cognitive style, which includes somatization disorder, factitious disorders, and Munchausen syndrome.

The controversies concerning somatoform disorders have not been resolved, and in fact, probably no area in psychiatry immediately elicits such strong feelings and opinions as "hysteria." Every psychiatrist and psychologist seems to know exactly what he or she means by the term *hysteria* and also seems to have a clear idea of the etiology of this disorder. It is amusing, and perhaps somewhat unfortunate, that one person's opinion rarely coincides with that of another.

The descriptions of the four major groups of somatoform disorders discussed in this chapter accord with the descriptions in the DSM-III-R. There is an attempt to keep these disorders as distinct as possible, as defined by the phenomenological features of each, and to cover as comprehensively as possible the various treatments proposed for each of these disorders.

SPECIFIC DIAGNOSTIC AND DEVELOPMENTAL CONSIDERATIONS

Each of the various somatoform disorders is the subject of a large body of psychiatric literature. This literature describes the phenomenology, including the typical personal background and/or developmental factors that are believed to be important in the genesis of each diagnostic entity. Each disorder will be discussed separately although, as noted above, there is overlap among them.

Conversion Disorder

Although the official diagnostic term is *''conversion disorder*,'' Ford and Folks (1985) suggested that conversion phenomena should be more properly regarded as a symptom. These conversion symptoms occur in a wide variety of situations among different psychiatric diagnoses, including schizophrenia, neuropsychiatric disorders, and personality disorders. These symptoms are also found in relatively normal people. In brief, there is too little specificity in the phenomenon for it to be identified as a ''diagnosis.''

Some investigators have further proposed that there may be a neuropsychological-physiological substrate that predisposes people to conversion symptoms (Ludwig, 1972; Whitlock, 1967). Many patients with conversion symptoms have had a prior head injury or some other type of central nervous system disease (Whitlock, 1967). Detailed neuropsychological testing of persons prone to repetitive conversion symptoms indicates an increased frequency of cerebral dysfunction, particularly of the dominant hemisphere (Flor-Henry, Frown-Augh, Tepper, & Schopflocher, 1981). There is also some preliminary evidence of subtle differences in the patterns of evoked potentials (Gordon, Kraiuhin, Meares, & Howson, 1986).

A number of factors have been associated with a propensity to develop conversion symptoms, including such features as gender (increased incidence with women) and rural and lower socioeconomic backgrounds (Ford & Folks, 1985). Other features associated with the development of conversion symptoms include a previous experience with someone who has had a similar symptom (modeling) and a recent psychological stress (Raskin, Talbott, & Meyerson, 1966).

In persons who have apparent conversion symptoms, but who have none of the aforementioned risk factors, the possibility of an undiagnosed organic disease must be seriously entertained. Multiple studies have suggested that a significant proportion of those diagnosed as having ''conversion'' later show evidence of an organic disease that could account for the previously misdiagnosed symptoms (Slater & Glithero, 1965; Watson & Buranen, 1979).

Somatization Disorder

This disorder, officially listed as an Axis I diagnosis in the DSM-III-R, in many respects can be more appropriately regarded from a clinical perspective as an Axis II (characterological) diagnosis. These patients repeatedly use somatic symptoms as a coping mechanism, particularly at times of stress. The disorder is similar to what was once called *grand hysteria*. From a statistical standpoint, persons with somatization disorder (Briquet's syndrome) exhibit many common features. These patients frequently come from backgrounds that include a chaotic childhood, including broken marriages and situations in which one or both parents have abused alcohol or drugs (Ford, 1983). Their family histories include a higher proportion of female relatives with Briquet's syndrome than in the general population and a higher percentage of sociopathic personalities and alcoholism in male relatives than would be expected by chance (Woerner & Guze, 1968). Further, many of these patients themselves have characteristics that could be interpreted as at least ''softly'' sociopathic (Guze, Woodruff, & Clayton, 1971). Guze (1983) suggested that Briquet's syndrome and sociopathy are the same disorder with different symptomatic presentations determined by gender. Many patients with somatization disorder also have histrionic personality features. It must be stressed, however, that somatization disorder is *not* synonymous with histrionic personality, which is not a part of the diagnostic criteria for somatization disorder.

Many somatization patients also have a concurrent psychiatric disorder. They may have been incorrectly diagnosed as having somatization disorder because of a large number of physical complaints that may have resulted from either major depression or panic attacks (Liskow, Othmer, Penick, & DeSouza, 1986; Sheehan & Sheehan, 1982). It is common for patients with somatization disorder to be seen in psychiatric clinics because of their suicidal gestures, symptoms of anxiety or depression, substance abuse, and/or marital discord (Ford, 1983). A possible relationship between somatization disorder and Munchausen syndrome was noted by Livingston (1987). Recognition of the disorder in childhood was also proposed by Livingston and, if further studied, may be of major assistance in the prevention of unnecessary medical intervention later in life (Livingston & Martin-Cannici, 1986).

One psychiatric diagnostic group that may be confused with somatization patients are those who have atypical depression of the ''hysteroid dysphoria'' type. This particular group of patients is characterized by symptoms that include a high degree of mood reactivity, substance abuse, difficulty with weight control, and histrionic or flamboyant personalities (Liebowitz & Klein, 1979).

Psychogenic Pain (Somatoform Pain Disorder)

Patients who develop pain syndromes are a heterogeneous group. No common features characterize all members of this group. However, among these patients, a number of major subgroups do have common features and require similar therapeutic interventions.

One major group of pain patients are described as having ''pain-prone'' personality traits. In his classic description of these patients, Engel (1959) described them as frequently depressed, pessimistic individuals, who unconsciously do not believe that they deserve success or happiness. Their life histories are marked with instances of being hurt, defeated, or humiliated, even though in retrospect, it would appear that the patient could have avoided many of these situations. The developmental backgrounds of pain-prone patients often include reports of aggression, pain, and suffering during childhood. The childhood home may also have been marked by alcoholism and/or illness. Pain-prone patients often have a medical or surgical illness they believe accounts for their pain. Commonly, their pain is out of proportion to the underlying disorder.

Blumer and Heilbronn (1981) also found many common psychological characteristics in patients who later developed pain syndromes. They described these pain-prone patients as frequently alexithymic (unable to describe feelings through words), stoic, overly controlled, and action-oriented.

In contrast to a comparison of a group of patients with major depressive disorder and a group with chronic pain disorder, Blumer and Heilbronn (1987) identified traits of pain patients, suggesting that they are on a continuum of depressive disease. These patients demonstrated many biological markers (including failure to suppress on the dexamethasone suppression test and shortened latency for rapid-eye-movement sleep) of depressed patients, although the biological markers were less pronounced in the chronic pain patients. Blumer and Heilbronn labeled this subset of pain patients as having "dysthymic pain disorder."

Depression is a frequent finding in the patient with somatoform pain. However, pain is also common in major depression (Mathew, Weinman, & Mirabi, 1981), and it is important to differentiate major depression or dysthymia disorder from a somatoform pain syndrome in which depression may be a secondary phenomenon. France, Krishnan, Houpt, and Maltbie (1984) found that approximately 21% of patients with chronic pain had a positive dexamethasone-suppression test (failure to suppress), and that these patients' symptoms correlated well with the diagnostic criteria for major depression with melancholia.

Chaturvedi and Michael (1986) studied the coincidence of depressive features and chronic pain retrospectively. A predominance of dysthymic disorder rather than major depression was noted in their patients with chronic pain. This study also reported less frequent pain in the laboring class, contradicting the previous belief that chronic pain is more prominent among those in unskilled occupations.

Other characteristics of patients with pain syndromes that have been reported include narcissism (Blazer, 1980), drug abuse (Swanson & Maruta, 1980), and interpersonal alienation and manipulation (Timmermans & Sternbach, 1974).

Hypochondriasis

Like patients with idiopathic pain, hypochondriacs are a very heterogeneous group. Pilowsky (1970) divided Hypochondriasis into two major categories: primary hypochondriasis (the "crock") and secondary hypochondriasis.

Patients with primary hypochondriasis are often obsessive, emotionally constricted people who bore physicians as they present their litanies of physical complaints and worries. Their developmental backgrounds suggest that they often come from homes which had little emotional warmth and that one or both parents may have had problems with chronic illness and/or hypochondriasis. It is not uncommon for these patients to be self-sacrificing and committed to the care of others, such as an alcoholic spouse or a chronically ill parent (Lipsitt, 1970). Hypochondriacs are also often described as alexithymic in that they have little capacity to talk about their feelings and are not psychologically minded.

The secondary hypochondriacal states are secondary to another psychiatric disorder, a physical illness, or environmental stresses. One of the most common forms of secondary hypochondriasis occurs when there is a preoccupation with physical symptoms secondary to an underlying depression (e.g., masked depression; Katon, Kleinman, & Rosen, 1982a,b).

The monohypochondriacal states (e.g., dysmorphophobia, delusions of bromhidrosis, and delusions of parasitosis) are rare but dramatic. In these disorders, the patient is preoccupied with a physical complaint at a delusional or nearly delusional level (Bishop, 1980). Monosymptomatic hypochondriasis is probably a variant of true paranoia (Hopkinson, 1973).

FREQUENT CLINICAL PROBLEMS

As mentioned above, patients with somatoform disorders rarely enter into psychotherapy with enthusiasm. The therapist is continuously faced with resistance to the concept of psychotherapy and/or the administration of psychotropic medications. During treatment, patients frequently develop new symptoms that require reevaluation and/or referral back to their medical-surgical physician to determine that a new physical disease has not developed. Compliance with treatment becomes a problem because patients frequently cancel appointments or prematurely drop out of therapy. To reduce resistance, the therapist must avoid arguments with the patient about whether the physical complaints are real. It can be acknowledged, quite genuinely, that indeed the patient is in distress and that the discomfort is experienced as a physical problem. A direct confrontational approach, as a rule, increases the resistance and may precipitate a patient's discontinuation of therapy. Instead, it is more useful to listen patiently to the patient's physical complaints and at appropriate times to provide gentle suggestions about their associations with life events. Gradually, the patients recognize that there is a certain predictability in the development of their physical symptoms.

One clinical problem in the treatment of these patients with somatoform disorders is that they induce boredom and angry feelings in the psychotherapist. This is particularly true of patients who are hypochondriacal or who have an idiopathic pain disorder. Therapy sessions with these patients are frequently repetitive recitations of the patients' physical complaints. Their lack of psychological-mindedness and of affect makes it difficult to relate to them. Therapeutic gains are usually slow and are not appreciated, by either the patient or the physician, except when reviewed retrospectively in terms of the patient's decreased use of medical services.

TREATMENT APPLICATIONS

Irrespective of the type of somatization, several general principles need to be observed (Ford, 1986). First, invasive medical-surgical procedures should be undertaken only on the basis of objective evidence, not on the basis of subjective complaints. Consistent with this principle in the outpatient setting, medications (psychotropic medications included) should be prescribed only for specific indications. In general, the use of medications tends to reinforce the patient's concept of physical illness. A second principle is that there should be no argument with the patient about whether the symptom is "in the head" or not. To the patient, the physical symptom is real, and the patient's perceptions should not be challenged. Rather, there can be a subtle change over time, so that the patient becomes aware of the relationship between psychological events and somatic symptoms. Somatizing patients do require periodic reassurances that they do not have a physical disease (every new complaint must be individually evaluated), and the patient's primary-care physician must remain a central part of the treatment plan. Obviously, the best treatment occurs when there is early diagnosis. Management is optimal when the primary-care physician and the psychotherapist have a good working relationship.

Specific treatment techniques for each of the somatoform disorders are considered separately on the following subsections.

Conversion Disorder

A wide variety of successful treatment modalities have been suggested for conversion disorder. One of the first treatments reported was a cathartic treatment of Anna O by Josef Breuer. This particular case, which was of such great interest to Freud, proved to be seminal in many of the early ideas of psychoanalysis (Hollender, 1980). Psychotherapy—provided by a variety of techniques, including brief interventions—has also been reported to be remarkably effective in alleviating symptoms (Dickes, 1974; Folks, Ford, & Regan, 1984).

Physical therapy techniques may be very valuable in treating the patient with conversion disorder in that they represent a physical modality and active intervention. Therefore, the patient is allowed to discard the symptom in a face-saving manner over a period of several days.

Other therapies, based largely on suggestion, are hypnosis and amytal interviews (Maris, 1945). In amytal interviews, patients who have had paralysis or are mute may clearly demonstrate return of function during the period of narcosis. Information may also be obtained at that time that will provide some understanding of the psychological etiology of the symptom. It should be stressed, however, that conversion symptoms tend to be transient and to respond to suggestive therapy with or without the provision of insight into what the symptom may mean symbolically and/or into its psychological determinants. Hafeiz (1980) effectively treated conversion patients whom he saw at Khartoum General Hospital by passing an electric current through the affected area, in conjunction with the suggestion that the symptom would remit. There was a surprisingly low rate of symptom recurrence or substitution.

On occasion, a conversion symptom may be persistent, lasting for days or months. In such a situation, there are usually reinforcing factors within the environment that serve to perpetuate the symptom. An example of such a factor is secondary gains like disability payments from an accident or increased attention from a spouse or a family member. Symptoms that persist longer than 1 month are particularly resistant to treatment (Andrews, 1985). To treat persistent symptoms, it is often necessary to use a behavior modification program to extinguish the symptom (Blanchard & Hersen, 1976).

Secondary gains and conversion are often closely connected, and it is often difficult to distinguish conversion from malingering. In fact, the two are on a continuum, and the difference is the degree of the patient's conscious knowledge concerning the production of the symptom (Cameron, 1945). For example, conversion disorders are common in military populations. In one clinical illustration (C. V. Ford) a recruit during basic training, on bending over to pick up a cigarette butt, was unable to straighten up. He was admitted to the orthopedic surgery service, where it was apparent that there was no organic disease, and that in fact, he could lie flat on his back in bed. When he was seen in psychiatric consultation, it was apparent that he was highly dependent on his parents, from whom he had never been separated, that he had minimal ego strength with which to handle the stresses of military training, and that he was terrified by the prospect of having to become a "fighting man." Because of the persistence of the symptom, the man was transferred to a psychiatric unit, where he was treated primarily with "benign neglect." It was suggested to him that he was not quite ready for military training and that he would be discharged from the military service. However, it was "hinted" that it would not be possible to return him to his parents until he was able to stand up straight. Over the period of a week, the patient's posture became progressively more erect until he was asymptomatic.

Conversion symptoms may also occur during the course of psychotherapy as a "transference" phenomenon. An example is the patient reported by Ford (1983) who developed a "paraplegia" during the vacation of her therapist. The patient's symptom remitted within hours of the therapist's return from his vacation and his interpretation to her that she felt that she could not "stand on her own two feet" without his assistance.

As a rule there is no place for pharmacological therapy in the treatment of conversion disorder unless the symptom is serving as a defense against an underlying depression and/or psychosis. The use of a pharmacological agent carries with it the subtle implication that the problem is medical.

Conversion symptoms occur within a social-psychological matrix and may represent a strain within the system. Therefore, conjoint and/or family therapy may, at times, be the indicated therapeutic intervention.

The prognosis for the treatment of conversion symptoms is variable according to different authors. For example, Slater and Glithero (1965) reported that a large percentage of patients diagnosed as having conversion disorder later developed severe psychiatric disorders and/or neurological-physical disorders that explained the original symptom. It should be kept in mind, however, that their experience was from National Hospital (Queen Square, London), a tertiary referral hospital that accepts patients with severe and/or persistent problems. In contrast to the experience of Slater and Glithero was the aforementioned experience of Hafeiz (1980), who, in an acute-care setting, found that the overwhelming majority of patients responded quickly and did not have a recurrence of their symptoms.

There has been a fairly consistent finding that approximately 20% of patients with conversion disorder will develop a physical disease to account for their symptoms (Watson & Buranen, 1979). However, most authors have reported that conversion symptoms remit fairly quickly, and that, in the majority of cases, the symptoms do not recur.

Somatization Disorder

The management of patients with somatization disorder is a complex and frequently frustrating endeavor. The reason is not only that patients repeatedly present with dramatic physical symptoms, but that, in addition, the style of their lives is often characterized by instability, mood changes, and acting-out behavior. As mentioned above, the disorder may best be conceptualized as characterological. The degree of overall psychopathology is sufficiently great that management, rather than cure, should be the primary goal. In contrast to patients with single conversion symptoms, patients with somatizing disorder seem to have a much lower incidence of undiscovered illness (Zoccolillo & Cloninger, 1986).

Smith, Monson, and Ray (1986) indicated that some simple techniques can markedly reduce these patients' use of medical services. This ''therapeutic'' intervention consists of a psychiatric consultation followed by a letter to the patient's primary-care physician in which the nature of the disorder is described and recommendations are made for its management. These recommendations include regularly scheduled appointments every 4–6 weeks, physical examinations each visit so that symptoms will not be discounted, and avoidance of hospitalization, diagnostic procedures, surgery, and laboratory assessments unless clearly indicated. The physicians are also advised *not* to tell the patients that the symptoms are ''all in their heads.''

In addition to necessary ongoing medical management by the primary-care physicians, these patients are also frequently followed in psychiatric outpatient settings because of their multiple psychological problems. Recommendations similar to those above, made to the primary-care physician, are also applicable to outpatient psychiatric treatment. Psychotropic drugs are generally contraindicated for these patients because they have no specific symptoms for which drugs are effective and because these patients are at risk for habituation. The patient's symptoms, such as depression and/or anxiety, are usually highly situationally determined and respond to environmental manipulation or support, so that the use of pharmacological agents is unnecessary.

The University of Colorado has demonstrated improved care of somatizers by the use of a special clinic. Although the clinic (called Med H unit) is located in the medical-surgical outpatient area, it is staffed by psychiatrists and psychiatric residents. Somatizing patients are seen at regularly scheduled appointments and require significantly less hospitalization than other patients in the primary-care clinic (Ritvo & Thompson, 1986).

Psychotherapy techniques for somatization-disordered patients should emphasize a supportive approach that enables them to look at their difficulties from a problem-solving perspective instead of engaging in their usual emotional, acting-out behavior. As has been pointed out by Murphy (1982), these patients do not need encouragement to ''let it all out''; instead, techniques should be used to help them control their emotionality. The psychotherapy technique should consistently point out the relationship between life events and the development of symptoms as well as confront them with the self-defeating nature of their dramatic emotional and acting-out responses to these stresses. Crisis therapy techniques that emphasize having the patient look at alternative ways of handling life stresses are helpful, but insight-oriented therapy of an uncovering nature may be contraindicated because of the potential for regression and/or the provocation of anxiety.

Involvement with the family of the patient with somatization disorder may be necessary (Ford, 1983). From a realistic standpoint, these patients do come from chaotic backgrounds and frequently have made poor marriages. Children often have behavioral problems and/or school difficulties. The degree of stress that these patients experience should not be underestimated, and it may be helpful at times to make environmental changes and/or to give advice about how to handle a life problem, such as dealing with an alcoholic and abusive spouse.

Group therapy may prove to be an effective intervention for somatization disorder. A report by Valko (1976) indicates that women with Briquet's syndrome who were put into an educative, supportive group did very well, showing a marked diminution of both psychiatric and physical symptoms. The techniques of this group were to spend the initial sessions describing the characteristics of the disorder. Subsequent group meetings consisted of the patients' confronting each other with their behavior, providing group support, and learning new techniques for handling the stresses in their lives.

Hypochondriasis

As discussed above, hypochondriasis is actually a heterogeneous group of disorders. However, when people talk of hypochondriacs, they generally mean those with the form known as *primary hypochondriasis*, or "crocks." As in conversion disorders and somatizing disorder, the existence of underlying disease must be reasonably ruled out. It has been suggested that the hypochondriac is actually searching for a relationship with a physician, who is perceived unconsciously as a parent surrogate (Wahl, 1964). The "ticket" for admission to the physician's office is a somatic complaint. Therefore, one of the first techniques of dealing with the hypochondriac is to schedule regular appointments so that it is not necessary for the patient to have a new symptom in order to see the physician. This technique is similarly used in the treatment of somatization disorder.

To a large extent, hypochondriacs are alexithymic and have difficulty in expressing their internal distress in terms other than physical symptoms. They are uncomfortable in talking about their personal lives and the psychological stresses they are experiencing. Unlike the patients with somatization disorder, hypochondriacs are emotionally constricted, and they may require encouragement to express and/or communicate their emotions. They often have a history of self-defeating behavior that suggests an underlying masochistic personality structure. As a consequence, there must be no expectation by the physician nor promise to the patient that symptoms will be completely removed (Lipsitt, 1970). In a perverse way, the patients' symptoms are comforting to them, as if they function in accordance with the old Yiddish proverb "When things are too good, that is bad" (Wahl, 1964). Rather than cure, one can offer encouragement to persevere *despite* the symptoms.

A therapeutic technique that is basically behavior modification (Kutcher & Ford, 1985) is to allow patients to express somatic complaints but to respond with increased interest when they talk about personal issues, especially when such talk revolves around the expression of feelings or longings. Such "rewards" make it clear to the patient that the physician is interested in more than the somatic symptoms and that somatic symptoms are not necessary to perpetuate the relationship.

As a general rule, psychotherapeutic techniques, particularly those of a psychodynamic variety, have not been effective with hypochondriacal patients. One form of psychotherapy, reported by Kellner (1982), suggests initial good results. The techniques include repeated reassurance, explanations, multiple physical examinations, and "suggestions" to the effect that the patient is not physically ill. The patients studied were noted to be of the higher socioeconomic class, and this class affiliation may have affected the prognosis of psychotherapy in a favorable direction (Kellner, 1983).

As for Briquet's syndrome, group therapy has been suggested as a cost-effective modality for treating hypochondriacs (Ford & Long, 1977; Mally & Ogston, 1964; Schoenberg & Senescu, 1966). In fact, patients' emergency-room and medical-surgical-clinic visits have been shown to decrease dramatically with the institution of group therapy.

The techniques of group therapy for somatizing hypochondriacal patients do not emphasize the acquisition of psychological insight; instead, they provide a setting for social support and catharsis. The topics discussed in group therapy often center on several recurrent themes, including a sense of suffering that is not understood by others and anger at physicians for failing to tend to the patient's needs. Somatizing patients frequently imply that, because of their illness, others are responsible for taking care of them or making them feel better. Perhaps because of their lack of psychological-mindedness, hypochondriacal group members are not likely to confront other patients who display obvious displacement of psychological problems onto physical symptoms. As in the techniques of individual therapy suggested above, the group leader can suggest that cure is probably impossible, but that one can learn to live with the symptoms. Group therapy for hypochondriacs can be interpreted as providing an alternative and more appropriate form of social support than repeated diagnostic investigations.

Techniques that increase the acceptability of group therapy to hypochondriacal patients include arranging several individual visits to the therapist before referral to the group, scheduling group meetings in the medical-surgical clinic area instead of in a psychiatric setting, and using of educative techniques that focus on themes such as ways to adjust to chronic illness (Ford, 1984).

For patients with hypochondriasis that is secondary to acute stress (e.g., during convalescence from a myocardial infarction), there is a limited role for psychotropic medications. Patients who are experiencing concurrent symptoms of anxiety that may interfere with optimal recovery (e.g., tachycardia or premature ventricular contractions in a post-myocardial-infarction patient) may benefit from a time-limited course of benzodiazepines. Often, and perhaps more important, these patients require repetitive reassurance (Sapira, 1972) and, at times, psychotherapy. The goals of such psychotherapy might be to assist the patient to accept a new self-image and/or to examine his or her life values.

When symptoms of major depression underlie the hypochondriacal mask, the patients should be treated with the appropriate antidepressant medication. Some hypochondriacal patients fit into the pattern of "atypical" depression. The symptoms of atypical depression include hypochondriacal concerns, pseudo personality changes (passive-aggressive or passive-dependent) and a reversal of the usual vegetative changes of depression (e.g., hypersomnia instead of insomnia and increased appetite instead of anorexia). Monoamine oxidase inhibitors (MAOIs) have been reported to be especially effective with this syndrome (West & Dally, 1959), although there may be less specificity for MAOIs in the treatment of atypical depression than was originally believed (Silberman & Sullivan, 1984).

Patients with monosymptomatic hypochondriasis are rarely seen in psychiatric clinics because of their strong rejection of any implication that their concerns have any psychological basis. A few of these patients have psychotic depression (with somatic delusions) and respond favorably to a combination of neuroleptics and antidepressants if they can be induced to take these medications. The large majority have what amounts to true paranoia, and their delusions are not responsive to the usual neuroleptics. The responses of monosymptomatic hypochondriacal patients to pimozide, a diphenylbutylpiperidine available in the United States only for limited indications (Munro, 1978), have been promising.

With the exception of treating depression, the attempt to treat hypochondriacal patients with medication usually leads to frustration because of the patient's complaints about side effects. These patients, who are sensitive to all physiological symptoms, amplify such sensations (Barsky, 1979) and are exceedingly aware of all side effects of medications. It is not at all unusual that the patient's previous physicians have prescribed multiple medications for them, and hypochondriacal patients often recount long lists of side reactions that they have experienced. Thus, it is not advisable to prescribe medication for the hypochondriacal patient unless there are specific indications.

Somatoform Pain

Pain is probably the most common symptom for which patients seek medical assistance. There are, however, distinct differences between acute and chronic pain. Chronic pain is a symptom for which patients repeatedly seek medical care (''doctor-shop'') for various syndromes (e.g., abdominal pain and low back pain) that apparently have little or no known physical cause.

Because of the large number of these patients, and probably because of the patients' aversion to seeking overt psychiatric treatment, there has been a proliferation of ''pain clinics'' (Bonica, 1974b; Brena, 1983). Typically, these pain clinics have a multidisciplinary focus that incorporates both physical and psychological perspectives. Chronic pain patients are more accepting of psychological evaluation and treatment when it is a routine part of the treatment program for all patients. Pain clinics, in addition, use a variety of somatic modalities, such as nerve blocks, physical therapy, and/or transcutaneous nerve stimulation as a part of the treatment plan. Educative sessions discussing the nature of the pain and analgesics for both patients and family members are a useful part of the treatment program, as is group therapy. Selected patients may receive more extensive psychiatric interventions, as described below. The focus of many pain clinics is to diagnose and alleviate conditions that may be contributing physically to the pain symptom, to detoxify the patient from multiple habituating analgesics and/or other drugs, to redirect the focus from total symptom relief to rehabilitation, and to help the patient accept responsibility for the management of the illness. Many of these patients are dependent and have placed the responsibility for their care and their medical management on others, particularly physicians.

Although pain clinics have an advantage in their ability to attend to the special and multiple needs of chronic pain patients, many of the principles that these clinics use should also be used by the individual practitioners who care for these patients.

Individual psychotherapy is not usually helpful for patients with chronic pain. The reason is most likely that the patients are not psychologically minded and because the symptom of pain is multidetermined. There is often a nidus of organic dysfunction to initiate painful stimuli, concurrent intrapsychic and interpersonal conflicts, and reinforcers from the environment.

There are a few dramatic exceptions where insight-oriented psychotherapy is helpful, but these tend to be situations in which the pain has had an important symbolic meaning to the patient. An example is the case reported by Ford (1983) in which a woman had an acute, severe disabling back pain that had started simultaneously with the news of the death of her mother. The mother had died of metastatic breast carcinoma and had experienced severe back pain during her terminal illness. Psychotherapy revealed that the patient's chronic back pain was related to feelings of guilt about her mother and her need for punishment following her mother's death. There was complete relief of pain after the patient had worked through her unresolved grief and had obtained insight into the symbolic function of the symptom.

Although individual therapy has not proved, on the whole, to be an effective treatment for these patients, group therapy has been somewhat more promising. The reason is that the group apparently helps patients to become more competent in social activities and to begin a more active life, whether or not the pain itself is changed. The group experience seems to facilitate the emergence of more self-reliance and independence (Hendler, 1984; Herman & Baptiste, 1981; Pinsky, 1978).

Consistent with the systems-theory formulation of pain, it is becoming increasingly obvious that the patient's symptom of pain may represent a strain within the family or other social situation (Bokan, Ries, & Katon, 1981; Ford, 1983). As a consequence, family therapy is beginning to emerge as one of the more effective methods of treating the pain patient. Hudgens (1979) reported that 75% of patients treated with a short-term, family-centered behavioral approach were returned to normal. The approach required that family members be taught operant conditioning techniques, and the family members were regularly involved in patient care. Patients with addiction or litigation proceedings were excluded from the study.

As demonstrated in the above-mentioned study, behavioral modification techniques are important in the treatment of chronic pain (Fordyce, 1974). The goal is to extinguish pain behaviors and to encourage new behaviors that are pain-incompatible. One helpful technique for initiating behavior modification is to have the patient maintain a 1- or 2-week diary that includes periods of pain, periods of down-time, and all activities (Chapman, 1983a). Patients are also encouraged to include information in the diary about what was concurrent in their lives at the time they experienced the pain. The behavior therapist can use this diary to suggest new behaviors at certain times during the patient's day. Physical therapy and exercise can also be used as a form of behavior modification. Patients are encouraged to progressively increase the amount of time spent in physical activities and are provided verbal praise for time spent in activities other than those that were previously related to pain.

It is beyond the scope of a book on psychiatric treatment to intelligently discuss somatic interventions such as nerve blocks, but one should keep in mind that they are frequently a useful adjunct in the treatment of regional pain problems (Bonica, 1974a). Their effectiveness may be due partially to the placebo effect and partially to physiological changes. With some relief of physical pain, patients can increase their activity, thereby, changing and reducing their pain behaviors. A dramatic procedure, such as a nerve block, can also provide the patient with a face-saving way to discard the symptom. Another somatic treatment is the use of transcutaneous electrical nerve stimulation (TENS) units (Loeser, Bluck, & Christman, 1975). These units provide an electrical stimulus to nerve root areas. Their apparent effectiveness lies in providing competitive inhibition of the pain fibers by stimulating other nerve fibers. TENS units tend to be helpful for short periods of time, but as with most somatic interventions in the treatment of chronic pain, effectiveness is lost over a period of weeks to months.

Similarly, biofeedback techniques that encourage either the production of brain alpha rhythms or muscle relaxation are often well accepted by patients. Not only do patients obtain some immediate symptom relief, but the use of such procedures often allows the patient to become amenable to the general idea of psychological intervention. For example, there may be the provision of supportive psychotherapy by the person operating the biofeedback equipment during the period before, during, and after the actual procedure itself (Chapman, 1983b).

In a report of chronic pain management from the Auckland Pain Clinic in New Zealand (Large, 1980), where a psychiatrist sees 15%–20% of all referrals, there was a 68% success rate with EMG feedback and 43% recovery or improvement with psychotropic medication (mostly tricyclic antidepressants with "occasional" phenothiazine or anticonvulsants). Brief psychotherapy usually accompanied other modalities.

Narcotic analgesics and habituating drugs, such as the benzodiazepines, have not been useful in the treatment of chronic pain. Many patients have become habituated to these drugs because of chronic use and are reluctant to discontinue them. But, in fact, their pain has continued without significant change. This point should be made to patients when they are reluctant to discard such agents; for example, if the medication were truly effective, they wouldn't have the pain. One of the first treatment principles for patients with chronic pain is to detoxify them from the habituating drugs because the addictions have created secondary problems.

Medications that have been helpful in the treatment of chronic pain syndromes include the tricyclics and neuroleptics. However, there is an increasing reluctance to prescribe neuroleptics for patients with benign conditions because of the danger of their developing tardive dyskinesia. There are two groups of patients with pain for whom tricyclics may be indicated. In the first group are those patients who have concurrent major depression. These patients should be treated with the usual dosage of tricyclics that is indicated for major depression. In the second group are those patients who have pain without major depression. For these patients, dosages of tricyclic antidepressants lower than those used for the treatment of major depression are often helpful in diminishing the perception of pain and increasing the quality of sleep. A typical dose would be 75 mg of amitriptyline per day.

Although an overall rate of 60% response to tricyclics has been suggested, there is a possibility that trials of other antidepressants may increase the responsiveness to medication (Lindsay & Wyckoff, 1981). Blumer and Heilbronn (1987) preferred a more sedating antidepressant in pain patients with insomnia and tended to avoid noradrenergic antidepressants. Lithium carbonate or a small amount of neuroleptic was added to the tricyclic regimen if the patient had not responded to a maximum dose of tricyclics in 3–4 weeks. The Blumer and Heilbronn study supports the common finding of high dropout rates. Among the nonresponders, a majority were disabled male blue-collar workers.

SUMMARY

The outpatient treatment of somatoform disorders is frequently difficult because of the resistance of patients to the idea that psychological issues may be related to their symptoms. Somatizing patients should, as a rule, be conceptualized from the standpoint of management rather than of cure.

Goals for treatment should be modest, without the expectation of complete symptomatic relief. A realistic objective is for the patients to obtain increased insight into the psychological factors that influence their lives and their corresponding emotional and physiological responses. Language that explains stress management is frequently more acceptable to these patients than psychiatric jargon. A second objective is to decrease inappropriate use of medical facilities by providing an alternative social support system (e.g., group therapy). A third objective is to increase the patient's function as a spouse or a parent in order to help prevent the multigenerational effects of somatization. In summary, the overall goal is not so much symptom relief as it is assisting the patient in reentering life as an active participant.

With increased understanding of the dynamics that produce the somatoform syndromes, the therapist obtains a feeling of increased competency, and as a consequence, there is greater enjoyment in working with these difficult patients.

REFERENCES

Adams, F. (1844). *The Seven Books of Paulus Aegineta: Vol. 1*. London: Sydenham Society.

American Psychiatric Association. (1980). *Diagnostic and statistical manual of mental disorders* (3rd ed., DSM-III). Washington, DC: Author.

American Psychiatric Association. (1987). *Diagnostic and statistical manual of mental disorders* (3rd ed., rev.; DSM-III-R). Washington, D.C.: Author.

Andrews, G. (1985). Treatment outlines for the management of the somatoform disorders. *Australian and New Zealand Journal of Psychiatry, 19,* 397–407.

Barsky, A. J. (1979). Patients who amplify bodily sensations. *Annals of Internal Medicine, 91,* 63–70.

Bishop, E. R. (1980). Monosymptomatic hypochondriasis. *Psychosomatics, 21,* 731–741.

Blanchard, E. B., & Hersen, M. (1976). Behavioral treatment of hysterical neurosis: Symptom substitution and symptom return reconsidered. *Psychiatry, 39,* 118–129.

Blazer, D. G. (1980). Narcissism and the development of chronic pain. *International Journal of Psychiatry in Medicine, 10,* 69–79.

Blumer, D., & Heilbronn, M. (1981). The pain-prone disorder: A clinical and psychological profile. *Psychosomatics, 22,* 395–402.

Blumer, D., & Heilbronn, M. (1987). Depression and chronic pain: Depressive symptoms in medical and other psychiatric disorders. In O. G. Cameron (Ed.), *Presentations of depression*. New York: Wiley.

Bokan, J. A., Ries, R. K., & Katon, W. J. (1981). Tertiary gain and chronic pain. *Pain, 10,* 331–335.

Bonica, J. J. (1974a). Current role of nerve blocks in diagnosis and therapy of pain. *Advances in Neurology, 4,* 445–453.

Bonica, J. J. (1974b). Organization and function of a pain clinic. *Advances in Neurology, 4,* 433–443.

Brena, S. F. (1983). Pain control facilities: Roots, organization and function. In S. F. Brena & S. L. Chapman (Eds.), *Management of patients with chronic pain* (pp. 11–20). Jamaica, NY: Spectrum.

Cameron, N. A. (1945). *The Psychology of Behavior Disorders*. Boston: Houghton Mifflin.

Chapman, S. L. (1983a). Behavior modification. In S. F. Brena & S. L. Chapman (Eds.), *Management of patients with chronic pain* (pp. 145–159). Jamaica, NY: Spectrum.

Chapman, S. L. (1983b). Relaxation, biofeedback and self hypnosis. In S. F. Brena & S. L. Chapman (Eds.), *Management of patients with chronic pain* (pp. 161–172). Jamaica, NY: Spectrum.

Chaturvedi, S., & Michael, A. (1986). Chronic pain in a psychiatric clinic. *Journal of Psychosomatic Research, 30,* 347–354.

Dickes, R. A. (1974). Brief theory of conversion reactions: An in-hospital technique. *American Journal of Psychiatry, 131,* 584–586.

Engel, G. L. (1959). "Psychogenic" pain and the pain-prone patient. *American Journal of Medicine, 36,* 899–918.

Flor-Henry, P., Frown-Augh, D., Tepper, M., & Schopflocher, D. (1981). A neuropsychological study of the stable syndrome of hysteria. *Biological Psychiatry, 16,* 601–626.

Folks, D. G., Ford, C. V., & Regan, W. M. (1984). Conversion symptoms in a general hospital. *Psychosomatics, 25,* 285–295.

Ford, C. V. (1983). *The somatizing disorders: Illness as a way of life*. New York: Elsevier.

Ford, C. V. (1984). Somatizing disorders. In H. B. Robach (Ed.), *Helping patients and their families cope with medical problems* (pp. 39–59). San Francisco: Jossey-Bass.

Ford, C. V. (1986). The somatizing disorders. *Psychosomatics, 27,* 327–337.

Ford, C. V., & Folks, D. G. (1985). Conversion disorders: An overview. *Psychosomatics, 26,* 371–383.

Ford, C. V., & Long, K. D. (1977). Group psychotherapy of somatizing patients. *Psychotherapy and Psychosomatics, 28,* 294–304.

Fordyce, W. E. (1974). Pain viewed as learned behavior. *Advances in Neurology, 4,* 415–422.

France, R. D., Krishnan, K. R. R., Houpt, J. L., & Maltbie, A. A. (1984). Differentiation of depression from chronic pain with the dexamethasone suppression test and DSM-III. *American Journal of Psychiatry, 141,* 1577–1579.

Gillespie, R. D. (1928). Hypochondria—Its definition nosology and psychopathology. *Guy's Hospital Reports, 78,* 408–460.

Gordon, E., Kraiuhin, C., Meares, R., & Howson, A. (1986). Auditory evoked response potentials in somatization disorder. *Journal of Psychiatric Research, 20,* 237–248.

Guze, S. G. (1983). Studies in hysteria. *Canadian Journal of Psychiatry, 28,* 434–437.

Guze, S. G., Woodruff, R. A., & Clayton, P. J. (1971). Hysteria and antisocial behavior: Further evidence of an association. *American Journal of Psychiatry, 127,* 957–960.

Hafeiz, H. B. (1980). Hysterical conversion: A prognostic study. *British Journal of Psychiatry, 136,* 548–551.

Hendler, N. H. (1984). Chronic pain. In H. B. Roback (Ed.), *Helping patients and their families cope with medical problems* (pp. 79–106). San Francisco: Jossey-Bass.

Herman, E., & Baptiste, S. (1981). Pain control: Mastery through group experience. *Pain, 10,* 79–86.

Hollender, M. H. (1980). The case of Anna O: A reformation. *American Journal of Psychiatry, 137,* 797–800.

Hopkinson, G. (1973). The psychiatric syndrome of infestation. *Psychiatric Clinics, 6,* 330–345.

Hudgens, A. (1979). Family-oriented treatment of chronic pain. *Journal of Marital and Family Therapy, 5,* 67–78.

Katon, W., Kleinman, A., & Rosen, G. (1982a). Depression and somatization: A review, Part 1. *American Journal of Medicine, 72,* 127–135.

Katon, W., Kleinman, A., & Rosen, G. (1982b). Depression and somatization: A review, Part 2. *American Journal of Medicine, 72,* 241–247.

Kellner, R. (1982). Psychotherapeutic strategies in hypochondriasis: A clinical study. *American Journal of Psychotherapy, 36,* 146–157.

Kellner, R. (1983). Prognosis of treated hypochondriasis. *Acta Psychiatrica Scandanavia, 67,* 69–79.

Kutcher, M., & Ford, C. V. (1985). Diagnosis and management of the hypochondriacal patient. *Comprehensive Therapy, 11,* 54–58.

Large, R. (1980). The psychiatrist and the chronic pain patient: 172 anecdotes. *Pain, 9,* 253–263.

Liebowitz, M. D., & Klein, D. F. (1979). Hysteroid dysphoria. In H. Akiskal (Ed.), *Affective disorders: Special clinical forms. Psychiatric Clinics of North American,* 2(3), 555–579.

Lindsay, P. G., & Wyckoff, M. (1981). The depression-pain syndrome and its response to antidepressants. *Psychosomatics, 22,* 571–577.

Lipsitt, D. R. (1970). Medical and psychological characteristics of "crocks." *Psychiatry in Medicine, 1,* 15–20.

Liskow, B., Othmer, E., Penick, E. C., & DeSouza, C. (1986). Is Briquet's syndrome a heterogenous disorder? *American Journal of Psychiatry, 143,* 626–629.

Livingston, R. (1987). Maternal somatization disorder and Munchausen syndrome by proxy. *Psychosomatics, 28,* 213–217.

Livingston, R., & Martin-Cannici, C. (1985). Multiple somatic complaints and possible somatization disorder in prepubertal children. *Journal of the American Academy of Child Psychiatry, 24,* 603–607.

Loeser, J. D., Bluck, R. G., & Christman, A. (1975). Relief of pain by transcutaneous stimulation. *Journal of Neurosurgery, 42,* 308–314.

Ludwig, A. M. (1972). Hysteria: A neurobiologic theory. *Archives of General Psychiatry, 27,* 771–777.

Mai, G. M., & Merskey, H. (1981). Briquet's concept of hysteria: An historical perspective. *Canadian Journal of Psychiatry, 26,* 57–63.

Mally, M. A., & Ogston, W. D. (1964). Treatment of the "untreatables." *International Journal of Group Psychotherapy, 14,* 369–374.

Maris, D. P. (1945). Intravenous barbituates: An aid in the diagnosis and treatment or conversion hysteria and malingering. *Military Surgeon, 96,* 509–513.

Mathew, R. J., Weinman, M. L., & Mirabi, M. (1981). Physical symptoms of depression. *British Journal of Psychiatry, 139,* 293–296.

Munro, A. (1988). Monosymptomatic hypochondriacal psychoses: A diagnostic entity which may respond to Pimozide. *Canadian Psychiatric Association Journal, 23,* 497–500.

Murphy, G. E. (1982). The clinical management of hysteria. *Journal of the American Medical Association, 247,* 2559–2564.

Nadelson, T. (1979). The Munchausen spectrum. *General Hospital Psychiatry, 1,* 11–17.

Phillips, M. R., Ward, N. G., & Reis, N. K. (1983). Factitious mourning: Painless patienthood. *American Journal of Psychiatry, 140,* 420–425.

Pilowsky, I. (1970). Primary and secondary hypochondriasis. *Acta Psychiatrica Scandanavia, 46,* 273–285.

Pinsky, J. S. (1978). Chronic, intractable, benign pain: A syndrome and its treatment with intensive short-term group psychotherapy. *Journal of Human Stress, 4,* 17–21.

Purtell, J. J., Robins, E., & Cohen, M. E. (1951). Observations on clinical aspects of hysteria: A quantative study of 50 hysteria patients and 156 control subjects. *Journal of the American Medical Association, 146,* 902–909.

Raskin, M., Talbott, J. A., & Meyerson, A. T. (1966). Diagnosed conversion reactions: Predictive value of psychiatric criteria. *Journal of the American Medical Association, 1997,* 530–534.

Ritvo, J., & Thompson, T., II. (1986). A 49-year-old clinic for chronically ill somatizers. *Hospital and Community Psychiatry, 37,* 631–633.

Sapira, J. D. (1972). Reassurance therapy: What to say to symptomatic patients with benign diseases. *Annals of Internal Medicine, 77,* 603–604.

Schoenberg, B., & Senescu, R. (1966). Group psychotherapy for patients with chronic multiple somatic complaints. *Journal of Chronic Diseases, 19,* 649–657.

Sheehan, D. V., & Sheehan, K. H. (1982). The classification of anxiety and hysterical states: 1. Historical review and empirical delineation. *Journal of Clinical Psychopharmacology, 2,* 235–244.

Silberman, E., & Sullivan, J. (1984). Atypical depression. *Psychiatric Clinics of North America, 7,* 535–547.

Slater, E., & Glithero, E. (1965). A followup of patients diagnosed as suffering from hysteria. *Journal of Psychosomatic Research, 9,* 9–13.

Smith, G., Jr., Monson, R., & Ray, D. (1986). Psychiatric consultation in somatization disorders. *New England Journal of Medicine, 314,* 1407–1413.

Swanson, D. W., & Maruta, T. (1980). Patients complaining of extreme pain. *Mayo Clinic Proceedings, 55,* 563–566.

Timmermans, G., & Sternbach, R. A. (1974). Factors of human chronic pain: An analysis of personality and pain reaction variables. *Science, 184,* 806–808.

Valko, R. J. (1976). Group therapy for patients with hysteria (Briquet's disorder). *Diseases of the Nervous System, 37,* 384–487.

Veith, I. (1965). *Hysteria: A history of disease.* Chicago: University of Chicago Press.

Wahl, C. W. (1964). Psychodynamics of the hypochondriacal patient. In C. W. Wahl (Ed.), *New dimensions in psychosomatic medicine* (pp. 201–214). Boston: Little, Brown.

Watson, C. G., & Buranen, C. (1979). The frequency and identification of false positive conversion reactions. *Journal of Nervous and Mental Disease, 167,* 243–247.

West, E. D., & Dally, J. P. (1959). Effects of iproniazid in depressive syndromes. *British Medical Journal, 1,* 1491–1494.

Whitlock, F. (1967). The aetiology of hysteria. *Acta Psychiatrica Scandanavia, 43,* 144–162.

Woerner, P. I., & Guze, S. B. (1968). A family and marital study of hysteria. *British Journal of Psychiatry, 114,* 161–168.

Zoccolillo, M., & Cloninger, C. (1986). Excess medical care of women with somatization disorder. *Southern Medical Journal, 79,* 532–535.

14

Borderline Disorders

PAUL H. SOLOFF

INTRODUCTION

The diagnosis of borderline disorder is among the most controversial in modern psychiatry. It is a concept whose origins extend into the last century; yet it has only recently achieved official status as a psychiatric disorder in the third edition of the American Psychiatric Association's Diagnostic and Statistical Manual of Mental Disorders (APA, 1980) (DSM-III). Controversy continues over the reliability and validity of the construct and the criteria used to define it. Despite the academic debate, the popularity of the clinical concept continues to grow. Estimates of the prevalence of the borderline diagnosis range from 7.8% of admissions to the psychiatric ward of a general teaching hospital (Mack, 1975) to 25% of admissions to a psychoanalytic psychiatric institute (Andrulonis, Glueck, Stroebel, Vogel, Shapiro, & Aldridge, 1981).

Borderline patients are among the most difficult patients to treat. They present with affective, schizotypal, and impulsive behavioral symptoms in bewildering combinations. Their episodic decompensations appear to be related to the stress of everyday life but present with such severity as to raise questions concerning biological dysregulation of affect, thought, and action. The response to treatment may be diagnostic more than therapeutic, as the patient endeavors to involve the therapist in his or her conflicts. Psychological modalities appear inadequate to manage the symptomatic states of the borderline patient, and medication fails to address the learned traits of behavior that render the patient chronically maladaptive. Although psychiatric schools of thought have staunchly defined their perspectives on the borderline patient, none can claim a superior understanding or method of management. In short, the diagnosis and treatment of the borderline patient remain the focus of considerable debate and controversy. This unresolved controversy is best appreciated through an exploration of its conceptual origins.

PAUL H. SOLOFF • Western Psychiatric Institute and Clinic, University of Pittsburgh, Pittsburgh, Pennsylvania 15213.

The concept of a borderline disorder evolved from efforts to define and to more clearly separate delimited neurotic and psychotic disorders. The "borderline case" was one that had attributes of both neurotic and psychotic functioning, a patient occupying the symptomatic "borderland" between these two organizing principles of psychiatric classification (Mack, 1975). Over 30 descriptive terms have been applied to patients who demonstrate a vulnerability to psychotic experience under stress but function in a neurotic, odd, or merely eccentric fashion in their everyday lives. Both descriptive and psychoanalytic schools of thought have contributed to the evolution and definition of the concept, as each has grappled with these patients from their own unique perspectives.

The descriptive, empirical school, especially under the influence of Bleuler (1950) described chronically maladaptive, odd, eccentric personalities who bore a resemblance to schizophrenic spectrum disorders but did not actually develop clinical psychosis. These "near-psychotic" individuals demonstrated a "soft" thought disorder, manifested by distortions of thinking (without overt looseness); magical, noncausal, illogical thoughts; and micropsychotic episodes (especially under emotional duress). They tended to be isolative, odd individuals, with superficial interpersonal relations, severe widespread anxiety, chaotic sexual adaptation, anhedonia, and ambivalence. The development of Rorschach's projective techniques gave additional definition to this group of patients, who demonstrated mildly disordered thinking on the inkblot test without dysfunction on more structured tests of cognition. The diagnostic formulations of *latent schizophrenia, borderline schizophrenia,* and *ambulatory schizophrenia* described individuals who were felt to have a *formes frustes* of the more severe psychotic disorder (Bleuler, 1911/1950; Knight, 1954; Zilboorg, 1941).

Hoch and Polatin (1949) and Hoch and Cattell (1959) described one such group as "pseudoneurotic schizophrenics." These patients were characterized by a multiplicity of neurotic symptoms ("pan-neurosis"), free-floating anxiety ("pan-anxiety"), and distorted interpersonal relationships, including primitive sexual adaptations ("polymorphous perverse sexuality"). Many had "soft" thought disorders—especially under duress—leading Hoch to classify his pseudoneurotic patients within the schizophrenic spectrum. (Hoch and Polatin, 1949).

The longitudinal study of individuals with odd-eccentric lifestyles and mild distortions of thinking led to a better understanding of the long-term stability of this pattern and, ultimately, to the definition of the schizotypal personality disorder as a separate diagnostic entity in the DSM-III. Although longitudinal studies indicate no clinical deterioration of schizotypal patients into schizophrenic psychosis, individuals in this group (e.g., borderline schizophrenics) may have a familial link to the psychotic disorder, and they may share some biological markers (Siever, 1981, 1985; Siever & Gunderson, 1979). Within a spectrum of borderline disorders, the schizotypal group represents the "border" with schizophrenia.

The second major conceptual contribution to the borderline diagnosis came from the work of the psychoanalytic school. Where the descriptive tradition typically defined "near-psychotic" disorders in a hospital or a clinic setting, psychoanalysts described a more functional outpatient population complaining of a multiplicity of neurotic and affective symptoms in the context of intensive psychoanalysis. As therapeutic work progressed with these patients, their defensive and symptomatic manifestations typically became more primitive. They tended to lose a "sense of reality" and to regress in the unstructured analytic setting, "uncovering" a vulnerability to psychosis (Frosch, 1964). Reality testing was not lost, as in the case of the schizophrenic psychosis, but "suspended" and contingent on external support of ego functioning. Transference reactions were rapid and primitive, often bordering on the psychotic. The patient's multiple neurotic complaints represented defensive operations against a more primitive disorganization of thinking and behavior. Regression in the analytic setting mimicked stress-related responses occurring elsewhere in the patient's life in response to emotional upset or rejection. External limits and structure were necessary for the reorganization of function.

Patients who demonstrated serious regression in the psychoanalytic setting often presented with predominantly affective symptoms, emotional instability, and hysterical character traits (Easser & Lesser, 1965; Marmor, 1953; Zetzel, 1971). These patients, termed *primitive oral hysterics* or *emotionally unstable character disorders*, constituted a group arising from the "border" with affective disorders. Such patients were typically highly social, impulsive, and emotionally labile, with frequent but brief and intensive depressive crashes. Under stress, these individuals could develop transient referential thinking, paranoid ideation, and dissociative experiences, which established an overlap of symptom presentation with the borderline patients from the schizotypal end of the spectrum. From this largely psychoanalytic experience has come the definition of the unstable borderline personality disorder of the DSM-III.

The heterogeneity of the clinical presentations in borderline patients, including affective, schizotypal, and impulsive-behavioral symptoms, has led to many theoretical efforts to unify the group of borderline disorders around some common organizing principle. These theoretical constructs focus on the patients' vulnerability to loss of reality testing when faced with significant interpersonal stress (e.g., Frosch's psychotic character, 1964) and on the dynamics of the unstable interpersonal relationships formed by these patients (e.g., Masterson, 1976; Rinsley, 1978). Perhaps the most widely applied theoretical system is that of Otto Kernberg (1967, 1975), who defined the borderline personality as a metapsychological *organization* of personality functions, with specific deficits determining the patient's adaptational style. Borderline personality organization is, in Kernberg's terms, a *structural* diagnosis, a specific organization of ego and superego functioning around which develop secondary traits that comprise specific character types (i.e., Axis II diagnoses). Latent borderline-personality organization is made manifest by specific deficits in reality testing under duress, by a syndrome of identity diffusion, and by the use of primitive defenses such as splitting and projective identification. This theoretical construct allows for heterogeneity in the manifest character presentation (e.g., descriptive diagnosis), as the structural diagnosis defines the underlying adaptational level of the patient's personality. Borderline personality organization may be conceptualized as the steel infrastructure of a building over which can be built any of a variety of stylized facades representing the manifest character type.

SPECIAL DIAGNOSTIC AND DEVELOPMENTAL CONSIDERATIONS

Empirical Studies

Empirical efforts to develop reliable psychiatric criteria for the borderline diagnosis began with the work of writers such as Robert Knight (1954) and Roy Grinker (Grinker, Werble, & Drye, 1968), who formulated specific inclusion criteria for their concepts. The work of Grinker, in particular, was instrumental in turning the study of borderline disorders toward empirical research. Grinker developed a cluster-analytic technique to define subtypes of the borderline syndrome using prospectively collected observational data from hospitalized patients. This method defined a group of patients at the "psychotic border" (Group I), a core borderline syndrome (Group II), an adaptive but affectless "as-if" group (Group III), and a group of patients at the "neurotic border" (Group IV) (Grinker, Werble, & Drye, 1968). Following in Grinker's footsteps, more recent researchers have focused on the development of reliable and valid diagnostic criteria and objective assessment measures for this group of disorders.

To define a valid psychiatric diagnosis, one must first develop criteria of inclusion and exclusion that separate the disorder from similar conditions. Gunderson and Singer (1975) reduced the extensive lists of diagnostic criteria in the descriptive literature into six categories that they felt characterized borderline patients: (1) an intense affect, usually hostile or depressed; (2) a history of impulsive behavior; (3) social adaptiveness in the face of a chaotic, emotional interpersonal style; (4) brief psychotic experiences; (5) unstable interpersonal relationships characterized by superficiality or, conversely, intense dependence; and (6) evidence of thought disorder on unstructured psychological tests (e.g., the Rorschach inkblot technique), but not on structured tests of cognitive functioning (e.g., the WAIS). Gunderson and associates (Gunderson & Kolb, 1978; Gunderson, Kolb, & Austin, 1981) incorporated these clinical criteria for borderline disorder into a semistructured Diagnostic Interview for Borderlines, which was shown to discriminate borderline from depressed and schizophrenic patients and borderline from nonborderline patients with a high degree of sensitivity and specificity (Kolb & Gunderson, 1980). The most discriminating features of the borderline disorder proved to be a history of impulsive-destructive behavior and a pattern of intense chaotic and pathological interpersonal relations (Gunderson, 1982).

Perry and Klerman (1978) reviewed the extensive psychiatric literature on borderline disorders, comparing the diagnostic systems proposed by Knight (1954), Kernberg (1975), Grinker (1968), and Gunderson and Singer (1975). There was little overlap among the criteria derived from mental status, personal history, interpersonal relationships, defensive style, or overall personality functioning, a finding suggesting that the borderline spectrum was too heterogeneous to provide reliable diagnostic criteria. Perry and Klerman then conducted their own prospective clinical study of borderline patients in a psychiatric emergency room using an ego functions inventory derived from their earlier literature review (Perry & Klerman, 1980). Patients defined clinically as borderline were compared to control patients with schizophrenia, personality disorder, neurosis, or adjustment disorder, and they were shown to differ significantly in nine major content areas: (1) anxiety intolerance; (2) self-destructive dyscontrol of impulses and anger; (3) regression in the context of treatment; (4) over-dependence in close relationships; (5) anger and hostility in close relationships; (6) unstable perception of others; (7) disturbance in self-perception and identity; (8) chronic feelings of emptiness; and (9) behavioral regression during crises.

Subsequent studies using Gunderson's Diagnostic Interview for Borderlines (e.g., Soloff & Ulrich, 1981), Perry's Borderline Personality Scale, or related symptom checklists (e.g., Sheehy, Goldsmith, & Charles, 1980) have replicated the discrimination of borderline from schizophrenic, neurotic, and nonborderline personality-disorder patients. The reliability and validity of the diagnostic criteria for borderline disorders have been tested by means of structured and unstructured interview methods, checklists, and psychological test batteries, in both inpatient and outpatient settings. In each instance, statistical studies by analysis of variance and discriminate-function analyses have demonstrated the separation of borderline from nonborderline patients, most notably from those with depressed, schizophrenic, and other personality disorders. Despite great differences in method, sample, and setting, these studies concur on the diagnostic criteria for borderline disorder and its discriminating features (Gunderson, 1982).

In the development of the DSM-III, Spitzer, Endicott, and Gibbon (1979) chose to preserve the historical dichotomy between schizotypal and affective dimensions of the borderline disorder and then developed two separate checklists for an "unstable" and a schizotypal borderline variant. The diagnostic criteria for these two subtypes were found to be statistically independent dimensions of the borderline concept; however, half of borderline patients met the criteria for both (Spitzer & Endicott, 1979). The diagnostic considerations discussed in this chapter follow the Gunderson model and use the DSM-III definitions as a means of subtyping the borderline into its unstable and schizotypal variants (Table 1).

Developmental Origins

The borderline diagnosis defines a heterogeneous group of patients with affective, schizotypal, and impulsive-behavioral symptoms. Although statistical reliability has been achieved for sets of diagnostic criteria, the long-term stability and validity of the borderline disorder as a discrete diagnostic entity remain to be clearly established. Given the heterogeneity of symptom presentation and the absence of a common natural history, it is no wonder that the developmental origin of the borderline disorder remains a matter of theoretical conjecture. Students of developmental process generally begin with subtype classifications based on adult psychopathology and then infer developmental origins retrospectively by using genetic, psychodynamic, and neurobehavioral theoretical models. Given our rudimentary understanding of the borderline disorder, we assume that these hypothetical origins are neither all-inclusive nor mutually exclusive. Questions of comorbidity among related disorders and inclusion within the borderline concept of special symptom disorders (e.g., bulimia) make a single developmental origin unlikely or, if present, difficult to isolate. Proposed subtypes of the borderline disorder include (1) the unstable affective borderline; (2) the schizotypal borderline; (3) the "organic" borderline; and (4) the "core" characterological borderline. For patients in the affective and schizotypal borderline subtypes, a genetic-familial etiology is generally proposed on the basis of their close association with the parent disorders.

The Affective Borderline

The etiology of the unstable borderline subtype is inseparable from the question of discrimination from its next neighbor, depression. Empirical surveys of patients with DSM-III borderline personality disorder indicate a prevalence of major depression in 14%–50% of patients, depending on the survey method (Kroll, Sines, & Martin, 1981; Pope, Jonas, Hudson, Cohen, & Gunderson, 1983). From a different perspective, Akiskal (1981) reported up to 39% of a similarly defined sample of borderline outpatients with subaffective or atypical affective disorders. Family studies of DSM-III borderline patients report a higher incidence of affective disorders in the first-degree relatives of borderline probands (Baron, Gruen, Asnis, & Lord, 1985; Loranger, Oldham, & Tulis, 1982 Soloff & Millward, 1983; Stone, 1981). This frequent comorbidity with affective disorder begs

Table 1. Diagnostic Criteria for Borderline Disorders

Source: Diagnostic Interview for Borderline Patients, Gunderson, Kolb, and Austin (1981) Method: Semistructured interview, 29 scored statements in 5 sections.	Source: Symptom Checklist, Sheehy, Goldsmith, and Charles (1980). Method: 16 items in 6 sections.	Source: Borderline Personality Disorder Scale—II, Perry and Klerman (1980) Method: Structured interview, 36 items in 9 sections	Source: DSM-III Checklist, Spitzer, Endicott, and Gibbon (1979). Method: 8 items
1. Social adaptiveness (includes stability at work or school, social life, appropriate behavior with peers). 2. Impulse action patterns (includes suicide threat, gesture, self-mutilation, drug abuse, promiscuity, etc.). 3. Affect (depressed or hostile, demanding, entitled, chronic dysphoria, anhedonia, emptiness, loneliness). 4. Psychosis (includes derealization, depersonalization, brief paranoid experience, transient psychosis in psychotherapy, regression in hospital). 5. Interpersonal relations (includes intolerance of being alone, intense unstable relations, social isolation, manipulation, idealization, devaluation, dependency).	1. Thought (includes episodic distortion of reality, dissociation, periodic use of projection with an imparied sense of reality). 2. Feelings and impulses (excessively strong impulses and feelings with difficulty in managing impulses, anhedonia, limited capacity to tolerate unpleasant affect). 3. Identity (difficulty maintaining a stable sense of self). 4. Neurotic symptoms (includes periodic phobias, obsessions, compulsions, hypochondriasis, abuse of drugs and/or alcohol). 5. Sexual behavior (unstable sexual behavior, promiscuity, bizarre sexual fantasies). 6. Interpersonal relationships (overidealization, excessive derogation of others, periodic withdrawal into partial or complete isolation).	1. Anxiety intolerance (includes episodic depersonalization, transient psychotic episodes). 2. Self-destructive dyscontrol of impulses and anger. 3. Regression in the context of psychiatric treatment (includes psychotic episodes developed or exacerbated by psychotherapy or psychiatric hospitalization). 4. Overdependency in close relationships (includes intolerance of being alone). 5. Anger and hostility arising in close relationships. 6. Unstable perception of others. 7. Disturbance in self-perception and identity. 8. Chronic feelings of emptiness. 9. Behavioral regression during crises (mental status items include anger at a variety of targets, devaluing, demanding, entitled).	A. (Unstable) borderline personality disorder 1. Impulsivity or unpredictability in self-damaging areas. 2. A pattern of unstable and intense interpersonal relationships. 3. Inappropriate, intense anger and lack of control 4. Identity disturbance. 5. Affective instability. 6. Intolerance of being alone. 7. Physically self-damaging acts (suicidal gestures, self-mutilation). 8. Chronic feelings of emptiness or boredom. B. Schizotypal personality 1. Magical thinking. 2. Ideas of reference. 3. Social isolation. 4. Recurrent illusions (including derealization-depersonalization). 5. Odd speech (not looseness). 6. Inadequate rapport in face-to-face interaction. 7. Suspiciousness or paranoid ideation. 8. Undue social anxiety or hypersensitivity to real or imagined criticism.

the question of whether the depressed borderline patient has one disorder or two. Indeed, Akiskal (1981) proposed that the borderline disorder itself be considered an atypical or "subaffective" disorder, noting that borderline patients share some biological markers with depressed patients, (e.g., they have the short REM-latency marker on EEG polysomnography studies, which is found in some borderline outpatients even when they are not depressed). Carroll, Greden, and Feinberg (1981) complicated this perspective by suggesting that borderline psychopathology may mask major depression, even of the endogenous subtype. The developmental origin of the affective borderline disorder appears to be very much linked to depression, whether the borderline itself is viewed as an affective disorder or as a frequent host to concurrent affective disorders. Gunderson and Elliot (1985) suggested that the two may arise from a common developmental *anlage* and that they differentiate according to life experience.

The Schizotypal Borderline

The relationship of the schizotypal borderline disorder to schizophrenia is based more on symptom similarity than on any clearly defined genetic or familial link. Carpenter, Gunderson, and Strauss (1977) found that 45% of their borderline sample had transient paranoid and depressive delusions, 20% had hallucinations, and 60% depersonalization or derealization on the Present State Examination. In the Danish adoption studies of Kety, Rosenthal, Wender, and Schulsinger (1968), the borderline schizophrenic was defined by a disorder of thinking, manifested by strange or atypical mentation, brief episodes of cognitive distortion, anhedonia, interpersonal behavior lacking in depth, chaotic sexual adjustment, multiple neurotic manifestations, and severe widespread anxiety. Among the relatives of the index schizophrenic adoptees were individuals with borderline schizophrenia. The pattern of schizophrenic spectrum disorders appearing among the biological relatives of index adoptees with borderline schizophrenia was not significantly different from that among the biological relatives of chronic schizophrenic index patients.

Siever and Gunderson (1979) reviewed the Danish adoption data and found significantly greater numbers of borderline patients among the biological relatives of chronic schizophrenics than among control patients. They suggested that borderline patients, as defined by the Kety *et al.* criteria, have less of a genetic loading for schizophrenia than chronic schizophrenics. Kendler (1985), also reanalyzing the Danish adoption data, applied the DSM-III criteria for schizotypal personality disorder (SPD) to interview data from the biological and adoptive relatives of the index schizophrenic adoptees and found a significantly higher prevalence of SPD in the biological relatives of schizophrenic adoptees than in the biological relatives of controls. Schizotypal disorder and borderline schizophrenia (Kety definition) were found to be related but not identical concepts. Nonetheless, Kendler supported a genetic link between schizophrenia and DSM-III SPD. To complete the circle, Spitzer *et al.* (1979), using the DSM-III criteria, found that 54% of clinically diagnosed borderline patients met the criteria for *both* SPD and BPD personality disorders.

Despite the overlap and the apparent relationship of SPD to borderline disorders, empirical studies of the families of borderline patients have found no increased incidence in the prevalence of schizophrenia among the relatives of borderline patients (Soloff & Millward, 1983). When a spectrum model is used, it is apparent that patients with DSM-III SPD lie close to the schizophrenic spectrum but that those with concurrent borderline disorder may not share the schizophrenic diathesis. Indeed, isolated, affectless schizotypes fail to meet the criteria for borderline disorder when that disorder is diagnosed by means of a structured interview such as Gunderson's Diagnostic Interview for Borderlines. The isolated, affectless SPD patient is therefore screened out of most studies of borderline disorder when the Gunderson criteria are used. To foreshadow a later discussion, pharmacological trials on patients with borderline disorder have demonstrated efficacy for low-dose neuroleptics against many schizotypal features of the borderline patient, a finding suggesting that these schizotypal features are state manifestations rather than enduring trait disorders. These features include the referential thinking, paranoid ideation, derealization, and depersonalization that accompany stress-related decompensations in the borderline patient. These symptoms contribute to the diagnosis of schizotypal disorder in cross-sectional evaluations but tend to remit with low-dose neuroleptics or the support and structure of a therapeutic setting. Our pharmacotherapy results challenge the validity of the association of SPD with borderline disorder.

The Organic Borderline

It has long been observed that patients with childhood histories of attention deficit disorder (ADD), encephalitis, epilepsy, and episodic dyscontrol syndromes manifest in adult life symptoms that overlap the phenomenology of borderline disorders. Thus, "classic" borderline symptoms such as impulsiveness, low frustration tolerance, labile affect, temper tantrums, defective sense of identity, low self-esteem, and manipulative behavior may be related to the deficits in inhibitory controls over attention, cognition, affect, and impulse that follow developmental or traumatic CNS insult (Hartocollis, 1979; Murray, 1979).

This theoretical perspective constitutes the neurobehavioral model of borderline development. The neurobehavioral model views the borderline style as an adaptation to childhood CNS dysfunction, which impairs integrative and inhibitory capacities. Andrulonis, Glueck, Stroebel, Vogel, Shapiro, and Aldridge (1981) described the frequent association of borderline personality disorder and childhood histories of ADD and learning disability in young male patients. Their female patients, more typical of the borderline pattern in general, did not share the high prevalence of CNS deficits. In systematically conducted surveys of consecutively admitted adult patients with borderline disorder, Soloff and Millward (1983) found no increased incidence of adverse medical conditions in childhood when they compared borderline with depressed and schizophrenic patients. In this study, there were no differences between groups for developmental milestones in childhood. Learning difficulties were more prevalent among schizophrenic than among borderline patients, who, in turn, had significantly more difficulties than depressed patients. Borderline patients did have a significantly higher incidence of childhood temper tantrums and a tendency toward more phobic behavior in childhood than the control groups. The bulk of the developmental evidence suggests that neurobehavioral deficits play a role in the development of borderline personality disorder among a very small number of borderline patients.

Examining the EEGs of consecutively admitted borderline adults produces a similar impression, namely, a very small number of significant abnormalities among borderline patients (Cornelius, Brenner, Soloff, Schulz, & Tumuluru, 1986). Although neurobehavioral factors may contribute to the development of borderline characteristics in selected populations (e.g., young males with attention deficit disorder), they are not a highly prevalent problem contributing to adult psychopathology in the predominately female borderline population.

The Core Characterological Borderline

The largest group of patients with borderline personality disorder provide unequivocal histories of long-standing maladaptive interpersonal relationships and impulsive self-destructive behavior patterns clearly related to meaningful psychodynamic events. Early life experience undoubtedly plays a pre-eminent role in the development of the psychopathology of these patients. The "core" borderline patients have been studied for many years by psychoanalytic writers, who have developed internally consistent theories on their psychological development and their manifestations of psychopathology. The work of Otto Kernberg (1975), James Masterson (1976), and Donald Rinsley (1978) is particularly valuable to the practicing clinician, as it provides a metapsychological framework within which to conceptualize the behavior of the borderline patient and a rational approach to treatment derived from theory. Building on the developmental theories of Mahler, Pine, and Bergman (1975), these authors have postulated a pathological outcome in the child's development in the resolution of the separation–individuation phase, occurring between 18 and 36 months of age. Developmental arrest in the separation–individuation phase has profound effects on the structural configuration of the entire personality. From the analytic perspective, borderline personality disorder is a structural diagnosis, a metapsychological construct defining the relationship between ego and superego functioning and instinctual drives. The borderline personality structure is viewed as a specific organization of these functions, with definable strengths and vulnerabilities.

Goldstein (1983) summarized the ego strengths of the borderline patient as the relative intactness of the reality testing of thought processes (i.e., *relative* to psychotic structure), of interpersonal relations, and of adaptation to reality. The patients' ego weaknesses are defined as a combination of poor impulse control and poor frustration tolerance, a proclivity to use primitive ego defenses, a syndrome of identity diffusion, and a characteristic affective instability. The borderline patients' superego is seen as overly punitive and the ego ideal as overly idealized. The instinctual drives of the patient suffer from a prevalence of aggression.

Failure to complete separation-individuation results in a failure to develop emotional object constancy. The inability of these patients to hold within themselves the image of a loving family and friends, with associated feeling states, leaves them in a state of object hunger, constantly driven to seek reassurance of the love of the significant others in their lives. This drive motivates much of these patients' manipulation and demandingness. The loss of relationship in the real world (or the threat of loss) leaves the patient feeling empty, hollow, and abandoned. Without emotional object constancy, there is no continuity or support for self-esteem from internally held objects. In a paniclike reaction, borderline patients manifest impulsive-destructive acts to end these intolerable affects. In the course of development, borderline patients typically resolve some of this need through the use of transitional objects. The security blanket or teddy bear of normal development becomes the model for relationships in the borderline adult.

Other important elements of adult borderline psychopathology are directly attributed to this developmental etiology. The borderline adult demonstrates a persistent splitting of aggressive from libidinal drives, a developmental separation of self and object representations into positively held aspects (associated with libidinal drive) termed *good self* or *good object*, and conversely, negatively held aspects (associated with aggressive drive) termed *bad self* or *bad object*. Kernberg (1975) conjectured that the splitting mechanism is a defensive operation that, in childhood, preserved some positive attachment to a "good mother" in the face of the overwhelming negative experience of the mothering caretaker. Together, the failure of object constancy and the persistence of defensive splitting dominate the quality of the interpersonal world of the borderline adults.

Although borderline patients share a set of structural personality vulnerabilities, the formal descriptive diagnosis (i.e., DSM-III) that is given to the patient depends on many factors unique to the individual, including specific childhood experience and acculturation. When Kernberg's definition is used, there are many patients with differing DSM-III personality diagnoses who have the same underlying structural borderline-personality organization. Because of the obvious relationship between personality organization and the potential for healthy adaptation, these DSM-III diagnoses are typically those of lower level character disorders such as schizoid, paranoid, or narcissistic types. For purposes of research, the absence of a direct correlation between structural and descriptive diagnoses makes difficult the definition of homogeneous samples. The structural diagnosis is made by analytic researchers on the basis of an open-ended "structural interview," assessing the adequacy of reality testing, the nature of defensive functioning, and the proof of identity diffusion (Kernberg, Goldstein, Carr, Hunt, Bauer, & Blumenthal, 1981). However, this search for the structural characteristics of borderline personality organization requires dynamic training, so that it is unsuitable as a vehicle for general use as an objective, structured research interview. Nonetheless, the excellent correlation between theory and behavior makes the analytic approach a useful tool for clinical practice if not for practical research application at the present time.

Empirical studies confirm the early deprivation and pathology of family life in borderline patients (Bradley, 1979; Frank & Paris, 1981). Studies by Soloff and Millward (1983) document parental loss due to divorce or death occurring in the childhood of borderline patients with a higher frequency than in the families of depressed or schizophrenic controls. Adult borderline patients tend to view their mothers in terms of a conflictual, hostile relationship and see their fathers as absent or distant. Family studies by Shapiro *et al.* (Shapiro, Zinner, Shapiro, 1975) suggest that the borderline child is identified as a target for the projection of conflicted hostile motives and covert expectations on the part of other members of the family. In this sense, the borderline patient "acts out" family pathology (E. Shapiro, Zinner, and R. Shapiro, 1975).

Many authors (e.g., Wolberg, 1982) have commented on the borderline characteristics of the mothers of borderline patients, suggesting that the patient's maladaptive behavior is conditioned to the mother's needs at an early age. The mother of the borderline patients is said to reward dependent behavior and to punish independence through the withdrawal of affection, creating a conflictual model of object relationships (Masterson, 1976). Further research is needed to support and extend these valuable insights into a comprehensive developmental etiology of "core" borderline disorders.

FREQUENT CLINICAL PROBLEMS

Historically, the borderline disorder has been variously defined as a syndrome, a state, or a structural organization of personality, depending on the perspective and school of thought of the writer. It may be conceptualized as a discrete diagnostic entity, as a series of disorders lying on a severity continuum between severe character pathology and psychosis, or, in a mixed model, as a syndrome with distinguishing signs and symptoms arising from a continuum of disordered ego functioning. (Carpenter *et al.*, 1977) As noted above, there have been many efforts to define diagnostic criteria for borderline disorders based primarily on clinical observation. Recent empirical studies have demonstrated the statistical reliability of a syndromal definition of borderline disorder that uses semistructured diagnostic interviews and clearly defined diagnostic criteria. The best studied of these semistructured diagnostic interviews, Gunderson's Diagnostic Interview for Borderlines, has been shown to discriminate borderline from depressed, schizophrenic, and other personality-disordered patients in a variety of inpatient and outpatient settings (Gunderson & Kolb, 1978; Soloff & Ulrich, 1981). This diagnostic system surveys the patient's behavior in the areas of social adaptation, impulse action patterns, affects, psychotic experiences, and interpersonal relationships. It provides an excellent framework for discussion of the clinical problems and the presentation of the borderline patient (Gunderson *et al.*, 1981).

Social Adaptation

Gunderson and Singer (1975) noted that the discrepancy between the patient's intact intellectual performance on structured psychological tests, such as the Wechsler Adult Intelligence Scale, and impairment on the unstructured Rorschach inkblot, is a diagnostic indicator of borderline functioning. Such a discrepancy in performance replicates the observation that borderline patients can show a remarkable stability in structured, nonaffective situations, such as work or school, but may become cognitively and emotionally disorganized with situational stress. It may be expected that borderline patients will function up to the full capability of their intelligence in highly structured, nonaffective situations. Their difficulty in consistently attending school or holding jobs is attributable to the practical consequences of emotional turmoil or impulsive behavior rather than poor academic or vocational performance due to disorganized thinking or affective instability on the job. Frequent hospitalizations and the physical sequelae of overdose, drinking, or drug use make consistent performance on the job or in school more difficult. Borderline patients are often able to use the structure of work or school to "forget" or avoid emotional conflict. Given their ability to perform in structured, nonemotional settings, borderline patients are capable of the same range of special achievements or job effectiveness found in the nonpsychiatric population. These patients are active socially, mix well, and behave appropriately with peers. Superficially, they may appear quite functional to casual acquaintances, creating an illusion of normality.

Impulse Action

It is the area of impulse action that generally brings the borderline patient to clinical attention and ends the superficial illusion of normality. In the statistical analysis of diagnostic criteria, impulsive behavior (along with pathological interpersonal relations) is one of the most discriminating diagnostic criteria of borderline disorder. Impulse action patterns generally appear in the context of a perceived rejection or the threat of object loss. When borderline individuals experience rejection or perceive the threat of loss or separation, they experience powerful and primitive feelings of rage, abandonment, and depression and a sense of inner emptiness (Masterson, 1976). The impulsive behavior that follows may directly express the patients' anger, such as in self-mutilation or aggression, and may simultaneously "fill the void" left by the loss of the external object. Excessive drinking, food binging, drug abuse, or sexual promiscuity may all serve to fill the emptiness that the patient feels internally. The concrete, primitive quality of this dynamic suggests the validity of its origin in early childhood. Impulse actions may include overtly self-destructive acts, such as wrist slashing and self-mutilation, as well as manipulative suicide threats or efforts. They may involve multiple overdoses with drugs or persistent and sustained drug abuse. They may include impulsive promiscuity, ego-dystonic homosexual acts, or sexual deviance. Impulsive aggression toward others may include assaults or antisocial acts.

In our culture, patients with borderline personality disorder express self-destructiveness in fairly stereotypical fashion. Female borderlines follow a cultural pattern and express their hostility more toward themselves than toward others. Wrist cutting and overdosing are found more in the female borderline than in the male, who, in our culture, typically expresses narcissistic rage outwardly with assault or antisocial acts. This cultural bias and sexual stereotyping of symptoms undoubtedly causes a distortion in research studies, as most of the borderline patients found in mental hospitals are female and most male borderlines may be found in prison settings. Nonetheless, the antisocial acts and external aggression that may characterize the male response to perceived loss express the same needs as the female equivalent, where the aggression is more self-directed.

Affect

The discrimination of borderline from depressive disorders is often a matter of one's perspective. It is the "characterological" quality of the borderline patient's affect that discriminates this presentation from more classic depressive syndromes. Grinker, Werble, and Drye (1968) noted that "anger is the main or only affect of the borderline patient" (p. 90). Although borderline patients complain of chronic depressive mood, anhedonia, emptiness, and loneliness, their affect is generally dominated by a demanding, angry, sarcastic quality that discriminates them from the more typically self-effacing depressive patient. Indeed, the narcissism of borderline patients is expressed in a demanding and entitled manner despite the complaints of chronic depression.

Descriptively, the quality of the depressed mood of borderline patients meets more of the "atypical" pattern, with preservation of reactivity to external events, a tendency to overeat and oversleep, and a loss of energy and motivation. Patients report lifelong low self-esteem, which gives a depressive quality to the entire character structure, and which confounds efforts to define specific episodes of depressed mood. The chronic low self-esteem, which is part of the underlying character structure, gives rise to the appearance of "double depression" when a discrete major depression occurs in these characterologically depressed patients. Because the mood of the borderline patient is highly reactive to external input, there are marked mood shifts from normal to depressed lasting several hours to days following clear psychodynamic stressors. Less well recognized is the phenomenon of brief-lived euphoria and hyperactivity, which may also present in borderline patients, clearly precipitated by dynamic events and time-limited to several hours. Some investigators have cited these brief euphoric periods of hyperactivity and high mood as indicating an underlying diathesis to hypomania or bipolar disorder, although borderline patients may manifest this pattern episodically without ever reaching the degree of severity or duration required for a formal diagnosis of bipolar I or bipolar II disorder.

The inappropriate, intense anger, the frequent displays of temper, and the affective instability are included in the DSM-III as diagnostic criteria for borderline disorder, along with chronic feelings of emptiness and boredom.

Psychosis

The inclusion of micropsychotic experience as part of borderline psychopathology reflects both a historical perspective and empirical evidence demonstrating transient, stress-related lapses of reality testing in the borderline syndrome. Most frequently, these symptoms consist of episodes of derealization, depersonalization, mood-congruent paranoid ideation, and referential thinking. Micropsychotic experiences typically occur when the patient is under significant emotional duress.

The dissociative experience (derealization or depersonalization) appears to be a defense against overwhelming anxiety. The patient complains that reality itself appears to have changed, the world appearing different, as though made of "papier-mâché." Some patients feel that they are separated from the real world by a pane of glass or a fog, detached from reality as though they are not part of it. Others experience depersonalization, describing themselves as feeling dead or lifeless. Out-of-body experience, the feeling that one is outside oneself, observing from a distance, is frequently reported. Some patients in this dissociate state are anesthetic to pain and may cut or burn themselves to terminate the unpleasant dissociated state. Paranoid experiences not related to drug abuse are common in borderline patients. These patients tend to project angry feelings outward and feel that people in the community talk about them, stare at them, or make gestures toward them. Such referential thinking is always mood-congruent, dynamically motivated, and generally easily interpreted. It is important to note that the micropsychotic experience of the borderline patient reflects a temporary "suspension" of reality testing rather than a true loss of ability, as in schizophrenia. In the context of a diagnostic interview, the patient should be able to test the reality of referential thinking and paranoid ideation using the structure of the therapist's questions.

One unusual empirical finding among borderline patients is their vulnerability to disinhibition by marijuana, amphetamine, or other psychedelic drugs. In small amounts, these drugs often uncover psychotic experience quite unlike the experience of normal individuals. These psychotic experiences may persist long after the chemical effects of alcohol, marijuana, or amphetamine have passed. This effect has been demonstrated experimentally by Schulz, Cornelius, Schulz, Brenner, and Soloff (1984) for single doses of amphetamine as low as 30 mg, taken orally in a double-blind placebo-controlled experimental design. Gunderson *et al.* (1981) proposed this vulnerability as a diagnostic criterion for the borderline disorder.

Borderline patients do not experience the typical Schneiderian signs or symptoms of schizophrenia. They do not experience widespread delusions or schizophreniform hallucinations. If the borderline individual reports hallucinations, they are typically very colorful and dramatic, and are often directly related to the specific events of the moment. (It is useful to recall that this primitive quality of hallucination falls within the definition of stress-related "transient psychotic symptoms" cited as an associated feature of borderline personality disorder in DSM-III.)

Regression in the course of psychotherapy has been cited as a feature of the borderline disorder so common as to be a valuable, although *post hoc*, criterion for the diagnosis. The psychotherapeutic setting offers a perfect medium for regression into a dependent relationship in which the patient attempts to manipulate and control the therapist in the same pathological manner that characterizes relationships outside treatment. Prolonged hospitalization, in particular, often leads to progressively primitive efforts on the part of the patient to involve hospital staff in intense but pathological relations. These efforts often result in the patient's coercing more and more attention through self-abuse. Rather than respond positively to staff time and attention, the patient becomes progressively demanding and manipulative, with marked worsening of behavior. In the context of intensive psychotherapy, this behavior may involve ''acting out'' in the office or intruding in the therapist's personal life. The primitive quality of the patient's transference and its inappropriate and early manifestation in the treatment are practically diagnostic of borderline disorder.

Interpersonal Relations

Borderline individuals relate to their partners in an exploitive, manipulative pattern, using the partner to meet functional needs rather than relating to that partner as a separate individual with wants and needs of his or her own. These relationships tend to be intense and highly unstable, characterized by dependency and hostility. This quality of interpersonal relationships is easily distinguished from that of the borderline patient's depressed and schizophrenic ''next neighbors'' and is one of the most discriminating criteria in empirical studies (i.e., along with impulse action patterns). Borderline patients generally avoid being alone and make insistent demands for attention and for proof of love and caring. They often seek to take care of others and easily identify with other individuals who are in need of care and nurturance. They are often able to lavish love or attention on disabled or disadvantaged people and to experience gratification vicariously as though they themselves were being cared for. Many borderline patients find themselves conflicted over giving or receiving care. Despite the intense drive to have someone take care of them, they also have the resentment of an individual who feels that enough is never enough. After several experiences of perceived rejection, many borderline patients are reluctant to place themselves in this dependent posture. Many view their ''neediness'' as pathological at an adult level and come to hate that aspect of themselves, going to great lengths to avoid accepting care from others.

The relationships of borderline patients are characterized by devaluation, manipulation, hostility, dependency, and masochism. Patients often report feeling unlovable and basically worthless as human beings. They will accept physical abuse (in a masochistic pattern) as a sign of caring and concern rather than experience neglect or abandonment.

The adult relationships of the borderline patient reflect the defensive use of splitting, a direct result of the defect in separation-individuation in childhood development. Patients engage others in dyadic relationships according to the roles assigned in the internal splitting process. In a hospital setting, this symptom is manifested by splitting of the staff into ''good'' and ''bad'' objects, with corresponding countertransference problems. Borderline patients typically create ''special'' relationships with some staff members, sharing confidences that are to be kept separate from others (Burnham, 1966; Main, 1957). The manipulation of "good" and "bad" objects into confrontation over the patient is the general consequence. This pattern of relatedness is diagnostic of the borderline patient in long-term care and reflects the nature of the patient's relationships in everyday life.

TREATMENT APPLICATIONS

Psychosocial Approaches

There is no treatment of choice for borderline patients. The heterogeneity of the disorder and the complex mix of state and trait symptoms make it impossible to define a uniform approach to this group of patients. It is clear that neither psychotherapy nor pharmacotherapy consistently produces improvement but that many patients with borderline disorders improve modestly using elements of both. Proponents of psychotherapy for borderline disorder argue the merits of an intensive versus a supportive approach, some favoring psychoanalysis (with important modifications) and others a highly structured, supportive strategy. Behavior therapy, group therapy, and family therapy have all been recommended by their respective proponents. There are few empirical studies on the outcome of psychotherapy for borderline patients; however, even the most intensive work has produced modest results. Waldinger and Gunderson (1984) reported that only 33% of borderline patients treated privately by experienced analysts completed treatment, and that only 10% of these patients achieved a satisfactory therapeutic outcome. In general, these patients went from "moderately severe impairment to modest impairment" (Gunderson, 1984a, p. 75).

A discussion of specific psychotherapy methods is beyond the scope of this chapter. All psychosocial therapies dealing with the borderline patient have a core of common principles. The therapy itself may provide a source of support and structure for the patient, whether it is individual therapy, group therapy, or family-based therapy. Paradoxically, therapy may also elicit regression and primitive transference, which lead to impulsive-destructive "acting-out" behaviors. Psychotherapy for the borderline patient is not without risk as well as benefit. Before embarking on an intensive course of outpatient treatment, it is important to assess the patient's ability to bear painful affect, to contain primitive impulses, and to test reality.

The therapy may be intensive and anxiety-provoking, with a focus on uncovering and resolving unconscious conflict or, conversely, focused on reinforcing the patient's defenses and encouraging more adaptive behavior. As applied to psychoanalytic psychotherapy, Kernberg (1978) differentiated the intensive, expressive approach from the supportive method by the therapist's position on technical neutrality, psychotherapeutic tools, and attitude toward transference interpretation. (Psychoanalytic psychotherapy differs from psychoanalysis in a selective rather than a systematic interpretation of the transference, keeping in focus the defined goals of the treatment and the patient's external reality.) The expressive approach is defined by the maintenance of technical neutrality on the part of the therapist, the use of clarification and interpretation as psychotherapeutic tools, and the selective interpretation of transference. Supportive psychotherapy is defined by the absence of technical neutrality in favor of direct intervention on behalf of better adaptation. The therapist uses suggestion and manipulation as therapeutic tools and monitors, but does not interpret, transference reactions. Kernberg (1978) asserted that the treatment must be either expressive or supportive, not a mixture of both. Other writers believe that supportive therapy may be moved toward expressive therapy as change occurs in treatment (Masterson, 1976).

The patient's external reality is always an important factor in what is done in the therapy. The acting out of conflicts in the real world, through impulsive, destructive behavior, may sabotage treatment and may require efforts on the part of the therapist to have the patient's life "structured" at times of difficulty in the treatment. In the extreme case, this may result in hospitalization if the therapeutic effort is to continue, or abandonment of an expressive approach in favor of supportive methods, or both.

Because of the borderline patient's potential for distortion of reality and regression in the context of psychotherapy, the structure of the therapeutic relationship must be made explicit at the beginning of treatment, covering the time of appointments, contacts outside office hours (e.g., phone calls), limits on behavior within the office, the payment of fees, and the handling of emergencies. Regardless of the theoretical approach to the content of the patient's dynamics, the structure of the therapeutic relationship must define limits on the borderline patient's manipulation, loss of affective control, and impulsive acting out.

The borderline patient may lose a sense of reality under duress, including the stress of interpersonal psychotherapy. The appearance of referential thinking, paranoid ideation, or dissociative experience in this context requires more attention to cognitive limits, clarification, and reality testing, and less to intensive, anxiety-provoking exploration. In this context, medication may be used to support psychotherapy. A psychoeducational approach in which therapist and patient share a commonality of language, defining symptoms or dynamics, provides a useful cognitive structure for the therapeutic work. Although such a commonality of concept is developed covertly in some therapies (i.e., analysis) and overtly in others (e.g., behavior therapy), the borderline patient often requires the structure provided by a classification of his or her behaviors. The psychoeducational approach provides cognitive limits on affective dyscontrol and, ideally, on impulsive destructive behavior. It may be argued that these elements of structure must be firmly in place before the real exploration of dynamic content begins. These elements represent part of the "therapeutic alliance" with the patient, the unspoken contract required before therapy begins. Adler (1979) challenged whether such an agreement is ever fully achieved with the borderline patient. Difficulty in engaging the borderline patient results in a high dropout rate in clinic settings, with frequent readmission during times of stress. Gunderson (1984b) found up to 38% attrition in a psychotherapy clinic in the first 15 weeks. In the private sector, the pattern of working with the borderline patient intermittently over the years may be more the rule.

For the more severely impaired patient, supportive therapy, coupled with vocational or academic training, may ideally result in decreased morbidity, hospitalization, and dysfunctional behavior. Successful adaptation in a highly structured social setting is the goal of this treatment. For the more functional borderline patient, expressive therapies may produce genuine change in the quality of interpersonal relationships and self-esteem. Termination is not a realistic goal; rather, the goal should be the completion of a piece of work, with the option to expand the scope of therapy into other areas as needed in the future. As noted by Gunderson (1984a), "Successfully treated borderline patients are not healthy . . . they are much more socially adaptive but they are still vulnerable persons" (p. 62).

Pharmacological approaches to the treatment of the borderline patient traditionally arouse heated debate and opposition from analytic psychotherapists. Medication is viewed, at best, as a temporary remedy for disruptive anxiety or loss of ego controls and, at worst, as a weapon for acting out hostile or self-destructive dynamics. This debate has been needlessly prolonged by the paucity of well-controlled drug trials in borderline patients. Disagreements over the definition of the borderline disorder and its separation from other related syndromes has delayed the systematic investigation of the efficacy of medication in borderline patients. The recent development of reliable diagnostic criteria and objective interview methods for diagnosing borderline disorders allows the definition of research samples for pharmacological treatment trials. Nonetheless, the central problem of studying borderline pathology from a pharmacological perspective is the heterogeneity of the presenting complaints and symptoms within the same patient. To deal with this diversity, analytic writers traditionally evolve clinical typologies around theoretical principles. Kernberg's construct (1975) of the borderline as an infrastructure of personality allows for the definition of multiple DSM-III personality diagnosis within the same structural diagnosis. Stone's typology (1977) adds a genetic dimension, including contributions from affective or schizophrenic inheritance, producing an unwieldy three-dimensional typology with axes defined on structural level, personality type, and genetic dimensions.

The pharmacologist's approach to a multidimensional syndrome is to define specific symptom clusters or traits as presumed targets for chemotherapy and to conduct controlled clinical trials to determine efficacy and specificity of treatment. Target symptoms for pharmacotherapy in the borderline disorders include all of the affective, cognitive, and impulsive behavioral manifestations of the syndrome. These symptoms generally present as state-dependent variables, symptoms reflecting acute reaction to current life stressors. The time frame used to measure the appearance and course of these symptoms (usually weeks to months) represents a cross-sectional view of the patient's pathology. From this cross-sectional perspective, it is difficult to separate the primary and enduring features of a disorder from secondary and transient reactions. In contrast, the analytic psychotherapist may view transient decompensations in the borderline patient as a superficial phenomenon, reflecting underlying dynamic conflicts. The overall organization of personality, style of interpersonal relatedness, identity diffusion, and use of primitive defenses are characteristics of the patient that provide the focus for psychotherapy. The psychotherapist wrestles with the concept of vulnerability to decompensation while the pharmacotherapist attacks symptom complexes as they become manifest. In actual practice, the dichotomy between symptom state and character trait is not always clear, given the chronicity of the pathology. The central role of "core" characteristics in defining borderline pathology is challenged by the responsiveness of some of these features to chemotherapy.

The current discussion is limited to recent, systematic drug trials involving criteria-defined borderline patients identified by modern definitions of the diagnosis. Recent drug trials have tested the efficacy of antidepressant, neuroleptic, and anticonvulsant medication, as well as the minor tranquilizers and lithium carbonate. A review of drug efficacy for the target symptom clusters of depression, anger-hostility, schizotypal symptoms, anxiety, and impulsive behavior offers general guidelines for treatment of the symptomatic borderline patient.

Depression

Antidepressant medications have been widely recommended for depression in borderline patients because of the well-recognized comorbidity of borderline disorders and major depression, including endogenous subtypes. Despite a wealth of case experience, there has been only one placebo-controlled study of the use of a tricyclic antidepressant for criteria-defined borderline patients. Soloff, George, Nathan, Schulz, Ulrich, and Perel (1986) tested the efficacy of amitriptyline against placebo (and haloperidol) in a double-blind study of symptomatic borderline inpatients. The patients received amitriptyline in a dose range of 100–175 mg in a total drug trial that lasted 5 weeks. Amitriptyline was found to be no better than placebo on an observer-rated measure of depression (the 17-item Hamilton Rating Scale) but did demonstrate significant antidepressant effects on a self-rated measure of depression (e.g., the Beck Depression Inventory). Contrary to expectation, the antidepressant effects of amitriptyline were not superior to those in a neuroleptic comparison group (haloperidol). There was no relationship between a concurrent diagnosis of major depression and the response to amitriptyline. Indeed, many patients who failed to respond to amitriptyline did significantly worse than patients on placebo. They made more suicidal and assaultive threats and were, in fact, more assaultive than placebo nonresponders. Rubin (1986) achieved better results with tricylic antidepressants (and lithium) in an uncontrolled treatment of patients with borderline disorder and concurrent major depression and bipolar illness.

Monoamine oxidase inhibitors (MAOIs) have been recommended for the atypical patterns of depression, including symptoms such as hypersomnia, hyperphagia, anergia, and rejection sensitivity. This pattern is found in hysteroid dysphoria, a borderline ''next neighbor'' diagnosis. Liebowitz and Klein (1979) conducted a study of phenelzine in patients with hysteroid dysphoria, most of whom also met the criteria for borderline personality disorder. In an open treatment design of 3 months' duration, phenelzine (in doses ranging from 15 to 75 mg per day), paired with intensive psychotherapy, produced significant improvement in the borderline diagnostic criteria used as outcome measures. These included ''problems being alone,'' ''complaints of chronic emptiness and boredom,'' and behavioral impulsivity. At the end of 3 months, the responding patients entered a double-blind, randomized, crossover study and were assigned to continue either phenelzine or placebo. The patients receiving active drugs continued to show a reduction in the borderline diagnostic criteria, and the patients switched to placebo seemed to worsen.

Cowdry and Gardner (1986) confirmed the usefulness of the MAOI antidepressants in borderline patients in a complex, multidrug, placebo-controlled crossover study using tranylcypromine (average 40 mg daily) in a randomized sequence. The patients in this study received either tranylcypromine, trifluperazine (average 7.8 mg a day), carbamazepine (average 820 mg. a day), alprazolam (average 4.7 mg a day), or placebo in a double-blind crossover trial, with each condition lasting 6 weeks. The response to tranylcypromine was multidimensional: decreases in depressed mood, anxiety, and experiences of rage, coupled with increases in euphoria and capacity for pleasure. The response to tranylcypromine was not correlated with a family history of affective disorder or any past history of major depression. (The patients in this study did not meet the criteria for major depression at the time of the study but suffered from a variety of atypical depressive features.)

In assessing the borderline outpatient for the possible use of antidepressant medication, the pattern of depressed symptoms defines the indication. The monoamine oxidase inhibitors are preferred if an atypical depression or hysteroid dysphoric pattern is present. A strongly endogenous pattern of depression (i.e., melancholia) warrants a cautious trial of tricyclic antidepressants.

Anger-Hostility and the Schizotypal Pattern

Neuroleptic medications have been widely used with borderline patients in the treatment of anger and hostility, referential thinking, paranoid ideation, derealization-depersonalization, and distortions in thinking. Empirical support for the use of low-dose neuroleptics against these target symptoms is derived from comparative drug studies using neuroleptic medications in criteria-defined borderline patients and several recent placebo-controlled trials.

In studies comparing chlorpromazine with loxapine and thiothixene with haloperidol, improvement occurred with these neuroleptic medications in a broad spectrum of symptoms in borderline outpatients, including anger and hostility, anxiety, somatic concerns, suspiciousness, confusion, and, surprisingly, depression (Leone, 1982; Serban & Siegel, 1984). Placebo-controlled trials by Goldberg, Schulz, Schulz, Resnick, Hammer, and Friedel (1986), using thiothixene in an outpatient population, resulted in significant drug effects against the cognitive symptoms of illusions, ideas of reference, and perceptual distortions (such as derealization and depersonalization), and with some effects on anger, hostility, and somatization. The more severely ill patients in this study showed the greatest response to the low-dose neuroleptic medication, which was given in an average of 8.67 mg over a 12-week period.

Soloff and associates (1986) conducted a double-blind, placebo-controlled trial using haloperidol in impaired borderline inpatients, defined by Gunderson's Diagnostic Interview. Medication was given in an average dose of 7.2 mg for a period of 5 weeks. Improvement was noted in both affective and cognitive symptoms, especially in areas of paranoid ideation and self-rated psychoticism. Although the low-dose neuroleptic strategy is clearly indicated for cognitive state symptoms such as suspiciousness, referential thinking, and paranoid ideation, improvement in depressed mood was also clearly demonstrated. These studies raise the interesting question of whether the depressed mood of borderline patients represents a primary or a secondary symptom, that is, a symptom reactive to and following the appearance of cognitive distortions.

Anxiety

The case of anxiety as a target symptom poses special difficulties. Some authors have recommended the use of minor tranquilizers for the rapid control of anxiety in borderline patients, though this practice is not without risk. Case experience with alprazolam, for example, suggests improvement in the severity of both cognitive and affective symptoms, including anxiety (Faltus, 1984). On alprazolam, patients are reported to be better able to withstand stress without developing schizotypal symptoms. In a double-blind crossover study, Reus and Markrow (1984) treated 18 hospitalized borderline patients with alprazolam and reported a favorable response in half of the patients. The symptoms predictive of favorable outcome included hostility, suspiciousness, cognitive disturbance, sleep disturbance, and pathological interpersonal relatedness. Gardner and Cowdry (1985) sounded a more pessimistic note and reported a significant increase in behavioral dyscontrol in borderline outpatients receiving alprazolam in a range of 1–6 mg, compared to placebo-treated controls. Furthermore, the drug was not associated with any significant improvement in anxiety compared to placebo. Although touted as an antianxiety drug with antipanic and antidepressive properties, alprazolam may have a paradoxical disinhibiting effect in borderline patients similar to the disinhibition of aggression reported for other benzodiazepines. Given the borderline patient's potential for abusing minor tranquilizers and the potential for the disinhibition of impulsive aggression, caution is recommended in prescribing these medications for anxiety.

Many clinicians routinely prescribe low-dose neuroleptic medication for anxiety in the borderline patient. Soloff and associates (1986) found no significant efficacy for low-dose haloperidol used for anxiety in their inpatient borderline population. Cowdry and Gardner (1986) found improvements in anxiety with trifluperazine (average daily dose 7.8 mg), carbamazepine (average daily dose 820 mg), and tranylcypromine (average daily dose 40 mg), though not with alprazolam.

These data suggest that the target symptom of anxiety may be a secondary feature of the disorder, that resolves when primary cognitive or affective features respond.

Impulsive Behavior Patterns

The impulsive behavior of the borderline patient, reflected in frequent and explosive episodes of aggression, self-destructive behavior, or interpersonal acting out, provides a most important target symptom for pharmacotherapy. Impulsiveness in the borderline patient may be conceptualized as secondary to affective distress and cognitive distortion, or as a primary characterological trait. Borderline patients are characterized by higher impulsivity trait scores than depressed and schizophrenic control groups (Soloff, 1981). The episodic nature of the borderline patient's distress at times resembles the dyscontrol syndromes found in attention deficit disorder or the sequela of head trauma, encephalitis, and epilepsy. Andrulonis and associates (1981) suggested that one subtype of borderline disorder owes its origin to early-life CNS-insult or attention deficit disorder, which results in difficulties in inhibiting impulsive aggression.

Empirical studies indicate some efficacy for low-dose neuroleptics and anticonvulsants in the treatment of the impulsive behavioral symptoms of borderline patients. In the study by Soloff and associates (1986), impulsive behavior was assessed on a Ward Scale derived from Gunderson's Diagnostic Interview for Borderlines. This scale assesses typical behavior patterns of borderline patients in inpatient care, including suicidal threat, suicidal gesture, manipulation, demandingness, and antisocial acts. Haloperidol was found to produce significant improvement over placebo on the Ward Scale. Cowdry and Gardner (1986) demonstrated an improvement in the symptoms of behavioral dyscontrol in their borderline outpatients on carbamazepine. They described the appearance of "a reflective delay" between impulse and action that contributed to improvement in the patients' behavior. The study suggests a possible neurobehavioral origin of impulsiveness in some borderline patients, although the stabilizing effect of carbamazepine on mood provides an equally plausible explanation for the control of impulse. Certainly, the patient with a history of attention deficit disorder, learning disability, or EEG abnormality may warrant a trial of carbamazepine in an effort to control impulsive aggression or self-destructive behavior.

The episodic nature of the borderline patient's affective and impulsive behavioral symptoms has long suggested a role for lithium carbonate. Early studies by Rifkin, Quitkin, and Carrillo (1972) suggested that female inpatients diagnosed with "emotionally unstable character disorders'' improved in mood stability on lithium carbonate. Lithium carbonate has been shown to decrease anger and aggressive behavior in studies conducted on adult male convicts, apparently by introducing a ''reflective delay'' between stimulus and behavioral response (Sheard, 1975; Tupin, Smith, Classon, Kim, Nugent, & Gaupe, 1973). Case experience confirms the antiaggressive effects of lithium in patients with severe impulse disorders and suggests its use in the borderline patient (Shader, Jackson, & Dodes, 1984).

The response to medication in the borderline patient tends to be multidimensional (i.e., it crosses affective, cognitive, and behavioral symptoms). Where one symptom complex dominates, the choice of medication is clearer. Thus, for the affective borderline subtype, MAOI drugs may be most useful. For the schizotypal borderline, the low-dose neuroleptic is recommended, and carbamazepine is suggested for impulsive patients with histories of attention deficit disorder or abnormal EEG patterns. However, the majority of borderline patients demonstrate a considerable overlap of many symptoms, enhancing the appeal of drugs with a broad spectrum of response and relative safety in short-term use. Low-dose neuroleptics, for example, appear to be useful against affective as well as cognitive and impulsive behavioral symptoms and are generally well tolerated by the patient.

The overall strategy for use of pharmacotherapy in borderline patients should be the short-term treatment of reactive state symptoms, although significant improvement in associated character traits often follows. Pharmacotherapy is an adjunct to ongoing psychotherapy and, in many cases, an essential prerequisite to successful engagement in psychotherapy. As in the case of psychotherapy, the results are modest at best, the patient improving from severe to moderately or mildly impaired. At the present time, there is no empirical support for long-term maintenance on any medication class for borderline patients.

The dangers of pharmacotherapy for borderline patients include the ever-present potential of abuse, overdose, noncompliance, or interactions of medication with alcohol or street drugs. These dangers are not unique to the treatment of the borderline patient. They must be addressed in the context of a supportive doctor–patient relationship. Further research is needed to provide us with a better understanding of the origin and the natural history of the borderline disorder, more accurate subtype definitions of the borderline disorder, and more refined empirical guidelines for the treatment of these patients.

SUMMARY

The borderline disorder has achieved official recognition as a reliable diagnostic entity. The validity of the construct remains to be proved through prospective longitudinal studies. Armed with a theoretical framework for understanding the individual borderline patient, a scheme for diagnosing the disorder and its subtypes, and some appreciation of the roles of psychosocial and pharmacological treatments, the practicing clinician can help borderline patients achieve a more stable adaptation to life. Questions to be addressed by future investigations include the relationship of borderline disorders to their next neighbors (i.e., the question of validity), the differential efficacy of supportive and expressive therapies in long-term outcomes, and the role of maintenance medication in preventing decompensation in borderline patients. The heterogeneity of the disorder means that no ''treatment of choice'' is likely to emerge until our basic understanding of the borderline diagnosis is refined. Clinical practice must remain flexible and responsive to ideas emerging from these and other studies.

ACKNOWLEDGMENT. This work is supported by NIMH grants MH35392 and MH00658, and by Clinical Research Center grant MH30915.

REFERENCES

Adler, G. (1979). The myth of the alliance with borderline patients. *American Journal of Psychiatry, 136*, 642–645.

Akiskal, H. S. (1981). Sub-affective disorders, dysthymic, cyclothymic and bipolar II disorders in the borderline realm. *Psychiatric Clinics of North America, 4*, 25–46.

American Psychiatric Association. (1980). *Diagnostic and statistical manual of mental disorders* (3rd ed.; DSM-III). Washington, DC: Author.

Andrulonis, P. A., Glueck, B. L., Stroebel, C. F., Vogel, N. G., Shapiro, A. L., & Aldridge, D. M. (1981). Organic brain dysfunction and the borderline syndrome. *Psychiatric Clinics of North America, 4*, 61–66.

Baron, M., Gruen, R., Asnis, L., & Lord, S. (1985). Familial transmission of schizotypal and borderline personality disorders. *American Journal of Psychiatry, 142*, 927–934.

Bleuler, E. (1950). *Dementia praecox, or the group of schizophrenias* (trans. by J. Zinkin). New York: International Universities Press. (Originally published 1911.)

Bradley, S. J. (1979). The relationship of early maternal separation to borderline personality in children and adolescents: a pilot study. *American Journal of Psychiatry, 138*, 424–426.

Burnham, D. L. (1966). The special-problem patient: Victim or agent of splitting. *Psychiatry, 29*, 105–122.

Carpenter, W. T., & Gunderson, J. G. (1977). Five year follow-up comparison of borderline and schizophrenic patients. *Comprehensive Psychiatry, 18*, 567–571.

Carpenter, W. T., Gunderson, J. G., & Strauss, J. S. (1977). Considerations of the Borderline Syndrome: A longitudinal comparative study of borderline and schizophrenic patients. In P. Hartocollis (Ed.), *Borderline personality disorders* (pp. 231–254). New York: International Universities Press.

Carroll, B. J., Greden, J. T., & Feinberg, M. (1981). Neuroendocrine evaluation of depression in borderline patients. *Psychiatric Clinics of North America, 4*, 89–99.

Cornelius, J. R., Brenner, R. P., Soloff, P. H., Schulz, S. C., & Tumuluru, R. N. (1986). EEG abnormalities in borderline personality disorder: Specific or nonspecific. *Biological Psychiatry, 21*, 977–980.

Cowdry, R. W., & Gardner, D. L. (1988). Pharmacotherapy of borderline personality disorder. *Archives of General Psychiatry, 45*, 111–119.

Easser, B. R., & Lesser, S. R. (1965). Hysterical personality: A re-evaluation. *Psychoanalysis Quarterly, 34*, 390–405.

Faltus, F. J. (1984). The positive effect of alprazolam in the treatment of three patients with borderline personality disorder. *American Journal of Psychiatry, 141*, 802–803.

Frank, H., & Paris, J. (1981). Recollections of family experience in borderline patients. *Archives of General Psychiatry, 38*, 1031–1034.

Frosch, J. (1964). The psychotic character: Clinical psychiatric considerations. *Psychiatric Quarterly, 38*, 81–96.

Gardner, D. L., & Cowdry, R. W. (1985). Alprazolam-induced dyscontrol in borderline personality disorder. *American Journal of Psychiatry, 142*, 98–100.

Gardner, D. L., & Cowdry, R. W. (1986). Positive effect of carbamazepine on behavioral dyscontrol in borderline personality disorder. *American Journal of Psychiatry, 143*, 519–522.

Goldberg, S. C., Schulz, C., Schulz, P. M., Resmick, R. J., Hammer, R. M., & Friedel, R. O. (1986). Borderline and schizotypal personality disorders treated with low-dose thiothixene vs. placebo. *Archives of General Psychiatry, 43*, 680–686.

Goldstein, W. N. (1983). DSM III and the diagnosis of borderline, *American Journal of Psychotherapy, 37*, 312–327.

Grinker, R. R., Werble, B., & Drye, R. C. (1968). *The borderline syndrome: A behavioral study of ego-functions*. New York: Basic Books.

Gunderson, J. G. (1982). Empirical studies of the borderline diagnosis. In L. Grinspoon (Ed.), *Psychiatry 1982: Annual Review* (pp. 415–435). Washington, DC: American Psychiatric Association.
Gunderson, J. G. (1984a). *Borderline personality disorder*. Washington, DC: American Psychiatric Association.
Gunderson, J. G. (1984b). *Research on the psychotherapy of borderline personality disorder: Patient recruitment and retention*. National Institute of Mental Health Workshop, November 8–9, Washington, DC.
Gunderson, J. G., & Elliott, G. R. (1985). The interface between borderline personality disorder and affective disorders. *American Journal of Psychiatry, 142,* 227–288.
Gunderson, J. G., & Kolb, J. E. (1978). Discriminating features of borderline patients. *American Journal of Psychiatry, 135,* 792–796.
Gunderson, J. G., & Singer, M. T. (1975). Defining borderline patients: An overview. *American Journal of Psychiatry, 132,* 1–10.
Gunderson, J. G., Kolb, J. E., & Austin, V. (1981). The Diagnostic Interview of Borderline Patients. *American Journal of Psychiatry, 138,* 896–903.
Hartocollis, P. (1979). Minimal brain dysfunction in young adults. In L. Bellak (Ed.), *Psychiatric aspects of minimal brain dysfunction in adults* (pp. 103–113). New York: Grune & Stratton.
Hoch, P., & Polatin, P. (1949). Pseudoneurotic forms of Schizophrenia. *Psychiatric Quarterly, 23,* 248–276.
Hoch, P. H., & Cattell, J. P. (1959). The diagnosis of pseudoneurotic schizophrenia. *Psychiatric Quarterly, 33,* 17–43.
Kendler, K. (1985). Diagnostic approaches to schizotypal personality disorder. *Schizophrenia Bulletin, 11,* 538–553.
Kernberg, O. F. (1967). Borderline personality organization. *Journal of American Psychoanalytic Association, 15,* 641–685.
Kernberg, O. F. (1975). *Borderline conditions and pathological narcissism*. New York: Jason Aronson.
Kernberg, O. F. (1978). Contrasting approaches to the psychotherapy of borderline conditions. In J. F. Masterson (Ed.), *New perspectives on psychotherapy of the borderline adult*. New York: Brunner/Mazel.
Kernberg, O. F., Goldstein, E. G., Carr, A. C., Hunt, H. F., Bauer, S. F., & Blumenthal, R. (1981). Diagnosing borderline personality. *Journal of Nervous Mental Disease, 169,* 225–231.
Kety, S. S., Rosenthal, D., Wender, P. H., & Schulsinger, F. (1968). The types and prevalence of mental illness in the biological and adoptive families of adopted schizophrenics. In D. Rosenthal (Ed.), *The transmission of schizophrenia* (pp. 345–362). New York: Pergamon Press.
Knight, R. P. (1954). Management and psychotherapy of the borderline schizophrenic patient. In R. P. Knight & C. R. Friedman (Eds.), *Psychoanalytic psychiatry and psychology* (pp. 110–122). New York: International Universities Press.
Kolb, J. E., & Gunderson, J. G. (1980). Diagnosing borderline patients with a semi-structured interview. *Archives of General Psychiatry, 37,* 37–41.
Kroll, J., Sines, L., & Martin, K. (1981). Borderline personality disorder: Construct validity of the concept. *Archives of General Psychiatry, 38,* 1021–1026.
Leone, N. F. (1982). Response of borderline patients to loxapine and chlorpromazine. *Journal of Clinical Psychiatry, 43,* 148–150.
Liebowitz, M. R., & Klein, D. F. (1979). Hysteroid dysphoria. *Psychiatric Clinics of North America, 2,* 555–575.
Loranger, A. W., Oldham, J., & Tulis, E. (1982). Familial transmission of borderline personality. *Archives of General Psychiatry, 39,* 795–802.
Mack, J. E. (1975). Borderline states: An historical perspective. In J. E. Mack (Ed.), *Borderline states in psychiatry* (pp. 1–29). New York: Grune & Stratton.
Mahler, M. S., Pine, F., & Bergman, A. (1975). *The psychological birth of the human infant*. New York: Basic Books.
Main, T. F. (1957). The ailment. *British Journal of Medical Psychology, 30,* 129–145.
Marmor, J. (1953). Orality in the hysterical personality. *Journal of American Psychoanalysis Association, 1,* 656–671.
Masterson, J. F. (1976). *Psychotherapy of the borderline adult*. New York: Brunner/Mazel.
Murray, M. E. (1979). Minimal brain dysfunction and borderline personality adjustment. *American Journal of Psychiatry, 33,* 391–403.
Perry, J. C., & Klerman, G. L. (1978). The borderline patient: a comparative analysis of four sets of diagnostic criteria. *Archives of General Psychiatry, 35,* 141–150.

Perry, J. C., & Klerman, G. L. (1980). Clinical features of the borderline personality disorder. *American Journal of Psychiatry, 137,* 165–173.

Pope, H. G., Jonas, J. M., Hudson, J. I., Cohen, B. M., & Gunderson, J. G. (1983). The validity of DSM-III borderline personality disorder. *Archives of General Psychiatry, 40,* 23–30.

Reus, V. I., & Markrow, S. (1984). *Alprozalam in the treatment of borderline personality disorder.* Presented at the Annual Meeting of the Society for Biological Psychiatry, May 2–6, Los Angeles.

Rifkin, A., Quitkin, F., & Carrillo (1972). Lithium carbonate in emotionally unstable character disorders. *Archives of General Psychiatry, 27,* 519–523.

Rinsley, D. R. (1978). Borderline psychopathology: A review of etiology, dynamics and treatment. *International Review of Psycho-Analysis, 5,* 45–54.

Rubin, A. L. (1986). *Pharmacotherapy in borderline personality disorder.* Presented at Annual Meeting of the American Psychiatric Association, May 13, Washington, DC.

Schulz, S. C., Cornelius, J., Schulz, P. M., Brenner, R., & Soloff, P. H. (1984). *Can amphetamine testing solve the heterogeneity of borderline disorders?* Presented at New Research, Annual Meeting of the American Psychiatric Association, Los Angeles.

Serban, G., & Siegel, S. (1984). Response of borderline and schizotypal patients to small doses of thiothixene and haloperidol. *American Journal of Psychiatry, 141,* 1455–1458.

Shader, R. I., Jackson, A. H., & Dodes, L. M. (1984). The antiaggressive effects of lithium in man. *Psychopharmacologia (Berl), 40,* 17–24.

Shapiro, E. R., Zinner, J., Shapiro, R. L., *et al.* (1975). The influence of family experience on borderline personality development. *International Review of Psycho-Analysis, 2,* 399–411.

Sheard, M. H. (1975). Lithium in the treatment of aggression. *Journal of Nervous and Mental Disease, 160,* 108–118.

Sheehy, M., Goldsmith, L., & Charles E. (1980). A comparative study of borderline patients in a psychiatric out-patient clinic. *American Journal of Psychiatry, 137,* 1374–1379.

Siever, L. J. (1981). Schizoid and schizotypal personality disorders. In J. R. Lion (Ed.), *Personality disorders: Diagnosis and management* (2nd ed.) (pp. 32–65). Baltimore: Williams & Wilkins.

Siever, L. J. (1985). Biological markers and schizotypal personality disorders. *Schizophrenia Bulletin, 11,* 564–575.

Siever, L. J. & Gunderson, J. G. (1979). Genetic determinants of borderline conditions. *Schizophrenia Bulletin, 5,* 59–86.

Soloff, P. H. (1981). Affect, impulse and psychosis in borderline disorders: A validation study. *Comprehensive Psychiatry, 22,* 337–350.

Soloff, P. H., & Millward, J. W. (1983). Psychiatric disorders in the families of borderline patients. *Archives of General Psychiatry, 40,* 37–48.

Soloff, P. H., & Ulrich, R. F. (1981). The diagnostic interview for borderlines: A replication study. *Archives of General Psychiatry, 38,* 686–692.

Soloff, P. H., George, A., Nathan, R. S., Schulz, P. M., Ulrich, R. F., & Perel, J. M., (1986). Progress in pharmacotherapy of borderline disorders. *Archives of General Psychiatry, 43,* 691–697.

Spitzer, R. L., & Endicott, J. (1979). Justification for separating schizotypal and borderline personality disorders. *Schizophrenia Bulletin, 5,* 95–104.

Spitzer, R. L., Endicott, J., & Gibbon, M. (1979). Crossing the border into borderline personality and borderline schizophrenia. The development of criteria. *Archives of General Psychiatry, 36,* 17–24.

Stone, M. H. (1977). The borderline syndrome: Evolution of the term, genetic aspects and prognosis. *American Journal of Psychotherapy, 31,* 345–365.

Stone, M. H. (1981). Psychiatrically ill relatives of borderline patients: A family study. *Psychiatric Quarterly, 58,* 71–83.

Tupin, J. P., Smith, D. B., Classon, T. L., Kim, L. I., Nugent, A., & Gaupe, A. (1973). Long-term use of lithium in aggressive prisoners. *Comprehensive Psychiatry, 14,* 311–317.

Waldinger, R. J., & Gunderson, J. G. (1984). Completed psychotherapies with borderline patients. *American Journal of Psychotherapy, 38,* 190–202.

Wolberg, A. R. (1982). *Psychoanalytic psychotherapy of borderline patients.* New York: Thieme-Stratton.

Zetzel, E. (1971). A development approach to the borderline patient. *American Journal of Psychiatry, 127,* 867–871.

Zilboorg, G. (1941). Ambulatory schizophrenia. *Psychiatry, 4,* 149–155.

15

Antisocial Personality Disorder

PHILIP H. BORNSTEIN, CAROLYN FORD, JOSEPH E. BIRON, BONNIE M. BREKKE, AND DAVID B. STUBE

INTRODUCTION

He opened the Rabelais to a page and began reading, walking to the kitchen doorway to serenade Alice with the flow. He read of Gargantua's arrival in Paris, his swiping of the Notre Dame Cathedral bells for his giant horse, and then his perching on the cathedral roof to rest while mobs of tiny Parisians stared up at him. And so he decided to give them wine.

''He undid his magnificent codpiece''—Jack read with mock robustness; his voice was not robust but of a moderately high pitch, excitable, capable of tremolos—''and bringing out his john-thomas, pissed on them so fiercely that he drowned two hundred and sixty thousand, four hundred and eighteen persons, not counting the women and small children.''

''My God, John,'' Alice said, ''do you have to read that?*''*

''Piss on 'em,'' Jack said. ''I always felt that way.'' And holding the book and talking to me, he said, ''You know what my full name is? John Thomas Diamond.'' And he laughed even harder. (Kennedy, 1975, Legs, *p. 44).*

This excerpt from William Kennedy's 1975 novel *Legs,* which revolves around the sordid life and times of one Jack ''Legs'' Diamond, a notorious Prohibition Era gangster (and bona fide antisocial personality), provides an illustrative look at the man and mentality residing behind the ''mask of sanity'' (Cleckley, 1964). Although in the third edition of the American Psychiatric Association's *Diagnostic and Statistical Manual of Mental Disorders* (DSM-III; APA, 1980) the definition of antisocial personality disorder (APD)

PHILIP H. BORNSTEIN, CAROLYN FORD, JOSEPH E. BIRON, BONNIE M. BREKKE, and DAVID B. STUBE • Psychology Department, University of Montana, Missoula, Montana 59812.

may lack some of the above "color," it does cite the official criteria to be used for diagnostic and classification purposes (see Table 1).

The DSM-III Axis II diagnosis of APD as a clinical entity is still very much in its formative stages. Currently, debate continues regarding the DSM-III emphasis on behavioral concomitants of crime as indicants of psychopathology (Millon, 1981). Indeed, a perusal of the long and arduous history of APD reveals its origins in, and continuing close association with, the concept of *criminal personality* (Yochelson & Samenow, 1976). Providing a counterpoint to the current DSM-III diagnosis of APD is Millon's nonevaluative, research-derived criteria for classification (1981). Couching his description in terms of an "active-independent" personality schema, Millon asserted:

> This pattern is typified by a self-assertive, temperamentally hostile and socially forceful and intimidating manner. There is pride in self-reliance, unsentimentality and hard-boiled competitive values. Malicious personal tendencies are projected outward, precipitating frequent outbursts of explosive anger. Vindictive gratification is obtained by humiliating and dominating others. A rash willingness to risk personal harm is notable as is a fearlessness in the face of threats and punitive action. Frank antisocial behaviors (e.g., truancy, non-traffic arrests, frequent fighting)

Table 1. Synopsis of DSM-III Diagnostic Criteria for Antisocial Personality Disorder

A. Current age at least 18

B. Onset before age 15 as indicated by a history of three or more of the following before that age:

1. Truancy
2. Expulsion or suspension from school for misbehavior
3. Delinquency
4. Running away from home
5. Persistent lying
6. Repeated sexual intercourse in casual relationships
7. Alcohol or other substance abuses
8. Thefts
9. Vandalism
10. School grades markedly below expectations
11. Chronic violations of rules at home and/or school
12. Initiation of fights

C. At least four of the following manifestations of the disorder since age 18:

1. Inability to sustain consistent work behavior
2. Lack of ability to function as a responsible parent
3. Failure to accept social norms with respect to lawful behavior
4. Inability to maintain enduring attachment to a sexual partner
5. Irritability and aggressiveness as indicated by repeated physical fights or assault
6. Failure to honor financial obligations
7. Failure to plan ahead, or behavioral impulsivity
8. Disregard for the truth
9. Recklessness

D. A pattern of continuous antisocial behavior in which the rights of others are violated

E. Antisocial behavior is not due to either severe mental retardation, schizophrenia, or manic episodes

are common among adolescent and post-adolescent aggressive personalities, as well as in certain socioeconomic sub-populations. However, the majority of these personalities do not exhibit flagrant antisocial behaviors, finding a sanctioned niche in conventional roles. (p. 197)

The reader will note that Millon's focus on the personality features of APD is in marked contrast to the DSM-III classification system, which emphasizes behavioral concomitants as indicators of the underlying disorder. Similarly, Hare (1983) compiled a comprehensive checklist of personality traits and behaviors that extend and expand on the earlier work of Cleckley (1976). This descriptive listing of criteria (see Table 2) correlates

Table 2. Checklist of APD Features[a]

1.	Glibness/superficial charm
2.	Previous diagnosis as psychopath (or similar)
3.	Egocentricity/grandiose sense of self-worth
4.	Proneness to boredom/low frustration tolerance
5.	Pathological lying and deception
6.	Conning/lack of sincerity
7.	Lack of remorse or guilt
8.	Lack of affect and emotional depth
9.	Callousness/lack of empathy
10.	Parasitic lifestyle
11.	Short-temperedness/poor behavioral controls
12.	Promiscuous sexual relations
13.	Early behavior problems
14.	Lack of realistic long-term plans
15.	Impulsivity
16.	Irresponsible behavior as parent
17.	Frequent marital relationships
18.	Juvenile delinquency
19.	Poor probation or parole risk
20.	Failure to accept responsibility for own action
21.	Many types of offenses
22.	Drug/alcohol abuse not direct cause of antisocial behavior

[a]From Hare (1983).

.66 with the DSM-III diagnostic schema and provides a useful tool in the clinical assessment of APD. Although the use of behavioral referents in the above systems is to be applauded, objectivity must not occur at the expense of an integrated conceptualization of the disorder. This chapter attempts to provide such a conceptualization across a variety of content areas. For this purpose, we discuss history, etiology, developmental considerations, assessment, and outpatient treatment programs. In order to assist the reader in understanding recent developments in the DSM-III Axis II definition of APD, we begin with a brief history of the diagnostic label.

HISTORY OF APD

Early Formations of APD

The conceptual controversy surrounding APD can be traced to the theory and practice of medicine in the early 1800s. Phillipe Pinel (1809), for example, in his "Medico-psychological Treatise on Mental Alienation," described a mania without delusions (*manie sans délire*). This disturbance was characterized by intact reasoning and sensory processes, with impairment in the affective faculties. In essence, Pinel described the disorder as resulting from either faulty parenting or a genetic-constitutional predisposition. The suggestion that individuals might be considered "insane" while maintaining intact intellectual faculties was clearly a radical notion. Previously, insanity had been considered a function of impaired reasoning. To conceive of psychological disorder without mental affliction was most certainly controversial.

During this same era, the American physician Benjamin Rush observed similar phenomena. Rush (1812) concluded, however, that the socially reprehensible behaviors engaged in by these lucidly thinking individuals were the result of moral depravity. A short time later, Esquirol (1838) extended the work of Pinel and Rush. He developed the conceptual categories of reasoning insanity and moral insanity to describe behaviors resulting from injuries to and/or impairment of "will and feeling" without apparent defect in intellectual faculties. Thus, we see these theoreticians still struggling with the problem of how an individual can be "sane" yet do "insane" things.

Meanwhile, in England, Grohman (1819; cited in Pichot, 1978) had characterized these individuals by creating the term *moral idiocy*. Yet, it was Pritchard who, in 1835, described "moral insanity" and "moral imbecility" as the socioethical equivalents of deficits in intellectual functioning. This notion of moral insufficiency remains a key concept in the definition of APD even to the present.

During the mid to late 19th century, early scientist-practitioners sought to explain the phenomenon of APD in a variety of ways. Whereas anthropologists and criminologists speculated that APD was the product of genetic determinism (Lombroso, 1872–1885; Gouster, 1878), Tuke (1892) and Maudsley, (1874) continued the morality–clinical-entity debate. Tuke (in the Pinelian tradition) referred to the syndrome as inhibitory insanity, attesting more to the clinical nature of the disturbance. Maudsley, on the other hand, hypothesized a seat of "natural moral feelings" subject to injury or congenital deficiency. Closely paralleling the development of the concept *moral depravity* in England was the doctrine of *moral degeneracy* in France. Operating from a distinctly Christian orthodox perspective, Morel (1857) indicated that "moral degeneracy" was a process of morbid deviation. His position was that the afflicted person, a victim of a genetically transmitted predisposition that exacerbated vulnerability to insult, was subject to a progressive psychological and moral decay. Morel developed a system for classifying all kinds and intensities of degeneracy and mental pathology according to the presence and proportion of endogenous (hereditary) and exogeneous (environmental-influence) causes. Included in Morel's system were four classes of psychopathology termed *hereditary insanities*. Two of these are germane to the historical development of APD. ''Manic instinctive'' was characterized by limited intelligence and a proclivity for ''evil.'' The second class was highly reminiscent of Pinel's ''reasoning insanity.''

Magnan and Legrain (1895) were next to attempt a reformulation of the APD. These authors were responsible for identifying and labeling many of the phobias and manias that are still in common usage today (e.g., claustrophobia and pyromania). Relevant to the evolution of APD is their description of the clinical pattern ''higher degenerate.'' They characterized these individuals as intelligent, expansive, changeable, given to excess, and weak-willed. Magnan and Legrain emphasized psychologically descriptive traits and indicated that such individuals often belonged to the highest classes of society (Pichot, 1978). Yet, 30 years later, Dupre (1925) was to move French psychiatry away from psychological description and back to the position of definition by manifestation of antisocial-amoral behavior.

Meanwhile, Koch (1891) was approaching the APD question from a slightly different perspective. He described a variety of innate constitutional inferiorities, three of which relate to the concept of APD: innate psychopathic disposition, innate psychopathic load, and innate psychopathic degeneracy. Kraepelin (1896) extended the work of Koch and further defined the notion of psychopathic personality. Using a comprehensive system of personality classification, Kraepelin's typology encompassed nearly all aspects of antisocial behavior. In fact, by 1915, Kraepelin had identified seven distinct types of psychopaths. He hypothesized that the condition was irreversible, originating in personality failure exacerbated by hereditary influences and unfavorable or unfortunate life circumstances. Many of the features of Kraepelin's system persist today as part of the International Classification of Disease (ICD) and DSM diagnostic codes.

Contemporary Developments in APD

Sociocultural upheaval, major world events (e.g., World War I), and scientists of genius (e.g., Freud) collectively modified the accepted conceptualization of APD. It is beyond our scope to explicate all of these in detail; however, we will attempt to highlight three major APD evolutionary trends. The first was a shift away from constitutional and hereditary explanations of APD and toward a more nondeterministic position of social causation. Birnbaum (1914) first proposed the term *sociopathic* as a more appropriate designation for APD. He postulated that APD was not the result of a preexisting constitutional defect, but the product of combined environmental and social influences. Thus, society was held accountable and ultimately responsible for the deviant behavior and actions of its citizenry. Further, Partridge (1927), theorizing from a psychoanalytic perspective, proposed that APD was the result of improper socialization. He postulated that sociopathic personalities failed to achieve normal developmental milestones and had resultant personality characteristics associated with their arrested stage of development. Partridge (1928, 1930) similarly criticized the diagnostic label *psychopathic personality* and recommended instead the use of Birnbaum's formulation, *sociopathic personality*.

The second major trend was the emergence of psychoanalytic thought and its emphasis on early environmental influences. Alexander (1923, 1935), for example, regarded antisocial behavior as being the direct result of unrestrained, primitive, unconscious impulses. However, Alexander was not content in ascribing APD strictly to unconscious processes. In an attempt to explain the disorder, he therefore continued to examine the complex interrelationships between environmental influences, genetic predispositions, and evolving personality dynamics. Other analytic writers described the phenomenological world of APD individuals and attributed APD's occurrence to a variety of developmental antecedents (Allen, 1950; Friedlander, 1945; Horney, 1945). More recently, Bursten (1972) recommended focusing less on lists of APD transgressions and more on the psychological underpinnings of the disorder.

The third trend has been the combined work of a variety of personality theorists and research psychologists (e.g., Bandura & Walters, 1959; Eysenck, 1967; Glueck, 1966; Megargee, 1972; Millon, 1969; Quay, 1964; Robins, 1966). The product of their efforts has been the integration of the available observational, assessment, and research data into a meaningful diagnostic picture of APD. Perhaps the most heuristic of these endeavors has been the work of Hervey Cleckley. His multiple-editioned volume, *The Mask of Sanity* (1941, 1950, 1955, 1964, 1976), is the product of a lifetime of diligent and thoughtful inquiry into the description and causation of APD. Cleckley believes that APD individuals mimic the genuine human personality and hide behind a "mask of sanity"; that the APD's perception of life is totally devoid of major emotional accompaniment; and that life experiences are not integrated into the personality in any meaningful fashion.

Even given the above developments, one notes that the concept of APD has changed little since World War II. The official terminology may have been modified, but the basic formulation remains the same. In the DSM-I (APA, 1952), sociopathic personality disturbance was listed under "personality disorders." This terminology reflected the then-current sentiment that APD was, by and large, a product of postnatal social influences. In the DSM-II (APA, 1968), the rather generic term *sociopathic personality disturbance* was withdrawn from usage. Instead, separate diagnostic categories, thought to more accurately represent distinct clinical entities of "antisocial" and "dyssocial" personality, replaced the term. Several other diagnostic categories descriptive of behavior (conduct) disorders of childhood and adolescence were also added. The DSM-III (APA, 1980) and DSM-III-R (APA, 1987) has, in reality, made few changes in the classification of APD. In fact, the diagnostic criteria have remained quite similar through all editions of the DSM. Thus, it seems, as work is now being conducted on the DSM-IV, that changes are in order. Certainly, behavioral descriptions have their place. However, by shifting the focus of attention to psychological substrates promoting antisocial behavior, we can simultaneously integrate theory, research, and treatment.

DEVELOPMENTAL ANTECEDENTS OF APD

In spite of the attention given APD in the literature, very little is actually known about the genetic or environmental factors that may predispose one to or may predict the development of the disorder. This curious situation exists despite the belief that the behavioral characteristics of adult APD are manifest during childhood (Morrison, 1978; Robins, 1978) and that a history of childhood problems is requisite for a diagnosis of the disorder (APA, 1980). Limitations that have hindered a clear definition of childhood correlates of adult antisocial personality disorder include the rarity of prospective or longitudinal studies; selective, biased data obtained through retrospective study; the heterogeneity of associated childhood diagnostic categories (e.g., conduct disorders, childhood or adolescent antisocial behaviors, and disorders of impulse control); and the tendency of investigators to identify children as subjects for study at the point of their entry into the mental-health or juvenile-justice system (Kazdin & Frame, 1983; Robins, 1978). As a result, the literature that addresses the developmental antecedents of APD quickly becomes the literature of childhood or adolescent delinquency. It is therefore necessary to review this work with caution, so that the often-stated conclusion that delinquency in childhood predicts adult psychopathology is not prematurely accepted as an explanatory model for the development of APD. In the absence of a theoretical framework for the etiology of APD, the variables that have been considered include those characterized as being environmental, neurophysiological, and/or genetic in nature.

Environmental Influences in the Development of APD

Among the earliest formulations of the etiology of APD was the notion that individuals so diagnosed had typically experienced early deprivation and/or the loss of parental care (Kaplan & Sadock, 1985; Morrison, 1978). Glueck and Glueck (1950), for example, considered the development of APD the result of inconsistent care by a primary caretaker (usually the mother) during the child's first 5 years of life. In addition, an ''incohesive'' family life that included lack of maternal discipline and affection was seen as a predictor of delinquency by 18 years of age. Rutter (1971) was among those who broadened the concept of deprivation to include deficits in maternal care and affection and childhood nonavailability of sustaining emotional ties with significant others. The general theme of these deprivation models was the child's lack of opportunity to experience affection, discipline, and interpersonal warmth. It was believed that antisocial personality characteristics (e.g., emotional distance in relationships, lack of empathy for others, and the failure to accept societal codes of conduct) were essentially the result of a failure to learn or internalize emotional closeness.

The psychoanalytic position also emphasized the importance of early parent–child relationships in the socialization of the child (Szurek & Berlin, 1969). Szurek (1969) stated that, for any child to conform his or her behaviors to socially approved standards, it was necessary to experience firm prohibition coupled with adequate reward for submission. He suggested that antisocial tendencies develop when the child is either consciously or unconsciously encouraged to act out the parents' amoral, neurotic fantasies. Because these behaviors vicariously gratify adult desires, the child learns to act without anxiety, guilt, or the need to delay or postpone actions. Further, Szurek speculated, it is unlikely that such parents would frequently support or reward socially approved behaviors. Thus, the child learns to meet the needs of the parent rather than the expectations of the culture or society.

The deprivation model (encompassing both inadequate and undesirable parenting) was generally accepted as an explanation for the development of APD (Morrison, 1978). It was not until the publication of the work of Robins (1966, 1978) and her colleagues (O'Neal & Robins, 1958; Robins, Murphy, Woodruff, & King, 1971) that more specific environmental antecedents of APD were identified. Although this work is dated, it still provides the most comprehensive information available.

Robins and her associates (Robins, 1966; Robins *et al.*, 1971) conducted two longitudinal studies designed to identify behavioral, family, and societal variables predictive of APD development. The first study (Robins, 1966), begun in 1924, compared data obtained through interviews and file reviews of 526 Caucasian children who had been referred to a child guidance clinic with "behavior problems" and 100 "normal" matched controls. These subjects were first seen during late childhood and were then followed into their 40s. The second study (Robins *et al.*, 1971) followed 235 "normal" black schoolboys from late childhood into their 30s. From these data, Robins (1978) described childhood behaviors identified as precusors of APD and delineated behavioral, family, and societal factors associated with the disorder.

In summary, Robins (1978) concluded that APD, more commonly seen among boys than girls, inevitably has its onset during childhood. Antisocial behaviors, which she described as precursors of the adult disorder, were characteristically identified either when the child first entered school or during early adolescence. Early "signs" of the personality disorder include, according to Robins (1978), "truancy, failure to perform well academically despite adequate IQs, stealing, and disciplinary problems in the classroom" (p. 259). Other behaviors commonly reported were theft, running away from home, violating curfew, incorrigibility, and associating with other delinquent children. Girls, more often than boys, were referred because of their sexual activities. Referral complaints also included fighting, recklessness, slovenliness, impulsivity, enuresis, lying, and being unloved. These descriptors, however, did not significantly differentiate those diagnosed as having APD from individuals with other psychiatric problems, including psychosis and alcoholism. The observant reader will recognize the above behaviors as those adopted as diagnostic criteria in the DSM-III (APA, 1980).

Although no one behavior or behavioral pattern consistently occurred among children later diagnosed as APD, Robins (1966) did propose that the single best predictor was the frequency, variety, and seriousness of juvenile antisocial behaviors. The data revealed that children diagnosed as APD most commonly had histories of thefts and/or aggressive acts directed against property or strangers. The results of these studies did not support the earlier beliefs that a "broken home" or association with other delinquent children increased the probability of APD development (Robins, 1978).

No family or societal variable was found to be predictive of adult APD (Robins, 1966, 1978; Robins *et al.*, 1971). There were, however, commonalities among families of children later diagnosed as having APD, including parental psychiatric disorder, excessive use of alcohol by parents, unemployment, poverty, absence of discipline, and lack of adult supervision. The fathers were most commonly diagnosed as having APD and/or as being alcoholic; the mothers were more frequently described as being psychotic, neurotic (having hysterical disorders), or mentally retarded. Many families had been abandoned by the father. For those fathers who did remain in the home, interactions with children were characterized as "cold" and passive. Further, Robins (1966) found that the child's likelihood of receiving an APD diagnosis was not reduced by the absence of an antisocial father. Dinitz (1980) suggested that the reason may be a single mother's lessened ability to exercise control over her child. Others (Robins, 1978) have speculated that such findings reflect genetic influences in the development of the disorder.

Reviews (Cloninger, Reich, & Guze, 1978; Morrison, 1978; Robins, 1978) generally acknowledge that the etiology of APD most likely lies in the interaction of genetic and environmental factors. The exact nature of the genetic or neurophysiological substrates, however, remains speculative.

Genetic and Neurophysiological Influences in the Development of APD

The notion of genetic influence in the development of APD finds support in data that reveal the greater incidence among males, the prevalence of parental psychiatric disorder (including fathers with APD), and the failure of the absence of an antisocial father to reduce children's APD risk. To date, there has been no evidence of direct genetic transmission (Cloninger *et al.*, 1978). Although parental reports that the child "has always been that way" (Robins, 1978) do suggest underlying child temperament or sensitivity to stimuli that may interact with the environment to produce the disorder, there have been no investigations that have examined this relationship. Twin and adoption studies have reported, however, that environmental-genetic information does have value in increasing knowledge about the etiology of APD, especially in those situations limited by a focus on delinquency and adult criminality.

In addition to unanswered questions regarding genetic transmission factors that may predispose the child to or increase the child's vulnerability to development of the disorder, there are also neurophysiological-dysfunction–immaturity concerns. This line of inquiry evolved from reports indicating abnormal EEG patterns among those diagnosed as having APD (Arthur & Cahoon, 1964; Hare, 1970). As would be expected, associated conditions (e.g., attention deficit disorder and specific learning disability) led researchers to consider this hypothesis further (Morrison, 1978; Satterfield, 1978). Unfortunately, these adjunct difficulties have been not limited to children later diagnosed as having APD, and research has not specifically addressed the neurophysiological correlates of the disorder.

DIAGNOSTIC AND ASSESSMENT CONSIDERATIONS

The decision of the DSM-III task force to establish APD criteria based on juvenile-delinquent and criminal behaviors rather than broader personality dimensions met with some criticism (e.g., Millon, 1983a, 1985; Wulach, 1983). Though the diagnostic category was empirically based on longitudinal research (Robins, 1966; Widiger, Williams, Spitzer, & Frances, 1985), more recent studies have indicated that the DSM-III classification may be overinclusive. That is, 75–80% of all criminals meet the Axis II APD diagnosis (Guze, 1976; Vaillant & Perry, 1980). This represents a 250% increase over those diagnosable as psychopathic personality by use of the DSM-II criteria (Wulach, 1983). Certainly, it is true that behaviorally operationalized diagnostic criteria do generate respectable levels of interrater agreement (Williams & Spitzer, 1980). Yet, diagnosis based on the sole use of explicit criteria leaves little room for gradations of the disorder (Wulach, 1983). Thus, the notion of a continuum of APD symptomatology no longer exists, and thought form and content is now basically irrelevant to APD diagnostic considerations.

Millon (1985) "unequivocally rejects" (p. 379) the DSM-III APD criteria, emphasizing that a strictly behavioral diagnosis is not particularly useful in cognitive and affective-interpersonal therapies. In fact, Millon implied that the diagnosis is underinclusive or lacking in specificity, as it fails to identify noncriminal clients who may be treatable as having "aggressive personality disorders" (his corollary of APD). In any case, a thorough assessment is the *sine qua non* of accurate diagnosis. Consequently, we will attempt to review a variety of assessment tools useful in the evaluation of APD.

Though it is a good practice to strive for social corroboration of any intake, the personality disorders and APD in particular make family and friend reports indispensable. Many of the diagnostic data for the DSM-III APD criteria can be gathered from a clinical interview supplemented by a work history, court records, and other public documents. The interviewer should elicit information regarding juvenile-delinquent and criminal behavior, past work history, and family background. The assessment should proceed with a keen eye on interpersonal process, seeking evidence of the client's ability to sustain relatedness; his or her anger control, self-management, and anxiety (or lack thereof); and the capacity for shared intimacy and closeness.

Behavioral Checklists

The DSM-III emphasis on explicit diagnostic criteria has provided further impetus for the use of behavioral checklists in the assessment of APD. Two such instruments are worthy of note. First, Hare's checklist for the assessment of psychopathology (Table 2) is based on descriptions provided by Cleckley (1976). This checklist includes both personality dimensions and behavioral indices. It has good internal consistency, high interrater reliability, and a demonstrated correlation with APD diagnoses in criminal populations (Schroeder, Schroeder, & Hare, 1983).

The Behavior Problem Checklist, a factor-analytic instrument, is also available for APD diagnoses (Peterson, Quay, & Cameron, 1959; Quay, 1964). Antisocial personalities can be differentiated into four types: inadequate-immature, neurotic-disturbed, socialized-delinquent, and unsocialized-psychopathic. In addition, checklists have also been developed by Craddick (1962), Jenkins (1964), and Ziskind (1978). However, most of these instruments have generated only limited empirical-validity studies.

Objective Personality Instruments

The Minnesota Multiphasic Personality Inventory and the Millon Clinical Multiaxial Inventory

The objective test profile most commonly associated with APD diagnosis has historically been the 4-9/9-4 code type of the Minnesota Multiphasic Personality Inventory (MMPI; e.g., Gilberstadt & Duker, 1965; Marks, Seaman, & Haller, 1974). A Scale 4 (Psychopathic Deviate) elevation is typically correlated with high scores on 9, F, and 8, depending on the degree of underlying schizophrenic thought process (Hedlund, 1977). Affective components are indicated by elevations on Scale 2 (Depression) during periods of remorse or incarceration. In addition, Scale 6 (Paranoia) may provide indications of whether hostility is repressed or is expressed directly (Green, 1980). Regrettably, the 4-9 profile has proved to be a poor differential-diagnostic tool, as 23% of all college students and 53% of all helping professionals exhibit this same profile (Hawk & Peterson, 1974). Indeed, the 4-9 profile is probably more descriptive of the DSM-II psychopathic personality than of the DSM-III criteria. New scales, however, are now being constructed to aid in determining DSM-III Axis II diagnoses (Morey, Waugh, & Blashfield, 1985).

The Millon Clinical Multiaxial Inventory (MCMI), a 175-item objective measure, was first introduced in 1977 as a clinical screening instrument. The original purpose was to correct for weaknesses of the MMPI while remaining consistent with the DSM-III diagnostic criteria (Millon, 1983b; Widiger *et al.,* 1985). Members of the DSM-III task force, however, have seriously questioned the similarity between the DSM-III Axis II categories and Millon's test scales (Widiger *et al.,* 1985). Millon (1985) indicated complete overlap between the criteria and the test scores. Regardless, in the 17 or 19 populations studied (total $N = 908$), Scale 6 (Antisocial) was revealed to be the highest mean scale. Furthermore, Millon provided information regarding the prototypical APD profile. Its characteristics are not surprising (see Millon, 1985).

Other Objective Instruments

One instrument of promise is Spielberger's Sociopathy Scale (SPY; Spielberger, Kling, & O'Hagen, 1978), an objective measure used to identify sociopathic personality styles for research purposes. Additionally, the California Psychological Inventory (CPI; Gough, 1957) has been used for diagnostic classification. Antisocial personalities tend to exhibit So (Socialization) scale depressions.

Intelligence Testing

Though the Wechsler Adult Intelligence Scale–Revised (WAIS-R) is not a measure of personality *per se,* APD individuals have shown identifiable test characteristics (Heilbrun, 1982; Rappaport, Gill, & Schafer, 1968). Typically, antisocial personalities exhibit significantly higher Performance than Verbal IQ scores. This finding is frequently attributed to an action orientation and to poor academic histories. Problem academic records also tend to be indicated by depressed Vocabulary, Arithmetic, and Information subtest scores. The APD individual may also show high scores on Picture Arrangement, indicative of a social facility or refined manipulative skills. Poor attention to detail may result in lower Picture Completion scores, as APDs do not always attend to the most salient details of their environment. Finally, deficits in Comprehension and Similarity may be reflective of limited social judgment and a tendency toward concrete rather than abstract problem-solving.

Projective Personality Tests

The Rorschach

It has been noted that personality disorders become readily apparent in intense interpersonal encounters (Vaillant, 1975). As a consequence, the Rorschach inquiry may serve as an excellent instrument for assessing APD. The work of Margaret Singer is especially relevant here. Singer (1977) adopted a transactional approach by treating the test situation as an opportunity to sample the client's interpersonal behavior. Antisocial personalities are usually alert and engaged during the assessment process, keeping responses short to provide a minimum of self-disclosure. The lack of structure may be particularly unnerving for the APD individual, and as a consequence, the total number of responses is apt to be limited. Few abstract responses and little elaboration are to be expected. Rather, popular responses tend to predominate. In addition, the *F%* tends to be low, and affectivity-anxiety is either constrained or absent. However, APDs may display hostility and discomfort, as exhibited by excessive card rotation or a high proportion of white-space responses. Color shock may result in delayed answers or responses indicative of immaturity and impulsivity. Finally, animal content usually predominates over human percepts.

Thematic Apperception Test

In a manner similar to the brief Rorschach protocol, the responses of the APD individual to the Thematic Apperception Test (TAT) tend to be short, poorly elaborated stories. Juvenile themes may arise, and aggressive imagery tends to be used, with little mention of appropriate consequation for antisocial malevolence. Frequently, when relating stories, the subject exhibits affect incongruous with the cruelty expressed. Relationships between characters tend to be instrumental, with little evidence of depth and intimacy. Blame or guilt is typically projected onto others or the environment and is rarely internalized (Bellak, 1975).

Other Projectives

The lack of structure inherent in all projective instruments tends to make the APD individual rather guarded and hostile, coupled with the highly interpersonal and interactive nature of the test situation. Therefore, projective techniques may be quite demanding on both the subject and the examiner. However, in addition to the Rorschach and the TAT, projective drawings have also been used, including the Kinetic Family Drawing to assess family dynamics, the Draw-A-Person test to examine self-image, and projective uses of the Bender-Gestalt (Carney, 1976). In our opinion, projective drawings are best used to substantiate hypotheses suggested by other test materials rather than being administered or interpreted in isolation.

CLINICAL PROBLEMS AND TREATMENT APPLICATION

We have chosen to combine sections on "clinical problems" and "treatment application" because the literature on APD clearly suggests that these topics are naturally integrative. That is, attempting to treat the APD individual operationally defines the term *clinical problem!* In fact, the general consensus among knowledgeable persons is that, to date, an effective treatment has not yet been developed (Turkat & Maisto, 1985). Further, the topic of APD treatment appears to be a stepchild to the historical emphasis on clinical description and etiological explanations of the problem. The interested reader will note, for example, that Cleckley's classical work devoted a mere seven pages to the topic; Hare (1970) discussed treatment for a grand total of eight pages; and the excellent work by Brantley and Sutker (1984) did not deal with treatment at all. Thus, our purpose here is threefold: First, we briefly examine the relevant treatment literature. Second, we present a series of therapeutic principles. Third, we discuss the 10 most common clinical problems encountered in work with APD individuals.

Treatment Literature

A complete review of the APD treatment-outcome literature is beyond the scope of this chapter. Moreover, an exemplary review has been provided by Suedfeld and Landon

(1978). We will, however, briefly comment on research methodology and clinical outcome studies to date.

Research Methodology

A review of the research in the area of APD treatment indicates that it is replete with methodological problems. The most obvious methodological problems are as follows:

1. APD nomenclature has changed dramatically over the years. Correspondingly, diagnostic criteria have also evolved over time. As a consequence, it is difficult to compare results across studies because populations vary as a result of differing diagnostic criteria.

2. A related methodological problem involves the explicitness of the criteria used for subject selection. Frequently, standards for subject inclusion are vague and poorly specified. Thus, the reader is unsure of the exact nature of the presenting problem or the diagnostic impression.

3. Limited information is often provided about therapeutic technique. Was treatment applied as part of a multicomponent package? Is the described treatment, in fact, identical to what was actually imposed? Can the reader clearly discern the therapeutic procedures used? Quite frankly, in a great many instances, clinical replication is a nearly impossible task.

4. Standards for the evaluation of outcome have been grossly inadequate. Change may occur, but the level of clinical significance remains virtually unknown.

5. Follow-up data are rarely provided. In those instances where such information is obtained, the reporting of mean scores is of scant help in describing the change processes within the individual client. In sum, APD experimental methodology most certainly leaves something to be desired.

Clinical Outcome

As already suggested in this chapter, successful clinical outcome is far from ensured when one is treating the APD individual. In fact, treatment variability arises from a number of factors: (1) the severity of the disorder; (2) the expertise of the therapist; (3) the appropriateness of the treatment modality used; and (4) the expectations of the referring parties who have encouraged the client to seek treatment. In any case, the most commonly used treatment methods include individual, group, and milieu approaches.

McCord and McCord (1956) reviewed psychoanalytic work over the course of 30 years. They expressed little optimism regarding psychoanalytic prospects when applied to APD. Though advocates exist (Dias, 1963; Schmideberg, 1949), no pervasive evidence attests to the successful treatment of APD by analytic procedures. Ferrari and Marticorena (1968) reported some positive results when using short-term individual therapy in conjunction with group approaches. In general, group therapy frequently contains a wide variety of treatment techniques (e.g., medication, psychodrama, Gestalt procedures, and behavior modification tactics), and therapeutic purity therefore becomes an impossibility. In any case, there are some supportive data regarding the efficacy of structured group therapy and milieu approaches (Craft, 1969). Chemotherapeutic interventions have not proved very successful (McCord & McCord, 1956), and psychosurgical methods are now generally frowned on. Behavior modification programs, on the other hand, have shown some promise. Unfortunately, long-term follow-up results have not been encouraging (Jesness, 1975). Nonetheless, the therapeutic principles elaborated below are an attempt to operationalize effective tactics that may be used in the outpatient treatment of APD.

Therapeutic Principles

A number of comments can be made about the treatment of APD. First, the client needs to commit to treatment on some recognizable level. This may be as simplistic as the statement "I need to change my behavior." Once having made such a commitment, the client must be challenged to decide what kind of behavior he or she wants to change. In fact, such challenging should continue throughout the course of treatment; otherwise, the therapist will be working to *make* the client change—a futile endeavor!

Second, clinicians must constantly guard against the client's need to manipulate. It is our contention that the therapist must assume that the information presented to him or her by the client is, in fact, distorted. In essence, individuals with APD are to be presumed guilty of distortion or lying unless it is proved otherwise. Clearly, it is not the task of the therapist to play detective. Rather, when confronted with obvious dishonesty, the therapist should simply state, "I find that hard to believe." Under such circumstances, evidence and alibis will most assuredly be forthcoming. A change in factual data is required to disprove the distortion or lie; words, by themselves, should hold little weight. In essence, the therapist is not a judge, and the provision of evidence is quite irrelevant. The client must learn that psychotherapy is not akin to criminal court proceedings. It is, instead, a means by which clients may examine their own behavior and receive honest feedback regarding the effect they have on others.

Third, the therapist's task is not to criticize and/or devalue the client's way of relating to the world. Rather, it is his or her job to challenge for "effective" functioning. This approach suggests a proactive stance by the therapist, so that the individual with APD is provided with an opportunity for self-examination and to explore the determinants of his or her own behavior. This goal is best accomplished by providing a therapeutic mirror. Clearly, the intent of such a mirror is that the client come to recognize the self-centered, self-defeating behavior patterns that he or she typically exhibits. Obviously, this recognition is difficult for the client as his or her tendency is to act on impulse without much insight or introspection.

Fourth, a variety of criteria should be used for the assessment of progress. These might include a demonstration that the client is able to envision the consequences of his or her own behavior; role taking and understanding the feelings of others; the development of intimacy and trust in others; an increased degree of comfort in discussing the past; and the diminution or eradication of secrets. Control of impulsiveness can also be evinced via the maintenance of a residence, a job, good health, and interpersonal relationships. Positive reconnections may be made with family, and other life areas may show similar qualitative improvements.

Finally, the clinician must remember that time is on his or her side. That is, APD prognosis improves as time passes (Craft, 1969). Such behavioral improvement is probably the result of "burnout." Alternatively, clients may simply become more sophisticated in their antisocial endeavors and therefore less likely to be apprehended and prosecuted.

Common Clinical Problems

Psychotherapy with the individual with APD can be a frustrating and difficult process even for the most skilled clinician. As a result of our clinical experience in working with such individuals, we have developed a list of frequent problems typically encountered with this population. In the discussion that follows, we attempt to note both the problem and the means by which the clinician can most effectively deal with the situation:

1. The individual with APD is frequently forced into treatment. Obviously, this circumstance may not be conducive to the development of a good working relationship. It is therefore recommended that this issue be directly confronted, preferably very early in the course of treatment. Specifically, the client should be asked what it is that he or she would like to get out of therapy regardless of why or by whom he or she was referred. In essence, the client is asked to explore how to benefit from the therapeutic relationship. Indeed, this issue may need to be addressed frequently throughout the treatment process, particularly when impasses are reached.

2. Given that the client with APD is often referred by a third party (e.g., a judge or a probation officer), solicited or unsolicited reports and information are frequently received by the therapist. Indeed, there may even be times when the therapist must provide information (assuming client permission has been obtained) to the referring agency. In such cases, the therapist must model open, forthright, and direct communication with the client. That is, details of the third-party conversation or written communication should be provided to and discussed with the client. Although therapist communication with third parties may initially arouse strong feeling in the client (e.g., anger and distrust), it can serve as an excellent tool for the establishment of more effective interpersonal relations.

3. Many individuals with APD attempt to provide the therapist with distracting crises or fascinating, scintillating stories that extol their many exploits. The information presented may be interesting but only tangentially related to the discussion at hand. Consequently, the therapist must understand the dynamics involved (e.g., self-agrandizement and sidetracking) and must maintain control by bringing the client back to a discussion of the more relevant issues. Thus, it would be quite appropriate to ask the following of the client: "I wonder what purpose is served when you share with me the explicit details of your many escapades?" In so doing, the therapist allows the opportunity for a here-and-now examination of the client's behavior.

4. In a manner similar to that noted above, the client will often attempt to misdirect the course of therapy by seizing on irrelevant and/or global topics for discussion (e.g., broad philosophical, religious, legal, political, or societal issues or psychological theories). Once again, the therapist must redirect the dialogue to more germane topics and must further comment on the interactional pattern that has emerged.

5. Early in treatment, the client is apt to lavishly and generously praise the therapist for his or her caring. At this point, such praise tends to be wholly disingenuous and merely an attempt at manipulation or emotional seduction. Consequently, a more reality-based interpretation of the relationship should be presented. Further, the therapist may openly comment that perhaps the client's intent is somewhat deceptive. The nature of the client's presumed perception can then be discussed as an appropriate treatment issue.

6. As therapy progresses, obvious lies or distortions on the part of the client will occur. The therapist must be sure to confront them immediately, not with anger, but as incidents that are simply worth examining more closely. The therapist should not argue with the client

regarding truthfulness in this specific instance. Rather, an attempt should be made to point out to the client that others cannot trust in him or her, and that he or she, in turn, cannot trust in others. The client must come to recognize the pervasiveness of this problem and the manner in which it contributes to and exacerbates his or her life dissatisfaction.

7. During the course of therapy, the client may experience strong feelings of anger. The clinician working with such individuals should therefore be prepared and should anticipate when these reactions are likely to occur. In fact, anger tends to be predictably encountered when the client finds that his or her long-standing maladaptive patterns of behavior no longer bring forth the expected results. Consequently, the client is apt to experience frustration and hostility toward himself or herself and toward those who thwart his or her misdirected endeavors. Retaliation and acting out are not at all uncommon at this time. This behavior must be confronted and dynamically explored in a nonjudgmental manner. The client needs to learn that his or her anger is controllable, justifiable, and capable of being expressed without destruction of persons or property.

8. In addition to anger, as manipulations prove no longer effective and behavior begins to change, the client may exhibit some degree of boredom and feelings of despair because life just is not as exciting as it used to be. This affective state must be questioned and some understanding achieved. Moreover, alternative socially appropriate forms of stimulation should be explored as possible means by which the client may find satisfaction with his or her newly developing lifestyle. Competition, games, and athletic activities are excellent outlets of appropriate sublimation.

9. When working with clients with APD, therapists must be prepared to set and enforce limits both inside and outside therapy. For example, a clinician cannot tolerate repeated missed appointments. If, after discussion and exploration, such behavior continues, the therapist must inform the client of the consequences. Namely, a hierarchy of consequences may be implemented with termination as the end point. Such action is prompted by our belief that great disservice is done by continuing to reinforce the client's irresponsible behavior. Financial obligations and the mechanics of payment serve as a case in point. We believe that, immediately on contracting for treatment, the client should be informed that payment is expected at the time the services are provided. Undoubtedly, there will be occasions when such payment does not occur. Clearly, these incidents are grist for the therapeutic mill, and the therapist must bring this issue up for discussion and attempt to examine its meaning within the therapeutic relationship. Later, as progress is achieved and mutual trust begins to develop, payment at the time of service may be modified. In fact, the client may be "rewarded" with traditional monthly billing statements as the APD symptomatology lessens in response to treatment.

10. Clarity must be achieved, maintained, and imparted both within the therapy room and in contact with referral agencies. If expectations differ among the concerned parties, therapeutic and administrative problems are bound to arise. These may involve the amount of time to be committed to therapy, the length of treatment, issues of privacy, the release of information, and/or the collection of research data. Failure to focus adequately on any of these potential problems will undoubtedly compromise the effectiveness of the treatment.

SUMMARY

This chapter has reviewed the concept of antisocial personality disorder (APD). After a brief historical overview, the DSM-III diagnostic criteria for the disorder were presented. Some distinction was made between early and contemporary formulations for APD. Developmental, environmental, genetic, and neurophysiological influences in the progression of APD were highlighted. A variety of assessment tools (e.g., interviews, checklists, and objective and projective personality instruments) were surveyed, and comments were made on their usefulness in the establishment of accurate diagnoses. Finally, selected remarks about the treatment literature, therapeutic principles, and common clinical problems were presented within the context of outpatient APD intervention programs.

REFERENCES

Alexander, F. (1923). *Psychoanalysis of the total personality* (English translation, 1930). New York: Nervous and Mental Disease Publications.

Alexander, F. (1935). *Roots of crime.* New York: Knopf.

Allen, F. (1950). The psychopathic delinquent child. *American Journal of Orthopsychiatry, 20,* 223–265.

American Psychiatric Association. (1952). *Diagnostic and statistical manual of mental disorders* (1st ed.; DSM-I). Washington, DC: Author.

American Psychiatric Association. (1968). *Diagnostic and statistical manual of mental disorders* (2nd ed.; DSM-II). Washington, DC: Author.

American Psychiatric Association. (1980). *Diagnostic and statistical manual of mental disorders* (3rd ed.; DSM-III). Washington, DC: Author.

American Psychiatric Association. (1987). *Diagnostic and statistical manual of mental disorders* (3rd ed. rev.; DSM-III-R). Washington, DC: Author.

Arthur, R. G. S., & Cahoon, E. B. (1964). A clinical and electroencephalographic survey of psychopathic personality. *American Journal of Psychiatry, 120,* 875–882.

Bandura, A., & Walters, R. H. (1959). *Adolescent aggression.* New York: Ronald.

Bellak, L. (1975). *The thematic apperception test and the senior apperception test in clinical use.* New York: Grune & Stratton.

Birnbaum, K. (1914). *Die psychopathischen verbrecker* (2nd ed.). Leipzig: Thieme.

Brantley, P. J., & Sutker, P. B. (1984). Antisocial behavior disorders. In H. E. Adams & P. B. Sutker (Eds.), *Comprehensive handbook of psychopathology.* New York: Plenum Press.

Bursten, B. (1972). The manipulative personality. *Archives of General Psychiatry, 26,* 318–321.

Carney, F. L. (1976). Psychological testing of the personality disorders. In J. R. Lion (Ed.), *Personality disorders: Diagnosis and management* (pp. 253–267). Baltimore: Williams & Wilkins.

Cleckley, H. (1964). *The mask of sanity* (4th ed.). St. Louis: Mosby.

Cleckley, H. (1976). *The mask of sanity* (5th ed.). St. Louis: Mosby.

Cloninger, C. R., Reich, T., & Guze, S. B. (1978). Genetic-environmental interactions and antisocial behaviour. In R. D. Hare & D. Schalling (Eds.), *Psychopathic behavior: Approaches to research* (pp. 225–237). New York: Wiley.

Craddick, R. (1962). Selection of psychopathic from nonpsychopathic prisoners within a Canadian prison. *Psychological Reports, 10,* 495–499.

Craft, M. J. (1969). The natural history of psychopathic disorder. *British Journal of Psychiatry, 115,* 39–44.

Dias, P. C. (1963). Symposium in psychopathology and neurosis: Therapeutic procedures. *Jornal Brasileiro de Psiquiatria, 12,* 69–80.

Dinitz, S. (1980). The antisocial personality. In W. J. Curran, A. L. McQuarry, & C. S. Petty (Eds.), *Modern legal medicine, psychiatry, and forensic science,* (pp. 799–813). Philadelphia: F. A. Davis.

Dupré, E. (1925). La doctrine des constitutions. In E. Dupré (Ed.), *Pathologie de l'imagination et de l'emotivité.* Paris: Payot.

Esquirol, E. (1838). *Maladies mentales* (2 vols.). Paris: Bailliere.

Eysenck, H. J. (1967). *The biological basis of personality.* Springfield, IL: Charles C Thomas.

Ferrari, H., & Marticorena, A. G. (1968). An experiment in short-term therapy. *Acta Psiquiatrica' y Psicologica de America Latina, 14,* 139–143.

Friedlander, K. (1945). Formation of the antisocial character. *Psychoanalytic Study of the Child, 1,* 189–203.

Gilberstadt, H., & Duker, J. (1965). *A handbook for clinical and acturial MMPI interpretation.* Philadelphia: Saunders.

Glueck, S., & Glueck, E. T. (1950). *Unraveling juvenile delinquency.* New York: Commonwealth Fund.

Glueck, S., & Glueck, E. (1963). *Criminal careers in retrospect.* New York: The Commonwealth Fund: Harvard University Press.

Gouch, H. G. (1957). *Manual for the California Psychological Inventory.* Palo Alto, CA: Consulting Psychologist Press.

Gouster, M. (1878). Moral insanity. *Review of Scientific Medicine, 38,* 115–131.

Green, R. L. (1980). *The MMPI: An interpretive manual.* New York: Grune & Stratton.

Guze, S. B. (1976). *Criminality and psychiatric disorders.* New York: Oxford University Press.

Hare, R. D. (1970). *Psychopathy: Theory and research.* New York: Wiley.

Hare, R. D. (1983). Diagnosis of antisocial personality disorder in two prison populations. *American Journal of Psychiatry, 140,* 887–890.

Hawk, S. S., & Peterson, R. A. (1974). Do MMPI psychopathic deviancy scores reflect psychopathic deviancy or just deviancy? *Journal of Personality Assessment, 38,* 362–368.

Hedlund, J. L. (1977). MMPI clinical scale correlates. *Journal of Consulting and Clinical Psychology, 45,* 739–750.

Heilbrun, A. B., Jr. (1982). Cognitive models of criminal violence based upon intelligence and psychopathy levels. *Journal of Consulting and Clinical Psychology, 50,* 546–557.

Horney, K. (1945). *Our inner conflicts.* New York: Norton.

Jenkins, R. L. (1964). Diagnosis, dynamics, and treatment in child psychiatry. *Psychiatric Research Reports, 18,* 91–120.

Jesness, C. F. (1975). Comparative effectiveness of behavior modification and transactional analysis programmes for delinquents. *Journal of Consulting and Clinical Psychology, 43,* 738–779.

Kaplan, H. I., & Sadock, B. J. (Eds.), (1985). *Comprehensive textbook of psychiatry, IV.* Baltimore, MD: Williams & Wilkins.

Kazdin, A. E., & Frame, C. (1983). Aggressive behavior and conduct disorder. In R. J. Morris & T. R. Kratochwill (Eds.). *The practice of child therapy* (pp. 167–192). New York: Pergamon Press.

Kennedy, W. (1975). *Legs.* New York: Penguin Books.

Koch, J. L. A. (1891). *Die psychopathischen Minderwertigkeiten. Erste Abteilung. Einleitung-Die angeborenen andauernden psychopathischen Minderwertigkeiten.* Ravensburg: Otto Maier.

Kraepelin, E. (1896). *Psychiatrie: Ein lehrbuch.* (5th ed.). Leipzig: Barth.

Kraepelin, E. (1915). *Psychiatrie: Ein lehrbuch.* (8th ed.). Leipzig: Barth.

Lombroso, C. (1872–1885). *L'Uomo delinquente.* Bocca: Torina.

Magnan, V. & Legrain, M. (1895). *Les degeneres (etat mental et syndromes episodiques).* Paris: Rueff et Cie.

Maudsley, H. (1874). *Responsibility in mental disease.* London: King.

Marks, P., Seeman, W., & Haller, D. (1974). *The actuarial use of the MMPI with adolescents and adults.* Baltimore: Williams & Wilkins.

McCord, W., & McCord, J. (1956). *Psychopathy and delinquency.* New York: Grune & Stratton.

Megargee, E. I. (1972). *California psychological inventory handbook.* San Francisco: Jossey-Bass.

Millon, T. (1969). *Modern psychopathology: A biosocial approach to maladaptive learning and functioning.* Philadelphia: W. B. Saunders.

Millon, T. (1981). *Disorders of personality, DSM-III: Axis II.* New York: Wiley.

Millon, T. (1983a). The DSM-III: An insider's perspective. *American Psychologist, 38,* 804–814.

Millon, T. (1983b). *Millon clinical multiaxial inventory manual* (3rd ed.). Minneapolis: National Computer Systems.

Millon, T. (1985). The MCMI provides a good assessment of DSM-III disorders: The MCMI-II will prove even better. *Journal of Personality Assessment, 49,* 379–391.

Mischel, W. (1968). *Personality and assessment.* New York: Wiley.

Morel, B. A. (1857). *Traite des degenerescences physiques intellectualles et morales: de l'espece humaine et des causes qui produisent ces varietes maladives.* Paris: Bailliere.

Morey, L. C., Waugh, M. H. & Blashfield, R. K. (1985). MMPI scales for DSM-III personality disorders: Their derivation and correlates. *Journal of Personality Assessment, 49,* 245–251.

Morrison, H. L. (1978). The asocial child: A destiny of sociopathy? In W. Reid (Ed.), *The psychopath: A comprehensive study of antisocial disorders and behaviors* (pp. 22–65). New York: Brunner/Mazel.

O'Neal, P., & Robins, L. N. (1958). The relation of childhood behavior problems to adult psychiatric status: A 30-year follow-up study of 150 subjects. *American Journal of Psychiatry, 114,* 961–969.

Partridge, G. E. (1927). A study of 50 cases of psychopathic personality. *American Journal of Psychiatry, 7,* 953–974.

Partridge, G. E. (1928). Psychopathic personality and personality investigation. *American Journal of Psychiatry, 8,* 1053–1064.

Partridge, G. E. (1930). Current conceptions of psychopathic personality. *American Journal of Psychiatry, 10* 53–99.

Peterson, D. R., Quay, H. C., & Cameron, G. E. (1959). Personality and background factors in juvenile delinquency as inferred from questionnaire responses. *Journal of Consulting Psychology, 23,* 395–399.

Pichot, P. (1978). Psychopathic behavior: A historical overview. In R. D. Hare & D. Schalling (Eds.), *Psychopathic behaviour: Approaches to research* (pp. 55–70). Chichester: Wiley.

Pinel, P. (1809). *Traite medico-philosophique sur l'alienation mentale* (2nd ed.). Paris: Brosson.

Potterfield, J. H. (1978). The hyperactive child syndrome: A precursor of adult psychopathy? In R. D. Hare & D. Schalling (Eds.), *Psychopathic behavior: Approaches to research* (pp. 329–346). New York: Wiley.

Pritchard, J. C. (1835). *A treatise on insanity and other disorders affecting the mind.* London: Sherwood, Gilbert, & Piper.

Quay, H. C. (1964). Personality dimensions in delinquent males as inferred from the factor analysis of behavior ratings. *Journal of Research in Crime and Delinquency, 1,* 33–37.

Rappaport, D., Gill, M. M., & Schafer, R. (1968). *Diagnostic psychological testing.* New York: International Universities Press.

Robins, L. N. (1966). *Deviant children grown up: A sociological and psychiatric study of sociopathic personality.* Baltimore: Williams & Wilkins.

Robins, L. N. (1978). Aetiological implications in studies of childhood histories relating to antisocial personality. In R. D. Hare & D. Schalling (Eds.), *Psychopathic behavior: Approaches to research* (pp. 255–271). New York: Wiley.

Robins, L. N., Murphy, G. E., Woodruff, R. A., Jr., & King, L. J. (1971). The adult psychiatric status of black schoolboys. *Archives of General Psychiatry, 24,* 338–345.

Rush, B. (1812). *Medical inquiries and observations upon the diseases of the mind.* Philadelphia: Kimber & Richardson.

Rutter, M. (1971). Parent-child separation: Psychological effects on the children. *Journal of Child Psychology and Psychiatry, 12,* 233–256.

Satterfield, J. H. (1978). The hyperactive child syndrome: A precursor of adult psychopathy? In R. D. Hare & D. Schalling (Eds.), *Psychopathic behavior: Approaches to research* New York: Wiley.

Schmideberg, M. (1949). The analytic treatment of major criminals: Therapeutic results and technical problems. *International Journal of Psychoanalysis, 30,* 197 (Abstract).

Schroeder, M. L., Schroeder, K. G., & Hare, R. D. (1983). Generalizability of a checklist for assessment of psychopathy. *Journal of Consulting and Clinical Psychology, 51,* 511–516.

Singer, M. T. (1977). The Rorschach as a transaction. In M. A. Rickers-Ousiankinn (ed.) *Rorschach Psychology, revised edition* (pp. 455–485). Huntington: Kreiger Publishing, Inc.

Spielberger, C. D., Kling, J. K., & O'Hagen, S. E. J. (1978). Dimensions of psychopathic personality. In R. D. Hare & D. Schalling (Eds.), *Psychopathic behavior: Approaches to research* (pp. 23–46). New York: Wiley.

Suedfeld, P., & Landon, P. B. (1978). Approaches to treatment. In R. D. Hare & D. Schalling (Eds.), *Psychopathic behavior: Approaches to research* (pp. 347–376). New York: Wiley.

Szurek, S. A. (1969). Childhood origins of psychopathic personality trends. In S. A. Szurek & I. N. Berlin (Eds.), *The antisocial child: His family and his community* (pp. 2–12). Palo Alto, CA: Science and Behavior Books.

Szurek, S. A., & Berlin, I. N. (1969). *The antisocial child: His family and his community.* Palo Alto, CA: Science and Behavior Books.

Tuke, D. H. (1892). *Dictionary of psychological medicine.* Philadelphia: Blakiston.

Turkat, I. D., & Maisto, S. A. (1985). Application of the experimental method to the formulation and modification of personality disorders. In D. H. Barlow (Ed.), *Clinical handbook of psychological disorders: A step by step treatment manual.* New York: Guilford Press.

Yochelson, S., & Samenow, S. (1976). *The criminal personality* (Vol. 1). New York: Jason Aronson.

Vaillant, G. E. (1975). Sociopathy as a human process: A viewpoint. *Archives of General Psychiatry, 32,* 178–183.

Vaillant, G. E., & Perry, J. C. (1980). Personality disorders. In H. L. Kaplan, M. Friedman, & B. J. Saddock (Eds.), *Comprehensive textbook of psychiatry* (3rd ed.). Baltimore: Williams & Wilkins.

Widiger, T. A., Williams, J. B. W., Spitzer, R. L., & Frances, A. (1985). The MCMI as a measure of DSM-III. *Journal of Personality Assessment, 49,* 366–378.

Williams, J. B., & Spitzer, R. L. (1980). DSM-III field trial: Interrater reliability and list of project staff and participants. In American Psychiatric Association, *Diagnostic and statistical manual of mental disorders* (3rd ed.). Washington, DC: author.

World Health Organization (1978). *Mental disorders: Glossary and guide to their classification in accordance with the ninth revision of the International Classification of Diseases.* Geneva: Author.

Wulach, J. S. (1983). Diagnosing the DSM-III antisocial personality disorder. *Professional Psychology: Research and Practice, 14,* 330–340.

Ziskind, E. (1978). The diagnosis of sociopathy. In R. D. Hare & D. Schalling (Eds.), *Psychopathic behavior: Approaches to research* (pp. 47–54). New York: Wiley.

16

Alzheimer Disease and Other Dementias

BENOIT H. MULSANT AND JOE E. THORNTON

INTRODUCTION

This chapter discusses the outpatient management of dementia, with a major focus on Alzheimer disease (AD) and other irreversible dementing disorders. Their epidemiology and the demographic characteristics of the American population threaten to make dementia one of the major medical, social, and economic problems of our society during the coming decades. Dementia is a markedly age-dependent condition affecting 5%–15% of the population over age 65 and 25% of those over 85, the fastest growing segment of the U.S. population. Recent epidemiological studies (e.g., Rocca, Amaducci, & Schoenberg, 1986) have predicted that, despite a constant incidence rate, the prevalence of severe AD will increase by 42% during the next 15 years; more than 8 million people could be affected by the year 2000. Dementia is one of the major determinants of institutionalization (Katzman, 1986), and 60%–70% of nursing-home patients suffer from a dementing disorder—AD in 50%–80% of cases (U.S. Congress, 1985). According to the U.S. Congress Office of Technology Assessment, the cost of institutional care for patients with dementia exceeded $25 billion in 1985 and will have escalated to $43 billion a year by 1990.

Outpatient psychiatrists and other mental-health workers have a major role to play in the battle to control the social and economic burden of dementia. Despite extensive research efforts, effective means of prevention or specific treatments are available for only a few (10%–30%) dementing disorders. Furthermore, no dramatic therapeutic advance is to be expected until several basic problems—the identification of both the etiological

BENOIT H. MULSANT and JOE E. THORNTON • Department of Psychiatry, Western Psychiatric Institute and Clinic, University of Pittsburgh, Pittsburgh, Pennsylvania 15213.

factors and accurate peripheral markers, as well as an understanding of the genetics and pathogenesis—are solved. Although intensive research efforts continue, immediate efforts should focus on the outpatient management of dementia.

Contrary to popular beliefs, families do not abandon their failing elderly relatives. Rather, families make up the largest group of caregivers, providing 80% of the long-term care received by the extremely impaired elderly (Brody, Johnsen, Fulcomer, & Lang, 1983; Shanas, 1979a). Once reversible or arrestable dementing disorders have been ruled out, the major goal of the outpatient clinician should be to support those who constitute the patients' caregiving system. At present, this is the most effective way to preserve the quality of life and the autonomy of the affected individuals (Brody, Poulshock, & Masciocchio, 1978; Shanas, 1979a). Because institutionalization rates are not linked to patients' characteristics but to family burden (Colerick & George, 1986; Gilhooly, 1984; Goldstein, Regnery, & Wellin, 1981; Kraus, Spasoff, Beattie, Holden, Lawson, Rodenburg, & Woodcock, 1976; Sanford, 1975), this is best accomplished first by providing support to the family caregivers and, second, by attempting to control the target symptoms and behaviors associated with physical and emotional strain for the caregivers (Lezak, 1978; Morycz, 1980; Thornton, Davies, & Tinklenberg, 1986; Zarit & Zarit, 1982).

HISTORICAL OVERVIEW

Dementia, derived from the Latin *de* (''out of'') and *mens* (''mind''), means literally, ''out of one's mind.'' In the revised third edition of the American Psychiatric Association's *Diagnostic and Statistical Manual of Mental Disorders* (DSM-III-R; APA, 1987), this term is restricted to a syndrome characterized by an acquired cognitive deterioration involving memory and at least one other high function, or by personality changes with significant impairment of social or occupational functioning. Alzheimer disease, first described in 1907, is currently the most prevalent cause of dementia, accounting for at least 50% of cases (Katzman, 1986), however, this was not always the case and many of the more than 60 recognized dementing disorders had already been identified by 1907. (Table 1 shows a breakdown of the relative frequencies of different dementing disorders.)

The Continuing Identification of Dementing Disorders

During modern times, the identification of the various causes of dementia started in 1735, when a Spanish physician described pellagra under the name *mal de la rosa* and attributed it to a poor diet. Characterized by a typical triad of dermatitis, diarrhea, and dementia (''the three D's''), it was shown to be prevented by the ingestion of nicotinic acid (niacin) in 1937. In his 1817 ''Essay on Shaking Palsy,'' James Parkinson (himself a victim) mentioned specifically ''the unimpaired state of the intellect'' (p. 45). However, he clearly reported neuropsychiatric disturbances in some of his cases, and this association has since been increasingly recognized (Boller, 1980). In 1822, Bayle characterized general paresis (chronic syphilitic meningoencephalitis) as a clinical and pathological entity; its relation to syphilis was first proposed in 1857. At the turn of the century, about 50% of the patients in state mental hospitals were suffering from syphilitic dementia paralytica. With the antibiotic treatment of syphilis and the subsequent prevention of its tertiary form, a major cause of dementia was eliminated during this century. Even though the CNS effects of vitamin B_{12} deficiency have mostly been ignored until recently,

Table 1. Estimated Relative Frequencies of Various Dementias[a]

Diagnosis	Percentage
Alzheimer disease	40
Mixed vascular and Alzheimer	25
Vascular	10
Alcoholic	5
Drug intoxication	3
Intracranial mass	2
Normal-pressure hydrocephalus	2
Huntington disease	1
Uncertain	3
Creutzfeldt-Jakob disease	1
Other (includes posttraumatic, postsubarachnoid hemorrhage, postencephalitic neurosyphilis, amyotrophic lateral sclerosis, Parkinsonism, Pick disease, thyroidopathy, pernicious anemia, hepatic failure, and epilepsy)	8

[a]After Blessed *et al.* (1968); Larson *et al.* (1985); Rocca *et al.* (1986); Wade *et al.* (1987); and Wells (1977).

Addison mentioned occasional "wandering of the mind" in his 1849 and 1855 descriptions of pernicious anemia.

In 1872, George Huntington reported on families with an incurable chorea and noted that "as the disease progresses, the mind becomes more or less impaired, in many amounting to insanity" (cited in Cummings & Benson, 1983); later on, the autosomal dominant transmission of Huntington disease was confirmed, and the German neurologist Alois Alzheimer demonstrated its organic basis. In 1873, Gull published a paper, "On a Cretinoid State Supervening in Adult Life in Women," named *myxedema* 4 years later. In 1881, Wernicke reported a clinical triad consisting of acute ophthalmoplegia, ataxia, and clouding of consciousness; 6 years later, Korsakoff described the co-occurrence of recent-memory deficit, confabulation, apathy, and progressive dementia. The syndrome, usually associated with alcohol abuse and a poor diet, can be reversed by the early administration of thiamine. In 1892, Arnold Pick first characterized the clinical and pathological features of a progressive senile dementia, often presenting as personality change and with a marked atrophy of the frontal and temporal lobes; again, Alzheimer delineated the associated histological changes in 1911, after having reported on a presenile dementia in 1907.

Other causes of dementia, such as the autosomal recessive hepatolenticular degeneration described by Wilson in 1912, have continued to be regularly identified; the most relevant are Creutzfeldt-Jakob disease (1921), the prototypical subcortical dementia; progressive supranuclear palsy (1963); normal pressure hydrocephalus (1964); the dementia syndrome of depression (Kay, Roth, & Hopkins, 1955); the various types of vascular dementias (Blessed, Tomlinson, & Roth, 1968; Freyhan, Woodford, & Kety, 1951; Hachinski, Lassen, & Marshall, 1974); and most recently the AIDS dementia complex (Navia & Price, 1987; Nielsen, Petito, Urmacher, & Posner, 1984).

In 1907, Alois Alzheimer reported a case of presenile dementia in an otherwise healthy 54-year-old female who presented with suspiciousness, memory impairment, spatial disorientation, and anomic aphasia. When she died 4 years later after a continuous deterioration, her brain autopsy demonstrated ''senile'' (neuritic) plaques and neurofibrillary tangles. In the 1920s, other case reports were published, followed by reports of families with presenile dementia or Alzheimer disease, as Kraepelin had called it (Amaducci, Rocca, & Schoenberg, 1986)

In 1952, Sjogren, Sjogren, and Lindgren wrote a series of papers entitled ''Morbus Alzheimer's and Morbus Pick's,'' a retrospective review of 84 cases of dementia seen in a Swedish state hospital. This study established the modern concept of AD: it suggested that (1) many cases arise in the senile age range; (2) about 10% of cases have a positive family history with an autosomal dominant pattern of transmission; and (3) three stages can be delineated: the confused, demented, and vegetative stages.

In 1962, Sim and Sussman's remarkable naturalistic study completed the clinical picture. They followed 21 patients longitudinally for 4 years and obtained, for 13, either a brain biopsy or an autopsy. They established the pattern of *a*mnesia (with, in particular, the difficulty of learning new material), preceding *a*phasia, *a*praxia, and *a*gnosia—the four A's of AD—and confirmed the occurrence of myoclonic jerks and seizures, particularly in the late stages of the disease. At that time, however, most cases of dementia were still attributed to either normal aging or cerebral arteriosclerosis. In 1951, Freyhan, Woodford, and Kety had documented decreased brain blood flow in a group of sufferers from senile organic psychosis. They attributed it to ''hardening of the arteries.'' This theory was refuted in 1968, when Blessed, Tomlinson, and Roth published their landmark prospective study entitled ''The Association between Quantitative Measures of Dementia and of Senile Changes in the Cerebral Gray Matter of Elderly Subjects.'' Using control groups, they clearly demonstrated that dementia is not part of normal aging but is associated with one of two specific cortical pathologies: either the changes characteristic of AD or, more rarely, multiple small infarcts. Atherosclerosis was not by itself predictive of dementia. Furthermore, the study established a strong correlation between scores on cognitive and function tests and either the number of neuritic plaques or the amount of infarcted tissue.

Associated findings are cerebellar signs (Huff, Boller, Luchelli, Querriera, Beyer, & Belle, 1987), sleep-disordered breathing (Hoch, Reynolds, Nebes, Kupfer, Berman, & Campbell, 1988), cardiovascular autonomic instability (Francheschi, Ferini-Strambi, Minicucci, Sferrazza-Papa, & Smirne, 1986; Rezek, 1987; Warner, Peabody, Flattery, & Tinklenberg, 1986), olfactory deficits (Knupfer & Speigel, 1986), visual field deficits (Steffes & Thralow, 1987), and hearing impairment (Grimes, Grady, Foster, Sunderland, & Patronas, 1985). Extrapyramidal reactions (EPRs) are not uncommon (Stern, Mayeux, Sano, Hauser, & Bush, 1987). The clinical conceptualization of AD, as it exists today, had been completed.

A Decade of Basic Science Advances and Clinical Trials

The late 1970s were marked by an increasing political and social awareness of the magnitude and clinical significance of AD, best illustrated by Katzman's paper (1976), ''The Prevalence and Malignancy of Alzheimer Disease,'' reporting that AD was probably the fourth leading cause of death for American adults. The time was ripe for a major research effort toward the understanding of the etiological and pathogenic mechanisms and the development of specific preventive and therapeutic modalities; the National Institute of Aging, founded in 1975, and other federal agencies were ready to support this effort.

In 1973 and 1974, advances in neurochemistry led to the identification of specific neurotransmitter deficiencies in Huntington and Parkinson disease patients (GABA and dopamine, respectively). Also in 1974, Drachman and Leavitt documented the role of the cholinergic system in human memory. Only 2 years later, two research groups demonstrated independently a specific cholinergic deficit and a loss of central cholinergic neurons in AD (Davies & Maloney, 1976; Perry, Perry, Blessed, & Tomlinson, 1977). A follow-up study (Perry, Tomlinson, Blessed, Gergmann, Gibson, & Perry, 1978) demonstrated a close topographical correlation between senile plaques and the cholinergic abnormalities. It confirmed that both morphological and biochemical pathological changes characteristic of AD are not diffuse but have a preferential topographical pattern in the cerebral hemispheres. It also established a strong quantitative correlation between the number of senile plaques, cholinergic abnormalities, and scores on structured cognitive tests.

By then, it had been established that (1) AD is a specific disease distinct from the process of normal aging; (2) it is characterized by specific neuropathological changes (i.e., neurofibrillary tangles and neuritic plaques, occurring in a preferential topographical pattern); (3) presenile and senile forms represent the same entity occurring in presenile and senile populations; (4) it is associated with a specific biochemical abnormality (i.e., a central cholinergic deficit); and (5) this abnormality may be causally linked to memory impairment, one of AD's clinical hallmarks.

Further advances (Cummings & Benson, 1983; Katzman, 1986) attributed the CNS cholinergic deficit to a presynaptic decrease in choline acetyltransferase, an enzyme controlling acetylcholine synthesis. A significant reduction of the neuropeptide somatostatin was also identified consistently in the brain of AD patients. Finally, investigations of the complex relation between neurofibrillary tangles, neuritic plaques, amyloid proteins, and the cytoskeleton have been undertaken and are still progressing. New evidence also suggests that cholinesterases may play a role in the pathogenetic development of plaques and tangles and that cholinesterase inhibitors, such as physostigmine and tetrahydro-5-aminoacridine (THA), may actually have different biological effects in the AD brain and in the normal aged brain (Mesulam, Geula, & Moran, 1987).

A major area of interest has been the search for biological markers or diagnostic tests specific for AD and related disorders (Cutler, 1987). Most studies have focused on neurotransmitter levels in blood and cerebrospinal fluid. Interesting markers include platelet membrane fluidity (Zubenko, Wusylko, Cohen, Boller, & Teply, 1987), the cerebrospinal fluid (CSF) protein A68 (Wolozin & Davies, 1987), and pharmacological challenges, such as the effects of scopolamine on cognitive performance (Sunderland, Tariot, Murphy, Weingartner, Mueller, & Cohen, 1985).

Other markers have included 20-minute EEG recordings (Brenner, Reynolds, & Ulrich, 1988), EEG spectral analysis (Brenner, Ulrich, Spiker, Sclabassi, Reynolds, Marin, & Boller, 1986), sleep EEG recordings (Leuchter, Spar, Walter, & Weiner, 1987; Reynolds, Kupfer, Houck, Hoch, Stack, Berman, & Zimmer, 1988), event-related potentials (e.g., P300; St. Clair, Blackburn, Blackwood, & Tyrer, 1988), cerebral blood flow studies and positron emission tomography (Cutler, 1987), and serial visual evoked potentials (Orwin, Wright, Harding, Rowan, & Rolfe, 1986).

Today, basic histopathological and biochemical studies of AD continue in parallel with the search for an etiological factor. Various etiological hypotheses—aluminum intoxication, viral infection, immune reaction, or genetically induced defects in microtubular function—have been supported by initial results, but none of these hypotheses has been subsequently confirmed. The recent focus on the possible genetic determinants of AD illustrates this process. Early observations revealed that almost all patients suffering from trisomy 21 (Down syndrome) who survive past the age of 40 develop AD. Furthermore, epidemiological studies of sporadic (i.e., nonfamilial) cases of AD showed that, if a proband develops symptomatic AD (eventually confirmed by autopsy) before the age of 70, his or her siblings have a relative risk of developing AD symptoms of about 2; that is, 10% will demonstrate symptoms of AD by age 70 and 45% by 84 (Heston, Mastri, Anderson, & White, 1981). Breitner (1987) summarized clinical data suggesting that AD is transmitted in an autosomal dominant fashion. In 1987, Delabar, Goldgaber, Lamour, Nicole, Huret, Grouchy, Brown, Gajdusek, and Sinet reported the presence of an extra copy of a small region of chromosome 21, coding for beta-amyloid protein, in three sporadic cases of AD. They speculated that it may be the central genetic defect in AD. However, a few months later, three replication studies involving 81 AD patients failed to confirm this result (St. George-Hyslop, Tanzi, Polinsky, Haines, Nee, Watkins, Myers, Feldman, Pollen, Drachman, Growdon, Bruni, Foncin, Salmon, Frommelt, Amaducci, Sorbi, Piacentini, Stewart, Hobbs, Conneally, & Gusella, 1987).

This continuing search for the etiological, histopathological, and biochemical defects underlying AD has inspired multiple attempts to identify a palliative or curative treatment specific for AD. These drug trials have been reviewed by Hollander, Mohs, and Davis (1986). See Table 2 for a listing of drugs tried in the treatment of the primary syndrome of dementia. Because of the early arteriosclerosis hypothesis of dementia, initial trials tested metabolic enhancers and vasodilators, such as Hydergine, a combination of ergot alkaloids. Once memory impairment was identified as the initial cognitive deficit in AD, various compounds shown to enhance learning in animals (e.g., naloxone and vasopressin) were tested.

The identification of the cholinergic deficit of AD shifted the focus toward acetylcholine augmentation. Four classes of compounds were used: (1) acetylcholine precursors such as choline and phosphatidylcholine, or lecithin; (2) physostigmine or tetrahydro-5-aminoacridine (THA), which inhibits the enzymatic degradation of acetylcholine by acetylcholinesterase; (3) betanechol, a cholinergic agonist acting on postsynaptic muscarinic receptors, which was given by intrathecal continuous infusion, and (4) lithium, which is known to increase red-blood-cell choline by inhibiting its transmembranous transport. The results of these trials were inconclusive. Some studies using lecithin and physostigmine showed a modest cognitive improvement or slowing of cognitive decline in some patients. However, it was insufficient to warrant the clinical use of these compounds. For a comprehensive review of cholinesterase inhibition in AD, see Becker and Giacobini (1988). The search for a curative treatment will continue. This search will probably encompass the use of neurotrophic factors and/or neuronal transplantation. These have been shown to reverse memory deficits associated with normal aging in rats (Gage, Bjorklund, Stenevi, Dunnett, & Kelly, 1984). However, many biological and ethical problems have to be addressed before these techniques can be applied in human subjects (Gash, Collier, & Stadek, 1985; Katzman, 1986).

An ideal drug-design study that would help support enthusiasm for treatment opportunities should meet certain criteria (Tinklenberg, Thornton, & Yesavage, 1984; Wolkowitz, Tinklenberg, & Weingartner, 1985). Such a study must identify and describe the subjects, in terms of both diagnosis (preferably with NINCDS-ADRDA criteria)

Table 2. A List of Drugs Tested for the Primary Memory Disorders[a]

Obsolete
Vitamins
Glutamic acid
Hormones—thyroid, adrenal, gonadal
Yeast RNA
Procaine (Gerovital)
Improve oxygen perfusion, i.e., hyperbaric oxygen, carotid endarterectomies
Stimulate central nervous system—amphetamines
Chelation agents
Vasodilators
Cyclandelate
Papaverine
Isoxuprine
Pentoxyfylline (Trental)
Cinnarizine
Isoxsuprine
Metabolic enhancers
Codergocrine mesylate
Piracetam and homologues
Nafronyl
Pentoxyfylline (Trental)
Alter cellular metabolism
Ergot alkaloids, e.g., dihydroergotoxine mesylate (Hydergine)
Methylxanthines, e.g., pentoxyfylline (Trental)
Piracetam derivatives, e.g., pramiracetam
Alter neurotransmitter functioning
Acetylcholine
Presynaptic, e.g., choline, phosphatidylcholine (lecithin), lithium (to enhance cholinergic uptake), 4-aminopyridine
Postsynaptic, e.g., arecholine, oxotremorine, bethanechol, RS-86
Acetylcholinesterase inhibitors, e.g., physostigmine or tetrahydroaminoacridine
Catecholamines, e.g., MAOIs
Serotonin, e.g., alaproclate, zimelidine
GABA, THIP
Dopamine, l-dopa
Alter neuromodulators
Adrenocorticotropic-hormone-like peptides, e.g., Org 2766
Vasopressin derivatives, e.g., DDAVP, DGAVP, lysine-8-vasopressin
Somatostatin 1363,586,msd, TRH
Other
Opiate antagonists; naloxone, naltrexone
S-Adenosine methyltransferase (SAM)

[a]Adapted from Hollister (1986); Dysken (1987); and Mohs and Davis (1987).

(McKhann, Drachman, Folstein, Katzman, Price, & Stadlan, 1984) and cognitive, affective, and behavioral measures of severity. The assessment measures must be sensitive to disease, age, and drug effects. The duration of the drug trial should be sufficient (months). Double-blind, parallel groups are necessary. Crossover studies are only suggestive and cannot account for carryover effects. Control groups should include a comparison drug with some known psychoactive properties in addition to a placebo group. A biological confirmation of drug effect should be demonstrated in terms of both drug levels and biological effect. There should be an understanding of the basic pharmacokinetics of the drug (i.e., the optimal dose range and schedule). Studies not meeting all of these requirements must be interpreted with skepticism.

SPECIAL DIAGNOSTIC CONSIDERATIONS

The outpatient clinician meeting an elderly patient with cognitive decline and without an obvious causative medical or psychiatric disorder has to engage in a two-step diagnostic process. First, the presence of a dementia syndrome has to be established and its severity assessed. Second, the contribution of a reversible dementing condition has to be ruled out. Going through these two steps will not only provide data essential to guide the selection of an optimal long-term management strategy but also establish a rapport with the patient and his or her family. Later, it will help them to accept the working diagnosis, particularly if it carries a grim prognosis. Except in a few cases, a diagnosis of dementia is not "final"; rather, it entails a dynamic process that includes longitudinal follow-up and, in many cases, therapeutic trials.

Establishing and Grading the Dementia Syndrome

The diagnostic principles presented in this section are based on the DSM-III-R criteria (APA, 1987) and the recommendations of two recent conferences sponsored by the U.S. Department of Health and Human Services and the National Institutes of Health (McKhann *et al.*, 1984; Consensus Conference, 1987).

According to the DSM-III-R, the diagnosis of a *dementia syndrome* is "based on clinical factors alone, and carries no connotations concerning prognosis" (p. 104). The diagnostic criteria emphasize three major aspects: (1) the presence of an acquired cognitive impairment involving memory and at least one other higher cognitive function (e.g., abstract thinking, judgment, language, or constructional abilities) or personality changes; (2) an impairment that is not due exclusively to delirium; and (3) an impairment severe enough to interfere with occupational or social functioning.

Cognitive Impairment

The cognitive impairment should be objectively and quantitatively documented with a validated "rating scale," assessing at least orientation, repeating and registration, attention, calculation, recent memory, naming, understanding, reading, writing, and the ability to draw or copy. We favor the use of the Folstein Mini-Mental State (MMS) (Folstein, Folstein, & McHugh, 1975), an 11-item scale that is widely used. Neuropsychological testing may help to detect a true cognitive deterioration in two or more aspects of cognition in highly intelligent patients presenting with incipient dementia and complaining of subjective difficulties in functioning at work or at home, or in patients with an uncommon cultural background or with a previously known cognitive impairment. Repeated testing may be useful in following these patients longitudinally.

Assessing for Delirium

Once global cognitive impairment has been objectively documented, the clinician must rule out the possibility that it is due exclusively to delirium. Whereas dementia may be conceptualized as chronic brain failure that may be assessed over a relatively extended period of time, delirium is equivalent to acute brain failure. Delirium is often caused by a significant organic problem, has a high morbid risk, and should be evaluated in an inpatient setting. Clinically, the two hallmarks of delirium are wandering of attention and clouding or a fluctuating level of consciousness. Trzepacz, Baker, and Greenhouse (1988) developed a rating scale for delirium. For more details on delirium, see Chapter 17.

Severity

To be called dementia, cognitive impairment has to be severe enough to interfere with occupational or social functioning. This last criterion enables us to differentiate dementia from the milder cognitive alterations experienced by most elderly individuals. In the past, these alterations have sometimes been referred to as *benign senescent forgetfulness*.

The DSM-III-R grades dementia as mild, moderate, or severe, entirely according to the level of independence that the patient can maintain. A mild dementia implies preserved "capacity for independent living"; in a moderate dementia, "independent living is hazardous, and some degree of supervision is necessary"; finally, with severe dementia, "activities of daily living are so impaired that continual supervision is required" (p. 107). The outpatient clinician is involved mainly with mild to moderate dementia.

Excluding a Reversible or Arrestable Dementing Condition

Theoretically, to establish a diagnosis of dementia, a specific causative organic disease must be identified; when no organic disease is identified, and if all the nonorganic mental disorders can be ruled out, a clinical diagnosis of "primary degenerative dementia of the Alzheimer type" (DAT) can be made by exclusion. McKhann *et al.*, (1984) proposed clinical criteria for a "positive" diagnosis of possible, probable, or definite AD. In the absence of peripheral markers for AD, a definite diagnosis requires a brain biopsy or autopsy and is rarely made except in a research setting. A probable diagnosis requires the presence of a dementia syndrome as defined in the previous section, with a typical insidious onset after age 40, progressive worsening, and "the absence of systemic disorders or other brain disease that . . . could account for the progressive deficits in memory and cognition" (p. 940; see below). Other clinical features may either support or be consistent with a probable diagnosis.

Becker, Huff, Nebes, Holland, and Boller (1988) reported that the most common cognitive changes in AD are deficits in recent memory and in lexical-semantic abilities. A progressive deterioration of language (aphasia), motor skills (apraxia), and perception (agnosia) constitutes, with amnesia, the classic four A's of AD and supports a probable diagnosis. Depression, psychosis, angry or hostile outbursts, incontinence, weight loss, neurological abnormalities, and seizures in the advanced stages are consistent with a probable diagnosis. Conversely, a sudden onset, focal neurological findings, seizures, and gait disturbance very early in the course of the disease make probable AD unlikely. A diagnosis of possible AD corresponds to an atypical presentation of progressive dementia, when other disorders have been reasonably excluded. Among the more than 60 recognized dementing disorders (Cummings, 1987), the following have to be specifically excluded: mood disorder, Parkinson disease, multi-infarct dementia (MID), drug intoxication, thyroid disease, pernicious anemia, syphilitic meningoencephalitis and other chronic CNS infections, normal-pressure hydrocephalus (NPH), subdural hematoma (SDH), Huntington disease, Creutzfeldt-Jakob disease, and brain tumors. Yesavage (1979) developed the mnemonic *DEMENTIA* to help in remembering the differential causes (see Table 3). In

Table 3. DEMENTIA: A Device for Recalling Reversible Causes of Organic Brain Syndrome[a]

Drugs
Psychoactive drugs, sedatives, hypnotics, anticholinergics, anti-Parkinsonians, antispasmatics, cardiac drugs, antihypertensives, diuretics, digoxin
Emotional disorders
Mood disorder, schizophrenia-spectrum disorders
Metabolic and endocrine disorders
Myxedema, hyperadrenocorticism, apathetic thyrotoxicosis
Hypoglycemia, hyperosmolar states
Electrolyte abnormalities
Hypercarbia with chronic obstructive pulmonary disease
Hypoxemia from a number of causes
Azotemia
Portosystemic encephalopathy
Eyes and ears
Nutritional deficiency and normal-pressure hydrocephalus
B_{12}, folate, thiamine
Other water-soluble vitamins
Anemia due to iron deficiency
Tumor and trauma
Chronic subdural hematoma
Primary or secondary neoplasm in brain
Infection
Syphilitic meningoencephalitis
Encephalitis, meningitis
Pneumonia, urinary tract infection
Arteriosclerotic complications
Strokes or transient ischemic attacks
Congestive heart failure

[a]Adapted from Yesavage (1979).

practice, the differential diagnosis process requires a systematic but relatively straightforward clinical and laboratory evaluation (Consensus Conference, 1987).

This complete "dementia workup" can usually be performed on an outpatient basis. Its usefulness goes beyond the diagnostic stage in that it provides management guidelines. Even in the absence of a reversible or arrestable dementing disorder, a thorough workup often detects a concurrent treatable condition that exacerbates dementia (Larson, Reifler, Sumi, Canfield, & Chinn, 1985). Reifler and Larson (1988) called this phenomenon the "rule of halves." Of their patients evaluated for dementia (200), 62% had coexisting illness, 28% had at least 1-month improvement with treatment, and 14% had improvement lasting over 1 year. Of the 200, 2 returned to normal (their dementia was due to alcohol and drug toxicity).

The clinical history is probably the single most important procedure in the diagnosis of dementia. It should be obtained from both the patient and an informant close to the patient. It is essential to characterize the mode of onset and the time course of the process. Typically, AD has an insidious onset, over several weeks, and a slow, continuous deterioration, over months. A sudden onset, followed by a stepwise deterioration, intertwined with plateaus and even some periods of improvement, is characteristic of MID. A rapid onset, over days, with a short, rapid deterioration, usually over less than 6 and even 3 months, suggests a dementia syndrome of depression. A recent onset, followed by a dramatic progression, over days, raises the possibility of delirium, or a systemic or neurological disease.

Often, families relate the onset of symptoms to a specific event: "Father has had trouble with his memory since his operation." The identification of such a "precipitant," at or around the time of onset, is also of great value. Some of these precipitants point directly to a specific cause or class of causes: a fall or an accident with or without a recognized head trauma may have caused a subdural hematoma; a hospitalization raises the possibility of the administration of general anesthesia, an intubation, or a major blood loss, associated with a hypoxic encephalopathy; the prescription of a new drug for any medical problem, even minor, may be responsible for a delirium or a chronic drug intoxication. Other stressors are less easily interpreted. In particular, it may be extremely difficult to assess whether certain events have precipitated a depression or whether they have been precipitated by an existing dementia. Early retirement or moving may have caused a depression; they may also have been required because of an incipient dementia. Similarly, the death of a caring spouse may make obvious to outsiders a long-standing inability to function independently.

The differentiation of the various dementing disorders, suggested by the mode of onset and the general time course of the process, may be further refined by the identification of specific clinical patterns of cognitive and behavioral impairment.

We have already discussed how the presence of a decreased level of consciousness and an attention deficit characterizes delirium, whereas the absence of an objective deficit documented with a rating instrument and/or neuropsychological testing may suggest a "worried well" or mildly depressed elderly person.

Attempts have been made to improve the validity of various rating instruments for the diagnosis of AD (Cummings & Benson 1986; Reisberg, Ferris, Anand, Buttinger, Borenstein, Sinaiko, & de Leon, 1984), but they always run into the problem of incorrectly classifying atypical cases of AD. Follow the rule that "atypical presentations of common disorders are more common than classic presentations of rare disorders" (Cutler, 1979, p. 17). Scales can be specific for only certain levels of severity of the disorder because early AD looks like benign senescent forgetfulness and late AD may look like many late dementias (Tierney, Snow, Reid, Zorzitto, & Fisher, 1987). For further discussion of cognitive screening instruments, see Chapter 22, as well as Nelson, Fogel, and Faust (1986) and Roca (1987). An assessment of sensory function is essential because hearing, olfaction, and vision (Hinton, Sadun, Blanks, & Miller, 1986; Steffes & Thralow, 1987) may all be affected as part of the AD process and may interfere with the interpretation of cognitive testing (Corbin & Eastwood, 1986).

Hachinski, Iliff, Zilhka, Du Boulay, McAllister, Marshall, Russell, and Symon (1975) recommended basing the positive diagnosis of multi-infarct dementia (MID) on their Ischemic Score (IS), calculated on a 13-item scale. A maximum scores of 18 indicates the presence of a dementia with abrupt onset (2 points), stepwise deterioration (1), fluctuating course (2), nocturnal confusion (1), relative preservation of personality (1), depression (1), somatic complaints (1), emotional incontinence (1), history of hypertension (1) or strokes (2), evidence of associated atherosclerosis (1), and focal neurological symptoms (2) and signs (2). Initially, a score above 7 was thought to be indicative of MID, but more recent studies have shown that the Hachinski IS is more reliably used to eliminate MID or a mixed dementia (MID and AD) when it is below 4 (Wade, Mirsen, Hachinski, Fisman, Lau, & Merskey, 1987).

Cummings and Benson (1983) based their etiological diagnosis of dementia on the identification of three distinct clinical patterns, named according to the topography of the pathological process. First, cortical dementias, such as AD and Pick disease, involve primarily the cerebral cortex; they present with the specific cognitive deficit described earlier (the four A's) and an almost normal neurological examination until the late stages. Pick disease can sometimes be distinguished clinically from AD by the predominance of personality changes in its early stage, occasionally manifested as a Kluver-Bucy syndrome (emotional blunting, hypersexuality, gluttony, hyperorality, hypermetamorphosis, and visual or auditory agnosia). Second, subcortical dementias include the extrapyramidal disorders (e.g., Parkinson, Huntington, or Wilson disease or progressive nuclear palsy), normal-pressure hydrocephalus, and toxic metabolic conditions. Subcortical dementias affect the basal ganglia, the thalamus, and the brain stem and are characterized by a forgetfulness, slowing of cognition, and depressed, apathetic, or, more rarely, manic mood. They also are associated with prominent neurological abnormalities. Finally, global dementias involve both cortical and subcortical structures and present with both types of features. They include MID and various infectious, traumatic, neoplastic, and anoxic dementias.

This classification is a useful theoretical conceptualization that may help to organize the systematic consideration of the various dementing disorders. Unfortunately, its clinical usefulness is greatly limited by a considerable overlap in the clinical presentation of cortical, subcortical, and mixed dementias.

The past psychiatric and medical history also plays a major role in the etiological diagnosis of a dementia. We have found that a past history of depression, treated or untreated, sometimes identified only because of a remote suicide attempt, is one of the most suggestive pieces of evidence supporting the diagnosis of a dementia syndrome of depression. A history of heavy and prolonged ingestion of alcohol may warrant a diagnosis of dementia associated with alcoholism (APA, 1987), if alcohol intake has been interrupted for at least 3 weeks (in order to rule out the transient effects of alcohol intoxication or withdrawal), and if all other causes of dementia have been excluded, in particular, alcoholic liver disease with hepatic encephalopathy, Wernicke-Korsakoff syndrome, or subdural hematoma associated with an unnoticed fall. Subdural hematoma may also be suspected in the presence of any recent trauma, and a remote history of head trauma is a statistical risk factor for AD. A history of intravenous drug abuse, blood product transfusion, or recurrent venereal disease should alert the clinician to the possibility of AIDS dementia-related complex, particularly in demented patients below 50 for whom human immunodeficiency virus infection is probably already one of the most common causes of dementia. Dementia can be the first and only manifestation of human immunodeficiency virus (HIV) infection, as demonstrated recently by Navia and Price (1987), who reported that dementia was the initial presentation in 29 of 112 patients (26%) diagnosed with AIDS dementia complex.

Many other medical disorders may be causally related to dementia. As discussed above, a history (or the presence) of hypertension or of cerebrovascular events (strokes or transient ischemic attacks) is very suggestive of MID. Severe pulmonary or cardiac diseases (e.g., acute heart failure associated with a myocardial infarction), a surgical intervention, or any major acute blood loss may be responsible for a hypoxic encephalopathy. A metabolic encephalopathy, due to hepatic or renal failure, may also occasionally present as a dementia. A remote partial or total gastrectomy may cause a vitamin B_{12} deficiency and its associated dementia. Repeated episodes of hypoglycemia should be ruled out in demented patients with treated diabetes mellitus. A history of thyroid disease, with or without treatment, may be the cause of current hypothyroidism. Finally, a history of venereal disease (including, obviously, syphilis), tuberculosis, or fungal infection should prompt the clinician to consider a diagnosis of chronic meningitis with dementia. In addition, the intake of any prescribed medication should be evaluated critically and may evoke the diagnoses of delirium and/or chronic drug intoxication.

When indicated, the personal history should include a rapid screening for occupational exposure to heavy metals and industrial solvents. Creutzfeldt-Jakob disease in neurosurgeons, neuropathologists, and morticians, as well as dementia pugilistica in retired professional boxers, represent other rare examples of occupationally related dementia.

A family history of dementia may be elicited for several dementing disorders, most notably the autosomal dominant Huntington disease, some familial forms of AD and Pick disease, or the rare autosomal recessive Wilson disease. A family history of mood or other psychiatric disorders may also contribute to the etiological diagnosis of a dementia syndrome.

The physical examination may confirm the information obtained during the history or may sometimes reveal some etiological clues, such as an elevated blood pressure, tender and thickened temporal arteries, a stiff neck, a goiter, a carotid or cardiac murmur, or an abdominal scar. A thorough neurological examination, including an assessment of vision and hearing, is essential. It may detect focal neurological signs compatible with previous strokes and MID or multiple sclerosis, or it may suggest an unsuspected space-occupying lesion. An extrapyramidal movement disorder is more difficult to interpret: in the presence of a characteristic Parkinson disease that clearly antedated the dementia, a diagnosis of dementia of Parkinson disease may be made. However, a brain autopsy of demented patients presenting with marked Parkinsonian manifestations often demonstrates pathological changes characteristic of both Parkinson disease and AD (Boller, 1980). As discussed earlier, gait disturbance very early in the course of a dementia makes a diagnosis of AD unlikely and should prompt the diagnostician to search for a neurological dementing disorder, in particular normal-pressure hydrocephalus and subdural hematoma. Conversely, Huff, Boller, Luchelli, Querriera, Beyer, and Belle (1987) reported that the presence of release signs, olfactory deficit, impaired stereognosis or graphesthesia, a short-stepped bradykinetic gait, or abnormalities on cerebellar testing differentiated patients in the early stages of AD from healthy controls. Finally, a cranial or peripheral neuropathy may be an important clue in the identification of some toxic or metabolic dementing disorders, for instance, Wernicke-Korsakoff syndrome, vitamin B_{12} deficiency, recurrent hypoglycemia, or heavy-metal intoxication (Cummings & Benson, 1983).

Because of the high social and economic costs involved in the management of a demented patient, the customary etiological investigation of dementia includes a complete "battery" of diagnostic tests to exclude as definitely as possible a reversible or arrestable dementing disorder. The following laboratory exams are usually performed: serum electrolytes, glucose, BUN-creatinine, liver and metabolic profile including calcium level, thyroid function tests including TSH, vitamin B_{12} and folate levels, complete blood count, erythrocyte sedimentation rate, serology for syphilis, urinalysis, chest roentgenogram, and electrocardiogram. Testing for human immunodeficiency virus should now be performed systematically in the presence of identified risk factors for human immunodeficiency virus infection and probably in all demented patients below 60 without a clear etiology (Navia & Price, 1987).

A computerized tomography (CT) of the head is recommended for all demented patients (Martin, Miller, Kapoor, Karpf, & Boller, 1987). In the near future, magnetic resonance imaging (MRI) may replace CT scanning as the imaging procedure of choice, but Kent and Larson (1988) reported that at present, there is no clear superiority of MRI over CT (see also Council on Scientific Affairs, 1988). The increased use of MRI and the correlation of its results with neuropathological studies will help to clarify the clinical significance of radiological periventricular white-matter lucencies, named *leukoaraiosis*. At the present time, leukoaraiosis is associated with Binswanger disease, normal-pressure hydrocephalus, and AD (Roman, 1987).

The electroencephalogram (EEG) may provide helpful clues in the etiological evaluation of demented outpatients (Cummings & Benson, 1983). In rare cases, a pathognomonic EEG pattern establishes a diagnosis of Creutzfeldt-Jakob disease, heavy-metal poisoning, hepatic encephalopathy, or subacute sclerosing panencephalitis. EEG may also reveal an occult seizure disorder. Moreover, an epileptogenic focus (or focal slowing) may indicate a space-occupying lesion. The EEG also has considerable value in identifying delirium or metabolic or toxic dementia. Finally, a relatively normal EEG in a mildly demented patient supports the diagnosis of a progressive dementia (AD or Pick disease) or of a dementia syndrome of depression.

The role of lumbar puncture (LP) and cerebrospinal fluid (CSF) examination is more limited. It was addressed by two recent studies (Becker, Feussner, Mulrow, Williams, & Vokaty, 1985; Hammerstrom & Zimmer, 1985); both concluded that an LP should be performed only in demented patients with at least one of the following characteristics: age under 55, a rapid onset or progression of dementia, headache or signs and symptoms of meningeal irritation, fever, positive syphilis serology, leukocytosis or infiltrate on chest radiographs, other evidence of infection by *Mycobacterium tuberculosis, Cryptococcus neoformans,* or another fungus.

Other diagnostic tests are restricted to specific cases. For instance, dynamic radioisotope cisternography may demonstrate normal-pressure hydrocephalus. Brain biopsy is useful in planning the treatment of some CNS neoplasms and infections; it may also be justified in unusual clinical circumstances. The use of positron emission tomography and the study of various peripheral markers are, at present, limited to research settings (Cutler,

1987). Finally, the dexamethasone suppression test (DST) does not distinguish dementia from depression (Balldin, Gottfries, Karlsson, Lindstedt, Langstrom, & Walinder, 1983; Raskind, Peskind, Rivard, Veith, Barnes, 1982).

The Role of Longitudinal Follow-Up and Therapeutic Trials

Often, despite an initial thorough evaluation, the etiology of a dementia remains obscure and only the evolution of the patient's condition will reveal his or her dementing disorder. In many cases, this evolution is influenced by selective and careful therapeutic intervention. The outpatient psychiatrist is in a good position to solve these diagnostic puzzles because of his or her ability to follow patients longitudinally and to undertake therapeutic trials. A positive response to these therapeutic trials constitutes the ultimate confirmation of the reversible or arrestable character of the dementia.

It is probably in patients presenting with incipient dementia that the yield of the complete workup described above will be the greatest. Furthermore, most reversible dementing disorders are reversible only in their early stages. This is particularly true of dementia due to normal-pressure hydrocephalus, nutritional deficiency, alcohol, neoplasm, or infection. Meyer, Judd, Tawaklna, Rogers, and Mortel (1986) also showed that some vascular dementias may be arrested (and even sometimes reverted) by a careful control of the risk factors for cerebrovascular accidents. This control includes maintaining systolic blood pressure between 135 and 150 mm Hg (lower pressures may cause neurological and cognitive deteriorations), abstinence from smoking, limitation of alcohol ingestion, and, in selected cases, aspirin prophylaxis or surgical revascularization.

Dementia and Depression

In the elderly, not only may the syndromes of dementia and depression coexist, but their symptoms may overlap considerably. We conceptualize dementia and depression as interacting in four different ways: (1) a depression may mimic a dementia; (2) a depression may cause a dementia syndrome; (3) a depression may be superimposed on a dementia; and (4) a dementia may look like a depression.

1. A major depressive episode may mimic a dementia in an elderly patient complaining of incapacitating memory and attention problems that cannot be demonstrated by a structured cognitive examination or neuropsychological testing. Because depressed patients are apt to complain about memory difficulties, whereas ''memory-impaired patients defend vigorously against revelation of their deficits'' (Popkin, 1986, p. 17), this clinical presentation suggests the diagnosis of a major depressive episode. The elicitation of other depressive symptoms and, often, a personal or familial history of mood disorder establish this diagnosis. It is then confirmed by the joint resolution of the subjective mood and cognitive difficulties with proper antidepressant treatment. The authors recommend that the term *pseudodementia*—in keeping with its original use (Kiloh, 1961; Wells, 1979)—should be reserved for depressed patients without objective cognitive deficit; the corresponding DSM-III-R diagnosis is a major depressive episode.

2. More rarely, a depression causes a significant cognitive and functional impairment, which can be objectively demonstrated and will resolve totally with antidepressant treatment. The expression ''dementia syndrome of depression'' should refer to this dementia's resolving completely and durably with an antidepressant treatment; in that case,

a dual diagnosis of dementia and major depressive episode is probably warranted. The diagnosis of this reversible dementia syndrome of depression is suggested by several clinical factors: a past history of mood disorder, especially bipolar; a clear temporal relationship between a predominant mood disorder and a dementia; a serious psychosocial stressor preceding any cognitive decline; a dementia worsening rapidly over a short duration (usually less than 6 months); or inconsistent performances in repeated cognitive testing. Once delirium and dementing organic diseases have been ruled out, a suspected diagnosis of dementia syndrome of depression justifies aggressive antidepressant treatment. The clinician should consider electroconvulsive therapy (ECT) if the patient does not improve after an adequate trial with oral tricyclic antidepressants (TCA) or monoamine oxidase inhibitors (MAOIs) (Allen, 1982; Bulbena & Berrios, 1986; Liang, Lam, & Ancill, 1988).

3. During the early stages of a progressive dementia, a patient may remain aware of his or her cognitive decline and the ensuing deterioration in occupational and social functioning. At this stage, the patient may actively complain of a depressed mood. Often, this secondary depression, superimposed on a primary dementing disorder, exacerbates the dementia. Treatment with antidepressants and psychotherapy may significantly improve the patient's mood, cognition, and social functioning. In a study, 26% of a cohort of demented outpatients were given a secondary diagnosis of depression; with treatment, 14.5% of those (i.e., 4% of all demented patients) had a significant improvement of their cognition lasting more than 1 month (Larson *et al.*, 1985).

4. As dementia worsens, sleep and appetite problems, weight loss, marked apathy and psychomotor retardation, or anxiety and psychomotor agitation may mimic a depression. Furthermore, the patient's family may still focus on the initial depressive symptomatology and minimize his or her inability to perform, attributing it to depression with loss of interest and motivation. The emotional lability and crying episodes seen with some subcortical dementias may complicate the diagnosis further. However, at this later stage, the patient no longer complains of a depressed mood. An antidepressant therapeutic trial is still warranted in many cases. The chances of significant cognitive improvement are slim, but a decrease in the depressive symptomatology and an improvement of functioning in the activities of daily living are not unusual (Reifler, 1986). According to the DSM-III-R principle stating that an organic mental disorder preempts the diagnosis of any other disorder that could produce the same symptoms, patients with a depression superimposed on a dementia due to another condition should generally be given a diagnosis only of dementia; a diagnosis of primary degenerative dementia (i.e., AD) or multi-infarct dementia may be refined by specifying the subtype "with depression."

Drug Intoxication

Like depression, chronic drug intoxication may either cause or exacerbate dementia. Larson, Kukull, Buchner, and Reifler (1987) reported that 35 of 308 (11.5%) elderly outpatients with suspected dementia were found to have a chronic drug intoxication causing cognitive impairment without delirium. With modification of the drug regimen, the dementia resolved completely in 10 (3%); objective measures of cognition improved significantly and durably in all others, despite the coexistence of irreversible or unarrestable dementing disorders. The authors noted that, because of its rigorous design, their study probably underestimated the prevalence of chronic drug intoxication in demented outpatients. This study also illustrates the typical characteristics of drug intoxication in elderly demented patients. Most patients have used the offending drug for years, and cognitive impairment has developed insidiously; most often, there is no associated change in the level of consciousness (i.e., no delirium). The patient does not complain of specific "side effects"; her or his caretakers, expecting a benefit from the drug, are not able to distinguish its insidious adverse effects from dementia or cognitive decline due to normal aging. The risk of intoxication increases with the number of drugs taken. However, there is a strong tendency to treat the associated behavioral manifestations with the addition of other drugs, thus worsening the problem. In this study, the drug-intoxicated patients had been prescribed significantly more drugs than other demented patients (3.7 ± 2.3 vs. 1.7 ± 1.8; $p < .001$). Otherwise, they were not distinguished by age, sex, living arrangement, type of onset, duration, or severity of dementia. In contrast, they were also about three times more prone to falling, and most stopped falling when the offending drug was discontinued. This finding suggests that falling might be used as a sensitive (even though nonspecific) clinical indicator for chronic drug intoxication in the demented elderly (Buchner & Larson, 1987).

The drugs most commonly causing or exacerbating chronic cognitive impairment are, in an approximately decreasing order: sedative medications, in particular meprobamate, benzodiazepines, and neuroleptics; antihypertensives, in particular reserpine, alpha-methyldopa, clonidine, diuretics, and lipophilic beta-blockers that cross the blood–brain barrier; narcotic and nonsteroidal anti-inflammatory analgesics; other psychotropic medications with anticholinergic properties (e.g., tricyclic antidepressants); anti-Parkinsonians; anticonvulsants; insulin; cimetidine; lithium; and steroids.

In most cases, the offending drug(s) can and should be discontinued. A drug-free trial is necessary to confirm the diagnosis of drug intoxication. Despite the presence of a coexistent AD in nearly two thirds of their patients, Larson *et al.* (1987) reported that "the improvement . . . was usually surprising to family and caregivers" (p. 172). In the presence of a potential drug intoxication causing or exacerbating a dementia, we cannot imagine any situation justifying the continuation of meprobamate, a "sleeping pill," or a "routine" analgesic for mild arthritic pain. The authors were also able to discontinue most antihypertensives and neuroleptics. In rarer cases, when an offending drug plays an active therapeutic role, its dosage regimen should be modified, or better, it should be replaced by another drug with similar therapeutic effects but fewer potentially adverse effects. Thus, most hypertensives may be beneficially replaced by a calcium channel blocker (e.g., nifedipine or verapamil) or an ACE (angiotensin converting enzyme) inhibitor (e.g., enalapril). If a diuretic is needed, we avoid the thiazides and prefer furosemide. A hydrophilic beta-blocker (e.g., atenolol or nadolol) may be substituted for a lipophilic one. Acetaminophen is as useful as nonsteroidal anti-inflammatory drugs to treat the minor pain of osteoarthritis. In elderly patients, insulin may often be replaced by one of the modern oral hypoglycemiants (e.g., glyburide or glypizide), which cause hypoglycemia less frequently. Finally, sucralfate should be used rather than cimetidine or ranitidine.

FREQUENT CLINICAL PROBLEMS

Prognosis of Dementia

Predictors of the course of an illness are fraught with problems for determining which end points are most relevant and most related to the disease, for example, institutionalization and death (Kaszniak, Fox, Gandell, Garron, Huckman, & Ramsey, 1978; Knopman,

Kitto, Deinard, & Heiring, 1988), absolute cognitive decline (Stern *et al.*, 1987), rate of cognitive decline (St. Clair *et al.*, 1988), or global deterioration (Rubin, Morris, Storandt, & Berg, 1987). The main findings of these studies are the variability in progression and the apparent separation of cognition and noncognitive measures of self-care (Skurla, Rogers, & Sunderland, 1988). The primary symptoms that the clinician sees in the AD patient depend on the stage of the illness (Reisberg *et al.*, 1984) and were described in the section "The Evolution of the Concept of Alzheimer Disease." However, the trap is to believe that the stage of the illness has significant predictive value.

Careful longitudinal studies of patients with probable Alzheimer disease show that the course of the illness is relatively unpredictable not only in the rate of the change in cognitive performance, but also in the direction of the change in cognitive performance. Moreover, this change is not necessarily in the same direction if different instruments are used, that is, measures of cognition versus measures of function (Berg, Edwards, Danzinger, & Berg, 1987; Eastwood, Lautenschlaeger, & Corbin, 1983). At follow-up, patients are usually close to their initial exam, whether it be improved, indifferent, or worse, and therefore, patients who are severely demented on their initial visit are likely to be impaired on follow-up visits. Specific prognostic indicators are functional brain impairment (instead of CT atrophy) (Kaszniak *et al.*, 1978); global dementia rating (Hughes, Berg, Danziger, Cohen, & Martin, 1983; Reisberg *et al.*, 1984); psychosis and EPRs (extra-pyramidal reactions) (Stern *et al.*, 1987); and hearing impairment (Uhlmann, Larson, & Koepsell, 1986). Note that most case-control studies show that dementia has a high risk of mortality (Barclay, Zemcov, Blass, & McDowell, 1985; Christie & Wood, 1988; Martin, Miller, Kapoor, Arena, & Boller, 1987).

Psychiatric Symptoms in Alzheimer Disease

The relationship of specific symptoms to specific levels of impairment is of greater interest. If certain symptoms occur more frequently in certain stages of impairment, then those symptoms may be related to the pathophysiological process of the disease. Symptoms that occur independently of clinical severity may be less related to the primary disease process and may be more amenable to standard treatments. Psychiatric symptoms that seem to be related to disease severity include agitation, wandering, decreased self-care, disturbed sleep, perceptual disturbances (fragmented delusions and hallucinations), and the misidentification syndrome. Symptoms that are less related to disease severity include dysphoria-depression, irritability, restlessness, formed or systematized delusions, and paranoia (Berrilos & Brook, 1985; Breen, Larson, Reifler, Vitaliano, & Lawrence, 1984; Fisk & Pannill, 1987; Mayeux, Stern, & Spanton, 1985; Mayeux, Stern, & Sano, 1985; Merriam, Aronson, Gaston, Wey, & Katz, 1988; Reisberg & Ferris, 1985; Rubin, Morris, & Berg, 1987; Rubin, Morris, Storandt, & Berg, 1987; Rubin, Drevets, & Burke, 1988; Teri, Larson, & Reifler, 1988). Falling correlates more with medications than with diagnoses or severity of illness (Granek, Baker, Abbey, Robinson, Myers, Samkoff, & Klein, 1987).

Depressed mood, or at least dysphoria, is present in 30%–85% of patients examined (Merriam *et al.*, 1988; Reifler, Larson, & Hanley, 1982). When depression and dementia coexist, the depression seems to affect functional performance (Dementia Rating Scale) rather than cognitive performance (Weschler Memory Score) (Breen *et al.*, 1984; Fisk & Pannill, 1987; Reynolds, Perel, Kupfer, Zimmer, Stack, & Hoch, 1987).

Sleep is disturbed in AD patients, who exhibit markedly decreased sleep efficiency and an increasing incidence of sleep-disordered breathing with increasing disease severity (Hoch *et al.*, 1988; Reynolds *et al.*, 1988).

According to King (1986), active alcohol abuse occurs in about 12% of patients presenting to a dementia clinic. The detection of alcohol use in the elderly may be improved by the use of the Michigan Alcohol Screening Test (MAST) or its modified form, the unit scoring MAST (UMAST) (Willenbring, Christensen, Spring, & Rasmussen, 1987).

Other DSM-III-R Axial Problems

Axis II diagnoses are made much less frequently in geriatric patients in general (Mezzich, Fabrega, Coffman, & Glavin, 1987). Axis II disorders probably should not be diagnosed *de novo* after the onset of dementia, as there is a likelihood that any apparent personality disturbance may reflect either an organic personality syndrome or pathological defense reactions to a severe stressor. The clinician must not forget to diagnose any relevant Axis III disorders and to maintain eternal vigilance for treatable medical conditions, keeping in mind the rule of halves. Axis III is often overlooked (Maricle, Leung, & Bloom, 1987). The task on Axis IV is to rate the severity of the stress (or the combined stressors) and not the individual's response to it. Axis V grades the patient's overall level of functioning both now and in the past year and should prove to be a valuable marker for coping or therapeutic successes. Most patients with uncomplicated dementia have similar Axis V ratings for similar levels of dementia severity, but bear in mind that Axis V is also sensitive to impairment in premorbid functioning and the presence of concomitant disorders (such as depression with suicidal ideation), either of which would markedly lower the rating score. In general psychiatric patients, Axis IV and Axis V are related to the severity of the disorder on Axis I (Gordon & Gordon, 1987), but this relationship has not been systematically examined in geriatric patients or patients with dementia.

Alzheimer Disease Syndrome

The clinician deals primarily with the AD patient and must attempt to marshal and train the patient's informal caregiver system (U.S. Congress, 1985). This informal caregiving system is itself composed of individuals who may in turn require individual attention as a result of their role in the system (e.g., depression in the spouse). Gallagher (1985) reviewed the mental health problems in caregivers. The constellation of problems facing the Alzheimer disease patient and his or her family and their reaction to these problems constitute what has been called the *Alzheimer's disease syndrome* (Thornton *et al.*, 1986). However, there is no place for this syndrome to be noted on the DSM-III-R multiaxial system, and the clinician must classify each patient and family member separately.

ADAPTATION OF TREATMENT APPROACHES

This section addresses the outpatient treatment of AD. The principles presented may be applied to other irreversible dementias and, in fact, to most chronic, incurable, debilitating illnesses. We limit ourselves to AD, as the management of a reversible or arrestable dementia is based primarily on the identification and treatment of the specific underlying dementing disorder. The identification of these disorders is discussed in the section "Special Diagnostic Considerations." Specific information on the treatment of reversible or arrestable dementing disorders may be found in general textbooks on medical therapeutics.

Treatment of the Primary Symptoms

Drug Therapy

Many drugs have been tried to treat or palliate the cognitive deficit of AD (Table 2). Some cholinergic enhancers have shown a limited effect in some research studies; however, so far these results are insufficient to justify the clinical use of any of these compounds outside research settings.

The ergoloid mesylate compound Hydergine is the only drug approved by the FDA for the specific treatment of cognitive decline. Hydergine has been used for more than 30 years, and its effectiveness and safety have been demonstrated in more than 22 well-controlled studies (Yesavage, Tinklenberg, Hollister, & Berger, 1979). Patients displayed limited but detectable and significant improvement in mental alertness, orientation, recent memory, confusion, emotional lability, anxiety, fear, agitation, motivation, initiative, vertigo, locomotion, and, most of all, depression (Jenike, 1985a). Usually, no consistent clinically significant improvement is detected, but occasionally, some patients show a dramatic response to the drug (Hollister & Yesavage, 1984).

Hydergine is daily doses of 3.0–4.5 mg has often been used in American studies; the highest doses (greater than or equal to 4.5 mg/day) have produced the best results. A dose of 6 mg/day is commonly used in Europe and doses of 7.5 mg or 12 mg/day have been given without serious side effects (Dysken, 1987; Hollister & Yesavage, 1984). The manufacturer describes minimal adverse effects, limited to transient nausea and gastric irritation; we have seen some patients develop orthostatic hypotension. Hollister and Yesavage (1984) recommended a 6-month trial of 2 mg p.o. TID. If no improvement is documented after 6 months, the treatment should be discontinued.

Psychological Approaches

Yesavage (1985) reviewed the nondrug treatment of memory disorders. Evidence exists to support the strategies of mnemonic devices (verbal) and the method of loci (visual) for list learning; general performance may be improved by decreasing anxiety with relaxation training and improving the extent of material processing with verbal elaboration.

Group Therapy for Patients

Although many different types of group therapy modalities have reportedly been used with AD patients (reality orientation, reminiscence therapy, bibliotherapy, music therapy, and art therapy), few controlled studies exist (Burnside, 1984). Baines, Saxby, and Ehlert (1987) reported that reality orientation followed by reminiscence treatment improved both cognitive and behavioral measures, and that a combination treatment was superior to either modality alone. They also noted positive effects on staff morale and improved staff–patient interactions.

Depression

Controlled trials indicate that all antidepressants are equally effective. Minimizing unwanted side effects is the main factor guiding the selection of an antidepressant (Peabody, Whiteford, & Hollister, 1986; Plotkin, Gerson, & Jarvik, 1987). The authors prefer nortriptyline because of the availability and reliability of nortriptyline blood levels and the reduced incidence of orthostatic hypotension (and the associated falls) (Roose, Glassman, Giardina, Walsh, Woodring, & Bigger, 1987). Usually, a daily dose of 50 mg for 5 weeks produces therapeutic blood levels and good clinical results (Reynolds, Kupfer, Hoch, Stack, Houck, & Sewitch, 1986). If a tricyclic cannot be used, monoamine oxidase inhibitors (MAOIs) can be used successfully even in AD with depression (Jenike, 1985b). ECT may help some patients refractory to medication. (Allen, 1982; Liang *et al.*, 1988). Current data suggest that ECT does not significantly worsen cognition in mixed depression and dementia, but more research is required (Bulbena & Berrios, 1986). Poststroke mood disorders and Parkinsonism complicated by depression also respond to antidepressant treatment (Atre-Vaidya & Jampala, 1988; Lipsey, Robinson, Pearlson, Rao, & Price, 1984).

Agitation

In order to treat agitation, the clinician must first define what is meant by agitation. One investigator used the definition of ''inappropriate vocal and motor activity that cannot be explained by needs or confusion'' (Cohen-Mansfield, 1986, p. 722; Cohen-Mansfield & Billig, 1986). The same author noted that there are several dimensions of agitated behavior: agitation directed toward an object, the frequencies, the location, the context, and the social setting. Salzman (1987) described agitation in terms of subtypes of other types of behavior, for example, agitation associated with psychosis, anxiety, depression, or pain. No one rating scale adequately covers all of the behavioral disturbances manifested by patients with dementia, but some widely used and treatment-sensitive scales include the Brief Psychiatric Rating Scale (BPRS) for psychotic symptoms and the Sandoz Clinical Assessment Geriatrics (SCAG) scale for other behaviors (Overall & Gorham, 1962; Shader, Harmatz, & Salzman 1974). Once the actual behaviors are defined, the frequency of the behaviors should be determined. Frequently occurring behaviors (i.e., several times a day) are better targets for drug interventions than infrequent behaviors. Once a specific intervention (perhaps a drug or a behavioral technique) has been selected, the clinician should hypothesize the temporal course, benefits, and side effects of the intervention on the behavior. For example, she or he should not abandon a behavioral technique after only a few days because may repetitions are necessary for learning. She or he should be suspicious when a drug given orally works within a few seconds or minutes; in such situations, the effect is more likely a placebo effect on the patient or the caregiver. In cases in which agitated depression complicates dementia, antidepressants are the drugs of choice, but the patient may feel more uncomfortable during the first several days of treatment and may not show a resolution of symptoms until after several weeks of treatment.

There is general agreement that, for agitation in dementia, the efficacy of drug treatment is low (35%) and the incidence of side effects is high (50%). The choice of drug depends on a careful consideration of the patient and the situation, along with an estimate of the tolerance of side effects. In general, neuroleptics are minimally superior to benzodiazepines (Ayd, 1988; Barnes, Veith, Okimoto, Raskind, & Gumbrecht, 1982). Propranolol, lithium, carbamazepine, and other drugs are of interest but have not been rigorously studied (Raskind, Risse, & Lampe, 1987; Risse & Barnes, 1986; Salzman, 1987). There is some evidence that, in the later stages of AD, there is a physiological excess of noradrenergic activity (Raskind, Peskind, Halter, & Jimerson, 1984). For agitation secondary to anxiety, buspirone has not been well studied but shows promise. Buspirone has a favorable side effect profile compared to benzodiazepine: it causes less sedation, no amnesia, and no impairment of psychomotor performance (Shader, Kennedy, & Greenblatt, 1987).

Behavioral treatment paradigms, including time out, differential reinforcement, and visual screening, have been tried for disturbed behaviors and show promise (Burgio & Burgio, 1986; Burgio, Page, & Capriotti, 1985; Burgio, Burgio, Engel, & Tice, 1986). As will also be seen in the section "Interventions for Caregivers," much of the work with caregivers consists in teaching them simple behavioral interventions. In conclusion, the behavioral management of agitated behavior should be preferred to the often dismal and risky attempts of drug treatment.

Alcohol Abuse

Alcohol abuse in the elderly is amenable to treatment (Schuckit, 1982) but requires greater attention to medical complications. Older patients may benefit from being in separate groups from younger patients (Atkinson, 1987). No specific studies of treating demented patients who abuse alcohol have been reported.

Sleep Disturbance

Reynolds and Kupfer (1987) addressed the management of sleep disturbance in demented patients. They emphasized sleep hygiene, as AD patients have a higher incidence of sleep apnea and benzodiazepines are relatively contraindicated.

Conclusions on Direct Treatment

The clinician should keep in mind that no combination of psychosocial interventions and drugs works similarly in any two demented patients. As summarized in Blass (1986):

> The general rule is to individualize care. . . . As people get older, they tend to differ more and more from each other. Superimposed on the genetic and developmental differences they were born with are the effects of everything else that happened to them during their life. . . . The rational approach in the face of all this diversity is empiricism guided by theory. (p. 549)

Interventions for Caregivers

The authors defined the Alzheimer disease syndrome as the constellation of problems and reactions of the demented patient and his or her support system. Maintaining a demented patient in the community under the care of his or her family is probably the best way to preserve the patient's autonomy and well-being. However, this should not be accomplished at the cost of the family members' psychological and physical well-being. Furthermore, the family caregivers' burden has been shown to be the major determinant precipitating institutionalization (Morycz, 1985). In striking contrast, the patient's characteristics (e.g., the symptoms, duration, or severity of dementia) are not by themselves significant predictors of institutionalization (Colerick & George, 1986). Therefore, psychosocial interventions directed to the caregivers constitute the mainstay of the long-term management of demented outpatients (Drinka, Smith, & Drinka, 1987). General intervention strategies focus on caregiver instructions and education, particularly in the form of family meetings. Specific interventions include those designed to decrease the burden of caregiving (day care, home care, and respite care), psychotherapeutic interventions for caregivers to enhance coping or caregiving skills, and specific enhancements of social support (Gallagher, 1985; Morycz, 1985; Zarit & Zarit, 1982).

Psychoeducation of Caregivers

Printed materials may constitute an excellent source of information for appropriate families. We recommend, in particular, any of the following: *The 36-Hour Day* (Mace & Rabins, 1981); *Alzheimer's Disease: A Guide for Families* (Powell & Courtice, 1983); or *The Loss of Self* (Cohen & Eisdorfer, 1986). However, it remains essential to take time to inform caregivers and to answer their many questions about AD and dementia. Table 4 summarizes the general strategies that may be useful to caregivers. Table 5 lists many common problems and their corresponding management techniques. As stated in Thornton *et al.* (1986):

> There are no magic tricks for dealing with problem behaviors. The caregiver's task is to work on specific, solvable problems and yet to respond to problems within a general framework. By developing a pre-planned strategy for dealing with problems in advance, the caregiver gains control, does not have to approach each problem as a crisis, and establishes a consistency that helps to stabilize the environment for the patient. (p. 18)

Problem solving leads to environmental and behavioral modifications. Fairly simple ("low-tech") devices and environmental alterations may allow the patient to continue to

Table 4. General Strategies for Caregivers

Instructions to caregivers
1. Display patience, gentleness, calmness.
2. Avoid arguments.
3. Use distractors.
4. Touch.
5. Ignore unwanted behavior (if safe to do so).
6. Praise wanted behavior.
7. Respond to feelings, not just content.
8. Plan ahead.
9. Take time for yourself.

Table 5. Understanding and Managing Behavior Problems[a]

Common problems	Recommended management techniques
	I. Early dementia
Learning and recent memory deficit	Use memory aids and reminders: notes, logs, calendars, clocks.
Losing things	Establish "a place" for things such as keys and wallet.
Communication problems	Use reassurances; speak slowly, distinctly, and softly; avoid open-ended questions; communicate through nonverbal cues such as smiling and holding hands.
Attempts to "cover up"	Use respect in response to a person's denial as a coping skill, yet ensure safety.
Depression	Discuss feelings; seek professional help.
Lack of motivation or initiative	Suggest activities or plans.
Fear of losing control	Establish familiar and secure routines; encourage the person to do as much for himself or herself as is safely possible (e.g., simple meals using a microwave); give praise for accomplishments.
Problems in judgment or calculation	Simplify decisions or tasks; help with financial matters; avoid rationalizing or asking, "Why did you do that?"
	II. Moderate dementia
Confusion and disorientation	Minimize distractions; use repetition.
Safety concerns	Look for safety hazards in and around the home (cooking, bathing, using electrical appliances) and make needed changes; don't hesitate to restrict driving if necessary.
Difficulties with bathing, grooming	Use simple "one-step" directions; employ humor.
Changes in sexual behavior	Initiate intimate and affectionate exchanges; recognize impairments and limitations.
Sleep disturbances	Encourage regular exercise and sleep hygiene (i.e., discourage daytime naps); prevent boredom. Ask physician about medications.
Angry outbursts and agitation	Identify the precipitants and avoid them; respond in a calm, reassuring voice; smile and try touch if this doesn't upset the person further; use distractors; leave the room if necessary. Ask physician about exercises and medications.
	III. Severe dementia
Decreased recognition of family and familiar places	Use links from the past (photo albums, portraits, memories); ues reassurance and repetition.
Problems in dressing	First, offer help with choosing clothes, then with actual mechanics of dressing; use "one-step" direction; use special clothing (e.g., shoes with velcro bands instead of laces).
Eating problems	Do not rush mealtime; serve foods easily broken or eaten with one utensil; use "finger foods"; give one item at a time; instruct when to chew or swallow.
Incontinence	Inform physician; use routine toileting; restrict fluids after evening meal; use special clothing and adult diaper.
Falls	Eliminate throw rugs or other safety hazards; provide adequate lighting (e.g., night lights); use walker or cane; supervise ambulation; have a plan to pick up fallen person.

[a]Adapted with permission from M. Bozich and S. Housley (1985). Unpublished.

function at home. As illustrated in Table 5, the process of altering the environment has to be continuous because of the progression of the disease. These devices and alterations include written reminders and calendars, pill boxes, special "geriatric" chairs, a cane, a walker or a wheelchair, adult diapers, the improvement of lighting (e.g., on staircases), the installation of handle bars in the bathroom or on staircases, unplugging electric appliances and switching the gas off when the caregivers leave home, and the installation of locks or alarms on outside doors to prevent wandering (George, Binns, Clayden, & Mulley, 1988).

Because demented persons tend to respond to and mirror the affective behavior of those around them, behavioral modifications first involve the caregivers. They should act as role models by displaying patience, gentleness, and calmness. In every case, it is essential that they avoid arguments, which are counterproductive. Instead, they should learn to use nonverbal cues to communicate and distractors to redirect attention (Bartol, 1979). Smiling, touching, and holding hands are often the best ways to soothe the patient and to say, "I'm with you." Caregivers should praise desired behaviors, such as eating meals and bathing and should ignore undesired behavior when safely feasible.

The central role of psychological support is to improve the caregivers' well-being and to increase their coping skills. In many cases, problem solving and behavioral modifications are unsuccessful in suppressing a disturbing behavior. However, by becoming aware of the anxiety, frustration, or anger that such a behavior generates in them, caregivers can reduce its impact on them. Clinicians can help the caregivers to recognize that they are upset, not by the behavior itself but by how they evaluate it. Perseveration, inoffensive delusions or hallucinations, and failure to perform a simple daily task are examples of symptoms and behaviors that are commonly evaluated as "hostile."

Caregivers should also realize that the accumulation of minor stresses, rather than one particular problem, is often the source of their frustration; this realization may help them to identify when they need to take "time out" for themselves and to get some respite before tensions build too high. However, taking time out may engender guilt; understanding that they are the main resource for their demented dependent and that they must take care of themselves to be able to continue to provide good care will help them to take time for themselves without feeling guilty of neglect. As emphasized by Lezak (1978): "This very important issue must be brought up early and often, for the notion of enlightened self-interest runs counter to popular moral equations of self abnegation and duty taught by many religious and social institutions" (p. 595).

Family Meetings

Family meetings are a very effective way to educate the various family members involved in the care of a demented patient and to work with them through a crisis. It is also a natural way to foster support for the primary caregiver. Often, relatives and friends are willing and able to help but have no idea of how to do so, and the caregiver is hesitant or embarrassed to ask. The aims of a meeting are to bring the family's level of information up to that of the caregiver, to answer questions, to identify the caregiver's most pressing needs, to problem-solve with the family, and to strengthen or develop a family support system (Zarit & Zarit, 1982).

The authors recommend the organization of at least one family meeting on completion of the initial evaluation. As mentioned in the section "Special Diagnostic Considerations," this evaluation is usually conducted on an outpatient basis and most often requires several visits scheduled over a few weeks. These two or three visits offer an excellent opportunity to start educating the patient and her or his caregivers about dementia while establishing a trustful and empathic rapport with them. However, we avoid making any definite statement until the evaluation is completed and a diagnosis is established with a reasonable degree of certainty. If, during the first visit, a patient is obviously cognitively impaired, we explain the situation in the following way: "Obviously, you are having some problems with your memory. They may be due to a condition called dementia. Dementia can be caused by various diseases. A complete clinical evaluation, some blood tests, and some radiological tests are needed to determine which disease is responsible for your problem and what treatment is most appropriate." If the patient has been given a prior diagnosis of AD or if it is specifically mentioned, we also explain that AD is one of the possible causes of the patient's dementia and that other causes need to be ruled out.

Once the results of the diagnostic studies are available, we schedule a formal family meeting involving the patient, all the relatives willing to attend, and the health professionals who participated in the evaluation and who will be involved in the patient's future care (in our setting, a psychiatrist and/or an internist, a social worker, and occasionally a nurse practitioner). During this meeting, we present the results of the clinical evaluation and the diagnostic studies, explain the diagnosis, present a comprehensive treatment plan describing the interventions and their possible outcomes, and answer questions from the caregivers. This meeting also allows us to see the various persons involved in the patient's care and to assess the family dynamic. If we detect or suspect underlying family conflicts (e.g., a fight for control between a spouse and children from a previous marriage), we schedule follow-up family meetings to work on these conflicts. Usually, however, we schedule subsequent family meetings at the request of the caregivers or when we feel they may help to resolve a crisis.

Specific Interventions

In 1986, one of the authors (Thornton *et al.,* 1986) wrote that "the single most important intervention is a referral to a support group" (p. 21). The field has advanced so that the recommendation is now "Specific caregivers may benefit from specific interventions." Caregivers who are depressed or stressed may benefit from cognitive psychotherapy groups or counseling; patients with moderate dementia and their caregivers may benefit from a combination of hospital respite and caregiver skills training; and caregivers of patients who are severely ill and institutionalized may benefit from grief work (for anticipatory grieving). In line with the assertion of Lieberman, Yalom, and Miles (1973) that self-help groups have both great benefit and potential risks, the universal recommendation to seek help can now be modified by alternatives that have documented efficacy.

Caregiver characteristics, that is, the relationship of child or spouse (Snow, Davidson, Puterski, Tworkowski, & Sussman, 1987), race (Morycz, Malloy, Bozich, & Martz, 1987), or the health of the caregiver (Gallagher, 1985) influence the outcome of interventions. Efforts to decrease the burden of caregiving only with home health care or respite have not been effective (Davidson, 1987; Lundervold & Lewin, 1987). Hospital respite alone has no beneficial effect on the patient (Seltzer, Rheaume, Volicer, Fabiszewski, Lyon, Brown, & Volicer, 1988) or on the family (Pfeiffer, Cairl, Keller, & Doblas, 1987).

Zarit and Zarit (1982) described an individual and family counseling (IFC) program consisting of six individual sessions, including a family meeting during Session 5. Zarit and Zarit found no difference between IFC and traditional support groups. Supporter endurance training (Levine, Dastoor, & Gendron, 1983) has been described, but no outcome data are available (Gallagher, 1985). One center found no difference between a waiting list, a support group, and skills training in stress-management (cognitive) groups (Haley, Brown, & Levine, 1987). However, these authors suggested that, in their subjects with high pretreatment stress, both treatment groups were effective, and they recommended selecting for the group the people who are most likely to benefit.

Combined treatments have been much more encouraging. Day hospital for patients in conjunction with skills training for their families is beneficial, but there is a tendency for higher functioning people not to do as well as patients or as caregivers (Seltzer, Ivry, & Litchfield, 1987). The same is true of day care (Winogrond, Fisk, Kirsling, & Keyes, 1987) and respite (Berman, Delaney, Gallagher, Atkins, & Graeber, 1987).

Future studies on caregiver interventions should include, as a minimum, a description of the caregiver and the patient that includes age, sex, race, family relationship, cognition, mood, function, stress, the model for the intervention, measurements pre- and postintervention, a description of the specificity of the intervention, and a comparison with randomly assigned interventions (Gallagher, 1985). The knowledge that specific interventions are useful or hurtful for specific people makes these controlled studies not only ethical but most humane.

Table 6. Prevention of Dementia and Other Late-Life Disabilities[a]

Maintain physical health
Eliminate tobacco.
Control blood pressure, blood sugar, blood cholesterol.
Control weight: eat well-balanced meals, low fat, low salt.
Limit alcohol intake to less than two drinks/day.
Exercise (aerobics) 20 minutes three times/week.
Protect from overexposure to direct sunlight.
Practice dental hygiene.
Protect self from AIDS.
Maintain psychological health
Introspection.
Determine values, make choices.
Develop new skills; don't just add more information.
Use the skills you have.
Develop nondestructive coping skills for dealing with stress.
Maintain outlets for expression, autonomy, and accomplishment.
Maintain social networks
Plan for changes in situations, not just living but who you will see, and who will be your resources (e.g., health care, legal matters, insurance).
Prepare for loss of loved ones: What is the meaning? Where can you turn for sharing?
Develop sociability skills.

[a]Adapted from Fries and Crapo (1981) and Vaillant (1977).

Recall that almost 50% of dementias are caused by something other than AD and that almost 40% are related to vascular disease and alcohol, conditions that are potentially preventable (Table 1). Recall also the rule of halves, which states that the mental health of demented patients is markedly improved when they are in good medical condition. And finally, consider the hypothesis by John Breitner (1987) that, even if AD is autosomal dominant, if we had a better understanding of the expression of this gene and could delay that expression by as little as 5 years for the entire population, then millions of Americans would be spared dementia in their lifetime. Consider also the relevant reports that alcohol consumption is an underrecognized risk factor for stroke, that psychological deficits mimic normal aging prematurely in male social drinkers, and that patients with larger brain weights appear to have a larger reserve with which to maintain a normal mental status despite the pathological changes of AD in their brains (Mesulam *et al.*, 1987).

All these factors suggest that possibly half of all dementias can be prevented or delayed by maintaining good health. Some simple rules for maintaining good health are listed in Table 6 (Fries & Crapo, 1981).

Ultimately, prevention depends on more research (Butler, 1980). Patients and families should be offered the opportunity to participate in research studies and should be told the extreme importance of obtaining autopsy information; primary clinicians need to communicate research results to patients and family in the form of practical information. The routine annual assessment of patients with instruments such as the Folstein Mini-Mental State Exam, the Sandoz Clinical Assessment—Geriatric Scale, and the Brief Psychiatric Rating Scale (Overall, 1958) could be extremely valuable in documenting the disease's course. Researchers must attend to their public constituency with responsible conduct and reporting of research results. Research, service, and social support are inextricably linked in the treatment and prevention of dementia.

REFERENCES

Allen, R. M. (1982). Pseudodementia and ECT. *Biological Psychiatry, 17,* 1435–1443.

Amaducci, L. A., Rocca, W. A., & Schoenberg, B. S. (1986). Origin of the distinction between Alzheimer's disease and senile dementia: How history can clarify nosology. *Neurology, 36* 1497–1499.

American Psychiatric Association. (1987). *Diagnostic and statistical manual of mental disorders* (3rd ed. rev.). Washington, DC: American Psychiatric Association.

Atkinson, R. M. (1987). Alcohol problems of the elderly. *Alcohol and Alcoholism, 22,* 415–417.

Atre-Vaidya, N., & Jampala, V. C. (1988). Electroconvulsive therapy in Parkinsonism with affective disorder. *British Journal of Psychiatry, 152,* 55–58.

Ayd, F. J., Jr. (Ed.). (1988). Rational pharmacotherapy of agitation in dementia. *International Drug Therapy Newsletter, 23,* 13–14.

Baines, S., Saxby, P., & Ehlert, K. (1987). Reality orientation and reminiscence therapy: A controlled cross-over study of elderly confused people. *British Journal of Psychiatry, 151,* 222–231.

Balldin, J., Gottfries, C-G., Karlsson, I., Lindstedt, G., Langstrom, G., & Walinder, J. (1983). Dexamethasone suppression test and serum prolactin in dementia disorders. *British Journal of Psychiatry, 143,* 277–281.

Barclay, L. L., Zemcov, A., Blass, J. P., & McDowell, F. H. (1985). Factors associated with duration of survival in Alzheimer's disease. *Biological Psychiatry, 20,* 86–93.

Barnes, R., Veith, R., Okimoto, J., Raskind, M., & Gumbrecht, G. (1982). Efficacy of antipsychotic medications in behaviorally disturbed dementia patients. *American Journal of Psychiatry, 139,* 1170–1174.

Bartol, M. A. (1979). Nonverbal communication in patients with Alzheimer's disease. *Journal of Gerontological Nursing, 5,* 21–31.

Becker, J. T., Huff, J., Nebes, R. D., Holland, A., & Boller, F. (1988). Neuropsychological function in Alzheimer's disease: Pattern of impairment and rates of progression. *Archives of Neurology, 45,* 263–268.

Becker, P. M., Feussner, J. R., Mulrow, C. D., Williams, B. C., & Vokaty, K. A. (1985). The role of lumbar puncture in the evaluation of dementia: The Durham Veterans Administration/Duke University study. *Journal of the American Geriatrics Society, 33,* 392–296.

Becker, R. E., & Giacobini, E. (1988). Mechanisms of cholinesterase inhibition of senile dementia of the Alzheimer type: Clinical, pharmacological, and therapeutic aspects. *Drug Development Research, 12,* 163–195.

Berg, G., Edwards, D. F., Danzinger, W. L., & Berg, L. (1987). Longitudinal change in three brief assessments of SDAT. *Journal of the American Geriatrics Society, 35,* 205–211.

Berg, L., Miller, J. P., Storandt, M., Duchek, J., Morris, J. C., Rubin, E. H., Burke, W. J., & Coben, L. A. (1988). Mild senile dementia of the Alzheimer type: 2. Longitudinal assessment. *Annals of Neurology, 23,* 477–484.

Berman, S., Delaney, N., Gallagher, D., Atkins, P., & Graeber, M. P. (1987). Respite care: A partnership between a veterans administration nursing home and families to care for frail elders at home. *The Gerontologist, 27,* 581–584.

Bernios, G. E., & Brook, P. (1985). Delusions and the psychopathology of the elderly with dementia. *Acta Psychiatrica Scandinavia, 72,* 296–301.

Blass, J. P. (1986). Pragmatic pointers on managing the demented patient. *Journal of the American Geriatrics Society, 34,* 548–549.

Blazer, D. G., Federspiel, C. F., Ray, W. A., & Schaffner, W. (1983). The risk of anticholinergic toxicity in the elderly: A study of prescribing practices in two populations. *Journal of Gerontology, 38,* 31–35.

Blessed, G., Tomlinson, B. E., & Roth, M. (1968). The association between quantitative measures of dementia and of senile changes in the cerebral grey matter of elderly subjects. *British Journal of Psychiatry, 114,* 797–811.

Boller, F. (1980). Mental status of patients with Parkinson's disease. *Journal of Clinical Neuropsychology, 2,* 157–172.

Botwinick, J., Storandt, M., & Berg, L. (1986). A longitudinal, behavioral study of senile dementia of the Alzheimer type. *Archives of Neurology, 43,* 1124–1127.

Breen, A. R., Larson, E. B., Reifler, B. V., Vitaliano, P. P., & Lawrence, G. L. (1984). Cognitive performance and functional competence in coexisting dementia and depression. *Journal of the American Geriatrics Society, 32,* 132–137.

Breitner, C. S. (1987). Genetic factors in the etiology of Alzheimer's disease. In H. Y. Meltzer (Ed.), *Psychopharmacology: The third generation of progress* (pp. 929–938). New York: Raven Press.

Brenner, R. P., Ulrich, R. F., Spiker, D. G., Sclabassi, R. J., Reynolds, C. F., III, Marin, R. S., & Boller, F. (1986). Computerized EEG spectral analysis in elderly normal, demented, and depressed subjects. *Electroencephalography and Clinical Neurophysiology, 64,* 483–492.

Brenner, R. P., Reynolds, C. F., III, & Ulrich, R. F. (1988). Diagnostic efficacy of computerized spectral versus visual EEG analysis in elderly normal, demented and depressed subjects. *Electroencephalography and Clinical Neurophysiology, 69,* 110–117.

Brody, E. M., Poulshock, W., & Masciocchio, C. (1978). The family caring unit: A major consideration in the long-term support system. *The Gerontologist, 18,* 556–561.

Brody, E. M., Johnsen, P. T., Fulcomer, M. C., & Lang, A. M. (1983). Women's changing roles and help to elderly parents: Attitude of three generations of women. *Journal of Gerontology, 38,* 597–607.

Buchner, D. M. & Larson, E. B. (1987). Falls and fractures in patients with Alzheimer-type dementia. *Journal of the American Medical Association, 257,* 1492–1495.

Bulbena, A., & Berrios, G. E. (1986). Pseudodementia: Facts and figures. *British Journal of Psychiatry, 148,* 87–94.

Burgio, L. D., & Burgio, K. L. (1986). Behavioral gerontology: Application of behavioral methods to the problems of older adults. *Journal of Applied Behavior Analysis, 19,* 321–328.

Burgio, L. D., Page, T. J., & Capriotti, R. M. (1985). Clinical Behavioral pharmacology: Methods for evaluating medications and contingency management. *Journal of Applied Behavior Analysis, 18,* 45–49.

Burgio, L. D., Burgio, K. L., Engel, B. T., & Tice, L. M. (1986). Increasing distance and independence of ambulation in elderly nursing home residents. *Journal of Applied Behavior Analysis, 19,* 357–366.

Burnside, I. (1984). *Working with the elderly: Group process and techniques.* Monterey, CA: Wadsworth Health Sciences Division.

Butler, R. N. (1980). Research: The ultimate service. *Aging*, Jan-Feb Issue, 4–7.
Christie, A. B., & Wood, E. R. M. (1988). Age, clinical features and prognosis in S.D.A.T. *International Journal of Geriatric Psychiatry, 3,* 63–68.
Coblentz, J. M., Mattis, S., Zingesser, L. H., Kasoff, S. S., Wisniewski, H. M., & Katzman, R. (1973). Presenile dementia. *Archives of Neurology, 29,* 299–308.
Cohen, D., & Eisdorfer, C. (1986). *The loss of self: A family resource for the care of Alzheimer's disease and related disorders.* New York: Norton.
Cohen-Mansfield, J. (1986). Agitated behaviors in the elderly: 2. Preliminary results in the cognitively deteriorated. *Journal of the American Geriatrics Society, 34,* 722–727.
Cohen-Mansfield, J., & Billig, N. (1986). Agitated behaviors in the elderly: 1. A conceptual review. *Journal of the American Geriatrics Society, 34,* 711–721.
Colerick, E. J., & George, L. K. (1986). Predictors of institutionalization among caregivers of patients with Alzheimer's disease. *Journal of the American Geriatrics Society, 34,* 493–498.
Consensus conference. (1987). Differential diagnosis of dementing diseases. *Journal of the American Medical Association, 258,* 3411–3416.
Corbin, S. L., & Eastwood, M. R. (1986). Sensory deficits and mental disorders of old age: causal or coincidental associations?. *Psychological Medicine, 16,* 251–256.
Council on Scientific Affairs. (1988). Magnetic resonance imaging of the central nervous system. *Journal of the American Medical Association, 259,* 1211–1222.
Cummings, J. L., & Benson, D. F. (1983). *Dementia: A clinical approach.* London: Butterworth.
Cummings, J. L., & Benson, D. F. (1986). Dementia of the Alzheimer type: An inventory of diagnostic clinical features. *Journal of the American Geriatrics Society, 34,* 12–19.
Cutler, P. (1979). *Problem solving in clinical medicine: From data to diagnosis.* Baltimore: Williams & Wilkins.
Cutler, N. R. (1987). In vivo markers in Alzheimer's disease and related dementias. In H. Y. Meltzer (Ed.), *Psychopharmacology: The third generation of progress* (pp. 897–899). New York: Raven Press.
Davidson, J. K. (1987). Respite care and perceptions of burden among family caregivers of frail elderly living at home. *The Gerontologist, 27,* 197a.
Davies, P., & Maloney, A. J. F. (1976). Selective loss of central cholinergic neurons in Alzheimer's disease. *Lancet, 2,* 1403.
Delabar, J. M., Goldgaber, D., Lamour, Y., Nicole, A., Huret, J-L., Grouchy, J., Brown, P., Gajdusek, D. C., & Sinet, P-M. (1987). Beta-amyloid gene duplication in Alzheimer's disease and karyotypically normal Down syndrome. *Science, 235,* 1390–1392.
Drachman, D. A., & Leavitt, J. (1974). Human memory and the cholinergic system: A relationship to aging? *Archives of Neurology, 30,* 113–121.
Drinka, T. J. K., Smith, J. C., & Drinka, P. J. (1987). Correlates of depression and burden for informal caregivers of patients in a geriatrics referral clinic. *Journal of the American Geriatrics Society, 35,* 522–525.
Dysken, M. (1987). A review of recent clinical trials in the treatment of Alzheimer's dementia. *Psychiatric Annals, 17,* 178–191.
Eastwood, M. R., Lautenschlaeger, E., & Corbin, S. (1983). A comparison of clinical methods for assessing dementia. *Journal of the American Geriatrics Society, 31,* 342–347.
Fisk, A. A., & Pannill, F. C., III. (1987). Assessment and care of the community-dwelling Alzheimer's disease patient. *Journal of the American Geriatrics Society, 35,* 307–311.
Folstein, M. F., Folstein, S. E., & McHugh, P. R. (1975). "Mini Mental State": A practical method for grading the cognitive state of patients for the clinician. *Journal of Psychiatry Research, 12,* 189–198.
Folstein, M., Anthony, J. C., Parhad, I., Duffy, B., & Gruenberg, E. M. (1985). The meaning of cognitive impairment in the elderly. *Journal of the American Geriatrics Society, 33,* 228–235.
Francheschi, M., Ferini-Strambi, L., Minicucci, F., Sferrazza-Papa, A., & Smirne, S. (1986). Signs of cardiac autonomic dysfunction during sleep in patients with Alzheimer's disease. *Gerontology, 32,* 327–334.
Freyhan, F. A., Woodford, R. B., & Kety, S. S. (1951). Cerebral blood flow and metabolism in psychosis of senility. *Journal of Nervous and Mental Disease, 113,* 449–456.
Fries, J. F., & Crapo, L. M. (1981). *Vitality and aging: Implications of the rectangular curve.* San Francisco: W. H. Freeman.
Gage, F. H., Bjorklund, A., Stenevi, U., Dunnett, S. B., & Kelly, P. A. T. (1984). Intrahippocampal septal grafts ameliorate learning impairments in aged rats. *Science, 225,* 533–536.
Gallagher, D. E. (1985). Intervention strategies to assist caregivers of frail elders: Current research status and

future research directions. In M. P. Lawton & G. Maddox (Eds.), *Annual review of gerontology and geriatrics* (Vol. 5). New York: Springer.

Gash, D. M., Collier, T. J., & Stadek, J. R., Jr. (1985). Neural transplantation: A review of recent developments and potential applications to the aged brain. *Neurobiology of Aging, 6,* 131–150.

George, J., Binns, V. E., Clayden, A. D., & Mulley, G. P. (1988). Aids and adaptations for the elderly at home: Underprovided, underused, and undermaintained. *British Medical Journal, 296,* 1365–1366.

Gilhooly, L. M. (1984). The impact of care-giving on care-givers: Factors associated with the psychological well-being of people supporting a dementing relative in the community. *British Journal of Medical Psychology, 57,* 35–44.

Goldstein, V., Regnery, G., & Wellin, E. (1981, January). Caretaker role fatigue. *Nursing Outlook,* 24–30.

Gordon, R. E., & Gordon, K. K. (1987). Relating Axes IV and V of DSM-III to clinical severity of psychiatric disorders. *Canadian Journal of Psychiatry, 32,* 432–424.

Granek, E., Baker, S. P., Abbey, H., Robinson, E., Myers, A. H., Samkoff, J. S., & Klein, L. E. (1987). Medications and diagnoses in relation to falls in a long-term care facility. *Journal of the American Geriatrics Society, 35,* 503–511.

Grimes, A. M., Grady C. L., Foster, N. L., Sunderland, T., & Patronas, N. J. (1985). Central auditory function in Alzheimer's disease. *Neurology, 35,* 352–358.

Hachinski, V. C., Lassen, N. A., & Marshall, J. (1974). Multi-infarct dementia: A cause of mental deterioration in the elderly. *Lancet, 2,* 207–210.

Hachinski, V. C., Iliff, L. D., Zilhka, E., Du Boulay, G. H., McAllister, V. L., Marshall, J., Russell, R. W. R., & Symon, L. (1975). Cerebral blood flow in dementia. *Archives of Neurology, 32,* 632–637.

Haley, W. E., Brown, S. L., & Levine, E. G. (1987). Experimental evaluation of the effectiveness of group intervention for dementia caregivers. *The Gerontologist, 27,* 376–382

Hammerstrom, D. C., & Zimmer, B. (1985). The role of lumbar puncture in the evaluation of dementia: The University of Pittsburgh study. *Journal of the American Geriatrics Society, 33,* 397–400.

Heston, L. L., Mastri, A. R., Anderson, V. E., & White, J. (1981). Dementia of the Alzheimer type. *Archives of General Psychiatry, 38,* 1085–1090.

Hinton, D. R., Sadun, A. A., Blanks, J. C., & Miller, C. A. (1986). Optic-nerve degeneration in Alzheimer's disease. *New England Journal of Medicine, 315,* 485–487.

Hoch, C. C., Reynolds, C. F., III, Nebes, R. D., Kupfer, D. J., Berman, S., & Campbell, D. (1989). Clinical significance of sleep-disordered breathing (SDB) in Alzheimer's disease: Preliminary data. *Journal of the American Geriatrics Society, 37,* 138–144.

Hollander, E., Mohs, R. C., & Davis, K. L. (1986). Cholinergic approaches to the treatment of Alzheimer's disease. *British Medical Bulletin, 42,* 97–100.

Hollister, L. E. (1986). Drug therapy of Alzheimer disease: Realistic or not? *Progress in Neuropsychopharmacology and Biological Psychiatry,* 10, 439–446.

Hollister, L. E., & Yesavage, J. (1984). Ergoloid mesylates for senile dementia: Unanswered questions. *Annals of Internal Medicine, 100,* 894–898.

Huff, F. J., Boller, F., Lucchelli, F., Querriera, R., Beyer, J., & Belle, S. (1987). The neurologic examination in patients with probable Alzheimer's disease. *Archives of Neurology, 44,* 929–932.

Hughes, C. P., Berg, L., Danziger, W. L., Coben, L. A., & Martin, R. L. (1983). A new clinical scale for the staging of dementia. *British Journal of Psychiatry, 140,* 566–572.

Jenike, M. A. (1985a). *Handbook of geriatric psychopharmacology.* Littleton, MA: PSG Publishing.

Jenike, M. A. (1985b). Monoamine oxidase inhibitors as treatment for depressed patients with primary degenerative dementia (Alzheimer's disease). *American Journal of Psychiatry, 142,* 763–764.

Kaszniak, A. W., Fox, J., Gandell, D. L., Garron, D. C., Huckman, M. S., & Ramsey, R. G. (1978). Predictors of mortality in presenile and senile dementia. *Annals of Neurology, 3,* 246–252.

Katzman, R. (1976). The prevalence and malignancy of Alzheimer disease: A major killer. *Archives of Neurology, 33,* 217–218.

Katzman, R. (1986). Alzheimer disease. *New England Journal of Medicine, 314,* 964–793.

Kay, D. W. K., Roth, M., & Hopkins, B. (1955). Affective disorder arising in the senium. *Journal of Mental Science, 101,* 302–318.

Kent, D. L., & Larson, E. B. (1988). Magnetic resonance imaging of the brain and spine: Is clinical efficacy established after the first decade? *Annals of Internal Medicine, 108,* 402–424.

Kiloh, L. G. (1961). Pseudo-dementia. *Acta Psychiatrica Scandinavia, 37,* 336–351.

King, M. B. (1986). Alcohol abuse and dementia. *International Journal of Geriatric Psychiatry, 1,* 31–36.

Knopman, D. S., Kitto, J., Deinard, S., & Heiring, J. (1988). Longitudinal study of death and institutionalization in patients with primary degenerative dementia. *Journal of the American Geriatrics Society, 36,* 108–112.

Knupfer, L., & Speigel, R. (1986). Differences in olfactory test performance between normal aged, Alzheimer and vascular type dementia individuals. *Intl Journal of Geriatric Psychiatry, 1,* 3–14.

Kraus, A. S., Spasoff, R. A., Beattie, E. J., Holden, D. E. W., Lawson, J. S., Rodenburg, M., & Woodcock, G. M. (1976). Elderly applicants to long-term care institutions. *Journal of the American Geriatric Society, 24,* 117–125.

Larson, E. B., Reifler, B. V., Sumi, S. M., Canfield, C. G., & Chinn, N. M. (1985). Diagnostic evaluation of 200 elderly outpatients with suspected dementia. *Journal of Gerontology, 40,* 536–543.

Larson, E. B., Kukull, W. A., Buchner, D., & Reifler, B. V. (1987). Adverse drug reactions associated with global cognitive impairment in elderly persons. *Annals of Internal Medicine, 107,* 169–173.

Leuchter, A. F., Spar, J. E., Walter, D. O., & Weiner, H. (1987). Electroencephalographic spectra and coherence in the diagnosis of Alzheimer's-type and multi-infarct dementia. *Archives of General Psychiatry, 44,* 993–998.

Levine, N. B., Dastoor, D. P., & Gendron, C. (1983). Coping with dementia: A pilot study. *Journal of the American Geriatrics Society, 31,*12–18.

Lezak, M. (1978). Living with the characterologically altered brain injured patient. *Journal of Clinical Psychology, 39,* 592–598.

Liang, R. A., Lam, R. W., & Ancill, R. J. (1988). ECT in the treatment of mixed depression and dementia. *British Journal of Psychiatry, 152,* 281–284.

Lieberman, M., Yalom, I., & Miles, M. B. (1973). *Encounter groups: First facts.* New York: Basic Books.

Lipsey, J. R., Robinson, R. G., Pearlson, G. D., Rao, K., & Price, T. R. (1984). Nortriptyline treatment of post-stroke depression: A double blind study. *The Lancet, 1,* 297–300.

Lundervold, D., & Lewin, L. M. (1987). Effects of in-home respite care on caregivers of family members with Alzheimer's disease. *Journal of Clinical Experimental Gerontology, 9,* 201–214.

Mace, N. L., & Rabins, P. V. (1981). *The 36-hour day: A family guide to caring for persons with Alzheimer's disease, related dementing illnesses, and memory loss in later life.* Baltimore: John Hopkins University Press.

Maricle, R., Leung, P., & Bloom, J. D. (1987). The use of DSM-III axis in recording physical illness in psychiatric patients. *American Journal of Psychiatry, 144,* 1484–1486.

Martin, D. C., Miller, J. K., Kapoor, W., Arena, V. C., & Boller, F. (1987). A controlled study of survival with dementia. *Archives of Neurology, 44,* 1122–1126.

Martin, D. C., Miller, J., Kapoor, W., Karpf, M., & Boller, F. (1987). Clinical prediction rules for computed tomographic scanning in senile dementia. *Archives of Internal Medicine, 147,* 77–80.

Mayeux, R., Stern, Y., & Sano, M. (1985). Psychosis with dementia of the Alzheimer type. *Annals of Neurology, 18,* 144.

Mayeux, R., Stern, Y., & Spanton, S. (1985). Heterogeneity in dementia of the Alzheimer's type: Evidence of subgroups. *Neurology, 35,* 453–461.

McEvoy, J. P., McCue, M. Spring, B., Mohs, R. C., Lavori, P. W., & Farr, R. M. (1987). Effects of amantadine and trihexyphenidyl on memory in elderly normal volunteers. *American Journal of Psychiatry, 144,* 573–577.

McKhann, G., Drachman, D., Folstein, M., Katzman, R., Price, D., & Stadlan, E. M. (1984). Clinical diagnosis of Alzheimer's disease: Report of the NINCDS-ADRDA work group. *Neurology, 34,* 939–944.

Merriam, A. E., Aronson, M. K., Gaston, P., Wey, S-L., & Katz, I. (1988). The psychiatric symptoms of Alzheimer's disease. *Journal of the American Geriatrics Society, 36,* 7–12.

Mesulam, M-M., Geula, C., & Moran, M. A. (1987). Anatomy of cholinesterase inhibition in Alzheimer's disease: Effect of physostigmine an tetrahydroaminoacridine on plaques and tangles. *Annals of Neurology, 22,* 683–691.

Meyer, J. S., Judd, B. W., Tawaklna, T., Rogers, R. L., & Mortel, K. F. (1986). Improved cognition after control of risk-factors for multi-infarct dementia. *Journal of the American Medical Association, 256,* 2203–2209.

Mezzich, J. E., Fabrega, H., Coffman, G. A., & Glavin, Y-F. (1987). Comprehensively diagnosing geriatric patients. *Comprehensive Psychiatry, 28,* 68–76.

Molloy, D. W., Beerschoten, D. A., Borrie, M. J., Crilly, R. G., & Cape, R. D. T. (1988). Acute effects of exercise on neuropsychological function in elderly subjects. *Journal of the American Geriatrics Society, 36,* 29–33.

Morycz, R. (1980). An exploration of senile dementia and family burden. *Clinical Social Work Journal, 8,* 16–27.

Morycz, R. C. (1985). Caregiving strain and the desire to institutionalize family members with Alzheimer's disease: Possible predictors and model development. *Research on Aging, 7,* 329–361.

Morycz, R. K., Malloy, J., Bozich, M., & Martz, P. (1987). Racial differences in family burden: Clinical implications for social work. *Journal of Gerontological Social Work, 10,* 133–154.

Navia, B. A., & Price, R. W. (1987). The acquired immunodeficiency syndrome dementia complex as the presenting or sole manifestation of human immunodeficiency virus infection. *Archives of Neurology, 44,* 65–69

Nelson, A., Fogel, B. S., & Faust, D. (1986). Bedside cognitive screening instruments. *Journal of Nervous and Mental Disease, 174,* 73–83.

Nielsen, S., Petito, C. K., Urmacher, C. D., & Posner, J. B. (1984). Subacute encephalitis in acquired immunodeficiency syndrome: A post-mortem study. *American Journal of Clinical Pathology, 82,* 678–682.

Orwin, A., Wright, C. E., Harding, G. F. A., Rowan, D. C., & Rolfe, E. B. (1986). Serial visual evoked potential recordings in Alzheimer's disease. *British Medical Journal, 293,* 9–10.

Overall, J. E. (1985). Psychiatric rating scales: State of the art and directions for future research. In T. Crook, S. Ferris, & R. Bartus (Eds.), *Assessment in geriatric psychopharmacology* (pp. 69–79). New Canaan, CT: Mark Powley.

Overall, J. E., & Gorham, D. R. (1962). Brief psychiatric rating scale. *Psychological Reports, 10,* 799–812.

Peabody, C. A., Whiteford, H. A., & Hollister, L. E. (1986). Antidepressants and the elderly. *Journal of the American Geriatrics Society, 34,* 869–874.

Perry, E. K., Perry, R. H., Blessed, G., & Tomlinson, B. E. (1977). Necropsy evidence of central cholinergic deficits in senile dementia. *Lancet, 1,* 189.

Perry, E. K., Tomlinson, B. E., Blessed, G., Gergmann, K., Gibson, P. H., & Perry, R. H. (1978). Correlation of cholinergic abnormalities with senile plaques and mental test scores in senile dementia. *British Medical Journal, 2,* 1457–1459.

Pfeiffer, E., Cairl, R., Keller, D., & Doblas, R. (1987). Changes in caregiver characteristics as a function of service setting: A multipopulation comparison. *The Gerontologist, 27,* 195a.

Plotkin, D. A., Gerson, S. C., & Jarvik, L. F. (1987). Antidepressant drug treatment in the elderly. In H. Y. Meltzer (Ed.), *Psychopharmacology: The third generation of progress* (pp. 1149–1158). New York: Raven Press.

Popkin, M. K. (1986). Organic brain syndromes presenting with global cognitive impairment: Delirium and dementia. In G. Winokur & P. J. Clayton (Eds.), *The medical basis of psychiatry* (pp. 3–19). Philadelphia: W. B. Saunders.

Powell, L., & Courtice, K. (1983). *Alzheimer's disease: A guide for families.* Reading, MA: Addison-Wesley.

Raskind, M., Peskind, E., Rivard, M-F., Veith, R., & Barnes, R. (1982). Dexamethasone suppression test and cortisol circadian rhythm in primary degenerative dementia. *American Journal of Psychiatry, 139,* 1468–1471.

Raskind, M. A., Peskind, E. F., Halter, J. B., & Jimerson, D. C. (1984). Norepinephrine and MHPG levels in CSF and plasma in Alzheimer's disease. *Archives of General Psychiatry, 41,* 343–346.

Raskind, M. A., Risse, S. C., & Lampe, T. H. (1987). Dementia and antipsychotic drugs. *Journal of Clinical Psychiatry, 48* (Suppl.), 16–18.

Reding, M. J., Orto, L. A., Winter, S. W., Fortuna, I. M., di Ponte, P., & McDowell, F. H. (1986). Antidepressant therapy after stroke: A double-blind trial. *Archives of Neurology, 43,* 763–765.

Reifler, B. V. (1986). Mixed cognitive-affective disturbances in the elderly: A new classification. *Journal of Clinical Psychiatry, 47,* 354–356.

Reifler, B. V., & Larson, E. (1988). Excess disability in demented elderly outpatients: The rule of halves. *Journal of the American Geriatrics Society, 36,* 82–83.

Reifler, B. V., Larson, E., & Hanley, R. (1982). Coexistence of cognitive impairment and depression in geriatric outpatients. *American Journal of Psychiatry, 139,* 623–626.

Reisberg, B., & Ferris, S. H. (1985). A clinical rating scale for symptoms of psychosis in Alzheimer's Disease. *Psychopharmacology Bulletin, 21,* 101–104.

Reisberg, B., Ferris, S., Anand, R., Buttinger, C., Borenstein, J., Sinaiko, E., & de Leon, M. (1984). Clinical assessments of cognition in the aged. In C. A. Shamoian (Ed.), *Biology and treatment of dementia in the elderly.* Washington, DC: American Psychiatric Press.

Reynolds, C. F., III, & Kupfer, D. J. (1987). Neuropsychiatric aspects of sleep disorders. In R. E. Hales & S. C. Yodofsky (Eds.), *Textbook of neuropsychiatry*. Washington, DC: American Psychiatric Press.

Reynolds, C. F., III, Kupfer, D. J., Taska, L. S., Hoch, C. C., Sewitch, D. E., Restifo, K., Spiker, D. G., Zimmer, B., Marin, R. S., Nelson, J., Martin, D., & Morycz, R. (1985). Sleep apnea in Alzheimer's dementia: Correlation with mental deterioration. *Journal of Clinical psychiatry, 46,* 257–261.

Reynolds, C. F., III, Kupfer, D. J., Hoch, C. C., Stack, J. A., Houck, P. R., & Sewitch, D. E. (1986). Two-year follow-up of elderly patients with mixed depression and dementia: Clinical and electroencephalographic sleep findings. *Journal of the American Geriatrics Society, 34,* 793–799.

Reynolds, C. F., III, Perel, J. M., Kupfer, D. J., Zimmer, B., Stack, J. A., & Hoch, C. C. (1987). Open-trial response to antidepressant treatment in elderly patients with mixed depression and cognitive impairment. *Psychiatry Research, 21,* 111–122.

Reynolds, C. F., III, Kupfer, D. J., Houck, P. R., Hoch, C. C., Stack, J. A., Berman, S. R., & Zimmer, B. (1988). Reliable discrimination of elderly depressed and demented patients by electroencephalographic sleep data. *Archives of General Psychiatry, 45,* 258–264.

Rezek, D. L. (1987). Olfactory deficits as a neurologic sign in dementia of the Alzheimer type. *Archives of Neurology, 44,* 1030–1032.

Risse, S. C., & Barnes, R. (1986). Pharmacologic treatment of agitation associated with dementia. *Journal of the American Geriatrics Society, 34,* 368–374.

Roca, R. P. (1987). Bedside cognitive examination: Usefulness in detecting delirium and dementia. *Psychosomatics, 28,* 71–76.

Rocca, W. A., Amaducci, L. A., & Schoenberg, B. S. (1986). epidemiology of clinically diagnosed Alzheimer's disease. *Annals of Neurology. 19,* 415–424.

Roman, G. C. (1987). Senile dementia of the Binswanger type. A vascular form of dementia in the elderly. *Journal of the American Medical Association, 258,* 1782–88.

Roose, S. P., Glassman, A. H., Giardina, E. G. V., Walsh, B. T., Woodring, S., & Bigger, J. T. (1987). Tricyclic antidepressants in depressed patients with cardiac conduction disease. *Archives of General Psychiatry, 44,* 273–275.

Rubin, E. H., Morris, J. C., & Berg, L. (1987). The progression of personality changes in senile dementia of the Alzheimer's type. *Journal of the American Geriatrics Society, 35,* 721–725.

Rubin, E. H., Morris, J. C., Storandt, M., & Berg, L. (1987). Behavioral changes in patients with mild senile dementia of the Alzheimer's type. *Psychiatry Research, 21,* 55–62.

Rubin, E. H., Drevets, W. D., & Burke, W. J. (1988). The nature of psychotic symptoms in senile dementia of the Alzheimer type. *Journal of Geriatric Psychiatry and Neurology, 1,* 16–20.

Salzman, C. (1987). Treatment of the elderly agitated patient. In H. Y. Meltzer (Ed.), *Psychopharmacology: The third generation of progress* (pp. 1167–1176). New York: Raven Press.

Sanford, J. (1975). Tolerance of debility in elderly dependents by supporters at home: Its significance for hospital practice. *British Medical Journal, 3,* 471–473.

Schuckit, M. A. (1982). A clinical review of alcohol, alcoholism, and the elderly patient. *Journal of Clinical Psychiatry, 43,* 396–399.

Seltzer, B., Rheaume, Y., Volicer, L., Fabiszewski, K. J., Lyon, P. C., Brown, J. E., & Volicer, B. (1988). The short-term effects of in-hospital respite on the patient with Alzheimer's disease. *The Gerontologist, 28,* 121–124.

Seltzer, M. M., Ivry, J., & Litchfield, L. C. (1987). Family members as case managers: Partnership between the formal and informal support networks. *The Gerontologist, 27,* 722–728.

Shader, R. I., Harmatz, J. S., & Salzman, C. (1974). A new scale for clinical assessment in geriatric populations: Sandoz Clinical Assessment—Geriatric (SCAG). *Journal of the American Geriatrics Society, 22,* 107–113.

Shader, R. I., Kennedy, J. S., & Greenblatt, D. J. (1987). Treatment of anxiety in the elderly. In H. Y. Meltzer (Ed.), *Psychopharmacology: The third generation of progress* (pp. 1141–1148). New York: Raven Press.

Shanas, E. (1979a). The family as a social support system in old age. *The Gerontologist, 19,* 163–174.

Shanas, E. (1979b). Social myth as hypothesis: The case of the family relations of old people. *The Gerontologist, 19,* 3–9.

Shulman, K. I., MacKenzie, S., & Hardy, B. (1987). The clinical use of lithium carbonate in old age: A review. *Prog. Neuro-Psychopharmacol. & Biol Psychiat., 11,* 159–164.

Sim, M., & Sussman, I. (1962). Alzheimer's disease: Its natural history and differential diagnosis. *Journal of Nervous and Mental Disease, 135,* 489–499.

Sjogren, T., Sjogren, H., & Lindgren, G. H. (1952). Morbus Alzheimer and morbus Pick: A genetic, clinical, and pathoanatomical study. *Acta Psychiatrica Scandinavia, 34* (Suppl. 82).

Skurla, E., Rogers, J. C., & Sunderland, T. (1988). Direct assessment of activities of daily living in Alzheimer's disease: A controlled study. *Journal of the American Geriatrics Society, 36,* 97–103.

Snow, D. L., Davidson J. K., Puterski, D., Tworkowski, S., & Sussman, R. A. (1987). Perceptions of burden, informal support, and contexts of impairment among family caregivers of frail elderly. *The Gerontologist, 27,* 197a.

St. Clair, D., Blackburn, I., Blackwood, D., & Tyrer, G. (1988). Measuring the course of Alzheimer's disease: A longitudinal study of neuropsychological function and changes in P3 event-related potential. *British Journal of Psychiatry, 152,* 48–54.

St. George-Hyslop, P. H., Tanzi, R. E., Polinsky, R. J., Haines, J. L., Nee, L., Watkins, P. C., Myers, R. H., Feldman, R. G., Pollen, D., Drachman, D., Growdon, J., Bruni, A., Foncin, J-F., Salmon, D., Frommelt, P., Amaducci, L., Sorbi, S., Piacentini, S., Stewart, G. D., Hobbs, W. J., Conneally, P. M., & Gusella, J. F. (1987). The genetic defect causing familial Alzheimer's disease maps on chromosome 21. *Science, 235,* 885–890.

Steffes, R., & Thralow, J. (1987). Visual field limitation in the patient with dementia of the Alzheimer's type. *Journal of the American Geriatrics Society, 35,* 198–204.

Stern, Y., Mayeux, R., Sano, M., Hauser, W. A., & Bush, T. (1987). Predictors of disease course in patients with probable Alzheimer's disease. *Neurology, 37,* 1629–1653.

Sunderland, T., Tariot, P., Murphy, D. L., Weingartner, H., Mueller, E. A., & Cohen, R. M. (1985). Scopolamine challenges in Alzheimer's disease. *Psychopharmacology, 87,* 247–249.

Teri, L., Larson, E. B., & Reifler, B. V. (1988). Behavioral disturbance in dementia of the Alzheimer's type. *Journal of the American Geriatrics Society, 36,* 1–6.

Thornton, J. E., Davies, H. D., & Tinklenberg, J. R. (1986). Alzheimer's disease syndrome. *Journal of Psychosocial Nursing, 24,* 16–22.

Tierney, M. C., Snow W. G., Reid, D. W., Zorzitto, M. L., & Fisher, R. H. (1987). Psychometric differentiation of dementia: Replication and extension of the findings of Storandt and Coworkers. *Archives of Neurology, 44,* 720–722.

Tinklenberg, J. R., Thornton, J. E., & Yesavage, J. A. (1984). Clinical geriatric psychopharmacology and neuropeptides. In C. A. Shamoian (Ed.), *Biology and treatment of dementia in the elderly.* Washington, DC: American Psychiatric Press.

Trzepacz, P. T., Baker, R. W., & Greenhouse, J. (1988). A symptom rating scale for delirium. *Psychiatry Research, 23,* 89–97.

Uhlmann, R. F., Larson, E. B., & Koepsell T. D. (1986). Hearing impairment and cognitive decline in senile dementia of the Alzheimer's type. *Journal of the American Geriatrics Society, 34,* 207–210.

U.S. Congress, Office of Technology Assessment. (1985). *Technology and aging in America.* Washington, DC: U.S. Government Printing Office.

Vaillant, G. E. (1977). *Adaptation to life.* Boston: Little, Brown.

Verwoerdt, A. (1981). Individual psychotherapy in senile dementia. In N. E. Miller & G. D. Cohen (Eds.), *Clinical aspects of Alzheimer's disease and senile dementia* (pp. 184–208). New York: Raven Press.

Wade, J. P. H., Mirsen, T. R., Hachinski, V. C., Fisman, M., Lau, C., & Merskey, H. (1987). The clinical diagnosis of Alzheimer's disease. *Archives of Neurology, 44,* 24–29.

Warner, M. D., Peabody, C. A., Flattery, J. J., & Tinklenberg, J. R. (1986). Olfactory deficits and Alzheimer's disease. *Biological Psychiatry, 21,* 116–118.

Wells, C. E. (1979). Pseudodementia. *American Journal of Psychiatry, 136,* 895–900.

Willenbring, M. L., Christensen, K. J., Spring, W. D., Jr., & Rasmussen, R. (1987). Alcoholism screening in the elderly. *Journal of the American Geriatrics Society, 35,* 864–869.

Winogrond, I. R., Fisk, A. A., Kirsling R. A., & Keyes, B. (1987). The relationship of caregiver burden and morale to Alzheimer's disease patient function in a therapeutic setting. *The Gerontologist, 27,* 336–339.

Wolkowitz, O. M., Tinklenberg, J. R., & Weingartner, H. (1985). A psychopharmacological perspective of cognitive functions. *Neuropsychobiology, 14,* 88–96.

Wolozin, B., & Davies, P. (1987). Alzheimer-related neuronal protein A68: Specificity and distribution. *Annals of Neurology, 22,* 521–526.

Yesavage, J. A. (1979). Pharmacotherapy of the aged central nervous system. *Clinical Neuropharmacology, 4,* 199–220.

Yesavage, J. A. (1985). Nonpharmacologic treatments for memory losses with normal aging. *American Journal of Psychiatry, 142,* 600–605.

Yesavage, J. A., Tinklenberg, J. R., Hollister, L. E., & Berger, P. A. (1979). Vasodilators in senile dementia. *Archives of General Psychiatry. 36,* 220–223.

Zarit, S., & Zarit, J. (1982). Families under stress: Interventions for caregivers of senile dementia patients. *Psychotherapy: Theory, Research, and Practice, 19,* 461–471.

Zubenko, G. S., Wusylko, M., Cohen, B. M., Boller, F., & Teply, I. (1987). Family study of platelet membrane fluidity in Alzheimer's disease. *Science, 238,* 539–542.

17

Selected Organic Brain Syndromes

JACK R. CORNELIUS

INTRODUCTION

Organic brain syndromes (OBSs) are a heterogeneous group that exhibit a wide range of symptoms. Thus, OBS may mimic a variety of "functional" disorders. For example, the primary symptom complex in the various OBSs may include global cognitive impairment, selected cognitive deficits, psychotic and affective symptoms, personality abnormalities, or alcohol- and substance-related disorders. No single collection of behavioral symptoms is pathognomonic of all OBSs. It can be difficult to distinguish OBSs from functional psychiatric disorders on the basis of psychiatric symptoms alone (Hall, Popkin, DeVaul, Faillace, & Stickney, 1978). The third edition of the American Psychiatric Association's *Diagnostic and Statistical Manual of Mental Disorders* (DSM-III; APA, 1980) describes the essential feature of OBS as a psychological or behavioral abnormality associated with brain dysfunction. This cerebral dysfunction may be either primary brain dysfunction or a secondary abnormality, such as one caused by a toxic agent or metabolic abnormality. The dysfunction must be demonstrated by the patient's medical history, physical exam or laboratory tests and must be etiologically related to his or her psychiatric symptoms.

There are eight categories of OBS: delirium, dementia, amnestic syndrome, organic hallucinosis, organic delusional disorder, organic affective syndrome, organic personality syndrome, and atypical or mixed organic brain syndrome. Dementia is discussed in Chapter 16 and will not be covered further in this chapter.

In the *Comprehensive Textbook of Psychiatry III* (Lipowski, 1980c), organic mental disorders are described as the "most neglected area of clinical psychiatry" (p. 1359). Similarly, a Task Force (1975) of the National Institute of Mental Health concluded that "of all mental illness, organic psychosis has been the most severely neglected by researchers."

JACK R. CORNELIUS • Western Psychiatric Institute and Clinic, Pittsburgh, Pennsylvania 15213.

Such neglect of OBS has occurred despite the widespread occurrence of these disorders. For example, Hall *et al.* (1978) found medical disorders productive of psychiatric symptoms in 9.1% of 658 consecutive psychiatric outpatients. Similarly, Koranyi (1979) reported that a medical condition was the sole cause of the psychiatric disorder in 7.7% of his 2,090 psychiatric outpatients. OBSs are a common finding in psychiatric inpatients and consult–liaison patients as well. For example, Herridge (1960) reported that 5% of 209 consecutive psychiatric inpatients suffered from a medical illness that was considered the cause of their psychiatric disorder. Thus, it seems clear that 5%–10% of patients presenting for mental health treatment have an organic mental syndrome.

Little is known of the pathophysiology of the different OBSs. Delirium and dementia are generally associated with widespread cerebral abnormalities. However, amnestic syndrome, organic personality syndrome, organic delusional syndrome, and organic hallucinosis are usually conceptualized as more focal disorders. The localization of pathology in organic affective syndrome is less well understood.

There is variation from disorder to disorder in the nature of the etiological role played by cerebral dysfunction. For example, a causal relationship is evident in some disorders, such as the classical association of a frontal lobe stroke leading to an organic personality disorder. However, in other OBSs, the relationship between the medical disorder and subsequent behavioral symptoms may be described more accurately as a precipitation of symptoms in a predisposed person. For example, Goodwin and Bunney (1971) showed that the patients who experienced a major depressive disorder as a side effect of reserpine were generally those who had a prior history of depression.

A number of other observations concerning the pathophysiology and symptomatology of OBS are not fully understood. For example, it is not clear why symptoms may vary from individual to individual within a particular OBS. For example, patients with delirium may or may not exhibit a variety of affective and psychotic symptoms in addition to their cognitive symptoms. Similarly, it is often unclear why one patient with a particular medical disorder exhibits psychiatric symptoms (such as delirium) and another patient with the same medical disorder does not display these behavioral symptoms. Further, it is not clear why a specific medical disorder can be associated with different OBSs in different patients. For example, Cushing's syndrome may be associated with depression, mania, or psychotic symptoms in different patients. Finally, a particular OBS may be associated with a variety of seemingly unrelated medical disorders. These observations may be explained in part by differences in the patients' physiology, past psychiatric history, personality style, education level, psychosocial stressors, physical environment, and/or social support network. However, the exact reason for the above-mentioned variations in symptoms is not always clear.

An outpatient evaluation of the patient should always focus on *both* psychiatric and medical problems. Details of the mental status evaluation are discussed later in the sections concerning the specific OBSs and will not be discussed further here. A careful medical evaluation should be conducted, including a history of neurological deficits, seizures, recent infections, medications, and drug and alcohol usage patterns. A physical examination should always be performed, focusing especially on focal neurological signs, endocrine signs, and cardiac signs. Some of the more common laboratory tests include serum electrolytes, a complete blood count and differential, a toxic blood and serum screen, thyroid function tests, a syphilis screen, vitamin B_{12} and folate levels, an EEG, a CT scan, a lumbar puncture, and neuropsychological testing. Nonmedical therapists should collaborate with psychiatrists and with internists or family practitioners to fully evaluate all medical disorders. Hospitalization is required in some cases, as for patients with prominent suicidal or homicidal ideations, delirium, inability to care for themselves, or acute serious medical disorders. Hospitalization may also be required for some of the more sophisticated laboratory tests, for the close observation of patients with an unclear psychiatric diagnosis, and for the institution of certain treatments that may have significant side effects.

The general recommendation for the treatment of the OBSs has been to treat the underlying medical problem rather than to focus on the specific behavioral syndrome. This strategy is most useful in treating delirium, though, even in these patients, either sedative or antipsychotic medication may be helpful. In OBS other than delirium the underlying medical disorder may be less amenable to treatment, so psychotropic agents or psychotherapeutic interventions play a larger role. In general, psychotropic medications should be initiated at the lowest standard dosage because of the increased risk of paradoxical behavioral reactions or side effects (Ban, 1976). This note of caution about dosage is particularly important in geriatric patients. Medical treatment of the underlying medical problem is frequently used in conjunction with psychotropic medications for the behavioral symptoms. The patient's behavioral symptoms may run a course independent of the medical problems. Therefore, adjustments in psychotropic medications may not parallel the adjustments in other medications. It is difficult to make further generalizations about the treatment of OBS because of the wide variety of disorders and treatments and because of the scarcity in the literature of large, well-designed pharmacotherapy studies in this area. More specifics concerning the pharmacotherapy of specific OBSs will be discussed later in this chapter.

HISTORY

Two of the OBSs, delirium and dementia, have been recognized since antiquity; the others have been more recently acknowledged. Specifically, Lipowski (1980c) noted that Celsus introduced the terms *delirium* and *dementia* in the first century in his work entitled *De Medicina*. Thus, throughout most of recorded history, clouding of consciousness was considered a necessary feature of OBS. However, over the last 150 years, a body of literature has slowly accumulated in which a variety of psychiatric disturbances have been reportedly caused by medical disorders without the necessary presence of a clouded sensorium (Lipowski, 1980b). The first edition of the *Diagnostic and Statistical Manual of Mental Disorders* (DSM-I; APA, 1952) divided organic brain disorders into acute and chronic forms. The DSM-II (APA, 1968) subsequently divided organic brain syndromes into psychotic and nonpsychotic types but recommended that the terms *acute* and *chronic* also be used. These disorders were described as manifesting the following symptoms: lability and shallowness of affect and impairment of orientation, memory, intellectual function, and judgment. It was stated that most of these basic symptoms are generally present to some degree regardless of whether the syndrome is mild, moderate, or severe. The distinction between psychotic and nonpsychotic disorders was made according to the severity of the functional impairment, rather than on the basis of the presence of hallucinations or delusions.

Criticisms of the DSM-II classification system of OBS helped shape the DSM-III system. One such criticism was that the DSM-II system did not do justice to the variety of behavioral manifestations of cerebral disorders. A second criticism was that use of the terms *psychotic* and *nonpsychotic* to describe functional impairment was vague and offered little practical information (Lipowski, 1980b). A third criticism was that the terms *acute* and *chronic* were often difficult to distinguish on initial clinical presentation and did not invariably correspond to whether the disorder was reversible or irreversible. A final criticism noted that the DSM-II assertion that OBSs were caused by "diffuse" pathology excluded many psychiatric disorders associated with focal CNS lesions (Fauman, 1983).

The DSM-III classification of OBS differs from the DSM-II system in several important ways. One of the most important changes is the acknowledgment that OBSs are a heterogeneous group with a wide variety of symptomatology. The symptom spectrum of OBS has been broadened beyond the global cognitive deficits and emotional lability described in the DSM-II. Specifically, the DSM-III system also includes symptoms such as personality changes, a broader range of affective symptoms (including depression and mania), focal cognitive impairments (such as memory impairment without other cognitive abnormality), and use of the term *psychosis* to refer to the presence of hallucinations and delusions rather than to the level of functional impairment.

The DSM-III classification of OBS also differs from the DSM-II system in several other important ways. For example, the terms *acute*, *chronic*, and *psychotic* have been eliminated. Also, this edition recognizes that a systemic illness (as opposed to a primary disease of the brain) may secondarily affect the brain. For example, a number of endocrine disorders are associated with OBS. Further, the DSM-III acknowledges that focal cerebral pathology may be associated with OBS, thus abandoning the DSM-II requirement that such cerebral abnormalities be "diffuse." It is hoped that these changes will improve the correlation between clinical observation and the diagnostic criteria for OBS and thus will lead to improvements in the treatment of these disorders. It is also hoped that this classification system will stimulate research in OBS, especially in outpatient clinical issues, which previously has been lacking.

DELIRIUM

Specific Diagnostic Considerations

Many definitions have been given to the term *delirium*, some of which include all varieties of acute, organic behavioral disorders. The DSM-III diagnostic criteria for this disorder are more restrictive and therefore allow for a clearer distinction from other OBSs. The essential feature of delirium as defined in the DSM-III (APA, 1980) is a clouded state of consciousness manifested by a reduced capacity to sustain attention. At least two of the following must also be present: perceptual disturbance, incoherent speech, disturbance in the sleep–wakefulness cycle, and increased or decreased psychomotor activity. The perceptual disturbances may include hallucinations, delusions, or illusions. Other associated clinical features include disorientation, memory impairment, disordered cognition, frequent emotional disturbances, and occasional neurological signs. These emotional features may consist of anxiety, fear, depression, or anger, and the neurological signs may include tremor, asterixis, multifocal myoclonus, or generalized seizures. Signs of autonomic nervous system overactivity may also be seen in the more severe cases, such as tachycardia, tachypnea, hypertension, diaphoresis, flushing, and pupillary dilatation.

Patients' diagnosis may not always be immediately obvious if their affective changes, psychotic symptoms, or inappropriate behavior is initially more prominent than their cognitive impairment and medical problems. In that situation, patients may be misdiagnosed as schizophrenic, manic, or depressed on the basis of the most prominent behavioral symptoms, particularly if they have a history of prior psychiatric disorder. Dementia must also be ruled out. Delirium is distinguished from these other disorders by rapid onset, fluctuating course, clouding of consciousness, signs of autonomic hyperactivity, and generalized slowing shown EEG. In addition, delirium involves a clouding of consciousness rather than the global cognitive impairment in a normal state of consciousness that occurs in dementia.

The distinctiveness of the course of the illness in delirium should help the outpatient practitioner to distinguish it from other medical or mental disorders. The onset is brief, varying from almost instantaneous (as following stroke or head trauma) to a few days. Brief prodromal symptoms may include sleep disturbance, irritability, poor appetite, tremulousness, difficulty in concentrating, restlessness, hypersomnolence, and nightmares. The symptoms of delirium exhibit a fluctuating course. These symptoms are often worse after sundown, presumably because of decreased sensory input and fatigue. Lucid intervals may occur, during which the patient's symptoms seem transiently to resolve. The duration of the disorder is usually a few days, but in rare cases, it may last for weeks or longer. Recovery is usually complete if the syndrome is recognized and appropriately treated.

The pathogenesis and pathophysiology of delirium is incompletely understood. It has been suggested that the occurrence of hallucinations in delirium may represent an intrusion of dreams into wakeful awareness. Other proposed explanations of the hallucinations in delirium involve a reduction in cerebral oxidative metabolism, serotonin imbalance, inhibition of the cholinergic system, reduced or excessive cortical activation, or abnormal stimulation or disinhibition of the temporal lobes (Lipowski, 1985).

Few data are available on the incidence of delirium in psychiatric outpatients. Hall *et al.* (1978) found an incidence of delirium (which they called "organic brain disorder") of approximately 1%. This 1% consisted of 6 patients out of 658 consecutive psychiatric outpatients. The medical causes of delirium in these patients included pneumonia, carcinoma, liver dysfunction, congestive heart failure, emphysema, anemia, and pancreatitis. However, one would suspect that any medical disorder that may cause delirium in inpatients may also do so in outpatients. A list of these disorders may be found in Table 1. In this author's experience, the most common causes of delirium in psychiatric outpatients are an excessive dosage of psychotropic or other medication (through central anticholinergic mechanisms) and adverse interactions between medications. Patient groups at higher risk include the elderly, patients with significant medical problems (particularly cerebral and endocrine abnormalities), patients on high doses of antidepressant or neuroleptic medication, and patients on multiple medications.

The evaluation of an outpatient who clinically exhibits delirium should generally involve immediate hospitalization. Only the mildest cases may be treated entirely on an outpatient basis, when medical complications and suicidal ideations are absent, and when a strong support network is available. Laboratory tests to identify the cause of the delirium should always include a complete blood count with differential, a urinalysis, and blood chemistries such as sodium, potassium, chloride, bicarbonate, glucose, calcium, magnesium, liver enzymes, and blood urea nitrogen. Other tests that are often done include an electroencephalogram; a urine or blood drug screen; blood levels of antidepressant, neuroleptic, anticonvulsant, or other medications; an electrocardiogram; a chest X ray; and blood tests for syphilis. Further tests that are needed for some patients are a blood alcohol

Table 1. *Reported Medical Etiologies of Delirium*[a]

1. Intoxication by drugs and poisons
   a. Drugs: anticholinergic agents, sedative-hypnotics, digitalis derivatives, opiates, corticosteroids, salicylates, antibiotics, anticonvulsants, antiarrhythmic and antihypertensive drugs, antineoplastic agents, cimetidine, lithium anti-parkinsonian agents, disulfiram, indomethacin, bismuth salts, phencyclidine
   b. Alcohol: ethyl and methyl
   c. Addictive inhalants: gasoline, glue, ether, nitrous oxide, nitrites
   d. Industrial poisons: carbon disulphide, organic solvents, methyl chloride and bromide, heavy metals, organophosphorus insecticides, carbon monoxide
   e. Snakebite
   f. Poisonous plants and mushrooms
2. Withdrawal syndromes
   a. Alcohol: delirium tremens
   b. Sedatives and hypnotics: barbiturates, chloral hydrate, chlordiazepoxide, diazepam, ethchlorvynol, glutethimide, meprobamate, methyprylon, paraldehyde
   c. Amphetamines
3. Nutritional, hormonal, and metabolic disorders
   a. Hypoxia
   b. Hypoglycemia
   c. Hepatic, renal, pancreatic, and pulmonary insufficiency (encephalopathy)
   d. Avitaminosis: nicotinic acid, thiamine, cyanocobalamine (vitamin B_{12}), folate
   e. Hypervitaminosis: intoxication by vitamins A and D
   f. Hormonal disorders: hyperinsulinism, hyperthyroidism, hypothyroidism, hypopituitarism, Addison's disease, Cushing's syndrome, hypoparathyroidism, hyperparathyroidism
   g. Disorders or fluid and electrolyte metabolism
      i. Dehydration, water intoxication
      ii. Alkalosis, acidosis
      iii. Hypernatremia, hyponatremia, hyperkalemia, hypokalemia, hypercalcemia, hypocalcemia, hypermagnesemia, hypomagnesemia
   h. Errors of metabolism
      i. Porphyria
      ii. Carcinoid syndrome
      iii. Hepatolenticular degeneration (Wilson's disease)
4. Infections
   a. Systemic: pneumonia, typhoid, typhus, acute rheumatic fever, malaria, influenza, mumps, diphtheria, brucellosis, infectious mononucleosis, infectious hepatitus, malaria, subacute bacterial endocarditis, bactremia, septicemia, Rocky Mountain spotted fever, legionnaires' disease
   b. Intracranial: acute, subacute, and chronic
      i. Viral encephalitis; aseptic meningitis; rabies
      ii. Bacterial meningitis—meningococcal, pneumococcal, *Hemophilus influenzae,* etc.
      iii. Postinfectious and postvaccinial encephalomyelitis
      iv. Tuberculous meningitis
      v. Neurosyphilis
      vi. Fungal infections: cryptococcosis, coccidioidomycosis, histoplasmosis, moniliasis, mucormycosis
      vii. Protozoal infections: toxoplasma encephalitis, cerebral malaria
      viii. Trichinosis

5. Head trauma: concussion, contusion
6. Epilepsy: ictal and postictal automatism
7. Vascular disorders
    a. Cerebrovascular disorders
        i. Transient ischemic attacks
        ii. Hypertensive encephalopathy
        iii. Thrombosis, embolism
        iv. Polyarteritis nodosa
        v. Systemic lupus erythematosus
        vi. Rheumatoid vasculitis
        vii. Temporal arteritis
        viii. Subarachnoid hemorrhage
        ix. Wegener's granulomatosis
        x. Neuro-Behcet's disease
        xi. Pulseless disease
    b. Cardiovascular disorders
        i. Myocardial infarction
        ii. Congestive heart failure
        iii. Cardiac arrhythmias
    c. Migraine
8. Intracranial space-occupying lesions
    a. Tumor
    b. Abscess
    c. Subdural hematoma
    d. Aneurysm
    e. Parasitic cyst
9. Cerebral degenerative disorders
    a. Multiple sclerosis
    b. Alzheimer's disease and senile dementia
10. Extracranial neoplasm, e.g., bronchogenic carcinoma
11. Disorders of the hematopoietic system
    a. Pernicious anemia
    b. Erythremia
    c. Thrombotic thrombocytopenic purpura
12. Injury by physical agents
    a. Heatstroke
    b. Radiation
    c. Electrocution
13. Disorders due to hypersensitivity
    a. Serum sickness
    b. Food allergy

[a]From Z. J. Lipowski, *Delirium,* pp. 110–111, 1980. Courtesy of Charles C Thomas, Publisher, Springfield, Illinois.

level; thyroid function tests (including thyroid-stimulating-hormone level); a lumbar puncture for opening and closing pressure, cell count, and glucose, protein, culture, serology, and protein electrophoresis; a head CT scan; arterial blood gases; a heavy-metal screen; cortisol levels; vitamin B_{12} and folate levels; skull X rays; brain scans; Holter monitoring; sedimentation rate; urinary porphobilinogen and delta-aminolevulinic acid; and serum protein electrophoresis.

Treatment Applications

The treatment of patients with delirium involves appropriate medical care and psychological measures coupled with pharmacotherapy as needed. A cardinal rule in the treatment of delirium is to treat the underlying medical problem. Additional supportive medical care should be provided as needed, such as intravenous fluid and electrolytes.

A variety of psychological measures are important in the treatment of delirium. The delirious patient should be carefully evaluated for suicidal ideations and should be observed closely by the nursing staff. Constant nursing observation is necessary for delirious patients who are suicidal, agitated, or psychotic. Repeated reassurance should be provided, and the patient should be frequently and tactfully reoriented. A calendar and a clock in the patient's room will also aid in this reorientation. Every procedure should be patiently explained, including such basic procedures as taking the patient's vital signs. The patient's room should be well lighted without being overly bright. A night light is often helpful after sundown. The patient's room should be relatively quiet, and the same staff should attend him or her as much as possible. The presence of family members is often reassuring to the patient. The family should be reassured that the patient's unusual behavior is not willful but is a symptom of his or her delirium. If these measures are followed and psychotropic medication is used appropriately, physical restraint only rarely becomes necessary (Detre & Jarecki, 1971).

Pharmacotherapy is often useful in the treatment of delirium. However, psychotropic medications may mask organic signs or may cause side effects of their own, such as seizures or hypotension. Consequently, sedative medications should not be used unless clear target symptoms, such as agitation or psychosis, are present. Also, the dosage of sedative medication should be the lowest amount necessary to adequately control the patient's symptoms.

The antipsychotic haloperidol is frequently the drug of choice in the treatment of delirium because of its therapeutic effectiveness, its relative lack of side effects, and its relative lack of interactions with other medications (Ayd, 1978; Heller, 1976; Kiely, 1976; Moore, 1977). Specifically, haloperidol has been shown to be an effective treatment for the agitation, hallucinations, and delusions associated with delirium (Ayd, 1978; Heller, 1976; Moore, 1977). This medication generally does not cause adverse cardiovascular effects except for occasional mild hypotension (Ayd, 1978). The incidence of severe, potentially life-threatening hypotension is substantially lower with haloperidol than with chlorpromazine (Man & Chen, 1973). Also, it rarely produces electrocardiographic changes, unlike many phenothiazines (Ayd, 1978). Haloperidol has only mild anticholinergic side effects and minimal sedative effects, and its extrapyramidal side effects are easily treatable with medications such as benztropine mesylate (Baldessarini, 1980). Interactions with other medications are infrequent and seldom serious. One such drug–drug interaction involves the use of haloperidol and lithium, in which CNS neurotoxicity or severe extrapyramidal reactions may occur. Haloperidol also blocks the antihypertensive effects of guanethidine (Ayd, 1978), although this interaction would not be a major concern in an emergency situation.

The dosage of haloperidol used in treating delirium depends on the patient's age, medical health, level of agitation, and history of previous use of neuroleptics. One of the most common dosage strategies involves giving 5 mg/hr intramuscularly or by mouth as needed (Man & Chen, 1973; Moore, 1977). The intramuscular route has a more rapid onset, which is useful in the more agitated patient (Moore, 1977). Geriatric patients usually require smaller doses, in the range of 0.5–3 mg. Patients with chronic psychiatric disorders such as schizophrenia and with a history of previous use of neuroleptics may require somewhat higher doses than the standard. The total daily dose required to achieve symptomatic control is usually no more than 30 mg (Moore, 1977).

Haloperidol is not the treatment of choice for certain groups of patients with delirium. For example, a delirium associated with a withdrawal syndrome is more appropriately treated with a benzodiazepine (Heller, 1976; Thompson, Johnson & Maddey, 1975). Also, some practitioners prefer chlorpromazine to haloperidol in severely agitated patients who do not exhibit sedation, hypotension, or other cardiovascular abnormalities (Heller, 1976). Benzodiazepines are reportedly preferable to haloperidol in the treatment of delirium associated with hepatic encephalopathy because of the stupor and EEG slowing reported with neuroleptics (Editorial, 1977). Finally, haloperidol is generally avoided in the treatment of anticholinergic delirium because of its own anticholinergic effects.

AMNESTIC SYNDROME

Specific Diagnostic Considerations

Amnestic syndrome is defined as a deficit in short-term and long-term memory occurring in an unclouded state of consciousness. Immediate recall, such as the ability to repeat a series of numbers, is intact in this syndrome. Memories of the recent past are generally more severely impaired than those of the remote past. The patient's short-term memory impairment often results in disorientation. Confabulation, which is a fabricated account of events, is present in most cases but tends to decrease over time. The diagnosis of this disorder also requires that the level of consciousness and general intellectual capacity remain intact in order to differentiate an amnestic syndrome from delirium and dementia, respectively.

The course of amnestic syndrome varies according to the etiology. The course of alcohol amnestic disorder, also called *Korsakoff's psychosis*, is used here as an example of an amnestic syndrome, as alcohol-related thiamine deficiency is by far the most common etiology of this syndrome in outpatients. The discussion of the course of alcohol amnestic disorder starts with a description of Wernicke's disease, as these two disorders are not separate diseases but different stages in the same disease process, with Werniche's disease coming first (Malamud & Skillicorn, 1956; Victor, Adams, & Collins, 1971). Werniche's disease displays a triad of clinical features, including confusion, ophthalmological abnormalities, and ataxia. The ophthalmological abnormalities are the most distinctive diagnostic features. These ophthalmological findings include ophthalmoplegia (particularly palsy of the lateral rectus muscle, resulting in double vision), horizontal and vertical nystagmus, and diminished conjugate gaze. Other common clinical features include orthostatic hypotension, tachycardia, dyspnea on exertion, minor EKG abnormalities, slowing on the EEG, peripheral neuropathies, and malnutrition. Death results in 15%–20% of acutely hospitalized patients with this syndrome. The most common cause of death in Werniche's disease are infection and hepatic failure, though sudden death via cardiovascular mechanisms may also occur.

Following thiamine administration, the first clinical abnormalities to show improvement are the ocular palsies, which may occur within hours. Confusion and ataxia resolve more slowly (usually over a matter of days to months) and incompletely. A memory deficit is noted more clearly as the patient's confusion clears. This memory deficit is the alcohol amnestic disorder. In some patients with Werniche's disease who do not exhibit much confusion, alcohol amnestic disorder may be prevented by early recognition of the condition and treatment with large doses of thiamine. However, once Korsakoff's syndrome has become apparent, complete recovery of memory occurs in only 20% of patients. Slow, incomplete resolution of symptoms is noted in the others. Chronic hospitalization is necessary in the most severely affected individuals (Adams & Victor, 1985; Victor & Adams, 1983), although many individuals with milder impairments can now be managed in community settings provided that they can abstain from further alcohol use.

Amnestic syndrome may result from any pathological process that affects certain medial-temporal-lobe and diencephalic structures, including the mammillary bodies, the paraventricular regions of the thalamus and the hypothalamus, the floor of the fourth ventricle, the superior vermis of the cerebellum, and the periaqueductal region of the midbrain. Alcohol-related thiamine deficiency is the most common reason for this kind of cerebral pathology. However, a number of other etiologies may be associated with this syndrome, including cerebral anoxia, head trauma, epilepsy, infarction in the distribution of the posterior cerebral artery, electroconvulsive treatment, herpes simplex encephalitis, infiltrating tumors or granulomas, vascular lesions, and bilateral medial-temporal surgical excisions. The amnestic syndrome may also be seen early in the course of dementia, Alzheimer type, though generally not as the only cognitive deficit (Whitty & Zangwill, 1966).

After the initial diagnosis of an amnestic disorder or Werniche's disease is made in the outpatient setting, further evaluation on an inpatient unit is warranted. For patients with suspected amnestic disorder, close inpatient observation is useful to confirm the diagnosis and to rule out delirium and dementia. An EEG and a CT scan are generally warranted. Neuropsychological testing of some patients may be warranted once their clinical status has stabilized in order to quantitate memory impairment and other cognitive deficits.

Treatment Applications

The treatment of amnestic syndrome depends on its etiology. The treatment of alcohol-related amnesia is discussed here in detail, because it is the most common etiology. For the best results, treatment with thiamine should begin at the first sign of Werniche's disease, before cognitive symptoms become prominent. Such prompt treatment will help to minimize subsequent long-term amnesia. A standard thiamine regimen for Werniche's disease is 50 mg intravenously, with an additional 50 mg intramuscularly or orally for five days or until a normal diet is resumed (Adams & Victor, 1985). Alcoholic patients are often treated with thiamine prophylactically whenever they enter a hospital, even though they are not demonstrating memory loss or symptoms of Werniche's disease. In that situation, the patients may receive 50 mg by mouth for 5 days. Patients with chronic amnestic disorder are often treated with a multivitamin tablet and a well-balanced, nutritious diet. Acute treatment of dehydration, electrolyte abnormalities, or infection are also necessary in some cases. Sedative medication is occasionally needed. Treatment with digitalis preparations should occur if alcohol-related cardiac failure ensues.

Individual outpatient psychotherapy is important in the management of amnestic syndrome. Insight-oriented psychotherapy is not of benefit in treating the amnesia. However, supportive therapy plays an important role in the treatment of anger, depression, suspiciousness, and worthlessness, which may occur as a reaction to the patient's amnesia. Supportive therapy may minimize the tendency for the patient's anger to be displaced onto his or her caregiver, who may unintentionally serve as a frequent reminder of the patient's dependency and decreased functioning. Behavior therapy, in conjunction with family members, may also be necessary in some cases to control the negativism and acting out that sometimes accompany the patient's anger and sadness. An example of this type of behavior therapy technique is to have the caregiver (e.g., the spouse) ignore the patient's tantrums and to reward his or her appropriate behavior with undivided attention and verbal praise.

The outpatient psychotherapy of amnestic syndrome should focus on the patient's family as well as on the patient. Family members often feel sadness and anger in response to the patient's disorder. They may experience guilt for having failed the patient, for being angry with the patient, or for wishing for the patient's early demise. They may initially have unrealistically high expectations of the patient, which may be followed by disappointment and then unrealistically low expectations. The primary caregiver (often the spouse) is especially apt to feel exhausted, overwhelmed, socially isolated, and abandoned by the extended family. The spouse may also be verbally abused by the patient because of the frustration resulting from memory loss and dependence.

There are several goals for family therapy to help family members deal with the patient's amnestic syndrome. The therapy should help family members to readjust their expectations of the patient. It should provide management advice and remind family members of their own needs. It should provide a catharsis for the family's sadness, anger, and guilt and should show family members their own limitations in being able to help the patient. Also, it should help family members work through their divided loyalties to the patient, to the children, and to their own social lives (Lezak, 1978).

A variety of other interventions and other therapies are sometimes appropriate for the management of amnestic syndrome. For example, marital counseling, mutual support groups, or rehabilitation and vocational counseling may be appropriate. Referrals to psychiatrists, internists, or other medical specialists are often indicated. Visiting nurses may be helpful in dealing with psychiatric and medical problems. Social workers may be indicated to assist in obtaining day care, financial assistance, and placement services. Also, the assistance lawyers and financial counselors may be appropriate (Lezak, 1978).

ORGANIC DELUSIONAL SYNDROME

Specific Diagnostic Considerations

Organic delusional syndrome is distinguished by the presence of delusions that are attributed to some specific organic factor in a patient with a normal state of consciousness. This diagnosis is not made in the presence of a clouded sensorium, as in delirium, or in the presence of significant generalized intellectual dysfunction, as in dementia.

There are four types of organic delusions: simple persecutory delusions, complex persecutory delusions, grandiose delusions, and delusions associated with neurological impairments. Organic delusions are most commonly persecutory in nature. The complex persecutory delusions include the Schneiderian first-rank symptoms, the Capgras syndrome, the Fregoli syndrome, the intermetamorphosis syndrome, delusional jealousy, delusions of infestation, werewolfism, heutoscopy, and erotomania. Delusions associated with neurological deficits may include denial of blindness, denial of hemiparesis, reduplication of body, and reduplicative paramnesia (Cummings, 1985).

A wide range of clinical features may be associated with organic delusional syndrome, including cognitive, affective, and bizarre behavioral symptoms. One of the more common syndromes in which organic delusions play a major role appears in the so-called schizophrenialike illnesses. In these disorders, organic delusions are associated with hallucinations and other clinical features. The schizophrenialike illnesses are often chronic disorders associated with medical disorders such as epilepsy or brain trauma (Davison, 1983). Much speculation and controversy have arisen concerning the relationship of these schizophrenialike psychoses and "functional" schizophrenia. For example, one topic of debate has been whether the symptoms of organic schizophrenialike psychoses differ from

Table 2. Reported Medical Etiologies of Organic Delusional Syndrome[a]

1. Systemic illness: uremia, dialysis dementia, hepatic encephalopathy, pancreatic encephalopathy, hyponatremia, prophyria, hypercalcemia, hypoglycemia
2. Endocrinopathies: Addison's disease, Cushing's disease, hypothyroidism, hyperthyroidism, hypoparathyroidism, hyperparathyroidism, panhypopituitarism
3. Deficiency states: Wernicke-Korsakoff syndrome, vitamin B_{12}, folate, niacin
4. Inflammatory disorders: systemic lupus erythematosus, temporal arteritis
5. Drug intoxication: anti-Parkinsonian drugs, antituberculous drugs, antimalarials, anticonvulsants, anticholinergics, antidepressants, antihypertensive drugs, hallucinogens
6. Miscellaneous drugs: amphetamines, cimetidine, disulfiram, corticosteroids, benzodiazepines, digitalis, pentazocine, bromide
7. Metal toxicity: mercury, arsenic, manganese, thallium
8. Extrapyramidal disturbances: idopathic Parkinson's disease, postencephalitic Parkinson's disease, Huntington's disease, Sydenham's chorea, Wilson's disease, spinocerebellar degenerations, idiopathic basal ganglia calcification, carbon monoxide poisoning
9. CNS infections: herpes encephalitis, other acute viral encephalitides, Jakob-Creutzfeldt disease, cerebral malaria, syphilis, trypanosomiasis
10. Diseases affecting myelin: multiple sclerosis, metachromatic leukodystrophy, adrenoleukodystrophy, Marchiafava-Bignami disease
11. Miscellaneous: hydrocephalus, temporal lobe epilepsy, posttraumatic encephalopathy, neoplasma (temporal lobe, deep hemispheric), cerebrovascular disease, Alzheimer's disease, Pick's disease, cerebral anoxia, phenylketonuria

[a]Courtesy of Jeffrey L. Cummings (1985). "Organic Delusions." *British Journal of Psychiatry, 146*, 185.

the symptoms of "functional" schizophrenia. It has been reported that these disorders differ from schizophrenia in that they display a preservation of affect, a relative lack of thought disorder, a lack of family history of schizophrenia, and an older age of onset (63.7 years) (Cummings, 1985; Davison, 1983; Davison & Bagley, 1969).

The course of organic delusional syndromes may show considerable variation, depending on the medical etiology. For example, most cases of amphetamine delusional disorder resolve within a week, whereas the prognosis for recovery from chronic interictal psychosis is poor (Davison & Bagley, 1969). The organic delusions sometimes respond to treatment of the underlying medical problem, but many such psychoses follow a course independent of the medical disorder (Davison, 1983).

The major medical disorders resulting in organic delusional disorder are listed in Table 2. The most common medical etiologies involve abuse of substances such as amphetamine and amphetaminelike drugs, hallucinogens, and cannabis. Some such amphetaminelike drugs may be bought without a prescription in the form of diet capsules, cough syrups, and nasal sprays, despite the psychotic symptoms and dangerous behavior that sometimes result (Cornelius, Soloff, & Reynolds, 1984).

The pathology in this disorder has been reported to frequently involve the temporal lobe and the diencephalon of the brain (Davison, 1983). However, the pathophysiology of these abnormalities is poorly understood.

Treatment Applications

The therapy for organic delusional disorders involves both the treatment of the underlying medical disorder and the symptomatic treatment of the accompanying behavioral symptoms. This two-factor therapeutic approach is necessary because many such organic psychoses do not respond adequately to treatment of the underlying medical condition. A common method of treating the patient's psychotic symptoms involves the use of antipsychotic medications (Davison, 1983; Davison & Bagley, 1969). The dose of antipsychotic medication used in the outpatient treatment of organic delusional disorders is usually smaller than the dose used in treating schizophrenia, and the length of treatment is also generally shorter. As the patient's delusions decrease, she or he often develops concerns about the reasons for the psychotic symptoms, accompanied by fear of relapse and embarrassment over her or his previous condition. Supportive therapy is indicated to assist the patient in dealing with these concerns.

ORGANIC HALLUCINOSIS

Specific Diagnostic Considerations

Organic hallucinosis is a mental disorder in which persistent or recurrent hallucinations that are attributable to some specific organic factor occur in an individual with an unclouded sensorium (APA, 1980). This diagnosis is not made if a significant loss of intellectual capacities has occurred or if the predominant symptom complex involves a mood disturbance or delusions. Hallucinations may occur in any sensory modality but are most commonly visual, auditory, and tactile. The type of hallucination depends primarily on the underlying medical etiology.

Hallucinogen-related and alcohol-related hallucinations are described here in detail, as these are the two most common etiologies of organic hallucinosis seen in outpatient practice. Hallucinogen-induced hallucinations are primarily visual. They may vary in form, color, and movement. The form may appear as random blobs or simple designs such as lines, webs, checkerboards, spirals, or kaleidoscopes. Complex patterns may also occur, such as people, animals, or landscapes. These forms may occur in a wide variety of colors and may show different kinds of movement. Changes may occur from one visual image to another, or distortions may occur within an image. Images may also combine, duplicate themselves, or overlay other images. They may occur singly or in groups or panoramas and may appear enlarged or shrunken (Siegel & Jarvik, 1975). Occasionally, synesthesias occur, in which stimuli from one sensory modality produce sensations in another modality, such as colors being heard. These symptoms are sensitive to the expectations of the patient before drug use and to the patient's immediate surroundings.

Alcoholic hallucinosis differs from hallucinogen-induced hallucinosis in that the hallucinations are primarily auditory rather than visual. These alcoholic hallucinations commonly consist of human voices, which are often threatening or disturbing to the patient. Hallucinosis usually develops within 48 hours after cessation of drinking. The hallucinations may be more prominent at night. They generally last for hours or days but occasionally may last for weeks or months. These auditory hallucinations are sometimes accompanied by other types of hallucinations, especially visual hallucinations.

A variety of etiologies other than hallucinogens and alcohol may also cause different types of hallucinations. For example, occipital lobe tumors may be associated with visual hallucinations, and temporal lobe tumors may be associated with auditory, visual, or olfactory hallucinations. Migraine headaches may be associated with simple visual hallucinations, though sometimes complex visual hallucinations or auditory hallucinations may occur. Seizures are sometimes associated with hallucinations, the type of hallucination being determined by the location of the seizure focus. Amphetamine and similar sympathomimetic drugs may cause visual and auditory hallucinations accompanied by paranoid ideations in a clinical picture that may be indistinguishable from paranoid schizophrenia. Other medical conditions that are sometimes associated with hallucinations include neurosyphilis, porphyria, Huntington's chorea, systemic lupus erythematosus, narcolepsy, encephalitis, pernicious anemia, and a variety of endocrine disorders (Cornelius, Soloff, & Miewald, 1986; Lishman, 1978).

A variety of symptoms may accompany the patient's hallucinations. Additional behavior features may include delusions, fear, anxiety, dysphoria, derealization, depersonalization, illusions, or euphoria. A variety of physical symptoms may also accompany the hallucinations, including tachycardia, tachypnea, diaphoresis, palpitations, pupillary dilation, tremor, hyperreflexia, blurred vision, piloerection, incoordination, and hyperthermia. The patient may or may not have insight into the fact that the hallucinations are not real. If little insight is present, the patient is more likely to react physically to the hallucinations, usually by trying to flee.

The course of the organic hallucinosis depends on the underlying medical disorder. Alcoholic hallucinosis generally resolves in hours or days but may occasionally continue for weeks or months. Hallucinogen hallucinosis often lasts for hours or days but may sometimes last longer. Untreated seizures, brain tumors, syphilis, cataracts, or otosclerosis may cause a chronic hallucinosis. Flashbacks may also occur following hallucinogen hallucinosis; these consist of brief hallucinations weeks or even years after drug use. Such flashbacks usually decrease in frequency over time. They are more likely to occur if cannabis or other substance use continues.

The pathogenesis of organic hallucinosis is poorly understood. It has been suggested that these hallucinoses result from sensory deprivation in some patients. This hypothesis may explain hallucinations associated with blindness or deafness. Alternatively, hallucinations may result from the general arousal or stimulation of specific cerebral sites (DeVaul & Hall, 1980; Hartmann, 1975). A variety of biochemical mechanisms have been postulated to explain these mechanisms, involving substances such as endogenous opiates, dopamine, and serotonin. However, little proof is available to support any of these hypotheses.

The medical evaluation of patients with organic hallucinosis varies with the presenting medical complaints. Hospitalization is generally warranted. Some of the more common diagnostic tests include urine or blood drug screens, a CT scan, an electroencephalogram, and a lumbar puncture, in addition to the standard admission blood work.

Treatment Applications

The therapy for non-substance-related organic hallucinosis involves both the treatment of the underlying medical disorder and the symptomatic treatment of the accompanying behavioral symptoms. This two-factor approach to therapy is similar to that used in the treatment of patients with organic delusional syndrome. This approach is often necessary because organic psychoses do not necessarily respond to treatment of the associated medical problem. Antipsychotic medications are a common method of acutely treating many types of these organic hallucinoses (Davison, 1983; Davison & Bagley, 1969); the strategy used is the one discussed earlier for the delusional syndrome. The specific details of treatment of these disorders depend on the underlying medical condition.

The treatment for substance-related organic hallucinosis differs somewhat from that for other organic hallucinoses. For example, the psychotic symptoms often resolve spontaneously fairly quickly, so antipsychotic medication may not be necessary, and supportive measures may be sufficient. The specific details of the pharmacological treatment of these substance-related hallucinoses depends on the specific substance involved. For example, haloperidol in moderate doses has been suggested for treating amphetamine psychoses, and diazepam or haloperidol has been suggested for the treatment of hallucinogen hallucinosis (Ellinwood, 1976; Strassman, 1984). Marijuana psychosis has been treated with either neuroleptics, such as chlorpromazine (25–50 mg intramuscularly every hour as needed), or with oral dosages of minor tranquilizers, such as diazepam (20 mg followed by 10 mg doses every hour as needed) (Talbott, 1976). Finally, phencyclidine (PCP) psychosis is generally treated with haloperidol or minor tranquilizers rather than with phenothiazines because phenothiazines have not been shown to speed recovery and because they may produce severe, prolonged hypotension in PCP patients (Burns & Lerner, 1976). The nonpharmacological treatment of these disorders is similar to the treatment of delirium, as discussed earlier in this chapter, with an emphasis on diminishing stimulation and on reorientation, reassurance and close supervision.

ORGANIC PERSONALITY SYNDROME

Specific Diagnostic Considerations

The organic personality syndrome is defined by the DSM-III (APA, 1980) as a marked change of personality caused by a specific organic factor. Such personality changes may include emotional lability, impulsivity, apathy, and suspiciousness. These symptoms must occur in an unclouded sensorium, and evidence of a specific causative organic factor must be demonstrated from the history, a physical examination, or laboratory tests.

A variety of pathological behavior patterns are associated with organic personality syndrome, which are determined primarily by the location and nature of the abnormality. The frontal lobe syndrome is one of the most common examples of this disorder. The frontal lobe syndrome is characterized by impulsivity, emotional lability, inattentiveness, impersistence, poor social judgment, inappropriate jocularity, irritability, apathy, and a lack of initiative and spontaneity. The symptoms are more pronounced with large cerebral lesions than with small lesions. Bilateral cerebral lesions result in substantially more behavioral abnormalities than unilateral abnormalities. The prefrontal areas of the frontal lobe are particularly associated with these symptoms. A variety of etiological factors may cause frontal lobe damage and thus produce the above-mentioned symptoms.

Common medical etiologies of the organic personality syndrome include vascular disease, head trauma, and neoplasms. Subarachnoid hemorrhage is a common example of a vascular disease that may lead to organic personality syndrome. The most common personality change following subarachnoid hemorrhage is an increase in irritability and anxiety, as well as the loss of vitality associated with brain damage at any site (Storey, 1970). Professional boxers provide an example of organic personality syndrome caused by head trauma. Some boxers reportedly suffer diffuse brain damage, which is associated with "explosive" personality, morbid jealousy, occasional psychosis, and a chronic amnestic state (Johnson, 1969). Finally, ventromedial hypothalamic cancer provides an uncommon example of organic personality syndrome resulting from a neoplasm. Such neoplasms have been associated with aggressiveness, hyperphagia, and eventual dementia (Reeves & Plum, 1969).

There are a number of less common medical etiologies of organic personality syndrome. These include multiple sclerosis, Wilson's disease, neurosyphilis, endocrine disorders, encephalitis lethargica, neurosyphilis, Huntington's chorea, arteritis, mercury and manganese poisoning, and chronic substance intoxication, such as with amphetamine or LSD (Lishman, 1978).

The course and pathophysiology of organic personality disorder depend on the location and nature of the pathology. The evaluation of this disorder varies widely according to the patient's psychiatric and medical history and physical findings. Tests that are commonly used for this disorder include an EEG and a CT scan, among others. Evaluation and treatment may or may not necessitate hospitalization.

Treatment Applications

Whenever possible, the management of organic personality syndrome should involve treatment of the underlying medical disorder. Psychotropic medication may be appropriate for some patients. For example, neuroleptic medication may help control agitation. However, the effectiveness of these medications is unclear. Psychotherapy has also been used with some patients, but its effectiveness has not been sufficiently documented. The counseling of family members may facilitate their adjustment and their care of the patient (Lezak, 1978). The use of visiting nurses, rehabilitation, and other community services is often helpful. Further suggestions for nonpharmacological outpatient management are similar to those for the treatment of amnestic syndrome, as described earlier in this chapter.

Specific Diagnostic Considerations

This discussion of organic affective syndrome is divided into a section on organic mania and a section on organic depression. This division of the organic affective syndrome is in keeping with the nomenclature suggested in the *DSM-III-R In Development* (APA, 1985). This division allows for greater diagnostic precision than the DSM-III system (APA, 1980), which does not have separate diagnoses for organic mania and organic depression.

Organic affective disorder, manic type, may be defined as a manic episode due to an organic dysfunction. The psychological criteria for an organic manic episode are the same as the DSM-III criteria for a functional manic episode. A specific organic etiological factor must also be demonstrated by history, physical examination, or laboratory tests. The exclusionary criteria for this diagnosis include substantial intellectual impairment, a clouded sensorium, persistent hallucinations, and predominant delusions (APA, 1980). It has been suggested that an additional exclusionary criterion should be any clear past history of affective disorder (Krauthammer & Klerman, 1978).

Several criteria differentiate organic mania from functional mania and thus support the validity of organic mania as a distinct nosological entity. The first such factor is the presence of a specific organic insult in relatively close temporal proximity to the subsequent mania. The second factor is a negative family history for affective illness. The third factor is a later age of onset of organic mania (median age of 41 versus 25 in functional mania). The fourth factor is a negative past history for affective illness (Cummings & Mendez, 1984; Krauthammer & Klerman, 1978).

The course of organic mania is variable and is partially dependent on the underlying medical disorder. Treatment of the medical disorder often, but not always, leads to an improvement in the patient's manic symptoms. The pathophysiology explaining these variations in clinical course is poorly understood.

Table 3. Reported Medical Etiologies of Organic Affective Disorder, Manic[a]

1.	Drugs: corticosteroids, isoniazid, procarbazine, levodopa, bromide, procyclidine, phencyclidine
2.	Metabolic disturbance: hemodialysis, postoperative state, Grave's disease
3.	Infection: influenza, Q fever, post–St. Louis Type A encephalitis, neurosyphilis, AIDS, herpes simplex encephalitis
4.	Neoplasm: meningioma (parasagittal, medial frontoparietal, or right intraventricular), oat cell carcinoma (paraneoplastic encephalopathy), diencephalic glioma, suprasellar diencephalic tumor, benign spenooccipital tumor, subtemporal bone tumor, right temporoparietal-occipital metastases, hypothalamic teratoma, hypothalamic craniopharyngioma, brain-stem neoplasm, suprasellar neoplasm
5.	Epilepsy: right temporal focus
6.	Miscellaneous: hemidecortication, thalamotomy, hypothalamic surgical traction, temporal lobe trauma, temporal lobe hemorrhage, left- or right-hemisphere infarction, multiple sclerosis, Pick's disease

[a]Courtesy of Charles Krauthammer, and Gerald L. Klerman (1978). "Secondary Mania" (an updated version), *Archives of General Psychiatry, 35*, 1335.

A variety of medical disorders may result in organic manias. These disorders include brain neoplasms, cranial trauma, cerebral hemorrhage or infarction, epilepsy, infection, metabolic disturbance, neurosyphilis, Grave's disease, extrapyramidal syndromes, and Pick's disease. A more complete list of medical etiologies is provided in Table 3 (Cummings & Mendez, 1984; Gabel, Barnard, Norko, & O'Connell, 1986; Kermani, Borod, Brown, & Tunnell, 1985; Krauthammer & Klerman, 1978; Mapelli & Bellelli, 1982; Stasiek & Zetin, 1985; Villani & Weitzel, 1979).

The evaluation of the patient's underlying medical disorder should start with a careful history, including recent infections, seizures, neurological deficits, medications, and substance ingestion. In many cases, a reliable history cannot be obtained from the patient, so it is absolutely essential to interview family members or significant others. If at this point an organic affective syndrome is suspected, hospitalization should be considered, depending on the individual circumstances. A physical examination should be performed, focusing especially on focal neurological signs. The tests used to further evaluate the underlying medical disorder vary with the findings from the history and the physical examination. Some of the more common tests are electrolytes, EEG, CT scan, CBC and differential, BUN and creatinine, and toxic screen.

Treatment Applications

Initially, the treatment of organic mania should be directed at its underlying medical cause. However, the manic symptoms do not always resolve as the medical disorder is treated, the medical disorder may not be treatable, and/or the patient may be very agitated. In these clinical situations, a trial of neuroleptics or lithium may be warranted. Lithium should be used with special care in these individuals because of their underlying medical disorders. Specifically, BUN and creatinine levels should not be above the normal range before the institution of lithium, and lithium and electrolyte levels should initially be monitored three times a week. Lithium should be instituted at low doses, such as 300 mg p.o. BID, and may be increased by 300-mg increments once or twice a week. The patient's serum lithium concentration should range between 0.6 and 1.0 mEq/l. The patient's psychiatric and medical condition should be evaluated frequently, and initially, a mental status evaluation should be conducted daily. One would not expect long-term medication to be needed unless the organic mania is secondary to an irreversible medical disorder (Krauthammer & Klerman, 1978; Rosenbaum & Barry, 1975).

ORGANIC AFFECTIVE SYNDROME, DEPRESSED TYPE

Specific Diagnostic Considerations

Organic affective syndrome, depressed type, is defined as a disturbance in mood and behavior resembling a major depressive episode that is attributable to a specific organic factor. This diagnosis is not made in the presence of a clouded sensorium, significant intellectual impairment, persistent or recurrent hallucinations, or predominant delusions, (APA, 1980).

The course of organic depression varies somewhat with the nature and location of the underlying etiology. However, in some cases, the underlying medical disorder may run a course independent of the depressive symptoms once both problems have begun. For example, the depressive syndrome may respond to treatment while the underlying medical disorder cannot be fully treated. On the other hand, the depressive symptoms may persist in some cases after the associated medical disorder has been successfully treated.

Medical etiologies of these so-called organic depressions include antihypertensive medications, various other medications, endocrine disorders, degenerative neurological disorders, other neurological disorders, infectious disorders, metabolic and electrolyte disorders, cancer, immunological disorders, nutritional deficiencies, and sleep disorders. See Table 4 for further details (Anderson, 1979; Cornelius, Payton, & McGonigle, 1985; Hall, 1980b; Lishman, 1978; Whitlock, 1982). Nonorganic depressions that are thought to occur as a psychological reaction to the stress of illness are not included in this diagnostic category.

The pathophysiology of organic affective disorder, depressed, is unclear. However, one might assume that the pathophysiology of this disorder is similar to that of functional major depression. Several biochemical hypotheses have been proposed to explain the pathophysiology of major depression. For example, the biogenic amine theory emphasizes the role of deficiencies of cerebral catecholamines and serotonin. Alternatively, it

Table 4. Reported Medical Etiologies of Organic Affective Syndrome, Depressed

1. Medications and toxins: antihypertensive medications, antipsychotic medications, minor tranquilizers, alcohol, steroids, oral contraceptives, disulfiram, barbiturates, amphetamine withdrawal, cocaine discontinuation, anti-inflammatory medications, digitalis, sulfonamides, bromides, isoniazid, L-dopa, alpha-methyl dopa, ethambutol, cycloserine, lead poisoning, carbon disulfide

2. Endocrine disorders: Cushing's syndrome, hypothyroidism, Addison's disease, hyperthyroidism, hyperparathyroidism, primary hyperaldosteronism (Conn's syndrome), menopause, premenstrual syndrome, postpartum syndrome

3. Degenerative neurological disorders: Parkinsonism, Alzheimer's disease, Huntington's disease, multiple sclerosis, Pick's disease, Jakob-Creutzfeld disease

4. Other neurological disorders: epilepsy, brain tumor, chronic subdural hematoma, cerebral vascular accident, normal-pressure hydrocephalus, Wernicke-Korsakoff's syndrome, postconcussion syndrome

5. Infectious disorders: neurosyphilis, tuberculosis, viral encephalitis, mononucleosis, viral hepatitis, influenza, postencephalitic states, brucellosis, malaria, sarcoidosis, viral pneumonia, subacute bacterial endocarditis

6. Metabolic and electrolyte disorders: hypokalemia, hypocalcemia, hyperkalemia, hypomagnesemia, hyponatremia, increased plasma bicarbonate, decreased plasma bicarbonate, uremia, diabetes mellitus, hepatic disease, Wilson's disease, porphyria, amyloidosis, gout

7. Cancer: brain metastasis, paraneoplastic encephalopathy, pancreatic carcinoma, primary cerebral tumor, leukemias, lymphomas

8. Immunological disorders: systemic lupus erythematosus, rheumatoid arthritis, temporal arteritis, periarteritis nodosa, regional enteritis, ulcerative colitis, psoriasis

9. Nutritional deficiencies: pernicious anemia, severe iron-deficiency anemia, folate deficiency, pyridoxine deficiency, thiamine deficiency, pellagra, protein deficiency, ascorbic acid deficiency

10. Sleep disorders: Kline-Levin-Critchley syndrome, narcolepsy, sleep apnea syndrome

has been suggested that an imbalance between adrenergic and cholinergic activity may affect mood. Others have suggested that dopamine, sodium, calcium, endorphins, or enkephalins may be involved. The exact mechanism is not yet clear (Whitlock, 1982).

The evaluation of the patient with organic depression should start with a careful history, including previous use of medications, neurological deficits, endocrine-related symptoms, recent infections, symptoms of lung or pancreatic cancer, nutritional deficiencies, and symptoms of immunological disorders. If an organic depression is suspected, hospitalization may be warranted. For example, hospitalization is often necessary for patients with significant suicidal or homicidal ideations, for inability to care for oneself, for depression that is refractory to outpatient treatment, or for initiation of medication in patients who are especially sensitive to side effects. The patient's physical examination should focus especially on neurological and endocrine signs. Subsequent tests may include electrolytes, EEG, CT scan, CBC and differential, toxic screen, thyroid function tests and cortisol levels, syphilis screen, and sedimentation rate.

Treatment Applications

The initial management of organic depression involves treatment of the underlying medical disorder when possible. However, the depressive symptoms do not always resolve as the medical disorder is treated, or the patient may be very agitated, or the medical problem may not respond to treatment. In these clinical situations, a trial of antidepressant medication, electroconvulsive therapy (ECT), or psychotherapy may be useful. Antidepressant medication and supportive psychotherapy are often the initial treatment of choice, particularly in patients with prominent sleep and appetite disturbance. Desipramine or nortriptyline is often the initial treatment of choice because these medications are relatively less likely to cause orthostasis, cardiac rhythm disturbances, anticholinergic effects, and sedation. An appropriate initial dose of desipramine is 50 mg p.o. qD, which may then be increased by 25-mg or 50-mg increments on a weekly basis to an eventual dose of approximately 150 mg p.o. qD. Ascertaining the blood levels of the antidepressant may then be helpful to confirm that the antidepressant level is within the therapeutic range. The patient should be seen at least once a week while the medication is being adjusted for an evaluation of clinical effectiveness and side effects. ECT is generally not recommended for the treatment of organic depression on an outpatient basis unless it has been previously successful without serious complications on an inpatient basis. The effectiveness of these different therapies for organic depression has not yet been tested in large double-blind studies. Instead, these recommendations for therapy are based on case reports, personal experience, and inference from treatment studies on major depression (Klein, Gittelman, Quitkin, & Rifkin, 1980; Whitlock, 1982).

ORGANIC ANXIETY SYNDROME

Specific Diagnostic Considerations

Earlier, this chapter described organic mental disorders that correspond to a wide range of functional disorders, such as psychotic or depressive disorders. However, there is no DSM-III organic mental disorder that corresponds to the functional anxiety disorders.

Specifically, the DSM-III lists no diagnosis of organic anxiety syndrome. This omission implies that there are no organic mental disorders in which anxiety is the predominant symptom. However, there are several medical disorders in which anxiety is the principal symptom, such as pheochromocytoma and hyperthyroidism. Under the current diagnostic system, these organic anxiety symptoms must be coded as atypical organic mental disorders. Such imprecise terminology hinders research into the accurate diagnosis and treatment of these disorders (Mackenzie & Popkin, 1983).

Recently, the diagnosis of organic anxiety syndrome has been proposed to help clarify this imprecise terminology. The essential feature of this disorder is recurrent or persistent anxiety or panic attacks that are due to a specific organic factor. This diagnosis is precluded in the presence of clouding of consciousness, significant intellectual deterioration, hallucinations, delusions, or prominent mood disturbance. Evidence of a specific organic cause of this disorder must be shown in the patient's history, physical examination, or laboratory tests (Mackenzie & Popkin, 1983). This new diagnostic term, *organic anxiety syndrome,* has been included in a draft of the *DSM-III-R in Development* (APA, 1985).

The course of the organic anxiety disorder depends to some extent on the nature of the underlying medical disorder. The onset may be acute or insidious. In many but not all cases, the course of the medical disorder parallels that of the organic anxiety disorder. The anxiety not uncommonly persists for some brief period of time after the underlying medical disorder has responded to treatment. However, in other cases, the anxiety may respond to psychotropic medication or to other therapy even though the underlying medical disorder has not responded to treatment.

There are a variety of medical disorders in which anxiety may be a principle behavioral symptom. These include endocrine and metabolic disorders, secreting tumors (such as pheochromocytoma), neurological disorders, cardiovascular disorders, drug-related disorders, and an immunological disorder (see Table 5 for a summary of those disorders in which anxiety is an integral part of the disease process). Anxiety disorders caused by the psychological awareness of a medical disorder are not classified here as an organic disorder (Hall, 1980a; Lishman, 1978; Rosenbaum, 1979).

The pathogenesis of organic anxiety disorders varies with the underlying medical

Table 5. Reported Medical Etiologies of Organic Anxiety Syndrome

1. Endocrine and metabolic disorders: hyperthyroidism, hypothyroidism, Cushing's disease, Addison's disease, menopause, premenstrual syndrome, hypoglycemia, diabetes mellitus, hyperparathyroidism, hypoparathyroidism, Wilson's disease, fructose-1,6-diphosphatase deficiency
2. Secreting tumors: pheochromocytoma, insulinoma, carcinoid
3. Neurological disorders: temporal lobe seizures, multiple sclerosis, brain tumors, neurosyphilis, postconcussive syndrome, postencephalitic disorders, cerebral vascular disorders, Huntington's chorea
4. Cardiovascular disorders: arrhythmias, mitral valve prolapse, coronary insufficiency, anemia
5. Drug-related disorders: stimulants, akathesia from neuroleptics, withdrawal syndromes
6. Immunological disorders: systemic lupus erythematosus

etiology. Medical disorders resulting in anxiety states may be etiologically divided into three groups:

1. Those interfering with stimulus discrimination, such as degenerative brain disorders or toxic states
2. Those producing sympathetic nervous system disruption, such as tumors
3. Those producing direct end-organ changes, such as hypoglycemia or hyperthyroidism (Hall, 1980a)

In some cases, hereditary biochemical disorders may predispose some persons to organic anxiety disorders. For example, in one case, an organic anxiety disorder was found to be caused by a hereditary deficiency of fructose-1,6-diphosphatase. This substance is a rate-limiting enzyme in gluconeogenesis that is essential for the maintenance of normal blood sugar during fasting. A deficiency in this enzyme resulted in repeated profound hypoglycemic episodes, which in turn resulted in an organic anxiety syndrome (Cornelius, Payton, & McGonigle, 1985).

The evaluation of organic anxiety disorders should start with a thorough medical history and physical examination. Several laboratory tests may then be appropriate, depending on the results of the history and physical examination. Such tests may include thyroid function tests, cortisol levels, blood glucose levels, follicle-stimulating-hormone and luteinizing-hormone levels, calcium levels, copper and ceruloplasmin levels, an EEG, a syphilis screen, an EKG, a drug screen, an eosinophil sedimentation rate, a CT scan, and a 24-hour urine screen for free catecholamines, vanillyl mandelic acid, the metanephrines, and 5-HIAA levels. Hospitalization may or may not be necessary. The criteria for determining the need for hospitalization are similar to those described previously for organic effective syndrome, depressed type.

Treatment Applications

Little is known about the treatment of organic anxiety syndrome. Whenever possible, the disorder should be managed by treating the underlying medical disorder. In addition, medications such as minor tranquilizers or propranolol may be needed in some cases. The effectiveness of different therapies for this disorder has not been systematically evaluated (Mackenzie & Popkin, 1983).

SUMMARY

The wide variety of OBSs was not formally acknowledged until 1980, when the DSM-III was published. Since that time, no comprehensive review of the outpatient management of these disorders has been published. This chapter discusses the outpatient diagnosis and treatment of the DSM-III organic brain syndromes, excluding dementia. The history, epidemiology, etiology, and pathophysiology of these disorders is also briefly reviewed. Much research in this area remains to be done.

ACKNOWLEDGMENTS. The author thanks Charles F. Reynolds III, M.D., Paula Trzepacz, M.D., and Paul H. Soloff, M.D., for their comments and suggestions concerning this chapter.

Adams, R. D., & Victor, M. (1985). *Principles of neurology*. New York: McGraw-Hill.
American Psychiatric Association. (1952). *Diagnostic and statistical manual of mental disorders* (1st ed.; DSM-I). Washington, DC: Author.
American Psychiatric Association. (1968). *Diagnostic and statistical manual of mental disorders* (2nd ed.; DSM-II). Washington, DC: Author.
American Psychiatric Association. (1980). *Diagnostic and statistical manual of mental disorders* (3rd ed.; DSM-III). Washington, DC: Author.
American Psychiatric Association. (1985). *DSM-III-R in Development*. Washington, DC: Author.
Anderson, W. H. (1979). Depression. In A. Lazare (Ed.), *Outpatient psychiatry* (pp. 257–260). Baltimore: Williams & Wilkins.
Ayd, F. J. (1978). Haloperidol: Twenty years clinical experience. *The Journal of Clinical Psychiatry, 39*, 807–814.
Baldessarini, R. J. (1980). Drugs and the treatment of psychiatric disorders. In A. G. Gilman, L. S. Goodman, & A. Gilman (Eds.), *The pharmacological basis of therapeutics* (pp. 391–447). New York: Macmillan.
Ban, T. A. (1976). Psychopathology, psychopharmacology, and the organic brain syndromes. *Psychosomatics, 17*, 131–137.
Burns, R. S., & Lerner, S. E. (1976). Management and treatment of acute phencyclidine intoxications. In P. G. Bourne (Ed.), *Acute drug abuse emergencies* (pp. 297–306). Washington, DC: Academic Press.
Cornelius, J. R., Soloff, P. H., & Reynolds, C. F. (1984). Paranoia, homicidal behavior, and seizures associated with phenylpropanolamine. *American Journal of Psychiatry, 141*, 120–121.
Cornelius, J. R., Payton, J. B., & McGonigle, J. J. (1985). Overanxious disorder with FDPase deficiency and developmental disability. *Psychosomatics, 26*, 680–682.
Cornelius, J. R., Soloff, P. H., & Miewald, B. K. (1986). Behavioral manifestations of paraneoplastic encephalopathy. *Biological Psychiatry, 21*, 686–690.
Cummings, J. L. (1985). Organic delusions: Phenomenology, anatomical correlations, and review. *British Journal of Psychiatry, 146*, 184–197.
Cummings, J. L., & Mendez, M. F. (1984). Secondary mania with focal cerebrovascular lesions. *American Journal of Psychiatry, 141*, 1084–1087.
Davison, K. (1983). Schizophrenia-like psychoses associated with organic cerebral disorders: A review. *Psychiatric Developments, 1*, 1–34.
Davison, K., & Bagley, C. R. (1969). Schizophrenic-like psychoses associated with organic disorders of the central nervous system: A review of the literature. *British Journal of Psychiatry*, Special Publication No. 4, 113–184.
Detre, T. P., & Jarecki, H. G. (1971). *Modern psychiatric treatment*. Philadelphia: J. B. Lippincott.
DeVaul, R. A., & Hall, R. C. (1980). Hallucinations. In C. W. Hall (Ed.), *Psychiatric presentations of medical illness* (pp. 91–103). Jamaica, NY: Spectrum.
Editorial (1977). Sedation in liver disease. *British Medical Journal, 1*, 1241–1242.
Ellinwood, E. H. (1976). Emergency treatment of acute adverse reactions to CNS stimulants. In P. G. Bourne (Ed.), *Acute drug abuse emergencies* (pp. 115–138). New York: Academic Press.
Fauman, M. A. (1983). The emergency psychiatric evaluation of organic mental disorders. *Emergency Psychiatry, 6*, 233–257.
Gabel, R. H., Barnard, N., Norko, M., & O'Connell, R. A. (1986). AIDS presenting as mania. *Comprehensive Psychiatry, 27*, 251–254.
Goodwin, F. K., & Bunney, W. E. (1971). Depressions following reserpine: A re-evaluation. *Seminars in Psychiatry, 3*, 435–448.
Hall, R. C., Popkin, M. K., DeVaul, R. A., Faillace, L. A., & Stickney, S. K. (1978). Physical illness presenting as psychiatric disease. *Archives of General Psychiatry, 35*, 1315–1320.
Hall, R. C. W. (1980a). Anxiety. In R. C. W. Hall (Ed.), *Psychiatric presentations of medical illness* (pp. 13–35). Jamaica, NY: Spectrum.
Hall, R. C. W. (1980b). Depression. In R. C. W. Hall (Ed.), *Psychiatric presentations of medical illness* (pp. 37–63). Jamaica, NY: Spectrum.
Hartmann, E. (1975). Dreams and other hallucinations: An approach to the underlying mechanism. In R. K. Siegel & L. J. West (Eds.), *Hallucinations* (pp. 71–80). New York: Wiley.
Heller, S. S. (1976). The organic patient and medical problems. In R. A. Glick, A. T. Meyerson, E. Robbins, & J. A. Talbott (Eds.), *Psychiatric emergencies* (pp. 135–146). New York: Grune & Stratton.

Herridge, C. F. (1960). Physical disorders in psychiatric illness. *The Lancet, 2,* 949–951.

Johnson, J. (1969). Organic psychosyndromes due to boxing. *British Journal of Psychiatry, 115,* 45–53.

Kermani, E. J., Borod, J. C., Brown, P. H., & Tunnell, G. (1985). New psychopathologic findings in AIDS: Case report. *The Journal of Clinical Psychiatry, 46,* 240–241.

Kiely, W. F. (1976). Psychiatric syndromes in critically ill patients. *Journal of the American Medical Association, 235,* 2759–2761.

Klein, D. F., Gittelman, R., Quitkin, F., & Rifkin, A. (1980). *Diagnosis and drug treatment of psychiatric disorders: Adults and children.* Baltimore: Williams & Wilkins.

Koranyi, E. K. (1979). Morbidity and rate of undiagnosed physical illnesses in a psychiatric clinic population. *Archives of General Psychiatry, 36,* 414–419.

Krauthammer, C., & Klerman, G. L. (1978). Secondary mania. *Archives of General Psychiatry, 35,* 1333–1339.

Lezak, M. D. (1978). Living with the characterologically altered brain injured patient. *Journal of Clinical Psychiatry, 39,* 592–598.

Lipowski, Z. J. (1980a). *Delirium.* Springfield, IL: Charles C Thomas.

Lipowski, Z. J. (1980b). A new look at organic brain syndromes. *American Journal of Psychiatry, 137,* 674–678.

Lipowski, Z. J. (1980c). Organic mental disorders. In H. I. Kaplan, A. M. Freedman, & B. J. Sadock (Eds.), *Comprehensive textbook of psychiatry (Vol. 3)* (pp. 1359–1392). Baltimore: Williams & Wilkins.

Lipowski, Z. J. (1985). Delirium (acute confusional state). In J. A. M. Frederiks (Ed.), *Handbook of clinical neurology* (pp. 523–559). New York: Elsevier Science.

Lishman, W. A. (1978). *Organic psychiatry.* Oxford, Blackwell.

Mackenzie, T. B., & Popkin, M. K. (1983). Organic anxiety syndrome. *American Journal of Psychiatry, 140,* 342–344.

Malamud, N., & Skillicorn, S. A. (1956). Relationship between the Werniche and the Korsakoff syndrome. *Archives of Neurology and Psychiatry, 76,* 585–596.

Man, P. L., & Chen, C. H. (1973). Rapid tranquilization of acutely psychotic patients with intramuscular haloperidol and chlorpromazine. *Psychosomatics, 14,* 59–63.

Mapelli, G., & Bellelli, T. (1982). Letter to the editor. *Archives of General Psychiatry, 39,* 743.

Moore, D. P. (1977). Rapid treatment of delirium in critically ill patients. *American Journal of Psychiatry, 134,* 1431–1432.

Reeves, A. G., & Plum, F. (1969). Hyperphagia, rage, and dementia accompanying a ventromedial hypothalamic neoplasm. *Archives of Neurology, 20,* 616–624.

Rosenbaum, A. H., & Barry, M. J. (1975). Positive therapeutic response to lithium in hypomania secondary to organic brain syndrome. *American Journal of Psychiatry, 132,* 1072–1073.

Rosenbaum, J. F. (1979). Anxiety. In A. Lazare (Ed.), *Outpatient psychiatry* (pp. 252–256). Baltimore: Williams & Wilkins.

Siegel, R. K., & Jarvik, M. E. (1975). Drug-induced hallucinations in animals and man. In R. K. Siegel & L. J. West (Eds.), *Hallucinations* (pp. 81–161). New York: Wiley.

Stasiek, C., & Zetin, M. (1985). Organic manic disorders. *Psychosomatics, 26,* 394–402.

Storey, P. B. (1970). Brain damage and personality change after subarachnoid hemorrhage. *British Journal of Psychiatry, 117,* 129–142.

Strassman, R. J. (1984). Adverse reactions to psychedelic drugs: A review of the literature. *The Journal of Nervous and Mental Disease, 172,* 577–595.

Talbott, J. A. (1976). Emergency management of marijuana psychosis. In P. G. Bourne (Ed.), *Acute drug abuse emergencies* (pp. 153–161). Washington, DC: Academic Press.

Task Force, National Institute of Mental Health. (1976). *Research in the service of mental health.* Washington, DC: Government Printing Office.

Thompson, W. L., Johnson, A. D., & Maddey, W. L. (1975). Diazepam and paraldehyde for treatment of severe delirium tremens. *Annals of Internal Medicine, 82,* 175–180.

Victor, M., & Adams, R. D. (1983). Deficiency diseases of the nervous system. In R. G. Petersdorf, R. D. Adams, E. Braunwald, & J. D. Wilson (Eds.), *Harrison's principles of internal medicine* (pp. 2112–2118). New York: McGraw-Hill.

Victor, M., Adams, R. D., & Collins, G. H. (1971). *The Werniche-Korsakoff syndrome.* Philadelphia: F. A. Davis.

Villani, S., & Weitzel, W. D. (1979). Letter to the editor. *Archives of General Psychiatry, 36,* 1031.

Whitlock, F. A. (1982). *Symptomatic affective disorders.* Sydney, Australia: Academic Press.

Whitty, C. W. M., & Zangwill, O. L. (1966). *Amnesia.* London: Butterworths.

18

Problem Drinking

Cognitive-Behavioral Strategies for Self-Control

ALAN R. LANG AND MICHAEL KIDORF

INTRODUCTION

As empirically oriented clinicians, we feel obligated to promote a broad and flexible, largely cognitive-behavioral, approach to the outpatient treatment of problem drinking. This obligation is predicated on a desire to discuss realistically what is known or is reasonable to infer about the nature and modifiability of maladaptive alcohol use and to suggest the best applications of this information to remediation of the relevant clinical problems. It should be noted at the outset, however, that our task is undertaken with a sense of frustration and perhaps even some trepidation. The frustration stems from the fact that similar expositions, incorporating key research and theoretical advances, have been offered repeatedly by others for more than two decades (see Lazarus, 1965, for an early example) with little more than a negligible impact on the method and setting that typifies standard alcoholism treatment. Moreover, there is every indication that the reluctance of the alcoholism treatment establishment to embrace a scientific approach to examining its own concepts and techniques or to developing and evaluating new ones reflects more than the usual amount of inertia that might impede change and progress in any area.

One unique feature of the alcoholism field that has probably contributed heavily to its conservatism is the fact that so many of its counselors have entered their vocation primarily because they are former (or ''recovering'') alcoholics and this job choice affords them an opportunity to taken another step in their rehabilitation. These individuals often lack the broad theoretical and scientific perspective more common among professionals

ALAN R. LANG and MICHAEL KIDORF • Department of Psychology, Florida State University, Tallahassee, Florida 32306.

working in other specialized problem areas. They rely instead on personal experiences, many feeling they owe their sobriety and perhaps their very lives to a particular view of problem drinking and to the specific treatment approach of which it is part and parcel. They "know" it worked for them, ergo it must be *the* way. Despite the best of intentions and unquestionable dedication, it is easy to see how a quasi-religious "I've made up my mind, don't bother me with facts" attitude might evolve under these circumstances. Hence, the frustration inherent in preparing a chapter such as this is the expectation that it will be ignored by many of those in the best position to use its contents to benefit problem drinkers.

Beyond dismay over the possibility that our message may fall on deaf ears is a vague concern that some traditionalists in the alcohol field may be more than just parochial in their views. Instead of simply practicing a policy of benign neglect where divergent positions are concerned, there has been a pernicious tendency toward the aggressive suppression of those with competing ideas. The ostracism, character assassination, and even personal threats experienced by scientists (e.g., Peele, 1986; Sobell & Sobell, 1984) who have been a bit too visible or vociferous in their suggestion that alternatives to the traditional goals and concepts of alcoholism treatment ought to be entertained and investigated bespeak the risks one takes when entering the fray. The point is that, over and above the facts about treatment approaches, one must be cognizant of the complex sociopolitical and economic context in which they are practiced. This seems particularly true in the United States, where institutionalized forces with a single-minded conceptualization of and treatment strategy for drinking problems have become so entrenched that they may be held partly responsible for effectively denying services to those who are unwilling to accept their rigid definitions, goals, and methods and for the apparent intractability of many who do.

Lest the reader be left (or leave us at this point) with a totally cynical and pessimistic outlook for the future, let us hasten to add that there is hope on the horizon. Ironically, some of the very same kinds of forces—economic forces in particular—that have permitted ideology to prevail over science in the treatment of problem drinking appear poised for a reversal. As pressure mounts to contain spiraling health-care costs through the development and/or simply the greater utilization of demonstrably effective, but relatively less expensive, outpatient interventions, the traditional month-long inpatient program for alcohol abuse and dependence should be among the most obvious targets. Demands for accountability should be further augmented by an influx of more broadly trained and empirically oriented professionals into the alcohol field. Although resistance to any change is likely to be intense, the potential benefits in the reduction of individual and societal difficulties due to drinking are considerable.

Our general plan in this chapter is to outline a conceptual, diagnostic-assessment, and treatment approach to problem drinking that is compatible with identified trends in health-care delivery and that we believe averts many of the shortcomings of the views and methods for remediation of alcoholism that currently dominate the field. Before embarking on this course, however, a brief overview of the magnitude of the alcohol problem and the effectiveness of the treatments addressing it is in order. In keeping with the theme of this volume, the potential and proper place for outpatient alcohol services is also highlighted. Finally, an analysis of the historical why's and how's of our evolution to the status quo is summarized in the hope that an understanding of the past will facilitate our movement forward.

THE COSTS OF THE ALCOHOL PROBLEM

The magnitude of the biomedical, psychosocial, and economic consequences associated with the problem use of alcohol is staggering. Government studies estimate that 10–15 million Americans have serious problems directly related to their own alcohol abuse and dependence, and they place the proportion of the population indirectly affected through personal relationships with the index cases as high as 1 in 3 (National Institute of Alcohol Abuse and Alcoholism—NIAAA, 1983). In the physical health arena, perhaps 10% of the total annual mortality rate of the United States is at least partly attributable to drinking. Many more experience nonfatal, but permanently disabling, birth defects, accidental injuries, and diseases in which alcohol is a significant component. Naturally, difficulties in coping with these losses and consequences as well as with alcohol-related crime and family disruption exact an additional toll in terms of psychological suffering and mental health problems. Even considering only the purely economic costs, the price is appallingly high. Cruze, Harwood, Kristiansen, Collins, and Jones (1981), for example, calculated that total expenditures related to alcohol problems were nearly $50 billion in the year 1977, with projections for 1987 as high as $120 billion. Lost work productivity accounts for a major portion of these dollar totals, but outlays for the direct treatment of problem drinking and its immediate medical consequences have been substantial. Indeed, alcohol abuse may be responsible for up to 15% of U.S. health-care costs—even though an estimated 85% of those with problems due to drinking receive no treatment for their condition (Saxe, Dougherty, Esty, & Fine, 1983).

Although the dimensions of the alcohol problem as outlined above leave little doubt that some intervention is needed, several key questions remain: (1) Why are the existing services so underutilized? (2) Are the treatments currently being provided effective? and (3) How can the cost-effectiveness of promising interventions be maximized? Speculation about the answer to the first question will be postponed until after a historical perspective on popular conceptions of problem drinking and its treatment implications has been offered. For the moment, then, let us address issues of treatment effectiveness and its cost.

THE EFFECTIVENESS AND COST OF ALCOHOLISM TREATMENT

Anything more than a brief summary of the vast literature on the effectiveness of the various drug, psychologically based, and group or community efforts to treat problem drinking is well beyond our present scope. Fortunately, there have been a number of excellent reviews and commentaries on the area, and the interested reader is referred to one particularly comprehensive contribution by Miller and Hester (1986a). These authors, among others (e.g., Sobell & Sobell, 1982), have noted that much of the research on the efficacy of treatments for alcohol-related problems has been of rather poor methodological quality. Moreover, interpretations and comparisons of even the best controlled studies are often complicated by inadequately managed but potentially critical factors such as sample composition and selection, definition and measurement of outcome criteria, time of evaluation, handling of dropouts or patients lost at follow-up, statistical methods, and a host of threats to internal validity (Emrick & Hansen, 1983). Nevertheless, there is general consensus (see Saunders, 1985, for a contrary opinion) that some treatment of problem drinking is better than none. Still, misleading claims of many alcoholism treatment programs notwithstanding, in the aggregate indications are that the advantage of the treated over the untreated is rather modest.

Most studies of the efficacy of treatments for alcohol abuse and dependence have not included the untreated control groups essential to an assessment of absolute effectiveness. Furthermore, although there is clear evidence (Maisto & McCollam, 1980) of a substantially less-than-perfect correlation between drinking status and the functioning in other life areas often presumed to improve with treatment (e.g., socioemotional, family, and vocational functioning), an almost exclusive focus on some form of ''drinking outcome'' continues. With these caveats in mind, it is remarkable that the largest and one of the most comprehensive and methodologically sound treatment-outcome studies to date (Polich, Armor, & Braiker, 1980) reported that only 7% of male alcoholics treated in NIAAA-funded programs maintained a stable pattern of abstinence throughout a 4-year follow-up period. An additional 12% could be classified as nonproblem drinkers across the same period. These figures square reasonably well with estimates by Miller and Hester (1980) of a 26% rate of abstinent or ''improved'' status in their review of studies with data on 1-year follow-up.

Such results are not particularly impressive and are perhaps even less so when juxtaposed with the available, although limited, data on ''spontaneous remission'' in problem drinkers who either have not sought or have dropped out of treatment (see Armor & Meshkoff, 1983, for a review). Analyses of outcomes experienced by these individuals indicate that their rates of remission, defined as abstinence or nonproblem drinking, are within about 10 percentage points of those enjoyed by treated patients. Furthermore, self-selection factors, such as the distinct possibility that persons who do not seek treatment or who depart after minimal contact are less likely to want to change their behavior, may account for a substantial portion of any apparent advantage of treatment.

Disconcerting as the comparisons of results for treated and untreated samples may be, attention to them may be very instructive. For instance, all the relevant studies challenge the popular notion that alcoholic remission cannot occur without formal treatment. Particularly noteworthy in this connection are the correlates and probable causes of observed changes in those not exposed to treatment. As summarized by Armor and Meshkoff (1983), these most frequently involve major changes in or threats to physiological or psychosocial well-being, including alterations of residential, health, occupational, and family or other social situations. The importance of such extratreatment, life-context factors as the interactive determinants of outcome for persons who do receive formal treatment has also been highlighted by several researchers (e.g., Billings & Moos, 1983; Marlatt & Gordon, 1980). Of course, the potency of environmental contingencies and other contextual variables has long been recognized by laboratory researchers and is amply documented where drinking behavior is concerned (Lang & Marlatt, 1982). The clear implication is that, if clinicians in the alcohol field are to increment their effectiveness, they must broaden their perspectives to integrate such life-context factors.

Is it also possible that alcoholism treatment programs could improve on their overall lackluster performance if only they would incorporate methods having demonstrated efficacy? The answer appears to be a qualified yes. As Miller and Hester (1986a) noted, a number of techniques have creditable track records of producing improvements for substantial groups of clients in a majority of controlled evaluations. Among these are (1) certain aversive counterconditioning procedures designed to reduce the attraction of alcohol and to directly suppress the drinking response by repeatedly pairing it with unpleasant experiences such as nausea, although changes associated with these methods are relatively short-term; (2) broad-spectrum behavior-therapy approaches that train social skills and stress management and/or control reinforcement contingencies so that clients are better able and more inclined to substitute adaptive coping responses for drinking; (3) marital and/or family therapy addressing important reinforcers and dynamics in this critical social milieu of some problem drinkers; and (4) instruction in specific self-control techniques to help clients moderate their drinking to nonproblem levels. To be sure, these methods are by no means foolproof or unequivocally effective, but they are among the most promising, and their discreet application might improve overall treatment success rates significantly.

Unfortunately, the vast majority of U.S. alcoholism-treatment programs use few, if any, of the tactics outlined above. Instead, they typically opt for a package including many of the following elements: (1) Alcoholics Anonymous (AA), the popular self-help approach whose reputed efficacy has unfortunately been evaluated in only two reasonably controlled, random-assignment comparisons with no treatment or alternative treatments (Brandsma, Maultsby, & Welsh, 1980; Ditman, Crawford, Forgy, Moskowitz, & MacAndrew, 1967)—neither of which supported its superiority or even a high level of absolute success; (2) disulfiram (Antabuse) treatment, which, unlike an aversive counterconditioning procedure that intentionally pairs negative physiological reactions with drinking on repeated trials, seeks simply to inhibit or prevent drinking through the threat of such reactions if alcohol is consumed while it is still in the system, but which has no demonstrable advantage over placebos (e.g., Fuller & Roth, 1979) and may have negative side effects; (3) poorly defined individual or group "psychotherapy," which has little or no documented impact on long-term drinking behavior (Emrick, 1975); and (4) alcoholism education, which, at least in its most common forms, has not been shown to add anything to the usual treatment regimen (e.g., Uecker & Solberg, 1973). Most of these treatments also incorporate aggressive and sometimes dramatic confrontation of client "denial" or refusal to be labeled "alcoholics," even though such methods may precipitate flight from treatment and other negative side effects. In sum, the "standard" treatment package is virtually without a research base to recommend it, may produce undesirable side effects, and fails to incorporate methods that do enjoy some empirical support (Miller & Hester, 1986a). Small wonder that remission rates following conventional treatment for drinking problems surpass those that occur naturally by only the smallest of margins.

Another critical liability of most treatment of problem drinking as it is currently practiced is its inattention to the burgeoning investigation of the role of individual-difference factors in problem drinking and treatment response. Beyond insistent adherence to the unsubstantiated claim that alcoholics are qualitatively different from nonalcoholics because of some ill-defined biological anomaly, the uniqueness of the afflicted persons has generally been ignored. Although there is some lip service to individualized treatment, the fact is that the typical alcoholism program is patterned after the "one-size-fits-all" approach of AA. Thus, it offers few variations from a standard treatment package and even fewer choices of or rationally determined assignments to those that do exist. Most places apparently just prescribe whatever package they have without regard for patient characteristics (Hansen & Emrick, 1983), revealing an implicit "uniformity" assumption. Relentless promotion, if not scientific pursuit, of the one best treatment reflects a similar mentality. Yet, as we have already implied, considerable heterogeneity in patient response to treatment should be expected. Indeed, research has demonstrated that the amount of shared variance between client and treatment factors is substantial (Cronkite & Moos, 1978).

Could it be, even without strong evidence that one treatment is superior to any other for all clients, that matching subgroups of individuals having particular characteristics with certain kinds of treatments would improve overall effectiveness? Although only limited research on this matching hypothesis is available, its intuitive appeal has received at least tentative support. A recent review of studies in this area (Miller & Hester, 1986c) concluded that clients improve more when (1) allowed to exercise some choice regarding treatment approach rather than having only a single approach or program offered (e.g., Kissin, Platz, & Su, 1971) and (2) matched with an approach consistent with their cognitive style (e.g., McLachlan, 1974). In addition, there is evidence to support the commonsense notion that the selective use of specific components of "broad-spectrum" interventions, depending on the extent to which the problem drinker manifests the particular type of difficulty each is designed to address, results in differential benefit to clients (Miller & Hester, 1986c). Finally, Miller and Hester (1986b) summarized data indicating that "Clients with more severe alcohol-related problems benefit differentially from more intensive (*though not necessarily inpatient*) treatment, whereas clients with less severe problems benefit *at least as much if not more* from a minimal intervention" (p. 195, italics added). Thus, it is obvious that treatment effectiveness stands to profit from more detailed assessments of client characteristics and a greater willingness to use them in connection with flexible prescriptions for change. The relative cost of any such services, however, is most closely related to the conclusions about intensity of treatment quoted above, and it is to that topic that we now turn.

Based on an analysis of the number and percentage of inpatient and outpatient hospital-based treatment units for alcoholism, Knowles (1983) concluded that there has been a modest shift toward increasing use of outpatient services. A desire for more flexibility and lower costs may underlie this trend, but the fact remains that reimbursement systems, apparently wed to the definition of any drinking problem as "alcoholism" and the uninformed expectation that a 30-day hospital stay is essential to its remediation, have encouraged the indiscriminate use of inpatient, medically based treatments that continue to consume the vast majority of the funds available for intervention. Even Skinner's observation (1981) that, under naturally occurring circumstances, the alcoholism services clientele referred and admitted to inpatient facilities tended to have quantitatively more severe problems than were found in outpatient alternatives is not cause for much optimism. The reason is that, of the no fewer than 10 well-controlled studies that randomly assigned clearly "alcoholic" patients (who ordinarily would have all been hospitalized) to either inpatient or outpatient care, *none* indicated superior outcomes for those in the more expensive residential treatment (Miller & Hester, 1986b). Indeed, all differences that did occur favored outpatient settings. A similar lack of advantage in extending the length of treatment has also been noted (Miller & Hester, 1986b). Thus, the available evidence seems to suggest that any initial use of hospitalization for alcohol-related problems ought to be restricted to circumstances in which there are extreme and immediate threats to the life or health of clients or to those around them—much like the conditions surrounding civil commitment. Otherwise, reimbursement and general social policy ought to encourage early intervention that uses minimally intrusive outpatient approaches, with the progressive use of more intensive or drastic residential treatment only if less expensive approaches fail. Cost-effectiveness data simply do not justify any other strategy (cf. Marlatt, 1987).

We believe that the preceding introduction has illustrated that—if not in terms of knowledge itself, then certainly in terms of the application of the available knowledge—current efforts to deal with problem drinking in the United States are in rather a sorry state. Why is this so? One plausible explanation can be derived from a historical analysis of the social meaning of alcohol use and societal reactions to its attendant problems. We start with the premise that consumption of alcoholic beverages is a behavior about which there is a great deal of ambivalence in contemporary American society and that, in many ways, this is a legacy of conflicting historical conceptions of drinking (cf. Levine, 1978). The general view of alcohol in these bygone eras was far more clear than it is today, and hence, logical responses to problems associated with drinking were more straightforward. In the present atmosphere of ambivalence, one would think that no single conception of drinking problems and prescription for their control would be dominant. Indeed, in the scientific community, considerable ambiguity and controversy surround these issues. However, societies do not long tolerate uncertainties about deviations from the social order and are quick to adopt simplistic explanations that conform to social, political, and economic exigencies if no more workable alternative is immediately available. It is our view, and a brief review of history should bear us out, that this is precisely how the popular disease-concept of alcoholism and the hospital-based treatment programs it has spawned were elevated to their present status.

In Colonial America, alcohol was generally regarded as a "good creature of God," praised for its medicinal value as well as its contributions to warmth, relaxation, and good fellowship. Taverns were the gathering places for families and even governments in the largely agrarian society, and drinking was part of the social fabric. This is not to say there were no problems associated with drinking. But, even if drunkenness was commonplace, the prevailing attitude was one of acceptance—people needed breaks and alcohol was ubiquitous, so what was the harm? The occasional religious leader who criticized habitual drunkards did so largely on the basis of their coincident idleness, regarded as one of the more telling signs of weak moral fiber. Alcohol was not seen as the cause of any social problem. Rather, the fault was in the moral laxity of the drinker, who needed only motivation and discipline to reform. Accordingly, problem drinkers were treated as "out-patients," by punishment, humiliation, and preaching until they saw the error of their ways (Levine, 1978).

As 19th-century America expanded and industrialized, the average father was more likely to work away from home and family, and he also spent more of his leisure time without his wife or children. Taverns became male-dominated institutions ripe for gambling and prostitution, and the more restrictive work schedules of their patrons encouraged binges. Taken together, these changes led to an association of drinking with the lack of both self-control and respectability. It was alcohol that soon came to be seen as the agent of immorality and irresponsibility, even if the social milieu of the tavern was the more likely culprit. Temperance groups, led by religious figures discontented with the lack of self-control that alcohol had come to symbolize and by women whose families were threatened by drinking and all that the new taverns represented, sprang up everywhere. This powerful movement turned 180 degrees from the good creature of God, ushering in an era of "demon rum." It was no longer the individual who was to blame for the problems associated with drinking. Instead, it was assumed that alcohol was an addicting poison for *anyone* who drank it and that even the most moderate and controlled of persons were at risk whenever a drink touched their lips. Quite naturally, the solution to problem drinking was the elimination of alcohol and the transformation of America into a nation of abstainers. National prohibition was the treatment (Levine, 1978).

Although moderately successful in reducing per capita alcohol consumption and rates of liver disease and other indicators of alcoholism, undesirable side effects due primarily to enforcement problems led to the repeal of prohibition in 1933 (Moore & Gerstein, 1981). A new perspective on alcohol and drinking problems had to be developed. What evolved was something of a compromise between the good creature and the demon. The popular disease-concept held that, for the vast majority of people, alcohol was the benign substance of Colonial America. This concept pleased both the politician, whose constituents generally favored drinking, and the alcoholic beverage industry, whose profits would be only fractionally limited. On the other hand, it was also maintained that, for an unfortunate minority, alcohol acted like the addicting poison of temperance America. This caveat placated religious groups and health experts, soothing the consciences of many but finessing the whole issue of etiology and the identification of who had a problem and who did not. We were left with a vague notion of a vulnerability due to some genetic anomaly or biological adaptation and the hope that someday it would all be made clear. In the meantime, medical and related approaches stressing the helpless dependency of the problem drinker were to supplant punishment or prohibition as the treatment of choice. The expediency of this resolution to the need for a new conceptualization of problem drinking has contributed heavily to its durability (Wiener, 1981).

Before proposing an alternative view that reflects a more general public-health perspective than is evident in the traditional disease-concept of alcoholism, three points emerging from this historical overview should be underscored. The first is that there are identifiable reasons for America's present ambivalence about alcohol and for its choice of response to alcohol problems. The second is that changes in attitudes, concepts, and treatments from one era to the next have depended heavily on the social, political, and economic climate—*not* on an important scientific discovery that significantly altered objective knowledge about drinking and its associated problems. Finally, it is critical that conscientious practitioners today look beyond treatment methods that are simply popular to those that show promise on a rational and empirical basis. Otherwise, we may be doomed to repeat or perpetuate the errors of history and to the resulting inability to cope adequately with the alcohol problem.

SPECIFIC DIAGNOSTIC AND DEVELOPMENTAL CONSIDERATIONS

The definition of alcohol-related problems is, of course, a prerequisite to their diagnosis and treatment. Ideally, a working conceptualization of their nature, their likely course, and their probable etiology would also underlie any intervention. It is time to address these issues more explicitly.

Alcohol addiction, alcohol dependence, alcoholism, alcohol abuse, problem drinking, and other similar terms have often been used, sometimes interchangeably, to describe alcohol-related problems. However, there is little consensus about what these labels mean. Such ambiguity is perhaps a by-product of societal ambivalence about drinking as well as of the very real complexities of the definitional issue. Clearly, it is not drinking *per se* that is to be regarded as a problem, as the majority of adult Americans who consume alcoholic beverages apparently do so without adverse consequences. Even "heavy drinking," defined in terms of quantity, frequency, and variability norms (Cahalan, Cisin, and Crossley, 1969), is neither necessary nor sufficient for every alcohol-related problem, although it obviously is at least correlated with many (Sadava, 1985).

Apparently recognizing the need to incorporate the *consequences* of drinking into any diagnostic criteria describing problems related to it, the widely used third edition of the American Psychiatric Association's *Diagnostic and Statistical Manual of Mental Disorders* (DSM-III; APA, 1980) lists two categories of disorder: alcohol abuse and alcohol dependence. In the DSM-III, "abuse" is characterized as a pathological pattern of alcohol use resulting in the impairment of social or occupational functioning, the disturbance having a duration of at least 1 month. The criteria for "dependence" include either a pathological use pattern or social-occupational impairment *and* evidence of either alcohol tolerance (more alcohol required to produce similar effects, or diminished effects experienced with repeated use of the same amount) or alcohol withdrawal (an assortment of mostly physical symptoms) on a cessation of or a reduction in prolonged heavy drinking.

Laudable as the contemporary psychiatric definitions may be in their attention to the possible concomitants and direct consequences of alcohol use, they are not free of serious defects. Principal among these is the implicit assumption that "normal" alcohol use, alcohol abuse, and alcohol dependence represent discrete entities. We would argue that, given the complexity of human behavior, the uniqueness of individual manifestations of it, and the uncertainties about its cause, no such categorical assumption is justified. Moreover, it is clear that virtually all the DSM-III diagnostic criteria for alcohol-related problems not only lack the specificity essential to a meaningful categorical classification, but themselves refer to continuous rather than discrete variations in behavior. Even tolerance and withdrawal, the most fundamental features of classical descriptions of addiction, are not all-or-none phenomena. Like impairment, they exist on a continuum.

With the above considerations in mind, we reiterate the broad concept of alcohol-related problems proposed by Lang and Marlatt (1982) and use the term *problem drinking* to denote *any* pattern of alcohol consumption associated with subjective discomfort and/or objective impairment in the drinker and/or those around the drinker. This definition allows for a wide and continuous range of problem severity. It also encompasses a multitude of possible interactions between drinking and problems, recognizing that a variety of biological, psychological, and social problems involving discomfort and/or impairment may precipitate drinking as well as result from it. This approach escapes the all-too-easy but ill-advised assumption of a undirectional, causal relationship between drinking and problems of the individual. Instead, both the clinician and the client are encouraged to adopt an investigative frame of mind and to emphasize problem specification, understanding, and remediation rather than simply the assignment of a diagnostic label. Moreover, by using the problem-drinking concept, one is more apt to get beyond an exclusive focus on alcohol and the person to one that includes a consideration of broad contextual and immediate situational determinants of behavior.

The inclusion of the external environment among the potential causes of problem drinking may also result in a less permanent assignment of individuals to diagnostic categories, thereby reducing the negative potential of labeling. The idea that every individual having difficulties associated with drinking must accept the label *alcoholic* as if it critically and succinctly described one's personality and defined a lifelong state of being may have virtue for some, but it just does not jibe well with the unpredictability of outcomes for alcohol-related problems and is certainly not a prerequisite for change. On the other hand, simply being asked to recognize that one has some problems associated with drinking and might benefit from doing something about them makes entry into treatment more palatable and, in turn, should increase the use of early interventions, which are known to be more effective than those applied when discomfort and impairment have become extreme. Ultimately, clients are also more inclined to be active participants in their own treatment if they do not view themselves as permanent victims of a disorder that is outside their control. We see all these characteristics of the problem-drinking approach as advantageous and hence endorse its broad use. This is not to say, however, that there is no rationale or utility in identifying subtypes of drinking problems and meaningful individual differences in the persons who present with any of them.

Numerous dimensions and subtypes have been proposed to capture the many faces of problem drinking. For instance, Schuckit (1979) pointed out the importance of distinguishing between primary and secondary ''alcoholism,'' noting that the likely course of each syndrome may differ markedly. He defined as ''primary'' those serious alcohol problems occurring in individuals with no preexisting major psychiatric disorder, whereas ''secondary'' denoted a severe drinking problem beginning after another psychiatric disturbance (usually antisocial personality or major affective disorder) was already evident. Indications are that the most destructive and problem-ridden course is followed by antisocial personalities having alcohol problems secondarily. A more benign history and prognosis are expected of problem drinkers with affective disorders as the primary disorder (although suicide risk is elevated). Primary problem drinkers occupy an intermediate, but highly variable, position. Obviously, careful attention to differential diagnosis is important to the formulation of the most appropriate treatment plan in each case.

A primary versus secondary ''alcoholic'' distinction was also proposed by MacAndrew (1981), but his was based largely on personality data. Using individual traits correlated with scores on the special MacAndrew (MAC) subscale of the Minnesota Multiphasic Personality Inventory (MMPI), he showed that a majority of severe problem drinkers were of the primary type characterized by strong and easily aroused emotionality, an early onset of heavy drinking without an identifiable precipitant, and a sensation-seeking orientation to the world. The secondary type, although also highly emotional and easily aroused, was more ''reactive'' in alcohol consumption, apparently using it to avoid or escape aversive experiences such as high anxiety. Thus, the former style could be described as characterological reward-seeking and the latter as neurotic punishment-avoiding. A strikingly similar dimensional subtyping was also discussed in a very recent neurobiological analysis of problem drinking behavior (Cloninger, 1987). The point again is that the diagnosis and treatment planning for problem drinking may risk inefficiency if not outright error by ignoring the obvious diversity of the population in question.

The age of the problem-drinking client is still another feature worth noting because it may be systematically related to problem etiology, prognosis, and choice of intervention. A longitudinal study by Fillmore (1987) indicated that the incidence of heavy drinking and acute alcohol-related problems (e.g., accidents, violence, and coma) is greatest among young men and declines with age. Chronicity and its associated problems (e.g., liver disease and neurological impairment), however, peak in the middle years, decreasing thereafter (independent of mortality). These findings, along with additional evidence that early drinking patterns and difficulties are only weakly correlated with later ones (Fillmore, 1975), suggest that a substantial portion of youthful problem drinking may best be construed as one of many possible transitional ''problem behaviors'' (cf. Jessor & Jessor,

1977) rather than anything approximating a chronic, progressive, irreversible disease. Consequently, diagnosis and treatment ought to be broadly based as opposed to alcohol-specific. At the other end of the age spectrum, most late-onset problem drinking probably reflects a similar response to the demands for adaptation, but at this point, the stresses are those associated with advanced age (e.g., illness, retirement, and loneliness). In contrast, middle-aged men with alcohol problems tend to report more symptomatic behavior and psychological dependence specific to alcohol (Lisansky-Gomberg, 1982). Obviously, such developmental factors are germane to the differential diagnosis and treatment of problem drinking.

Finally, we would be remiss if we did not at least mention the gender of the problem-drinking client as a potentially important diagnostic and developmental consideration. For a host of sociocultural and psychobiological reasons, the antecedents, patterns, and consequences of excessive alcohol use may be markedly different in women than in men (Wilsnack & Beckman, 1984). For instance, the greater social stigmatization of the female drinker may lead to more solitary or otherwise concealed drinking. The concomitant problems of alcohol misuse by women (e.g., depression and inadequate role functioning as a homemaker) are likewise less apt to be visible than those associated with excessive drinking by men (e.g., aggression and lower employment status). The precipitants of drinking episodes as well as of problem-drinking careers are also likely to contain some significantly different elements for men and women. Thus, although there is little evidence that the overall outcomes of treatment for alcohol misuse differ as a function of client gender, efforts to use broad and flexible assessment and treatment approaches capable of accommodating unique gender-related features of problem drinking seem advisable.

By now, it should be evident that our perspective is one that eschews the traditional, unitary concept of "alcoholism." Instead, we favor a multisyndrome, dimensional model that is consistent with contemporary scientific thinking on the complex and interactive "biopsychosocial" etiology of pathology in general (Engel, 1977) and drinking problems in particular (Cloninger, 1987; Tarter, Alterman, & Edwards, 1985). Our approach does not deny the role of biological factors in problem drinking; it simply insists that they are only partial determinants of vulnerability and are the least modifiable components at that. Thus, the focus of assessment and treatment is on the function that drinking serves for an individual, given what can be determined about his or her particular susceptibility to problems. More specifically, we view problem drinking as a maladaptive habit or coping response. Following the basic tenets of social learning theory (Bandura, 1977), we propose that such problem behaviors be analyzed in terms of their antecedents and consequences as affected by differential reinforcements, modeling, and cognitive mediation. Treatments may then be devised to address the specific problems identified in this assessment.

FREQUENT CLINICAL PROBLEMS

Regardless of one's conceptual orientation, there is little question that among the greatest impediments to the successful outpatient treatment of problem drinking is difficulty in engaging clients in the process in the first place and in sustaining their involvement once an entry has been made. We have already noted that only a small percentage of individuals with drinking problems ever receive any treatment for them. Furthermore, of those who do complete an initial screening interview for outpatient treatment, only about a third are still in treatment after four sessions (Baekeland & Lundwall, 1977). It is, of course, conceivable that this reluctance to enter or stay in therapy reflects appropriate skepticism about the efficacy of treatment and an unwillingness to accept the stigmatization that the popular dichotomous views of drinking problems may visit on the participants. However, the pervasive belief in the alcoholism treatment community is that avoidance of and escape from treatment are due to a lack of client motivation (Sterne & Pittman, 1965). More specifically, a personality disposition toward defensive "denial" of drinking problems and of personal inadequacies has been presumed to be basic to the character structure of the alcoholic, and so minimal motivation for change is an expected part of the problem drinking syndrome (e.g., DiCicco, Unterberger, & Mack, 1978). Accordingly, traditionalists hold that the alcoholic either must be allowed to deteriorate to the point where problems can no longer be denied (i.e., must "hit bottom") or must be stripped of all defenses through aggressive confrontation before he or she is "ready" for recovery.

Popular as the trait notion of denial and low motivation is as an explanation of the failure of clients to start, continue, comply with, and/or succeed in treatment, it is a construct almost entirely devoid of empirical basis. Problem drinkers have not been shown to have any consistent personality profile, let alone one with denial as a central feature (Lang, 1983). In a recent review of the literature relevant to motivation for treatment, Miller (1985) also noted that, although certain nonspecific client characteristics (e.g., distress, self-esteem, problem severity, and selected cognitive characteristics) were sometimes moderately correlated with treatment seeking and response, measures of client motivation and of recognition and acceptance of drinking problems were poor predictors of treatment outcome in problem-drinking populations. Of perhaps greater significance, however, was his finding that *therapist* characteristics and behaviors were correlated with client involvement and treatment response. In particular, therapists communicating hostility and pessimism with aggressive confrontation—as alcoholism counselors, convinced of the inherently low motivation of most problem drinkers, yet compelled to argue for client acceptance of the "alcoholic" label and a commitment to abstinence for life, are liable to do—were found to experience more dropouts and generally poorer outcomes. Moreover, clients exposed to such therapy approaches may well be led to accept stable internal attributions for their failures and consequently may be so discouraged and demoralized that they will be even more reluctant to seek help in the future. In contrast, the clients of therapists who are empathetic and who convey expectations of a good prognosis have been found to exhibit greater involvement in treatment and better response to it, even when empathy and expectancy have been systematically controlled or randomly manipulated (e.g., Leake & King, 1977). Thus, client motivation, defined as an inclination to participate in treatment, appears to be subject to change without the potentially counterproductive side effects of "hitting bottom."

Expanding on the conclusion that an exclusive attribution of motivation for treatment (or lack thereof) to intrapsychic determinism is ill-advised, Miller (1983, 1985) proposed that it is better conceived of as a dynamic interpersonal process. This means that, besides some client characteristics, motivation should be understood to involve therapist and even environmental determinants, such as the length of the client waiting period before initial consultation. Greater attention to motivation as a multiply determined phenomenon holds promise as a means of overcoming one of the critical impediments to the outpatient treatment of problem drinking. A more detailed discussion of specific interventions that enhance motivation and commitment to change is incorporated in the later section on treatment applications.

Like motivation, another clinical problem that is not unique to, but is probably more common in, the outpatient setting is the management of clients who do not control their drinking while in therapy or who may even be intoxicated at a treatment session. Most treatment programs are united in their response to this event: they terminate the client's treatment. This approach strikes us as irrational. It is a well-documented fact that the road to the control of problem drinking is often interrupted by detours. It is our position that these ought not to be regarded as evidence of poor motivation, as a failure of willpower, or as a reason for rejection. Instead, ''slips'' should be viewed as learning opportunities even when (perhaps especially when) they happen to coincide with scheduled appointments. As long as the client is sober enough to talk, sessions may go on and important data may be gathered. For instance, details of the antecedents of the lapse in control may be more accessible when drinking episodes are temporally proximal. Likewise, the perceived consequences of drinking and their correspondence to expected effects may be more salient at this time. Finally, the suggestion of possible strategies to *limit* drinking once it has begun may be especially timely under these circumstances, and the client may even benefit from state-dependent learning.

The point of managing lapses of control in the way we have suggested is not that drinking behavior should be encouraged. Indeed, if it were to continue unabated, we would reexamine our problem conceptualization and intervention plan in the particular case, perhaps even considering a more restrictive treatment setting for a time. Rather, we believe it is important to accept the client, to recognize the often precarious nature of remission, and to model an investigative effort to understand the problems that need to be addressed so that effective intervention strategies are devised. These, in fact, constitute the key principles underlying our general approach to treatment. Let us turn now to an outline of their application.

TREATMENT APPLICATIONS

To begin, we should be humble. Drinking problems are complex, and simple solutions should not be expected. Indeed, as we have seen, a careful examination of the outcomes resulting from many professional and other organized efforts to treat problem drinking have not been impressive. Yet, many people do succeed in arresting their alcohol problems with no formal intervention whatsoever. Moreover, the recent development of transtheoretical models of the essential elements, stages, processes, and levels of both assisted and unassisted changes in addictive and habitual behaviors (e.g., Prochaska & DiClemente, 1986) now places us on the threshold of a better understanding of the modifiability of problem drinking. Perhaps, an incorporation of some of these emerging insights into the formulation and application of treatment techniques for problem drinking will put us in a better position to help those who do come to us for assistance.

Returning to our earlier theme of the societal ambivalence about alcohol use, we believe it is imperative that therapists appreciate the dilemma of clients with drinking problems. They are in conflict. For any number of reasons, alcohol consumption has considerable incentive value for them. Furthermore, the gratification associated with drinking is very salient, in part because it is immediate. For these individuals, cessation or even moderation of alcohol use is typically not regarded as an inherently attractive or virtuous goal. Because of the gradual way in which the alcohol intake of many of them has escalated in almost imperceptible steps over extended periods of time, they may be barely cognizant of its level, let alone guided toward treatment by the potentially adverse long-term consequences that may result from it. Instead, most problem-drinking clients are in some sense forced into treatment by a crisis—of liver, lover, livelihood, or law, as the old saying goes. These life stressors are often perceived to be transient, and although it is probably true that most changes in drinking habits coincide with transitions, there is no guarantee that a crisis will provide sufficient impetus for a permanent change having sufficient power to overcome a well-established drinking habit. This is particularly true because clients are disinclined to attribute the crises they experience to their drinking for fear that they will be labeled "alcoholic" and will be exposed to all the ego-threatening stigmatization and other implications that accompany such a classification in this society. Thus, problem-drinking clients who present themselves for treatment, regardless of the nominal reason, represent little more than an *opportunity* for change. This opportunity must be managed carefully if the chances of success are to be maximized.

A first consideration in the management of problem drinking is the question of who the change agent will be. In our view, it must be the clients themselves. This is not to say that drinking behavior cannot be controlled by external change agents. There is, in fact, ample evidence that scientist-practitioners can effectively reduce alcohol consumption in problem drinkers through the announced systematic manipulation of reinforcers according to "contingency contracts." These methods work within both institutional settings (e.g., Griffiths, Bigelow, & Liebson, 1978) and the community (e.g., Azrin, 1976; Miller, 1975). Unfortunately, drinking tends to return to baseline or above when the contingencies are removed. As no one would support the continuous institutionalization of problem drinkers and the prospects of the widespread alteration of community attitudes regarding alcohol use and resource distribution seem dim, some other approach to maintaining and generalizing changes in drinking behavior is needed. The obvious alternative is to help clients, who ultimately choose their own environments and the reinforcement contingencies coincident with them anyway, to learn to control themselves.

The essential elements of a cognitive-behavioral approach to the self-control of problem drinking are twofold. In simple terms, treatment must involve attention to both motive and means, both the will and the way, or both thought and behavior. We borrow from Prochaska and DiClemente's model of change (1986) three central stages involved in effective therapy outcomes:

1. *Contemplation,* when individuals come to recognize a problem; gain insight; develop an understanding of its nature and relation to themselves through observation, analysis, and interpretation; and then make a commitment to change.
2. *Action,* when steps are actually taken to arrest or control the problem.
3. *Maintenance,* when efforts are made to sustain the gains that have been made.

Naturally, some individuals never progress beyond "precontemplation," others fail to make the transition from contemplation to action, and still others enjoy only temporarily successful self-control before relapsing. We believe that much of the ineffectiveness of treatments for problem drinking is attributable to a narrow focus on the action stage and/or to a failure to assist clients in developing both the motive and the means for change at every stage in the sequence.

For simplicity of exposition we structure the remainder of this chapter around the traditional topics of assessment and treatment. However, our coverage of these areas differs from the usual in several ways. First, we present assessment not only as an effort on the part of the therapist to outline the dimensions of the problem and to identify the characteristics of the client and his or her situation that may suggest a matching with certain treatments, but also as a critical time of contemplation when clients assess their commitment to change. Second, treatment is regarded as subsuming both action and maintenance stage inventions because, in our view, drinking behavior is easy to control and indeed, is naturally under control except when it is actually happening. The problem, therefore, is not so much producing sobriety or moderation as it is prolonging or maintaining it. Finally, our intention is primarily to portray the spirit of the cognitive-behavioral approach. For details of the specific techniques, the reader will be referred elsewhere.

One final point should be raised before we proceed. Inasmuch as we are discussing outpatient treatment, our assumption is that those clients who require detoxification and other medical care will already have been treated or will be receiving appropriate treatment concurrently (see Feldman, Pattison, Sobell, Graham, & Sobell, 1975, for a discussion of outpatient alcohol detoxification). Responsible clinical practice dictates, however, that every problem drinker not already under a physician's care be referred for a physical examination, with special attention to problems produced or complicated by alcohol use.

ASSESSMENT

The type of assessment we recommend reflects an interactionist model of the determination of behavior and of behavior change (cf. Endler & Magnusson, 1976). This means that problem-drinking behavior is viewed as resulting from the interaction of both person variables (e.g., biological reactivity and personality traits) and situational variables (e.g., models and reinforcement contingencies). The objective of assessment should be to describe the dimensions of the problem in terms of these variables and in a way that will facilitate treatment planning, client awareness and motivation, and outcome evaluation. This is a dynamic rather than a static process that typically begins with the initial client contact and continues throughout treatment.

The first appointment should be scheduled as soon as is practical after the request for service is received. This promptness communicates concern and caring, while taking advantage of whatever crisis led the client to treatment before its urgency has passed or the client has had an opportunity to prepare elaborate plans to minimize it or defend against it. The management of the initial interview is critical in a variety of ways. It clarifies the client's and the therapist's roles, sets the tone for the clinical relationship, and, by the expectations it creates, may determine whether a client will return for a second appointment. What should the interviewer do?

If clients are to be both the objects and the agents of change, then therapists must assume a receptive and respectful demeanor while enacting the role of expert consultant. Effective consultants do not browbeat ambivalent clients with authoritarian confrontations aimed at the imposition of a single-minded definition of the problem and one unequivocally right solution for it. Even if the label (*alcoholic*) and the simple prescription (lifelong abstinence) is appropriate in a particular case, any client with a modicum of ego strength would be likely to react with anger, resentment, and denial, if not outright rejection of the affront. In effect, the client would be forced into a defensive posture in response to the consultant's denial of the legitimacy of ambivalence (about drinking in this case). Recognition of this natural process led Miller (1983) to develop his system of "motivational interviewing'' in the hope that by eliminating hostile confrontation and insistence on dichotomous labeling, treatment could reach more of the majority of problem drinkers who never will hit a helpless, defenseless ''bottom''. His approach stresses client choice, responsibility, and potential for change. Specific information about problems is elicited and reflected, but the data are used carefully to promote a level of cognitive dissonance that gently helps tip the balance of ambivalence in the direction of a desire for change.

Change for problem-drinking clients is frightening, and the overall benefit of it may be unclear to them. Moreover, addiction may well be the end point of a series of failures and maladaptive efforts to cope, so instilling optimism is often not easy. Kanfer (1986) suggested that the problem-drinking client is grappling with two basic questions about change: ''Will I be better off if I do?'' and ''Will I be able to do it or will I fail?'' The first step is to convince the client that he or she should change, not through scare tactics, but through the promotion of an enhanced awareness of how drinking relates to what is going on in the client's life and of the relative attractiveness of new behavior patterns and lifestyles. The emphasis should be on ''reaching toward'' more than ''escaping from'' if motivation is to be cultivated and maintained. When clients are willing to consider the possibilities, they are also more ready to acquire and practice coping responses to deal with ''craving'' and situations in which relapse is a high risk. This readiness helps make the change process itself as easy as possible. Thus, the therapist in our approach to assessment should offer a stable and supportive partnership that is encouraging as it explores current problems, helps clients recognize them, and establishes a rationale and procedures for self-managed interventions to resolve them and to develop interesting and reinforcing alternatives.

Against the backdrop of the attitudes described above, assessment begins with a solicitation of client concerns and an empathetic response to them. Most clients acknowledge at least some alcohol-related problems when approached in this way. The expression of these concerns may be subtly reinforced, and clients should be encouraged to elaborate. Ambivalence, however, is to be expected and should not be denied. The idea is simply to let clients delineate their own problems and implicitly make their own case for wanting to change. This process is facilitated by a therapist who is receptive and understanding rather than one who seizes every self-disclosure as an opportunity to pronounce the client an ''alcoholic.'' The picture of current concerns may be broadened temporally by inquiring about earlier problems, by asking clients to recount the circumstances surrounding past relapses, and by encouraging clients to imagine or predict the possible precipitants of future problem drinking.

The therapist may wish to introduce self-monitoring early in this otherwise unstructured phase of assessment and contemplation. Typically, clients are asked to keep records of their drinking behavior or simply of their urges to drink, and also to note the surrounding thoughts, emotions, and environments. This exercise is helpful in several ways. First, it further heightens awareness of the problem. Second, it encourages clients to assume the role of detached observers. Third, it provides data on the antecedents and consequences of drinking that may facilitate an analysis of the probable functions of drinking for the individual. Finally, and perhaps most important in the context of motivation, self-monitoring is known to be ''reactive'' and often produces at least a temporary decline in the problem behaviors being observed (Sobell & Sobell, 1978). This effect should be affirmed to bolster the sense of self-efficacy of clients apt to question their ability to change. Similar attention to reinforcing personal responsibility and internal attribution for control should continue throughout therapy.

As a complement to the highly individualized data collected thus far, a battery of standardized assessment instruments is also recommended. The rationale is that this is the most efficient way to sample the widest possible range of indicators that may be relevant to a description of the client, the selection of change strategies, and a prediction of the outcome. Many alternative choices are possible, depending on the individual case and on the specific diagnostic and developmental considerations discussed previously. Among the most rigorously researched and widely used instruments are those developed at the Center for Alcohol Abuse Research and Evaluation in Denver (see Wanberg & Horn, 1983, for details). These include the Alcohol Use Inventory (AUI), the Life Situation Questionnaire (LSQ), and the Personality Assessment Survey (PAS). The AUI taps the client's view of the benefits, concomitants, and consequences of and the concerns about drinking as well as the level of acknowledgement of a drinking problem. Levels of childhood instability (including drinking problems in family members), along with the details of current instability and social, health, legal, employment, and marital problems, are measured by the LSQ. Finally, the PSA assesses key personality characteristics known to vary across subsamples of problem drinkers. Other objective testing of cognitive functioning and style may also prove useful. If a structured-interview format is preferred, many of the data mentioned above may also be obtained by means of the Comprehensive Drinker Profile (Miller & Marlatt, 1984), which contains more detail on drinking behavior *per se*. Whatever the specific choices of instruments, it is probably wise to cover the broad areas of symptoms and situations, cognitions, interpersonal conflicts, family-system conflicts, and intrapersonal problems, as the resulting information may be relevant to determining the best level of intervention as well as the optimal matching of client to treatment technique.

Finally, at a broader, perhaps more philosophical, level, we recommend an assessment of the client's general lifestyle. *Lifestyle imbalance* (Marlatt & Gordon, 1985) is a term used to describe the experience of persons who perceive their lives to be guided largely by external demands ("shoulds"), to the neglect of internal forces consonant with self-expression, fulfillment, or simple pleasure ("wants"). Whether measured rather formally by daily "hassles and uplifts" scales (Kanner, Coyne, Schaefer, & Lazarus, 1981) or by a simple tally of subjectively rated shoulds and wants collected over a brief period of self-monitoring, the identification of serious imbalances may be important. Problem drinkers may be at greater risk for bouts of excessive, self-indulgent alcohol use because their virtuous overrestraint of wants in favor of shoulds leads them to feel they have "earned" a drunk. Many clients readily recognize the dynamics of this erratic shifting from overcontrol to undercontrol and regard the seemingly random fluctuations as uncomfortable. Clarification of this process sets the stage for a more enthusiastic reception to suggestions for improving lifestyle balance through moderation and the introduction of alternative sources and schedules of nondestructive reinforcement.

A comment should be made at this point about our extensive reliance on self-reports in assessment. Obviously, clients can falsify information if they choose to and may even misrepresent facts unintentionally because they simply do not recall. Extensive research on the reliability and validity of self-reports by problem drinkers, however, indicates that, on the whole, these data are remarkably accurate (Marlatt, Stephens, Kivlahan, Brief, & Banajc, 1986). Moreover, if the proper atmosphere of trust and mutual respect has been created, clients should be inclined to try to be honest. Finally, although various direct observational techniques have been developed and refined in the laboratory, they are impractical in most outpatient settings, just as blood, breath, and urine testing would probably be. Perhaps the only viable alternatives for crosschecking self-reports are archival data (police, hospital, and other institutional records) and collateral reports (e.g., from spouses, friends, and employers), both of which are rather intrusive and are not altogether foolproof either. Indeed, if spouses are interviewed (and we believe they should be, if at all possible), the objective probably ought to be to get their perspective on the problem and their reaction to the proposed treatment strategy to determine the likelihood of their assistance or resistance to change—not to check up on the veracity of client self-reports. In the final analysis, we believe that clients, if properly approached, are the best sources of information about themselves. And if we do not communicate confidence in them during assessment, how can we hope to create a positive outcome expectancy for self-control?

After gathering all the data described above, including the results of medical tests such as liver function analysis, clients should be given feedback. This is particularly true where standardized instruments have been used, as their results are often not obvious. Again, a basic principle of our approach to assessment is to be informative, not argumentative, so that client consciousness can be raised without quashing motivation. Thus, the therapist presents facts and any information necessary for interpretation (e.g., cutoff scores and norms) but frees clients to draw their own conclusions. As consultants, therapists may give opinions when asked to and may call attention to information that may otherwise be overlooked, but they should not try to force issues or "prove" anything. In other words, therapists should act to facilitate self-discovery and self-evaluation. If this job has been done properly, clients who indeed have drinking problems should naturally achieve a level of problem awareness and concern that motivates them to consider change. How rapidly this point is reached depends on the client, the dimensions of the problem, and the skill of the therapists, but when it occurs, the client is ready to explore alternatives and their implications. Before discussing options, however, it is often helpful for the therapist to offer a summary of the assessment findings and to invite additions, corrections, and comments from the client. The purpose of this presentation is to consolidate progress to this point. Thus, it should accurately reflect what the client has said or otherwise reported and should call special attention to potentially self-motivating statements that have been made, without denying ambivalent ones.

Assuming that alcohol-related problems are the focus, and not some major psychiatric disorder that has been uncovered in screening, a good place to start the exploration of alternatives is with the clients themselves. Therapists should ask them what they think should be done, just as they were asked for their interpretations of the assessment data. This approach offers an opportunity for the reinforcement of self-initiated ideas for action and may provide valuable clues to what approaches particular clients feel comfortable with and/or have had some success with in the past. The possibility that drinking may continue unabated should also be raised, perhaps in connection with the client's construction of a "decision matrix," in which all the positive and negative, immediate and delayed consequences of either bridled or unbridled drinking are enumerated. This exercise could be accompanied by the client's preparation of a brief autobiography, including projections into the future, to describe life as a drinker or a nondrinker. The object is to help clarify values relevant to the determination to change and to identify possible impediments to proposed changes.

It is entirely possible that some clients will reach this point in the consultation and decide that they do not wish to change. Obviously, this decision is their prerogative, although efforts should be made to redirect such clients, perhaps through referrals for second opinions. Others may choose to change but may elect to do so without further therapist help. This option should not necessarily be discouraged because, as we have noted earlier, many people do arrest their drinking problems with little or no formal intervention. If the client has certain characteristics (e.g., is a socially stable white male over 40 with a severe physical dependence on alcohol, has an externally controlled personality style, is highly religious, or shows cognitive simplicity or a low conceptual level) known to be associated with AA affiliation (Ogborne & Glaser, 1981), exploration of that organization may be suggested. In fact, regardless of treatment decision, any client could be encouraged to visit AA, if only to sample this ubiquitous option, although some warnings of what to expect should be issued. Bibliotherapy is another alternative that may prove suitable for many clients inclined toward independent self-help. Manuals offering simple, self-directed instruction in ways to monitor and reduce drinking, to analyze the environmental and emotional correlates of drinking, and to develop alternatives to drinking (e.g., Miller & Munoz, 1976) appear to be particularly useful to individuals seeking to moderate their drinking (Miller & Hester, 1980).

Having touched on the moderation of drinking as an alternative to the goal of total abstinence, we must comment on this highly controversial option. The issue has been thoroughly aired in many books (e.g., Heather & Robertson, 1983) and articles (e.g., Marlatt, 1983) and is too involved for detailed review here. However, suffice it to say that numerous empirical studies have demonstrated that a substantial minority of both treated and untreated individuals with drinking problems, representing all levels of severity, exhibit long-term maintenance of nonproblem levels of alcohol consumption. Moreover, despite indications that the option of a moderation goal may be most suitable for less severe drinking problems, the only two controlled evaluations to assign clients at random to moderation or total abstinence did not find the problem's severity to be a strong predictor of outcome (Foy, Nunn, & Rychtarik, 1984; Sanchez-Craig, Annis, Bornet, & MacDonald, 1984). Thus, our position is that, although abstinence is the intuitively obvious choice for severe drinking problems in particular, it should not be insisted on for anyone who is not in acute medical distress that is liable to be aggravated by further drinking. Allowed to make an informed choice, most clients choose abstinence anyway, and those who do not tend to be the ones with less severe problems. In addition, it should be noted that any attempts at moderation should enthusiastically apply the best available methods so that the outcomes will provide valuable feedback to clients instead of leaving them to wonder or driving them away.

Assuming the client decides to pursue change with the help of a therapist, what is the next step? An overview of the change process and the general plan for traversing it is the place to start. In a cognitive-behavioral approach, this means calling attention to the need to acquire new coping skills to avoid and substitute for drinking, to foster more functional cognitions about the nature of habits and one's capacity to change them, and to develop an everyday lifestyle more rich in nondestructive sources of gratification. A key point to emphasize is that the motivation or desire to change is essential but is not enough. One must get beyond reliance on fragile "willpower." The goal is to learn how to do things differently and to have the confidence and optimism to apply that knowledge.

TREATMENT: ACTION AND MAINTENANCE

Given the breadth and the specificity of the assessment we have recommended, the resulting data may suggest that certain directions of treatment be divergent for different individuals. For instance, some clients may benefit greatly from vocational rehabilitation, whereas for others, it may be inappropriate to pursue such a course. Much the same may be said about any number of client-specific needs that may arise. Certainly, the matching of clients to all relevant treatments is desirable, but to the extent that the problem area to be addressed is one common to general clinical practice, we will not discuss it here. This is not to suggest that such problems are not potentially quite important to overall treatment success, but simply to acknowledge that a thorough coverage of the many possibilities is beyond the scope of this chapter. Miller and Mastria (1977), among others, have provided highly readable prescriptions for dealing with a variety of such particular areas of client difficulty as they relate to problem drinking. The interested reader is encouraged to consult these sources for a more comprehensive picture of treatment planning. For present purposes, we intend to restrict ourselves to strategies that are broadly applicable to a cross section of problem drinkers. Moreover, although we are cognizant of the importance of interpersonal factors in drinking and of the potentially critical role of spouses and families in the remediation of many alcohol-related problems (cf. McCrady, 1987), coverage of marital and family interventions will also be sacrificed for the sake of brevity. This exclusion will facilitate a clearer focus on self-control and the individual's perspective. Finally, it should be noted that, although the assessment and subtyping of problem drinkers has reached a fairly high level of empirical sophistication, the matching of clients to the best treatments has not. Thus, matching decisions must often be based on logic, intuition, and the preferences of the clients themselves.

To reiterate, the approach outlined here holds that, aside from relatively unalterable biological and personality dispositions, the probability of drinking in a particular situation is a function of (1) the accessibility of alcohol and the constraints on its use; (2) the individual's associations and expectations pertinent to the reinforcing effects of drinking, especially as they relate to the coping demands of the situation; (3) the availability of alternative coping responses relevant to the situational demands; and (4) the individual's interpretation of the options in the situation as they relate to self-control. In addition, the frequency and the specific nature of the "high-risk" drinking situations that individuals are likely to encounter are presumed to be determined, at least in part, by their general lifestyle. These assumptions suggest a number of broad intervention strategies. Each is evaluated here with respect to its logical and empirical underpinnings, its practicality, and its compatibility with a self-control approach.

Limiting the accessibility of alcohol and placing constraints on its use have considerable merit as societal-level strategies, and these methods have enjoyed some empirical support (Moore & Gerstein, 1981). For the problem drinkers in outpatient treatment, however, public policy manipulations lack practicality, and it is safe to predict that alcohol will probably continue to be widely available. Nevertheless, clients should be cautioned not to overlook the possibility that they can manage their drinking more easily if they use "stimulus control" tactics to minimize their exposure to alcohol cues. Becoming more sensitive to and avoiding apparently irrelevant decisions (cf. Marlatt & Gordon, 1985), like meeting a friend in a bar instead of at the theater or keeping beer in the refrigerator "in case friends drop over," may help to reduce temptations. Likewise, engaging in activities having minimal drinking cues and/or limited compatibility with drinking (e.g., gardening), instead of those in which alcohol consumption is well-conditioned response (e.g., watching a ball game), is also a useful tactic to recommend early in treatment. Finally, clients may be encouraged to make reasonable requests of relatives, friends, and other social contacts (e.g., asking them not to offer alcoholic drinks to or buy them for the clients) as a way of expanding stimulus control. Without depending on others, such requests also constitute an implicit public acknowledgement of a problem and a commitment to change that may have motivational value. Unlike therapist- or self-imposed abstinence rules or contingency contracts that rely heavily on external controls or willpower, these techniques represent active plans to avoid high-risk situations, and when applied properly, they tend to engender the increased sense of personal efficacy that is crucial to sustained self-control.

Aversive counterconditioning is another method of reducing an individual's attraction to alcohol (and thereby suppressing or reducing the drinking response) by pairing its consumption with a noxious stimulus or an unpleasant experience. As noted earlier, empirical tests of these methods provide encouraging, but not unequivocally supportive, results for at least short-term outcomes (Miller & Hester, 1986a). The use of emetics in a paradigm that parallels well-documented taste-aversion phenomena apparently produces the best results, but only ''covert sensitization'' procedures, attempting to associate images of drinking with disgusting senses of nausea and vomiting, would appear to be widely applicable in nonresidential settings. This approach has the advantage of greater client participation and the opportunity for self-directed practice at home. However, the vividness of the imagery is difficult to monitor, and the empirical results of covert sensitization have not been as positive as those of chemical aversion (e.g., Telch, Hannon, & Telch, 1984). Perhaps more important, the use of any aversive counterconditioning approach alone fails to address the need to fill the behavioral vacuum left by the elimination of drinking. Unless a more adaptive response is programmed in, one is courting disaster, as there is no guarantee that naturally occurring substitutes will be any better than problem drinking. Thus, covert sensitization may be helpful in ''taking the edge off'' a desire to drink but may be best regarded only as a short-term adjunct to other treatment.

Explanations about the effects of alcohol—often quite independent of specific physiological effects—have been shown to provide powerful motives for the initiation of drinking and to figure heavily in ''loss-of-control'' drinking episodes in persons with alcohol-related problems (for review, see Lang & Michalec, 1989; Marlatt & Rohsenow, 1980). These beliefs, where false or exaggerated in such a way that they contribute to problem drinking, may be dealt with in several ways. First, a special alcohol-education component may be made a part of a broader treatment package. Unlike conventional ''alcoholism'' education programs, which seem to focus on scare tactics and have not been shown to improve outcomes, the focus should be on what has been discovered scientifically that is relevant to the expectancies that may motivate or sustain drinking. For instance, information indicating that alcohol has an initial stimulating effect on physiological responding and is only a depressant as blood-alcohol level rises (Pohorecky, 1977) is often news to the average problem drinker. This information does not deny the subjective experience of a ''rush'' upon drinking, but it illustrates why although some alcohol may be good, more will not be better. Clients armed with such knowledge are in a better position to evaluate their reactions and to make informed choices.

Expectations may also be challenged directly. Although these procedures have not been widely tested in outpatient settings, clients have been given limited doses of alcoholic beverages in controlled situations to demonstrate that ''craving'' to continue drinking will dissipate within a session if the opportunity for more drinks is denied and will extinguish after repeated cue exposures with response prevention over repeated sessions (e.g., Rankin, Hodgson, & Stockwell, 1983). Marlatt and Gordon (1985) also suggested that a ''programmed relapse'' may be a useful experience for clients who insist on a return to drinking because of the effects they expect from or associate with alcohol. These individuals may be asked to meet with the therapist, to detail the expected effects before commencing to drink in the therapist's presence, and then to provide a narrative description of what they actually feel as drinking continues. The inevitable failure of the experience to live up to expectations under these controlled conditions may provide convincing evidence that the circumstances and the social meaning of drinking are more important than the alcohol itself. This recognition, then, may set the stage for behavior change. Other forms of *in vivo* alcohol education, of course, include programs in moderation rather than cessation of alcohol use, such as the one discussed earlier in connection with bibliotherapy (Miller & Munoz, 1976). As already noted, this method has been shown to produce marked improvements in the drinking status of outpatient clients.

One of the cornerstones of cognitive-behavioral approaches to self-control over drinking is coping-skills training. The application of this technique has its conceptual base in laboratory-experimental demonstrations of stress-induced drinking and observations of a positive correlation between problem-drinking episodes and stressful life events (see Tucker, 1985, for a review). More specific investigations of the concomitants of relapses into problem drinking after a period of control (Litman, Eiser, Rawson, & Oppenheim, 1979; Marlatt & Gordon, 1980) have indicated that certain classes of situations seem to be particularly dangerous in precipitating relapses. Among these high-risk situations are negative intrapersonal emotional states (e.g., boredom or depression over job loss), interpersonal distress or conflict (e.g., anger or social anxiety), and external events (e.g., social pressure to drink or exposure to drinking cues). Also implicated are reduced cognitive vigilance and control. These findings clearly suggest the potential utility of training to develop flexible, effective coping skills that are more adaptive than drinking, and of efforts to enhance clients' sense of self-efficacy. Theoretically, the individual faced with a high-risk situation, but lacking adaptive alternative coping responses and/or the confidence to use them, experiences decreased self-efficacy, which, coupled with unchallenged positive expectancies of the effects of drinking, may lead to an initial use of alcohol—a lapse that may ultimately result in a total relapse if drinking continues.

Chaney, O'Leary, and Marlatt (1978) developed a short-term, skill-training intervention to address high-risk situations in problem drinkers. They evaluated the technique on inpatient "alcoholics," but it is equally applicable to outpatient settings and can be individually or group-administered. Basically, clients were given a general problem-solving orientation; then, an array of high-risk situations was described and the clients' initial responses were assessed. The participants entered into detailed discussions of each situation, trying to generate coping options and trace their probable outcomes. The therapists then modeled various constructive coping responses appropriate to the situation, using interpersonal role plays whenever possible. Particularly for intrapersonal stressors, modeling emphasized internal thought processes, cognitive restructuring, and self-statements designed to illustrate a stepwise process of problem solving: define the problem, generate alternatives, evaluate the short- and long-term costs and benefits of each option, choose a solution, and outline the best way to implement the choice. After every modeling demonstration, the subjects chose a particular response, rehearsed and enacted it, and received feedback, instruction, and coaching for improvement. Responses could then be repeated until a mutually acceptable level of performance was reached. A summary and review of the methods used to generate the adequate responses followed. Compared with control groups receiving either no additional treatment or an insight-oriented discussion of high-risk situations, the skills-training group not only was more capable of enacting appropriate responses to the problem situations on predischarge testing, but also experienced fewer and less severe drinking relapses during a 1-year follow-up period.

The Chaney *et al.* (1978) study illustrates several points about skills-training approaches. First, despite being administered without a specific consideration of particular situations that were high risks for each individual treated, the effects were sufficiently potent to produce significant improvements in group outcomes. "Broad-spectrum" behavioral approaches involving a variety of other components that rely on active client learning and self-control (e.g., self-directed stimulus control, stress management, blood-alcohol-level discrimination training, and moderation training), instead of passive resignation and dependence, have enjoyed similar success (Miller & Hester, 1986a). Perhaps it is not the particular behavioral techniques that are solely responsible for these outcomes, but the general conceptualization that underlies their application. In other words, clients may respond in part to nonspecific effects of the general self-control approach. If so, this response underscores the importance of providing a rationale that makes sense or "feels right" in connection with any procedure that is introduced (cf. Frank, 1975). Naturally, attention to the specific needs of clients in selecting particular treatments for them should further serve to reduce resistance and should enhance the success of the treatments. Another potentially critical feature of skills training is that it is geared to generalization in a way that is impossible with interventions that attempt only to suppress drinking directly through the application of contingencies that do not occur naturally in the environment. Finally, because successes based on acquired skills tend to be reinforcing not only in a tangible way, but also in a symbolic way, because of the self-satisfaction and self-confidence they generate, the prospects for long-term control are brightened. Such cognitive features should not be overlooked when recommending treatments aimed primarily at symptom relief. For instance, presenting relaxation procedures (e.g., progressive muscular relaxation and meditation) in a way that accentuates their value as skills that foster perceptions of control may result in more successful applications than when they are recommended simply as a means of reducing anxiety (Klajner, Hartman, & Sobell, 1984). Again, the focus should be on client responsibility, not on creating dependency on the therapist.

Suppose that, despite all the best efforts at stimulus control, alcohol education, skills building, and efficacy enhancement, the client still lapses and takes a drink. What then? Statistics indicate that, far from being a remote possibility, such slips should be expected. This is not to say that they are inevitable, but responsible therapists should prepare clients for the possibility. The primary objective should be to limit the damage attendant to a lapse, to prevent it from becoming a full-blown relapse.

Contrary to popular alcoholism lore, one drink need not always lead to a drunk. Certainly, relapses occurring in the natural setting vary considerably in intensity and duration. In addition, studies of drinkers with very severe problems given access to essentially unlimited supplies of alcohol in inpatient "experimental drinking" programs have indicated that these individuals do not always drink themselves into oblivion or even drink all the alcohol available. Instead, during observations lasting several weeks, they sometimes maintained only mild intoxication for extended periods and were able to terminate drinking episodes spontaneously (Mello, 1972). Furthermore, laboratory analogue experiments (e.g., Marlatt, Demming, & Reid, 1973) investigating factors that influence "loss-of-control" drinking have brought the role of psychological variables in this phenomenon into sharper focus. These studies have shown that "alcoholics" drank significantly more in taste-rating tasks when they thought their beverages contained alcohol—regardless of actual beverage content. Thus, to some extent, the expectations surrounding initial returns to alcohol use may serve to make continued drinking a self-fulfilling prophesy.

At least as important as expectations about relapses are the cognitive-affective reactions that clients may experience on taking a first drink. Marlatt and Gordon (1980, 1985) used the term *abstinence violation effect* (AVE) to describe the dual-component process that may occur in the ill-prepared client. First, the person is likely to experience cognitive dissonance because the drinking behavior is incompatible with a definition of the self as an abstainer. This conflict is emotionally unsettling and tends to produce anxiety, depression, and other negative affective drive states that may push the individual to "give up" control efforts and to continue drinking. Meanwhile, vulnerability is exacerbated if the client attributes the lapse to an internal cause, such as lack of willpower, and consequently experiences guilt, self-blame, and a sense of failure that detracts from self-esteem and self-efficacy. In this weakened state, any recall of alcohol as a means of restoring perceived control or of elevating mood is liable to increase the probability of a severe relapse.

To combat the AVE, the client must be prepared for it. From a behavioral point of view, this preparation may include a formal contract to limit initial use, for example, by agreeing (1) to delay taking that first drink for 20 or 30 minutes to permit time for reflection on whether lapsing is really the choice the client wants to make; (2) to obtain only a single drink, that is, not to purchase a whole bottle of liquor or a six-pack of beer because that would increase the temptation to finish the remaining alcohol; and (3) to allow at least an hour to pass between a first and second drink and, during this time, to review the precipitating events, coping strategies, expected effects, actual effects, and alternatives before drinking anything more. Such contracts may prove useful to particularly insecure clients and may even include response costs (e.g., fines for noncompliance), but we discourage their use beyond the earliest stage of therapy because they foster dependency by transferring some responsibility for change to the therapist. Instead, clients are better helped to reduce the severity of relapses by the offer of a more functional way of cognitively framing the experience.

There is now considerable evidence that the emotional responses associated with threats to control may be altered through cognitive restructuring (e.g., Janis & Rodin, 1979). Based on an analysis of factors contributing to the AVE, Marlatt and Gordon (1985) suggested that teaching clients to view a lapse as a single, isolated event that represents a mistake rather than a catastrophe signifying impending doom helps to minimize the probability of severe relapses. Many clients also benefit from a revision of their overly harsh and punitive standards for success and a redefinition of the causes to which they attribute lapses. Through modeling and direct instruction, they may be taught that perfection is neither expected nor required. Moreover, through a detached and objective attitude, they may come to recognize that drinking lapses are often the result of specific, external, but ultimately controllable factors (e.g., the improper choice of a coping response, fatigue, or an unforeseen stressor) rather than global, internal, and largely unchangeable factors (e.g., deficient willpower or a genetic anomaly). This attitude permits a lapse to be reconceptualized as an opportunity to pinpoint and correct potential vulnerabilities in self-control strategies, an opportunity that therapists should also avail themselves of in debriefing relapsed clients. In addition, alerting clients to the fact that a lapse is merely a temporary discontinuity in control and that the client can quickly regain control simply by ceasing to drink more allows motivation and optimism to thrive in the face of temporary setbacks. A final cognitive measure suggested by the Marlatt and

Gordon relapse prevention model (1985) is the preparation of a client-specific ''reminder card,'' a sort of prosthetic memory device permitting ready access to a systematic cognitive-behavioral plan to follow if a lapse ''emergency'' should occur. This card, along with a programmed relapse as described earlier, and perhaps some simple covert rehearsal of intended actions when faced with high-risk situations, helps to galvanize ideas for averting or minimizing damage due to lapses and the AVE.

Now that we have discussed behavioral and cognitive action interventions for changing drinking patterns and for maintaining control in specific high-risk situations, it is time to return to the topic of motivation. The ultimate goal of treatment must be to establish a stable lifestyle in which there is no need to be preoccupied with resisting temptation. Before this can occur, the client must see and accept the advantages of an addiction-free existence. In other words, changes must be reinforcing. How does this outcome evolve? In the short run, the therapist will want to break the overall task of change into small, manageable pieces, to emphasize proximal goal-setting, to provide feedback and support, and to encourage self-reinforcement with either tangible or symbolic rewards for each successful step. Meanwhile, natural negative reinforcements, such as an end to hangovers or a cessation of family arguments over drinking, helps to sustain effort. However, the potency of self-reinforcement and negative reinforcement for nondrinking is liable to diminish with time. The client must learn to do something else.

The effect of general lifestyle modification as it applies to the maintenance of control over problem drinking is largely untested. Nevertheless, the intuitive appeal of pursuing a healthier and more balanced lifestyle through regular participation in noncompetitive physical exercise (e.g., jogging or aerobics), relaxation activities (e.g., meditation or progressive muscle relaxation), and scheduled self-indulgences of a nondestructive nature (e.g., massage or pursuit of hobbies) is considerable. Moreover, a few studies (Marlatt & Marques, 1977; Murphy, Pagano, & Marlatt, 1986) have lent support to the notion that initiating programs including activities such as these spontaneously produces decreases in alcohol consumption. Finally, anecdotal evidence of the successful long-term arrest of problem drinking by untreated persons and some AA members suggests that a change in life roles and routine environments may be a key factor in maintenance. These are lifestyles adjustments that should be as effective in maintaining change when chosen by clients as they are when they occur coincidentally. The point is that, given the scarcity of proven methods for the enduring control of drinking problems, it makes good sense to entertain many diverse possibilities. The objective of the therapist should be to help clients identify and pursue attainable goals consistent with their character and the accessible environments. Ideally, these should offer some of the same positive outcomes formerly associated with drinking.

SUMMARY

Indications are that the already extraordinarily high individual and societal cost of problem drinking has been unnecessarily elevated to an even higher level by continued reliance on conventional treatments that stress expensive inpatient medical interventions and other traditional regimens having little or no demonstrated efficacy. This state of affairs is apparently the product of historically based social, political, and economic forces that have permitted a rather narrow and largely unsubstantiated view of alcoholism as a progressive, irreversible disease to become entrenched and to dominate conceptualizations of problem drinking. Among the more pernicious consequences of the unitary disease model is its insistence on the dichotomous classification of drinkers into alcoholic and nonalcoholic categories when, in fact, considerable research indicates that a wide range of drinking problems, differentially responsive to a variety of interventions, exists. As a result, many potential clients are essentially deprived of help because they are not willing to accept the pejorative labels and restrictive prescriptions that are associated with traditional concepts.

Our alternative cognitive-behavioral, self-control view of problem drinking as a dysfunctional coping response has as its principal virtue its flexibility. It may be easily applied in outpatient settings, and by empathetically responding to unique individual needs and goals, the model may accommodate the diversity of problem drinkers and cultivate their motivation to change rather than precipitate denial and resistance through confrontation and labeling. The client remains autonomous, and the role of the therapist is that of an expert consultant who assists clients in becoming more aware of their problems, in acquiring alternative coping skills and the confidence to apply them when needed, and in cognitively reframing the meaning of lapses of control so that they are less likely to become devastating relapses. There is also attention to the modification of general life-style in recognition of the fact that long-term control depends on positive reinforcement from everyday experiences, not just relief from drinking problems. Clearly, there is still much to learn, particularly in the area of matching individual clients to optimal treatments, but this is all the more reason to remain flexible and open to new ideas and developments.

ACKNOWLEDGMENT. Preparation of this chapter was supported, in part, by National Institute of Alcohol Abuse and Alcoholism grant R01 AA 06267 to the first author.

REFERENCES

American Psychiatric Association. (1980). *Diagnostic and statistical manual of mental disorders* (3rd ed.; DSM-III). Washington, DC: Author.

Armor, D. J., & Meshkoff, J. E. (1983). Remission among treated and untreated alcoholics. In N. Mello (Ed.), *Advances in substances abuse: Biological and behavioral research* (Vol. 3) (pp. 240–267). Greenwich, CN: JAI.

Azrin, N. H. (1976). Improvements in the community reinforcement approach to alcoholism. *Behaviour Research and Therapy, 14,* 339–348.

Baekeland, F., & Lundwall, L. (1977). Engaging the alcoholic in treatment and keeping him there. In B. Kissin & H. Begleiter (Eds.), *Treatment and rehabilitation of the chronic alcoholic* (pp. 161–196). New York: Plenum Press.

Bandura, A. (1977). *Social learning theory.* Englewood Cliffs, NJ: Prentice-Hall.

Billings, A. G., & Moos, R. H. (1983). Psychological processes of recovery among alcoholics and their families: Implications for clinicians and program evaluators. *Addictive Behavior, 8,* 205–218.

Brandsma, J. M., Maultsby, M. C., & Welsh, R. J. (1980). *The outpatient treatment of alcoholism: A review and comparative study.* Baltimore, MD: University Park Press.

Cahalan, D., Cisin, I., & Crossley, N. (1969). American drinking practices: A national study of drinking behavior and attitudes (Monograph No. 6). New Brunswick, NJ: Rutgers Center of Alcohol Studies.

Chaney, E., O'Leary, M., & Marlatt, G. (1978). Skill training with alcoholics. *Journal of Consulting and Clinical Psychology, 46,* 1092–1104.

Cloninger, C. R. (1987). Neurogenetic adaptive mechanisms in alcoholism. *Science, 236,* 410–416.

Cronkite, R., & Moos, R. (1978). Evaluating alcoholism treatment programs: An integrated approach. *Journal of Consulting and Clinical Psychology, 46,* 1105–1119.

Cruze, A. M., Harwood, H. J., Kristiansen, P. L., Collins, J. J., & Jones, D. C. (1981). *Economic costs to society of alcohol, drug abuse, and mental illness.* Rockville, MD: Alcohol, Drug Abuse, and Mental Health Administration.

DiCicco, L., Unterberger, H., & Mack, J. E. (1978). Confronting denial: An alcoholism intervention strategy. *Psychiatric Annals, 8,* 596–606.

Ditman, K. S., Crawford, G. G., Forgy, E. W., Moskowitz, H., & MacAndrew, C. (1967). A controlled experiment on the use of court probation for drunk arrests. *American Journal of Psychiatry, 124,* 160–163.

Emrick, C. D. (1975). A review of psychologically oriented treatment of alcoholism: 2. The relative effectiveness of different treatment approaches and the effectiveness of treatment versus no treatment. *Journal of Studies on Alcohol, 36,* 88–108.

Emrick, C. D., & Hansen, J. (1983). Assertions regarding effectiveness of treatment for alcoholism. *American Psychologist, 38,* 1078–1083.

Endler, N. S., & Magnusson, D. (1976). Toward an interactional psychology of personality. *Psychological Bulletin, 83,* 956–974.

Engel, G. (1977). The need for a new medical model: A challenge for biomedicine. *Science, 196,* 129–136.

Feldman, D., Pattison, E., Sobell, L., Graham, T., & Sobell, M. (1975). Outpatient alcohol detoxification: Initial findings on 564 patients. *American Journal of Psychiatry, 132,* 407–412.

Fillmore, K. M. (1975). Relationships between specific drinking problems in early adulthood and middle age. *Journal of Studies on Alcohol, 36,* 882–907.

Fillmore, K. M. (1987). Prevalence, incidence, and chronicity of drinking patterns and problems among men as a function of age: A longitudinal and cohort analysis. *British Journal of Addiction, 82,* 77–83.

Foy, D. W., Nunn, B. L., & Rychtarik, R. G. (1984). Broad-spectrum behavioral treatment for chronic alcoholics: Effects of training controlled drinking skills. *Journal of Consulting and Clinical Psychology, 52,* 218–230.

Frank, J. (1975). *Persuasion and healing* (2nd ed.). Baltimore, MD: Johns Hopkins University Press.

Fuller, R. K., & Roth, H. P. (1979). Disulfiram for the treatment of alcoholism: An evaluation in 128 men. *Annals of Internal Medicine, 90,* 901–904.

Griffiths, R., Bigelow, G., & Liebson, I. (1978). The relationship of social factors to ethanol self-administration in alcoholics. In P. Nathan, G. Marlatt, & T. Lorberg (Eds.), *Alcoholism: New directions in behavioral research and treatment* (pp. 351–379). New York: Plenum Press.

Hansen, J., & Emrick, C. D. (1983). Whom are we calling "alcoholic"? *Bulletin of the Society of Psychologists in Addictive Behaviors, 2,* 164–178.

Heather, N., & Robertson, I. (1983). *Controlled drinking* (rev. ed.). London: Methuen.

Janis, I. L., & Rodin, J. (1979). Attribution, control, and decision making: Social psychology and health care. In G. Stone, F. Cohen, & N. Adler (Eds.), *Health psychology: A handbook.* San Francisco: Jossey-Bass.

Jessor, R., & Jessor, S. (1977). *Problem behavior and psychosocial development: A longitudinal study of youth.* New York: Academic Press.

Kanfer, F. H. (1986). Implications of a self-regulation model of therapy for treatment of addictive behaviors. In W. R. Miller & N. Heather (Eds.), *Treating addictive behaviors: Processes of change* (pp. 29–47). New York: Plenum Press.

Kanner, A. D., Coyne, J. C., Schaefer, C., & Lazarus, R. S. (1981). Comparison of two modes of stress measurement: Daily hassles and uplifts vs. major life events. *Behavioural Medicine, 4,* 1–39.

Kissin, B., Platz, A., & Su, W. H. (1971). Selective factors in treatment choice and outcome in alcoholics. In N. Mello & J. Mendelson (Eds.), *Recent advances in studies of alcoholism* (pp. 781–802). Washington, DC: U.S. Government Printing Office.

Klajner, F., Hartman, L. M., & Sobell, M. B. (1984). Treatment of substance abuse by relaxation training. *Addictive Behaviors, 9,* 41–55.

Knowles, P. L. (1983). Inpatient versus outpatient treatment of substance misuse in hospitals: 1975–1980. *Journal of Studies on Alcohol, 44,* 384–387.

Lang, A. R. (1983). Addictive personality: A viable construct. In P. Levison, D. Gerstein, & Maloff, D. (Eds.), *Commonalities in substance abuse and habitual behavior* (pp. 157–235). Lexington, MA: Lexington Books.

Lang, A. R., & Marlatt, G. A. (1982). Problem drinking: A social learning perspective. In R. Gatchel, A. Baum, & J. Singer (Eds.), *Handbook of psychology and health* (Vol. 1) (pp. 121–169). Hillsdale, NJ: Lawrence Erlbaum.

Lang, A. R., & Michalec, E. M. (1989). Expectancy effects in reinforcement from alcohol. In W. M. Cox (Ed.), *Why people drink: Parameters of alcohol as a reinforcer* (pp. 193–232). New York: Gardner Press.

Lazarus, A. (1965). Towards the understanding and effective treatment of alcoholism. *South Africian Medical Journal, 39,* 736–741.

Leake, G. J., & King, A. S. (1977). Effect of counselor expectations on alcoholic recovery. *Alcohol Health Research World, 11,* 16–22.

Levine, H. (1978). The discovery of addiction. Changing conceptions of habitual drunkenness in American history. *Journal of Studies on Alcohol, 39,* 143–174.

Lisansky-Gomberg, E. (1982). Alcohol use and alcohol problems among the elderly. *Alcohol and health monograph* (No. 4) *Special populations* (pp. 263–290). Rockville, MD: National Institute of Alcohol Abuse and Alcoholism.

Litman, G., Eiser, J., Rawson, N., & Oppenheim, A. (1979). Difference in relapse precipitants and coping behavior between alcohol relapsers and survivors. *Behavior Research and Therapy, 17,* 89–84.

MacAndrew, C. (1981). What the MAC scale tells us about alcoholic men: An interpretive review. *Journal of Studies on Alcohol, 42,* 604–625.

Maisto, S. A., & McCollam, J. B. (1980). The use of multiple measures of life health to assess alcohol treatment outcome: A review and critique. In L. Sobell, M. Sobell, & E. Ward (Eds.), *Evaluating alcohol and drug abuse treatment effectiveness: Recent advances.* New York: Pergamon Press.

Marlatt, G. A. (1983). The controlled-drinking controversy. *American Psychologist, 38,* 1097–1110.

Marlatt, G. A. (1987). Research and political realities: What the next twenty years hold for behaviorists in the alcohol field. *Advances in Behaviour Research and Therapy, 9,* 165–171.

Marlatt, G. A., & Gordon, J. R. (1980). Determinants of relapse: Implications for the maintenance of behavior change. In P. Davidson & S. Davidson (Eds.), *Behavioral medicine: Changing health lifestyles.* New York: Brunner/Mazel.

Marlatt, G. A., & Gordon, J. R. (Eds.). (1985). *Relapse prevention: Maintenance strategies in the treatment of addictive behaviors.* New York: Guilford Press.

Marlatt, G. A., & Marques, J. (1977). Meditation, self-control and alcohol use. In R. Stuart (Ed.), *Behavioral self-management.* New York: Brunner/Mazel.

Marlatt, G. A., & Rohsenow, D. (1980). Cognitive processes in alcohol use: Expectancy and the balanced-placebo design. In N. Mello (Ed.), *Advances in substance abuse: Behavioral and biological research.* Greenwich, CT: JAI.

Marlatt, G. A., Demming, B., & Reid, J. B. (1973). Loss of control drinking in alcoholics: An experimental analogue. *Journal of Abnormal Psychology, 81,* 233–241.

Marlatt, G. A., Stephens, R. S., Kivlahan, D., Brief, D. J., & Banajc, M. (1986). *Empirical evidence on the reliability and validity of self-reports of alcohol use and associated behaviors.* Paper presented at National Institute of Alcohol Abuse and Alcoholism Workshop on the Validity of Self-Report in Alcoholism Treatment Research, Washington, DC.

McCrady, B. S. (1987). Interpersonal contexts, alcohol consumption and alcoholism: Implications for treatment. *Advances in Behaviour Research and Therapy, 9,* 127–143.

McLachlan, J. (1974). Therapy strategies, personality orientation, and recovery from alcoholism. *Canadian Psychiatric Association Journal, 19,* 25–30.

Mello, N. (1972). Behavioral studies of alcoholism. In B. Kissin & H. Begleiter (Eds.), *Biology of alcoholism* (Vol. 2). New York: Plenum Press.

Miller, P. M. (1975). A behavioral intervention program for chronic public drunkenness offenders. *Archives of General Psychiatry, 32,* 915–918.

Miller, P. M., & Mastria, M. A. (1977). *Alternatives to alcohol abuse: A social learning approach.* Champaign, IL.: Research Press.

Miller, W. R. (1983). Motivational interviewing with problem drinkers. *Behavioural Psychotherapy, 11,* 147–172.

Miller, W. R. (1985). Motivation for treatment: A review with special emphasis on alcoholism. *Psychological Bulletin, 98,* 84–107.

Miller, W. R., & Hester, R. K. (1980). Treating the problem drinker: Modern approaches. In W. R. Miler (Ed.), *The addictive behaviors: Treatment of alcoholism, drug abuse, smoking, and obesity* (pp. 11–141). Oxford: Pergamon Press.

Miller, W. R., & Hester, R. K. (1986a). The effectiveness of alcoholism treatment: What research reveals. In W. R. Miller & N. Heather (Eds.), *Treating addictive behaviors: Processes of change* (pp. 121–174). New York: Plenum Press.

Miller, W. R., & Hester, R. K. (1986b). Inpatient alcoholism treatment: Who benefits? *American Psychologist, 41,* 794–805.

Miller, W. R., & Hester, R. K. (1986c). Matching problem drinkers with optimal treatments. In W. R. Miller &

N. Heather (Eds.), *Treating addictive behaviors: Processes of change* (pp. 175–204). New York: Plenum Press.

Miller, W. R., & Marlatt, G. A. (1984). *Manual for the comprehensive drinker profile.* Odessa, FL: Psychological Assessment Resources.

Miller, W. R., & Munoz, R. F. (1976). *How to control your drinking.* Englewood Cliffs, NJ: Prentice-Hall.

Moore, M. H., & Gerstein, D. R. (1981). *Alcohol and public policy: Beyond the shadow of prohibition.* Washington, DC: National Academy Press.

Murphy, T. J., Pagano, R. R., & Marlatt, G. A. (1986). Lifestyle modification with heavy alcohol drinkers: Effects of aerobic exercise and meditation. *Addictive Behaviors, 11,* 175–186.

National Institute of Alcohol Abuse and Alcoholism. (1983). *Alcohol and health: Fifth special report to the U.S. Congress.* Rockville, MD: Author.

Ogborne, A. C., & Glaser, F. B. (1981). Characteristics of affiliates of Alcoholics Anonymous: A review of the literature. *Journal of Studies on Alcohol, 42,* 661–675.

Peele, S. (1986). Denial—of reality and of freedom—in addiction research and treatment. *Bulletin of the Society of Psychologist in Addictive Behaviors, 5,* 149–166.

Pohorecky, L. (1977). The biphasic actions of ethanol. *Biobehavior Review, 1,* 231–240.

Polich, M., Armor, D., & Braiker, H. (1980). Patterns of alcoholism over four years. *Journal of Studies on Alcohol, 41,* 397–416.

Prochaska, J. O., & DiClemente, C. C. (1986). Toward a comprehensive model of change. In W. R. Miller & N. Heather (Eds.), *Treating addictive behaviors: Processes of change* (pp. 3–27). New York: Plenum Press.

Rankin, H., Hodgson, R., & Stockwell, T. (1983). Cue exposure and response prevention with alcoholics: A controlled trial. *Behaviour Research and Therapy, 21,* 435–446.

Sadava, S. (1985). Problem behavior theory and the consumption and consequences of alcohol use. *Journal of Studies on Alcohol, 46,* 392–397.

Sanchez-Craig, M., Annis, H. M., Bornet, A. R., & MacDonald, K. R. (1984). Random assignment to abstinence and controlled drinking: Evaluation of a cognitive-behavioral program for problem drinkers. *Journal of Consulting and Clinical Psychology, 52,* 390–403.

Saunders, B. (1985). Treatment does not work: Some criteria of failure. In N. Heather, I. Robertson, & P. Davies (Eds.), *The misuse of alcohol: Crucial issues in dependence, treatment, and prevention* (pp. 102–116). London: Croom Helm.

Saxe, L., Dougherty, D., Esty, K., & Fine, M. (1983). The effectiveness and costs of alcoholism treatment. (Office of Technology Assessment Case Study No. 22). Washington, DC: U.S. Government Printing Office.

Schuckit, M. A. (1979). Treatment of alcoholism in office and outpatient settings. In J. Mendelson & N. Mello (Eds.), *The diagnosis and treatment of alcoholism* (pp. 229–256). New York: McGraw-Hill.

Skinner, H. A. (1981). Comparison of clients assigned to inpatient and outpatient treatment for alcoholism and drug addiction. *British Journal of Psychiatry, 138,* 312–320.

Sobell, L. C., & Sobell, M. B. (1982). Alcoholism treatment outcome evaluation methodology. In *Prevention, intervention, and treatment: Concerns and models.* (Alcohol and Health Monograph No. 3; DHHS Publication No. [ADM] 82-1192). Washington, DC: U.S. Government Printing Office.

Sobell, M. B., & Sobell, L. C. (1978). *Behavioral treatment of alcohol problems.* New York: Plenum Press.

Sobell, M. B., & Sobell, L. C. (1984). The aftermath of heresy: A response to Pendery et al's (1982) critique of "Individualized behavior therapy for alcoholics." *Behavior Research and Therapy, 22,* 413–440.

Sterne, M. W., & Pittman, D. J. (1965). The concept of motivation: A source of institutional and professional blockage in the treatment of alcoholics. *Quarterly Journal of Studies on Alcohol, 26,* 41–57.

Tarter, R. E., Alterman, A. I., & Edwards, K. L. (1985). Vulnerability to alcoholism in men: A behavior-genetic perspective. *Journal of Studies on Alcohol, 46,* 329–356.

Telch, M. J., Hannon, R., & Telch, C. F. (1984). A comparison of cessation strategies for the outpatient alcoholic. *Addictive Behaviors, 9,* 103–109.

Tucker, J. (1985). Stressful events and human drinking behavior: The role of contextual variables. In E. Gottheil (Ed.), *Stress: Alcohol and drug interactions.* Springfield, IL: Charles C Thomas.

Uecker, A. E., & Solberg, K. B. (1973). Alcoholics' knowledge about alcohol problems: Its relationship to significant outcomes. *Quarterly Journal of Studies on Alcohol, 34,* 509–513.

Wanberg, K. W., & Horn, J. L. (1983). Assessment of alcohol use with multidimensional concepts and measures. *American Psychologist, 38,* 1055–1069.

Wiener, C. L. (1981). *The politics of alcoholism.* New Brunswick, NJ: Transaction Books.

Wilsnack, S., & Beckman, L. (1984). *Alcohol problems in women: Antecedents, consequences, and intervention.* New York: Guilford Press.

19

Eating Disorders

L. K. GEORGE HSU

INTRODUCTION

The eating disorders of anorexia nervosa and bulimia nervosa have been estimated to affect between .5% and 2% of young women in Western societies (Cooper, Charnock, & Taylor, 1987; Crisp, Palmer, & Kalucy, 1976) and are probably becoming more common. For anorexia nervosa, case register and hospital record studies as well as population surveys indicate that the increase in the number of patients is probably due to an increase in incidence rather than in case referral (Crisp *et al.*, 1976; Jones, Fox, Babigan, & Hutton, 1980; Kendell, Hall, Hailey, & Babigan, 1973; Szmukler, McCance, McCrone, & Hunter, 1986; Theander, 1970; Willi & Grossman, 1983). This finding has clear implications for our search for the etiology of the eating disorders. Some have dismissed the search for causes as being irrelevant on the grounds that the disorders represent interactional and thus circular processes (e.g., Moley, 1983). This attitude is unfortunate because it may lead to premature foreclosure on further discussion and research. And it is misguided for the simple reason that, even if the process is interactive, self-reinforcing, and circular, the question remains why such processes, presumably present in all families, become pathological (i.e., correlated with the presence of an eating disorder) in some families and not in others.

The eating disorders primarily affect young Caucasian females from middle to upper social-class backgrounds in developed countries, and they always occur in the context of dieting to control or lose weight. In non-Western cultures, the disorders are apparently common in developed countries such as Japan (Suematsu, Ishikawa, Kubocki, & Ito, 1985) but are rare in less developed countries such as Malaysia (Buhrich, 1981). In a survey of some 1000 London highschool students, Patton (1988) found dieting to be a

L. K. GEORGE HSU • Western Psychiatric Institute and Clinic, University of Pittsburgh, Pittsburgh, Pennsylvania 15213.

significant risk factor in the subsequent development of an eating disorder. It is therefore safe to assume that the prevalence of the eating disorders in a given community is directly proportional to the number of subjects in the general population who are engaged in dieting. Nevertheless, not everyone who embarks on a diet develops an eating disorder. Other factors such as personality characteristics (Garner, Olmsted, Polivy, & Garfinkel, 1984), a family history of eating disorders, of depression, and of alcoholism and substance abuse (Hudson, Pope, Jonas, & Yurgelon-Todd, 1983; Rivinus, Biederman, Herzog, Kemper, Harper, Harmatz, & Houseworth, 1984), competitiveness, and a need for control of weight and shape (Garner & Garfinkel, 1980; Szmukler, Eisler, Gillis, & Hayward, 1985) may also increase the risk of developing an eating disorder. The search for endocrine or metabolic causes has so far proved unfruitful. However, if the control of eating and weight is finally mediated through biological mechanisms, it should not be surprising if, eventually, some disturbance in these control mechanisms is found.

Two other issues deserve to be mentioned here because they are relevant to treatment. The first is the relentless cultural pressure on women and sometimes on men to be slim. The majority of young Caucasian women are unhappy about their size and weight and shape, and as a result, many are dieting rigorously (Garn & Clark, 1975; Huenemann, Shapiro, Hampton, & Mitchell, 1966; Johnson, Lewis, Love, Lewis, & Stuckey, 1983; Nylander, 1971). Unfortunately, the issue is further compounded by finding that, for the young Caucasian female, satisfaction with physical characteristics is highly correlated with self-esteem (Lerner & Karabenick, 1974; Tobin-Richards, Boxer, & Petersen, 1983) and that the current feminine physical ideal is a lean lithe figure (Faust, 1983; Furnham & Alibhai, 1983; Jourard & Secord, 1955). This cultural bias toward slimness is particularly unfortunate because it is occurring at a time when young people in the West are generally becoming fatter and heavier (Garner, Garfinkel, Schwartz, & Thompson, 1980). Further, there is some evidence that the young Caucasian female is particularly prone to develop low self-esteem and greater self-consciousness and may have more difficulty with identity achievement (Marsha & Friedman, 1970; Orlofsky, 1978). Some researchers have argued that such insecurity intensifies their efforts to control their shape and weight in order to seek external approval (Boskind-Lodahl, 1976; Orbach, 1985).

The second issue relevant to treatment is the effects of starvation. Keys, Brozek, Henschel, Michaelson, and Taylor (1950) conducted an experiment at the University of Minnesota Nutrition Laboratory during World War II to study the effects of starvation. Thirty-six healthy young men without much preoccupation with weight and dieting were subjected to a 24-week semistarvation diet of about 1,500 calories per day after a 12-week adaptation period during which they consumed, on average, 3,400 calories per day. During the semistarvation period, they were given two meals a day based on a 3-day rotation menu. Within a matter of weeks of being on the semistarvation diet, the subjects reported an increase in moodiness, irritability, insomnia, and lethargy, and a decrease in concentration and sexual interest. There was a dramatic increase in preoccupation with food and cooking and recipes, and some reported dreams about food, including one about cannibalism. The subjects either spent hours over their small meals or else gulped their food down all at once. Bizarre food combinations and unusual eating habits such as plate licking became common, and there was an increase in the consumption of food substitutes such as coffee and tea and chewing gum. Four men became very depressed; two had to be hospitalized, including one who self-mutilated. Several admitted to breaking their diet and binge eating, including one who ate food out of a garbage can and vomited. During the 12 weeks of partial rehabilitation in which the intake was somewhat increased, the symptoms were not entirely reversed. Twelve men then agreed to stay on for further rehabilitation, and on the days that their eating was unrestricted, splurges of up to 10,000 calories per day were common. Some men ate until they got sick. Some became concerned about the fat accumulation in their abdomen and buttocks. This experiment clearly demonstrates that many of the features of the eating disorders occur directly as a result of the semistarvation that the patients impose on themselves to lose weight.

HISTORICAL PERSPECTIVE

The account of Richard Morton (1694) of an 18-year-old woman who died from what he called the "nervous atrophy" is widely regarded as the first medical report of a case of anorexia nervosa, and it has been repeatedly quoted (e.g., Bliss & Branch, 1960; Halmi, 1980; Nemiah, 1950). In the same treatise, Morton reported more briefly on a case of nervous atrophy in a 16-year-old boy who subsequently recovered (see Bliss & Branch, 1960, p. 11). Sir William Withey Gull, a Guy's Hospital physician, who was also in charge of the hospital's lunatic ward and later became physician to Queen Victoria, coined the term *anorexia nervosa* in 1874. Ernest Charles Laseque, a professor of medicine in Paris, named the illness *anorexie hystérique* in 1873. Subsequently, in both France and Italy, the illness was called *anorexie mentale,* a term used by Henri Huchard in 1883. Gilles de LaTourette (1895) was perhaps the first clinician to distinguish primary anorexia from secondary "gastric" anorexia and saw that the former was characterized by a refusal to eat rather than by a loss of hunger. However, the term was subsequently loosely applied to various conditions of weight loss, although Dejerine and Gauckler (1913) continued to distinguish primary from secondary *anorexie mentale.* More confusion occurred when, in 1914, Morris Simmonds, a Hamburg pathologist, published the first of a series of articles on "fatal hypophyseal atrophy." As a result, anorexia nervosa became widely regarded as hypophyseal cachexia and was treated with pituitary extracts and implants. However, physicians such as Berkman (1930) and Ryle (1936) never lost sight of the basic disturbance of the disorder. In 1949, Sheehan and Summers published a definitive article distinguishing anorexia nervosa from pituitary insufficiency and set to rest, at least for most clinicians, the confusion between the two disorders.

However, anorexia nervosa was not to emerge as a distinct clinical entity until the early 1960s, when the concept of primary anorexia nervosa was rediscovered by clinicians such as Bruch (1962) and King (1963). Even in an otherwise remarkably comprehensive monograph on anorexia nervosa, Bliss and Branch (1960) defined anorexia nervosa as "a malnutrition due to deficient diet, in which the calorie restriction is entirely psychological" (p. 24). In part, this overextension of the concept of anorexia nervosa is related to the misconception that the patient's refusal to eat is due to a loss of appetite (i.e., anorexia). It was not until the cardinal feature of "relentless pursuit of thinness" (Bruch, 1962), "weight phobia" (Crisp, 1967), and "fear of fatness" (Russell, 1970) was clearly identified that anorexia nervosa finally achieved its own identity. Unfortunately, many researchers still regard anorexia nervosa as an appetitive disorder, and more recently, some have revived the idea that anorexia nervosa is a variant of an affective disorder (Cantwell, Sturzenberger, Burroughs, Salkin, & Green, 1977), a point we return to briefly later.

Overeating occurring in the context of anorexia nervosa was recognized by Gull himself (1874), and bulimia has been considered a sign of chronic anorexia nervosa by more recent researchers (Hsu, Crisp, & Harding, 1979; Morgan & Russell, 1975). Self-induced vomiting has also been found to indicate poor prognosis (Hsu *et al.*, 1979; Morgan & Russell, 1975; Theander, 1970). Although self-induced vomiting often follows bingeing, it is not always so, and anorectic patients may vomit even after a small intake of food. Some even spit out their saliva for fear that they may gain weight by swallowing it. Following on an early observation by Nemiah (1950) that those anorectics who vomited were phenomenologically different from those who simply refused food, Beumont, George, and Smart (1976) suggested that anorexia nervosa may be subdivided into two subgroups: restrictor and vomiter. At about the same time, it became increasingly recognized that binge–purge behavior may occur in individuals who are at normal (i.e., average) weight and that it may become the predominant feature, overshadowing other concomitant symptoms. Since then, the terms *bulimarexia* (Boskind-Lodahl, 1976; Bruch, 1982, described the term as a semantic atrocity), *kibarashi gui* (i.e., orgiastic gorging; Nogami & Yabana, 1977), *dietary chaos syndrome* (Palmer, 1979), *bulimia nervosa* (Russell, 1979), and *abnormal normal weight-control syndrome* (Crisp, 1981), among others, have been proposed for the syndrome. The third edition of the American Psychiatric Association's *Diagnostic and Statistical Manual of Mental Disorders* (DSM-III; APA, 1980) used the term *bulimia* to delineate the syndrome from anorexia nervosa, and the revised DSM-III (DSM-III-R; APA, 1987) changed it, appropriately, to *bulimia nervosa*. Despite the differences in clinical features, it is still unclear whether anorexia nervosa and bulimia nervosa are best regarded as distinct syndromes or as the two extremes of a continuous spectrum, a point we will discuss presently.

DIAGNOSTIC AND DEVELOPMENTAL PERSPECTIVES

Two issues underlie the problem of diagnosing the eating disorders. The first is whether the eating disorders occur on a continuum with "normal" dieting and preoccupation with weight, and the second is whether the two disorders are distinct from each other. These issues are somewhat academic to the clinician, but they are relevant to the concept of the eating disorders and their treatment.

Nylander (1971) seemed to suggest that anorexia nervosa and dieting occur on a continuum. His survey of over 2,000 Norwegian high-school students indicated that anorectic symptoms occur on a continuum of severity. Other surveys have also supported this view (Button & Whitehouse, 1981; Szmukler *et al.*, 1985). These findings are in keeping with the finding, already briefly reviewed, that eating disorders are more common among populations that diet to control weight (Garner & Garfinkel, 1980; Szmukler, 1985). However, both Bruch (1973) and Crisp (1980) have stated that anorexia nervosa is distinct from the dieting and preoccupation with weight that occur in "normal" young women. Bruch believed that anorectic patients show three basic psychological disturbances that set them apart from "normal" women: a disturbance of delusional proportions in body image and body concept, a disturbance in the accuracy of the perception or cognitive interpretation of stimuli arising in the body, and a paralyzing sense of ineffectiveness. Crisp conceptualized anorexia nervosa as a psychobiosocial retreat from the maturational crisis and the demands of adolescence and adulthood, expressed through starvation to achieve a prepubertal body. Thus, the "goal" of anorexia nervosa is distinct from that of "normal" dieting to achieve a low average weight. Although these arguments are persuasive, they have never been empirically tested.

Garner *et al.* (1984) used the Eating Disorder Inventory (EDI) to study the psychological traits of anorectic, weight preoccupied, and non-weight-preoccupied women. They found that anorectics and weight-preoccupied women were best differentiated by the subscales of ineffectiveness, interpersonal distrust, and lack of interoceptive awareness on the EDI. Further, by using cluster analysis, the weight-preoccupied women could be further divided into two subgroups on the basis of their subscale scores on the EDI—one characterized by elevated scores on all EDI subscales (i.e., a pathological weight-preoccupied group) and one by elevated scores on only the subscales of drive for thinness, body dissatisfaction, and perfectionism (i.e., a nonpathological weight-preoccupied group). The authors argued that these findings supported the view that some weight-preoccupied women displayed psychopathology similar to anorectic patients whereas others were similar only with respect to their concern about weight and dieting. However, unless it can be shown that the pathological weight-preoccupied group eventually develops anorexia nervosa, whereas few or none of those in the nonpathological weight-preoccupied group does, then the findings still indicate that anorexia nervosa and normal dieting occur on a continuum. Community surveys (e.g., Patton, 1988) and "high risk" studies (e.g., Szmukler, Eisler, Gillis, & Hayward, 1985) have found no clear demarcation between excessive dieting and subclinical or diagnosable eating disorders.

Diagnostic criteria are established, among other reasons, to delineate a "case" from a "noncase" and one disorder from another. Early writers regarded self-imposed starvation as nonspecific (Bliss & Branch, 1960; Kay & Leigh, 1954; Nemiah, 1950). Recent criteria reflect the current conceptualization of the disorders but are likely to change with further progress in the understanding of the two disorders. Broadly speaking, attempts to define anorexia nervosa may be divided into those that use a more conceptual approach and those that use a more operational approach. Russell (1970), Garrow, Crisp, Jordan, Meyer, Russell, Silverstone, Stunkard, and VanHallie (1975), and Crisp (1977) have used a conceptual approach. Minor variations aside, they have all included the following elements: self-inflicted weight loss, amenorrhea in the female, and the characteristic psychopathology of the fear of fatness. Although the amount of weight loss or the degree of starvation was not explicitly defined, the implication was that there had to be enough weight loss for the effects of starvation to occur. However, it must be stated that Russell (1970) and Garrow *et al.* (1975) implied that the hypothalamic disorder, including the amenorrhea, may have occurred for other reasons than the starvation. Dally (1969) was perhaps the first to use a more operational approach, and this was taken up by Feighner, Robins, Guze, Woodruff, Winokur, and Munoz (1972), the DSM-III (APA, 1980), and the DSM-III-R (APA, 1987). The DSM-III-R criteria emphasize the self-imposed low weight, the weight phobia, the disturbance in body concept, and amenorrhea in the female. For body weight, a level of 15% below normal was suggested, and for amenorrhea, absence of three consecutive cycles. Age of onset was deleted. These changes are welcome and avoid the pitfalls of the DSM-III criteria (Hsu, 1986).

Binge eating as defined by the DSM-III is probably common among young college women (Halmi, Falk, & Schwartz, 1981), and as already mentioned, binge–purge behavior was earlier regarded as a part of the anorectic syndrome. The DSM-III used the term *bulimia* to distinguish the disorder from anorexia nervosa. The DSM-III-R changed it to *bulimia nervosa,* eliminating the confusion of using a term both for the symptom of binge eating and the syndrome of the disorder. The criteria emphasize the presence of bulimic episodes, the subjective feeling of lack of control during a binge, the behavior intended to prevent weight loss, a minimum frequency of two episodes per week, and a persistent concern about shape and weight. In contrast to the DSM-III, the DSM-III-R makes no mention of the actual body weight.

The DSM-III-R, by using operational criteria, implies, perhaps unintentionally, that the difference between a case and a noncase is quantitative and not qualitative. It also implies that the two disorders are distinct, and that, in a low-weight bulimic, both diagnoses should be made. A residual category of ''eating disorder not otherwise specified'' is used for the diagnosis of cases not meeting the severity criteria of the two conditions. These approaches are certainly logical given the deficiencies in our knowledge, although, for research purposes, the residual category should perhaps further be divided into subclinical anorexia nervosa, subclinical bulimia nervosa, and a true category of eating disorder, not otherwise specified, so that the progress of the two subclinical categories can be studied more specifically.

The DSM-III-R criteria, because of the absence of age and sex stipulations, can be applied to patients of all ages as well as to males if one substitutes loss of sexual interest for amenorrhea. Many early writers observed that anorectic patients have a fear of growing up (e.g., Brown, 1931; Janet, 1909). Although their emphases have differed, many recent writers have also suggested that anorexia nervosa often occurs in response to the stress of adolescent development. This suggestion is certainly supported by the finding that illness onset most often occurs in adolescence. Bruch (1970), for instance, suggested that the main issue in anorexia nervosa is a struggle for control and for a sense of identity, competence, and effectiveness. Such struggles are, of course, regarded as adolescent developmental tasks (Erikson, 1955). Crisp (1967, 1977, 1980) has repeatedly stated that anorexia nervosa is a psychobiosocial regression in the face of mounting adolescent conflict both within the patient and within the family. From a different perspective, family therapists such a Palazzoli (1985) and Minuchin, Rosman, and Baker (1978) have conceptualized the disorder in terms of a series of interactive processes in which separation and individualization, again adolescent tasks, may be a problem for the ''anorectic family.''

The most common age of onset of bulimia nervosa is perhaps a few years later than that of anorexia nervosa. Many of the issues that these patients struggle with are similar to those for anorectic patients. In addition, many writers have emphasized that bulimic behavior serves to regulate affect, to provide self-nurturance, and to express impulsivity and rebelliousness (e.g., Johnson & Connors, 1987). Although the similarities between adolescent storm and stress and the ''meaning'' of eating-disorder symptoms are obvious, it is perhaps an oversimplification to conceptualize the disorders as simply being aberrations of adolescent development. First, much of what has been said about the dynamics of the eating disorders may apply to other psychiatric disorders occurring in adolescence, such as an obsessive-compulsive disorder or a major depression. (Twenty years ago, some writers understood schizophrenia in much the same terms.) Second, the disorders are apparently rare in developing countries where the process of adolescence also occurs. Thus, the ''choice'' of an eating disorder as a way of expressing or retreating from adolescent conflicts still needs to be explained. Third, this concept does not explain why some patients ''choose'' anorexia nervosa and others bulimia nervosa or both combined. If the uniqueness of anorexia nervosa as an adolescent developmental illness lies in the fact that it is expressed through regression to a prepubertal body, the same cannot be said of bulimia nervosa, at least not when the patient is at normal weight. As already stated, this author believes that adolescents are particularly vulnerable to social-cultural influences and hence many go on a diet to control weight. For an eating disorder to develop, other risk factors, such as personality characteristics and family history, must also occur

Table 1. Physical Manifestations of the Eating Disorders

System	Anorexia nervosa	Bulimia nervosa
Endocrine	Amenorrhea Low luteininzing hormone (LH) and Follicle-stimulating hormone (FSH) Blunted LH response to luteinizing hormone releasing hormone (LHRH) Low T_4 and T_3 Variable changes in growth hormone, prolactin, somatomedin and somatostatin, norepinephrine, TSH, cortisol, arginine, vasopressin, and others	Irregular cycles may show other endocrine disturbances similar to those in anorexia nervosa
Metabolic	Electrolytes usually normal but may show disturbances similar to bulimia nervosa Osteoporosis and retarded bone growth Low cholesterol (from fasting) or high cholesterol (mechanism unclear) Hypercarotenemia Abnormal glucose tolerance Abnormal temperature regulation	Low potassium Low sodium Low chloride High or low bicarbonate Other metabolic disturbances may occur similar to those in anorexia nervosa
Cardiovascular	Bradycardia Hypotension Heart failure EKG changes Refeeding edema	Cardiomyopathy Heart failure EKG changes
Pulmonary		Aspiration pneumonia
Gastrointestinal	Constipation Decreased gastric emptying Acute gastric dilatation Increased hepatic enzymes	Constipation Decreased gastric emptying Dental enamel erosion Parotid enlargement Esophagitis Bleeding or rupture of esophagus Acute gastric dilatation Gastric ulcers Increased amylase
Renal	Low blood urea nitrogen (BUN) (from fasting) Increased BUN (from renal function impairment) Decreased glomerular filtration rate (GFR) Renal calculi	Increased BUN Decreased GFR Nephropathy and renal failure
Neurological	Epileptic seizures	Epileptic seizures
Hematological	Anemia Low erythrocyte sedimentation rate	Anemia

to finally precipitate an eating disorder. It is unclear why some develop anorexia nervosa and others bulimia nervosa or both.

The issue of whether the eating disorders are related to affective illness has been thoroughly reviewed (Swift, Andrews, & Barklage, 1986). Despite the views of some (e.g., Hudson *et al.*, 1983) that the eating disorders are variants of affective illness, most researchers consider the relationship between the disorders a complex one. In summary, arguments are made that eating-disorder patients are often depressed; that there is an increase in familial affective illness in these patients; that these patients demonstrate many of the biological abnormalities of depressed patients, such as a positive response on the dexamethasone suppression test; and that these patients often respond to antidepressants. However, the depression in the eating-disorder patient may well be related to the self-imposed starvation and is not usually phenomenologically identical to that of an affectively ill patient. A positive family history of affective disorder may simply act as a predisposing factor for the development of an eating disorder, although the significance of the biological findings in eating disorders (and, for that matter, in affective illness as well) is still unclear. Finally, a positive response to antidepressants does not make the illness a depression; for instance, those with panic or obsessive-compulsive symptoms sometimes respond well to antidepressants. Whatever the nosological relationship between affective and eating disorders, the clinician should always record both diagnoses and, if an eating-disorder patient meets criteria, an affective disorder as well. Recently, there is increasing speculation that the eating disorders may be related to the obsessive compulsive disorders (e.g., Rothenberg, 1988), a point we will discuss briefly in the section on treatment with antidepressants.

Finally, as part of the diagnostic process, it must be mentioned that an evaluation of an eating-disorder patient must include a physical examination and some laboratory tests. Electrolyte imbalance occurring as a result of starvation and vomiting-purging may be life-threatening. Thus, an electrocardiogram, hematology, blood chemistry, and a urine analysis should be taken for every patient, and other studies should be ordered as indicated. The more common physical manifestations are listed in Table 1.

FREQUENT CLINICAL PROBLEMS

The first problem of the clinician interviewing an eating-disorder patient is making a diagnosis. If the presenting problem is related to eating difficulties, the diagnosis is generally not difficult provided the clinician adheres to the accepted criteria. Occasionally, one still encounters the diagnosis of anorexia nervosa as an obsessive-compulsive disorder with eating difficulties, but fortunately, this is rare. If the patient presents with other psychiatric symptoms, such as those of depression, and if the clinician fails to inquire systematically into problems related to weight and eating, an eating disorder may be undiagnosed, particularly bulimia nervosa in a normal-weight patient. In a chronic anorectic, the weight phobia may initially be denied and may not become apparent until the patient has actually gained some weight. In some older patients, an eating disorder may be associated with alcohol or substance abuse, affective disorder, or personality disorder. In these cases, the diagnosis should include all these conditions.

Engaging the patient as a collaborator in treatment is often difficult, particularly an anorectic patient who insists that everything is all right. In an outpatient setting, the clinician may attempt to overcome this resistance by affirming the patient's need and effort to be slim and special and at the same explaining the effects of starvation and the course and outcome of the disorder. A discussion of the sociocultural emphasis on slimness and its effects may also be helpful. This should be followed by an outline of the treatment options and the reasons for each option. For adolescent patients, a family session to answer questions and explain treatment is always necessary unless the patient objects to it. Family members may feel very guilty about the illness is their fault or else may place all the responsibility for change on the patient. This process of engagement may take a few sessions or even longer. Attendance at a support group for both patient and parents may help to break down some of the resistance.

Bulimic patients are often distressed by their symptoms and in general are more motivated for treatment. Some are intensely ashamed of their behavior and thus may not admit to the full extent of it. Others may be concerned that recovery will involve massive weight gain and may thus want to hold on to the binge–purge behavior so that they can eat as much as they want to without putting on weight. Some may realize that the bulimia is serving to divert their attention from some insurmountable interpersonal difficulties that they cannot bear to confront, and others may insist that they do not know why they binge or purge. Most are ignorant of the effects of starvation. The clinician should therefore discuss both the effects of starvation and the functions of a binge. Again, a meeting with the family to answer their questions and to explain treatment may gain the family's confidence and support.

The choice of outpatient or inpatient treatment may be made after the initial evaluation. For anorexia nervosa, inpatient treatment is usually recommended if the body weight is below 75% of average, if the patient is suicidal, if the patient is vomiting and purging, if there are suspected physical complications, or if outpatient treatment is deemed difficult or impossible. For bulimia nervosa, outpatient treatment is usually recommended unless the patient is suicidal or has physical complications, or if previous outpatient treatment has failed and a period of inpatient treatment is necessary to break the binge–purge cycle.

Many patients are concerned about what their "target" weight should be. For anorectics, most writers have used a low average weight for age (Casper, 1982; Garfinkel & Garner, 1982). On the grounds that exposure to avoided experiences is essential for recovery, Crisp (1967) advocated a target weight of matched population mean weight at the age of onset of the illness. Some clinicians negotiate the target weight with the patient, and others just decide and inform the patient of the target weight. For bulimia nervosa, the weight issue has seldom been discussed, although some authors (e.g., Garnet, Rockert, Olmsted, Johnson, & Coscina, 1985) have suggested that some weight gain may be necessary to prevent the body from crying out for more nutrition. Because the weight issue may become a constant source of tension between therapist and patient, some therapists have been content to trust that the patient will stay above a minimum weight (e.g., Orbach, 1985). In the absence of firm data, perhaps a clinician should consistently use the approach that he or she feels comfortable with.

A common difficulty is the failure to define the treatment goals. The needs of a patient may change over time, and the treatment goals must therefore be reviewed periodically. For instance, the mood state of an eating-disorder patient should be closely monitored, and if there is significant depression, antidepressants should be considered. In a resistant patient, it may initially be wise not to tackle the eating problem directly, but this approach should not be continued indefinitely without regular periodic review.

Some writers have described the ideal qualities of a therapist for the eating disorders (e.g., Strober & Yager, 1985). These discussions are clearly relevant for a clinician seeking to build a treatment team. However, there has been no research on this issue. More recently, individuals with a personal history of an eating disorder have sought to become therapists. It is unclear how such a personal history may affect their effectiveness. In an outpatient clinic, perhaps it is not quite as essential to have a treatment team as in an inpatient unit. However, the clinician should either be adept in providing a range of treatments or be able to work in close collaboration with another clinician specializing in a different approach. Patients with multiple diagnoses almost always require treatment by several clinicians. Open communication and a harmonious working relationship between clinicians are then essential.

TREATMENT APPLICATIONS

Anorexia Nervosa

As already mentioned, an anorectic patient who is not severely emaciated, is not suicidal, is not vomiting or purging, is not in danger of any immediate physical complications, is motivated, and has the support of the family to seek treatment may initially be treated as an outpatient. The treatment goals are usually normalizing the weight, establishing healthy eating habits, understanding the underlying psychopathology, changing the weight phobia, and dealing with other issues, such as mood disturbances and peer and family relationships.

In contrast to treatment in an inpatient unit, weight restoration in an outpatient setting has rarely been discussed. Nursing care is obviously impossible, and behavioral techniques are difficult to implement apart, perhaps, from the weekly or twice-weekly weight monitoring. Therefore, the clinician has to rely heavily on nutritional education if he or she wants to tackle the weight issue. This education should probably cover basic knowledge about good nutrition; the food groups; the effects of starvation and of vomiting, purging, diet pills, and emetic abuse; meal planning, shopping for food; and basic techniques of food preparation. Even though many writers have advocated nutritional counseling, its effects have rarely been studied. Hall and Crisp (1987) found dietary advice to be as effective as combined individual and family therapy in the treatment of anorexia nervosa, and the effects were maintained at 1-year follow-up.

An alternative approach to nutritional counseling is to make an agreement with the patient that she or he should not drop below a minimum weight; otherwise, outpatient therapy cannot continue (e.g., Orbach, 1985). In effect, this agreement makes the patient responsible for maintaining a minimum weight. Dare (1983) approached the weight issue by asking the family to take the responsibility of making the patient eat and gain weight. Invasive techniques (e.g., tube feeding) are obviously not applicable to the outpatient. Antidepressants may be used in the usual dosage, with monitoring of blood levels if necessary for patients who are depressed. In bulimic anorectics, antidepressants may occasionally be very effective in decreasing the urges to binge. In the absence of depression, the effectiveness of antidepressants in anorexia nervosa is unclear. It is my preliminary experience that serotonergic agents such as thioxetine may be effective in improving the patient's dysphoria incessant ruminations about weight. They may also prevent weight loss in patients who have been successfully treated as inpatients. It is of interest to note that these agents are effective for obsessive compulsive disorder (Fontaine, 1988).

The mainstay of outpatient treatment for anorexia nervosa is therefore psychotherapy. Many approaches have been advocated; none has been properly evaluated. Classical psychoanalysis has been found to be relatively ineffective by many writers (e.g., Bruch, 1970; Casper, 1982; Crisp, 1980; Garner & Bemis, 1982), although claims of its unique efficacy persist (e.g., Hogan, 1983; Thoma, 1967). In any case, the view that the disorder is a defense against unconscious wishes of oral impregnation (Waller, Kaufman, & Deutsch, 1940) has probably been abandoned by even the most ardent advocates.

More recent writings seem to reflect what may be broadly called an *object relations approach* (e.g., Goodsitt, 1985), and although other psychodynamic therapists have chosen to label their approaches differently, by and large the approaches are similar in that they emphasize the role of the therapist in containing, educating, modulating, supporting, evoking, encouraging, challenging, and role modeling. Interpretation is considered less important, probably because it may reinforce patients' notions that others know what they themselves do not (Bruch, 1970). Instead of emphasizing intrapsychic conflicts, sexual or otherwise, current writings describe the patients' inward emptiness, their denial and fear of needs and feelings, their sense of ineffectiveness, and their low self-esteem. The patient may actually present as an intelligent, competent, manipulative and angry or sometimes exceedingly compliant individual, and it may take weeks or months for the therapist to gain the patient's trust and confidence (Casper, 1987). Cognitive therapists (e.g., Garner & Bemis, 1982) have emphasized the more proximal distorted thoughts and perceptions of the anorectic patient and have described systematic attempts to evoke, define, and challenge them. The obnoxious cultural influence on slimness and, for the female patient, the complex role of women in modern society are also discussed, as they are obviously relevant to the patient's concerns (e.g., Garner *et al.*, 1985; Orbach, 1985). Because many anorectic patients are struggling with issues of identity and intimacy, these issues should always be addressed in psychotherapy. This does not mean that the therapist must believe that anorexia nervosa is an adolescent developmental disorder; it simply means that the therapist cannot afford to ignore these issues in any adolescent or young-adult patients, whatever their diagnosis. The cardinal feature of fear of fatness may decrease with weight gain, although it may persist even in those who are clinically recovered (Hsu, 1980). Some therapists ask patients to accept it as a part of their illness and to live with it (e.g., Garner *et al.*, 1985), whereas others use nonverbal experiential techniques to help patients overcome it (Wooley & Wooley, 1985).

Family therapy has been regarded by some as the treatment of choice for anorexia nervosa (e.g., Minuchin *et al.*, 1978). In an inpatient setting, Minuchin *et al.* (1978) used the family lunch session to challenge and unbalance dysfunctional family interaction patterns, such as enmeshment and conflict avoidance, that is, "to transform the issue of an anorectic patient to the drama of a dysfunctional family" (p. 120). As already mentioned, Dare (1983), perhaps in a less dramatic fashion, essentially also places the responsibility of eating on the family and, in so doing, forces the family to change its interaction pattern. These techniques can, of course, be used in an outpatient setting. Subsequent family sessions should continue to focus on the dysfunctional interaction pattern and on strategies for change. Russell, Szmukler, Dare, and Eisler (1987) compared family therapy with individual supportive therapy in 80 anorexic outpatients and found the former to be much more effective in young patients with less that 3 years' duration of illness. It was, however, not more effective than individual therapy in those with a longer duration of illness, in those with an older age of onset (greater than 18), or in those with bulimic symptoms. Clinicians usually find anorectic patients unsuitable for group therapy because of their denial of difficulties, their inability to verbalize feelings, their need to compete with each other, and their tendency to escape from issues by losing weight (Hall, 1985). Group therapy may be useful as a means of decreasing patients' isolation and withdrawal if used in conjunction with individual and/or family therapy.

One of the greatest difficulties in the treatment of anorexia nervosa is relapse prevention. Treating an anorectic patient who dutifully returns each week to the session and yet loses exactly 1 pound per week can be a harrowing experience. Russell (1977) advocated repeated inpatient admissions until the patient grows out of the illness. Others use the various approaches that have been described. There is no good research to guide the clinician here. The management of a chronic patient is another challenging task. Perhaps supportive therapy and the judicious use of inpatient treatment are the best approaches. Paradoxical intention may also be beneficial (Hsu & Lieberman, 1982), and we have already mentioned the apparent benefit of serotonergic agents for some patients.

Recent studies suggest that the 4- to 10-year outcome of anorexia nervosa is encouraging for one half to two thirds of the patients; mortality is generally under 5%, and 25% of the patients are chronically ill at this point (Hsu, 1987). A 20-year follow-up suggests that as many as 18% may eventually die from the illness (Theander, 1985). There is clearly no room for complacency, and more research on treatment is urgently needed.

Bulimia Nervosa

The goals of treatment for bulimia nervosa are the reduction or cessation of the bulimic behavior, the establishment of a regular eating pattern, and overcoming the issues that perpetuate or precipitate the bulimic behavior. Admittedly, some clinicians do not regard these goals as being of equal importance; some may emphasize the reduction of bulimic behavior, and others, the understanding of the underlying dynamics.

With regard to decreasing the bulimic behavior, two approaches are effective. Several double-blind controlled studies have established the efficacy of antidepressants in bulimia nervosa. Pope, Hudson, Jonas, and Yurgelun-Todd (1983), in a 6-week study of 22 bulimic patients, found imipramine at the usual dosage to be significantly better than placebo. Walsh, Stewart, Roose, Gladis, and Glassman (1984) found phenelzine to be significantly better than placebo in a 6-week study of 20 bulimic women; over 50% of those on phenelzine reached total cessation of their binge–purge behavior. Unfortunately, the side effects of phenelzine were substantial. Hughes, Wells, Cunningham, and Ilstrup (1986) found desipramine to be vastly superior to placebo in a 6-week study of 22 patients; over 50% of those on the active medication reached total abstinence. Mitchell and Groat (1984) found amitriptyline to be better than placebo in improving the patient's mood, but it was not more effective than placebo in improving the patients' binge–purge behavior. Sabine, Yonace, Farrington, Barratt, & Wakeling (1983) found no difference in patients treated with mianserin and those treated with placebo; however, the dosage of mianserin used may not have been adequate for the purpose of controlling the bulimic behavior. In summary, antidepressants at an adequate dosage are likely to benefit many bulimic patients, provided they can tolerate the side effects. Patients who improve usually indicate a decrease in the urges to binge and an improvement in their mood. It is unclear whether bulimic symptoms in the absence of a concurrent depression also respond to antidepressants. The study by Hughes *et al.* (1986) seems to suggest that they do.

The cognitive-behavioral treatment of bulimia nervosa consists basically of two components: nutritional counseling and cognitive therapy. Nutritional counseling is believed to be important because the patient's eating behavior is obviously abnormal and there is some evidence to suggest that the illness is related to strict and prolonged dieting. Evidence from the Minnesota study (Keys *et al.*, 1950) has already been briefly described. In experimental situations "restrained eaters" overate once they perceived that they had violated their dietary control (Polivy, Herman, Olmsted, & Jazwinski, 1984). Bulimia nervosa almost always occurs in the context of dieting to control weight, and some 40% of bulimics have a previous history of anorexia nervosa (Hsu & Holder, 1986). Eighty percent of bulimics eat only one meal or less a day (Mitchell, Hatsukami, Eckert, & Pyle, 1985). Nutritional counseling generally consists of basic nutrition education; advise on meal planning; instructions on the effects of starvation, bingeing, vomiting, and laxative and emetic abuse; and suggestions on basic techniques of food purchase and preparation. Although clinical experience suggests that a pattern of regular eating may ameliorate the bulimic behavior, the effectiveness of nutritional counseling has unfortunately never been studied.

Many researchers have also conceptualized bulimia nervosa as a set of dysfunctional behaviors that represent "a difficulty in coping with disturbed feelings and thoughts" (Fairburn, 1982, p. 631). Binge eating has been interpreted as a response to stress, a means of modulating dysphoric or anxiety states, a behavior that meets an unfulfilled emotional need, a way of controlling weight when one fails to control other events in the environment, or a release from the control imposed on oneself in efforts to be perfect. These interpretations of the meaning of bulimic behavior are consistent with patients' self-reports that the urge to binge is often triggered by emotional states such as dysphoria, anger, anxiety, and boredom, and that the overeating, particularly of fattening, forbidden foods, initially produces a sense of satisfaction, nurturance, oblivion, or liberation, although this is soon followed by a sense of defeat and guilt. Some researchers have emphasized the primary role of vomiting or purging as a maladaptive way of relieving the anxiety associated with eating (Rosen & Lietenberg, 1982), and most patients insist that they engage in such behavior only to get rid of the calories. Many, however, also enjoy the fact that they can eat whatever they want to without gaining weight, and a few find the purging to have a relaxing or cleansing effect. Johnson and Connors (1987) stated, in summary, that bulimic behavior may serve to regulate affect and to express oppositionality, and that it be a means of impulse expression and self-nurturance. Finally, many female patients relate their chronic dysphoria and frustration to their low self-acceptance and self-worth, a constant need to appear slim, and a fear of negative evaluation and rejection, particularly from men. These experiences have led writers such as Boskind-Lodahl (1976) and Orbach (1985) to postulate that bulimia nervosa is related to the complex and conflicting role of women in Western society.

Following the pioneering effort by Fairburn (1981), many studies have been published that used nutritional and cognitive-behavioral principles in the treatment of bulimia nervosa. Garner, Fairburn and Davis (1987) reviewed a total of 19 studies of acceptable methodology published between 1981 and 1986 and found that, on average, there was a 79% reduction in binge frequency from pre- to posttreatment. Although these studies differed in the details of their design, by and large they attempted to evaluate the effectiveness of cognitive-behavioral techniques such as cognitive restructuring of attitudes toward weight and body, self-monitoring of thoughts and feelings in relation to the bulimic episodes, discussion of the function of a binge, stimulus control of eating behavior, social skills or assertiveness training, relaxation training, self-distraction during high-risk times for bingeing, and problem-solving training for averting a binge. Several authors (Wilson, Rossiter, Kleifeld, & Lindholm, 1986; Ordman & Kirshenbaum, 1985) have used exposure and response (i.e., vomit) prevention specifically to counteract the vomiting.

Eight studies used a controlled design (Fairburn, Kirk, O'Connor, & Cooper, 1986; Freeman, Sinclair, Turnbull, & Annadale, 1985; Kirkley, Schneider, Agras, Bachman, 1985; Lacey, 1983; Lee & Rush, 1986; Ordman & Kirschenbaum, 1985; Wilson *et al.*, 1986; Wolchik, Weiss, & Katzman, 1986). Those that used a ''waiting-list'' group as a control condition found active treatment to be vastly superior (Lacey, 1983; Lee & Rush, 1986; Ordman & Kirshenbaum, 1985; Wolchik *et al.*, 1986). Cognitive treatment is somewhat more effective than short-term therapy (Fairburn *et al.*, 1986) and nondirective therapy (Kirkley *et al.*, 1985). Cognitive restructuring along with exposure and vomit prevention is more effective than the former alone (Wilson *et al.*, 1986). In sum, all these studies indicate that cognitive-behavioral treatment is effective in the control of the bulimic behavior.

Although bulimic patients are often more open and forthcoming than their anorectic counterparts, it is nevertheless also true that they are often usually sensitive and overcompliant. It therefore makes good clinical sense that, even when the clinician chooses to use either a pharmacological or a behavioral approach, he or she should not overlook the dynamic issues within the patient and within the treatment relationship. Patients may initially make good improvement, only to drop out of treatment if these issues are ignored. It is this author's preference to begin treatment with the cognitive-behavioral approach and, if no significant improvement occurs after 4–6 weeks, to add a tricyclic antidepressant. There is, however, no study to validate this approach. Some patients who improve in terms of their bulimia may want to seek further, more insight-oriented psychotherapy, and they should be encouraged. Antidepressants should probably be continued for at least 6 months after improvement occurs, but there are no maintenance treatment studies. Relapse is not uncommon even after a lengthy period of recovery, and strategies for relapse prevention are therefore very much needed.

SUMMARY

This chapter summarizes the recent findings on the outpatient treatment of the eating disorders, as well as on the etiology and diagnosis of the disorder. Some common clinical problems are also highlighted. It is evident that further research is needed in many areas, particularly in the area of relapse prevention.

REFERENCES

American Psychiatric Association. (1980). *Diagnostic and statistical manual of mental disorders* (3rd ed.; DSM-III). Washington, DC: Author.

American Psychiatric Association. (1987). *Diagnostic and statistical manual of mental disorders* (3rd ed. rev.; DSM-III-R). Washington, DC: Author.

Berkman, J. M. (1930). Anorexia nervosa, anorexia inanition and low basal metabolic rate. *American Journal of Medical Science, 180,* 411.

Beumont, P. J. V., George, G. C. W., & Smart, D. E. (1976). Dieters and vomiters and purgers in anorexia nervosa. *Psychological Medicine, 6,* 617–622.

Bliss, E. L., & Branch, C. H. H. (Eds.). (1960). *Anorexia nervosa: Its history, psychology and biology*. New York: Paul B. Hoeber.

Boskind-Lodahl, M. (1976). Cinderella's step-sister: A feminist perspective on anorexia and bulimia. *Signs: Journal of Women in Culture and Society, 2*(11), 342–356.

Brown, W. L. (1931). Anorexia nervosa. In L. Brown (Ed.), *Anorexia nervosa* (pp. 11–17). London: C. W. Daniels.

Bruch, H. (1962). Perceptual and conceptual disturbances in anorexia nervosa. *Psychosomatic Medicine, 24,* 187–194.

Bruch, H. (1970). Psychotherapy in primary anorexia nervosa. *Journal of Nervous Mental Disorders, 150,* 51–67.

Bruch, H. (Ed.). (1973). *Eating disorders*. New York: Basic Books.

Bruch, H. (1982). Anorexia nervosa: Therapy and theory. *American Journal of Psychiatry, 132,* 1531–1538.

Buhrich, N. (1981). Frequency of presentation of anorexia in malaysia. *Australian and New Zealand Journal of Psychiatry, 15,* 153–155.

Button, E. J., & Whitehouse, A. (1981). Subclinical anorexia nervosa. *Psychological Medicine, 11,* 509–516.

Cantwell, D. P., Sturzenberger, S., Burroughs, J., Salkin, B., & Green, J. K. (1977). Anorexia nervosa: An affective disorder? *Archives of General Psychiatry, 34,* 1087–1093.

Casper, R. C. (1982). Treatment principles in anorexia nervosa. *Adolescent Psychiatry, 10,* 86–100.

Casper, R. C. (1987). The psychopathology of anorexia nervosa: The pathological psychodynamic processes. In P. J. V. Beumont, G. D. Burrows, & R. C. Casper (Eds.), *Handbook of eating disorders: 1: Anorexia and bulimia nervosa* (pp. 159–179). Elsevier.

Cooper, P. J., Charnock, D. J., & Taylor, M. J. (1987). The prevalence of bulimia nervosa. A replication study. *British Journal of Psychiatry, 151,* 684–686.

Crisp, A. H. (1967). Anorexia nervosa. *Hospital Medicine, 1,* 713–718.

Crisp, A. H. (1977). Diagnosis and outcome of anorexia nervosa. *Proceedings of the Royal Social Medicine, 70,* 464–470.

Crisp, A. H. (1980). *Anorexia nervosa: Let me be*. London: Academic Press.

Crisp, A. H. (1981). Therapeutic outcome in anorexia nervosa. *Canadian Journal of Psychiatry, 26,* 232–235.

Crisp, A. H., Palmer, R. L., & Kalucy, R. S. (1976). How common is anorexia nervosa? A prevalence study. *British Journal of Psychiatry, 128,* 549–554.

Dally, P. (1969). *Anorexia nervosa*. London: Heinemann Medical.

Dare, C. (1983). Family therapy for families containing an anorectic youngster. In *Understanding anorexia nervosa and bulimia* (pp. 28–36). Report of the Fourth Ross Conference on Medical Research. Ohio: Ross Laboratories.

Dejerine, J., & Gauckler, E. (1913). *The psychoneuroses and their treatment by psychotherapy* Philadelphia: Lippincott.

Erikson, E. H. (1955). The problem of ego identity. *Journal of Psychoanalytic Association, 4,* 56–121.

Fairburn, C. G. (1981). A cognitive behavioral approach to the management of bulimia. *Psychological Medicine, 11,* 707–711.

Fairburn, C. G. (1982). Binge eating and its management. *British Journal of Psychiatry, 141,* 631–633.

Fairburn, C. G., Kirk, J., O'Connor, M., & Cooper, P. J. (1986). A comparison of two psychological treatments for bulimia nervosa. *Behavior Research and Therapy, 24,* 629–643.

Faust, M. S. (1983). Alternative constructions of adolescent growth. In J. Brooks-Gunn & A. C. Petersen (Eds.), *Girls at puberty* (pp. 105–125). New York: Plenum Press.

Feighner, J. P., Robins, E., Guze, S. B., Woodruff, R. A., Winokur, G., & Munoz, R. (1972). Diagnostic criteria for use in psychiatric research. *Archives of General Psychiatry, 26,* 57–63.

Fontaine, R. (1982). Fluoxetine in the treatment of obsessive compulsive disorder. Paper presented at the 141st Annual Meeting of the American Psychiatric Association, Montreal, Canada.

Freeman, C., Sinclair, F., Turnbull, J., & Annadale, A. (1985). Psychotherapy for bulimia: A controlled study. *Journal of Psychiatric Research, 19,* 473–478.

Furnham, A., & Alibhai, N. (1983). Cross-cultural differences in the perception of female body shapes. *Psychological Medicine, 13,* 829–837.

Garfinkle, P. E., & Garner, D. M. (1982). *Anorexia nervosa: A multidimentional perspective*. New York: Brunner/Mazel.

Garn, S. M., & Clark, D. C. (1975). Nutrition growth, development, and maturation findings from the ten-state nutrition survey of 1968–1970. *Pediatrics, 56,* 306–319.

Garner, D. M., & Bemis, K. M. (1982). A cognitive behavioral approach to anorexia nervosa. *Cognitive Therapy and Research, 6,* 1–27.

Garner, D. M., & Garfinkle, P. E. (1980). Social cultural factors in the development of anorexia nervosa. *Psychological Medicine, 10,* 647–656.

Garner, D. M., Garfinkle, P. E., Schwartz, D., & Thompson, M. (1980). Cultural expectations of thinness in women. *Psychological Report, 47,* 483–491.

Garner, D. M., Olmsted, M. P., Polivy, J., & Garfinkle, P. E. (1984). Comparison between weight-preoccupied women and anorexia nervosa. *Psychosomatic Medicine, 46,* 255–266.

Garner, D. M., Rockert, W., Olmsted, M. P., Johnson, D. L., & Coscina, D. V. (1985). Psychoeducational principles in the treatment of bulimia and anorexia nervosa. In D. M. Garner & P. E. Garfinkle (Eds.), *Handbook of psychotherapy for anorexia nervosa and bulimia* (pp. 513–572). New York: Guilford Press.

Garner, D. M., Fairburn, C. G., & Davis, R. (1987). Cognitive-behavioral treatment of bulimia nervosa. *Behavior Modification, 11*(4), 398–431.

Garrow, J. S., Crisp, H. A., Jordan, H. A., Meyer, J. E., Russell, G. F. M., Silverstone, T., Stunkard, A. J., & VanItallie, T. B. (1975). Pathology of eating, group report. In T. Silverstone (Ed.), Life Sciences Research Report. Berlin: Dahlem Konferezen.

Goodsitt, A. (1985). Self-psychology and the treatment of anorexia nervosa. In D. M. Garner & P. E. Garfinkle (Eds.), *Handbook of psychotherapy for anorexia nervosa and bulimia* (pp. 55–82). New York: Guilford Press.

Gull, W. W. (1874). Anorexia nervosa (apepsia hysterica, anorexia hysterica). *Transections of Clinical Society London, 7,* 22.

Hall, A. (1985). Group psychotherapy for anorexia nervosa. In D. M. Garner & P. E. Garfinkle (Eds.), *Handbook of psychotherapy for anorexia nervosa and bulimia* (pp. 213–238). New York: Guilford Press.

Hall, A., & Crisp, A. H. (1987). Brief psychotherapy in the treatment of anorexia nervosa outcome at one year. *British Journal of Psychiatry, 151,* 185–191.

Halmi, K. A. (1980). Anorexia nervosa. In H. I. Kaplan, A. M. Freedman, & B. J. Sadock (Eds.), *Comprehensive textbook of psychiatry* (Vol. 2, 3rd ed., pp. 18–87). Baltimore: Williams & Wilkins.

Halmi, K. A., Falk, J. R., & Schwartz, E. (1981). Binge-eating and vomiting: A survey of a college population. *Psychological Medicine, 11,* 697–706.

Hogan, C. C. (1983). Psychodynamics. In C. P. Wilson (Ed.), *Fear of being fat* (pp. 115–128). New York: Jason Aronson.

Hsu, L. K. G. (1980). Outcome in anorexia nervosa: A review of the literature (1954–1978). *Archives of General Psychiatry, 37,* 1041–1046.

Hsu, L. K. G. (1986). The treatment of anorexia nervosa. *American Journal of Psychiatry, 143*(5), 573–581.

Hsu, L. K. G. (1987). Are the eating disorders becoming more common in blacks? *International Journal of Eating Disorders, 6,* 113–123.

Hsu, L. K. G., & Holder, D. (1986). Bulimia nervosa: Treatment and short-term outcome. *Psychological Medicine, 16,* 65–70.

Hsu, L. K. G., & Lieberman, S. (1982). Paradoxical intention in the treatment of chronic anorexia nervosa. *American Journal of Psychiatry, 139,* 650–653.

Hsu, L. K. G., Crisp, A. H., & Harding, B. (1979). Outcome of anorexia nervosa. *Lancet, 1,* 61–65.

Hudson, J. I., Pope, H. G., Jonas, J. M. & Yurgelun-Todd, D. (1983). Family history study of anorexia nervosa and bulimia. *British Journal of Psychiatry, 142,* 133–138.

Huenemann, R. L., Shapiro, L. R., Hampton, M. C., & Mitchell, B. W. (1966). A longitudinal study of gross body composition and body conformation and then association with food and activity in a teenage population. *American Journal of Clinical Nutrition, 18,* 325–338.

Hughes, P. L., Wells, L. A., Cunningham, C. J., & Ilstrup, D. M. (1986). Treating bulimia with desipramine: A double-blind, placebo-controlled study. *Archives of General Psychiatry, 43,* 182–186.

Janet, P. (1909). *Les neuroses.* Paris: Ernest Flammarion.

Johnson, C., & Connors, M. E. (Eds.). (1987). Demographic and clinical characteristics. *The etiology and treatment of bulimia nervosa: A biopsychosocial perspective* (pp. 31–60). New York: Basic Books.

Johnson, C. L., Lewis, C., Love, S., Lewis, L., & Stuckey, M. (1983). A descriptive survey of dieting and bulimic behavior in a female high school population. *Report of the Fourth Ross Conference on Medical Research* (pp. 14–18). Ohio: Ross Laboratories.

Jones, D. J., Fox, M. M., Babigan, H. M., & Hutton, H. E. (1980). Epidemiology of anorexia nervosa in Monroe County, New York: 1960–1976. *Psychosomatic Medicine, 42,* 551–558.

Jourard, S. E., & Secord, P. F. (1955). Body-cathexis and the ideal female figure. *Journal of Abnormal and Social Psychology, 50,* 243–246.

Kay, D. W. K., & Leigh, D. (1954). The natural history, treatment and prognosis of anorexia nervosa based on a study of 38 patients. *Journal of Mental Science, 100,* 411–431.

Kendell, R. E., Hall, D. J., Hailey, A., & Babigan, H. M. (1973). The epidemiology of anorexia nervosa. *Psychological Medicine, 3,* 200–203.

Keys, A., Brozek, J., Henschel, A., Michaelson, O., & Taylor, H. L. (1950). *The biology of human starvation: Volume I.* Minneapolis: University of Minnesota Press.

King, A. (1963). Primary and secondary anorexia nervosa. *British Journal of Psychiatry, 109,* 470–479.

Kirkley, B. G., Schneider, J. A., Agras, W. S., & Bachman, J. A. (1985). Comparison of two group treatments for bulimia. *Journal of Consulting and Clinical Psychology, 53,* 43–48.

Lacey, J. H. (1983). Bulimia nervosa, binge eating, and psychogenic vomiting: A controlled treatment study and long-term outcome. *British Medical Journal, 1,* 1609–1613.

Laseque, C. (1873). On hysterical anorexia. *Medical Times and Gazette, 2,* 265, 367.

LaTourette, Gilles de (1895). *G.A.E.B.: Traite clinique et therapeutic de l'hysteric.* Paris: Plou, Nourit.

Lee, N. F., & Rush, P. A. J. (1986). Cognitive-behavioral group therapy for bulimia. *International Journal of Eating Disorders, 5,* 599–615.

Lerner, R. M., & Karabenick, S. A. (1974). Physical attractiveness, body attitudes and self-concept in late adolescents. *Journal of Youth and Adolescents, 3*(4), 307–316.

Marsha, J. E., & Friedman, M. L. (1970). Ego identity status in college women. *Journal of Personality, 38,* 249–263.

Minuchin, S., Rosman, B. L., & Baker, L. (1978). *Psychosomatic families.* Cambridge: Harvard University Press.

Mitchell, J. E., & Groat, R. (1984). A placebo-controlled, double-blind trial of amitriptyline in bulimia. *Journal of Clinical Psychopharmacology, 4,* 186–193.

Mitchell, J. E., Hatsukami, D., Eckert, E. D., & Pyle, R. L. (1985). Characteristics of 275 patients with bulimia. *American Journal of Psychiatry, 142*(4), 482–485.

Miyai, K., Yamamoto, T., Azukizawa, M., Ishibashi, K., & Kumahara, Y. (1975). Serum thyroid hormones and thyrotropin in anorexia nervosa. *Journal of Clinical Endocrinology and Metabolism, 40,* 334–338.

Moley, V. A. (1983). Interactional treatment of eating disorders. *Journal of Strategic and Systemic Therapies, 2,* 10–28.

Morgan, H. G., & Russell, G. F. M. (1975). Value of family background and clinical features as predictors of long-term outcome in anorexia nervosa: Four year follow-up study of 41 patients. *Psychological Medicine, 5,* 355–371.

Morton, R. (1694). *Phthisologia or a treatise of consumption.* London: Smith & Walford.

Nemiah, J. C. (1950). Anorexia nervosa. *Medicine, 29,* 225–268.

Nogami, Y., & Yabana, F. (1977). On kibarashi-gui. *Folia Psychiatry Neurology Japan, 31,* 159–166.

Nylander, I. (1971). The feeling of being fat and dieting in a school population: Epidemiologic interview investigation. *Acta Sociomedica Scandinavica, 3,* 17–26.

Orbach, S. (1985). Accepting the symptom: A feminist psychoanalytic treatment of anorexia nervosa. In D. M. Garner & P. E. Garfinkle (Eds.), *Handbook of psychotherapy for anorexia nervosa and bulimia* (pp. 83–106). New York: Guilford Press.

Ordman, A. M., & Kirshenbaum, D. S. (1985). Cognitive-behavioral therapy for bulimia: An initial outcome study. *Journal of Consulting and Clinical Psychology, 53,* 305–313.

Orlofsky, J. L. (1978). Identity formation, achievement, and fear of success in college men and women. *Journal of Youth and Adolescence, 7,* 49–62.

Palazzoli, M. S. (Ed.). (1985). *Self-starvation.* New York: Jason Aronson.

Palmer, R. L. (1979). The dietary chaos syndrome: A useful new term? *British Journal of Medical Psychology, 52,* 187–190.

Patton, G. C. (1988). The spectrum of eating disorder in adolescence. *Journal of Psychosomatic Research, 32* (6), 579–584.

Polivy, H. G., Herman, C. P., Olmsted, M. P., & Jazwinski, C. (1984). Restraint and binge eating. In R. C. Hawkins, W. J. Fremouw, & P. F. Clement (Eds.), *The binge-purge syndrome: Diagnosis, treatment and research* (pp. 104–122). New York: Springer.

Pope, H. G., Hudson, J. I., Jonas, J. M. & Yurgelun-Todd, D. (1983). Bulimia treated with imipramine: A placebo-controlled, double-blind study. *American Journal of Psychiatry, 140,* 554–558.

Rivinus, T. M., Biederman, J., Herzog, D. G., Kemper, K., Harper, G. P., Harmatz, J. S., & Houseworth, S. (1984). Anorexia nervosa and affective disorders: A controlled family history study. *American Journal of Psychiatry, 144,* 1414–1418.

Rosen, J. C., & Leitenberg, H. (1982). Bulimia nervosa: Treatment with exposure and response prevention. *Behavior Therapy, 13,* 117–124.

Rothenberg, A. (1988). Obsessive compulsive symptoms in anorexia nervosa. *Comprehensive Psychiatry, 29,* 427–432.

Russell, G. F. M. (1970). Anorexia nervosa: Its identity as an illness and its treatment. In J. H. Price (Ed.), *Modern trends in psychological medicine,* (Vol. 2, pp. 131–164). London: Butterworths.

Russell, G. F. M. (1977). The present status of anorexia nervosa. *Psychological Medicine, 7,* 353–367.

Russell, G. F. M. (1979). Bulimia nervosa: A ominous variant of anorexia nervosa. *Psychological Medicine, 9,* 429–448.

Russell, G. F. M., Szmukler, G. I., Dare, C., & Eisler, I. (1987). An evaluation of family therapy in anorexia nervosa and bulimia nervosa. *Archives of General Psychiatry, 44,* 1047–1056.

Ryle, J. A. (1936). Anorexia nervosa. *Lancet, 2,* 893.

Sabine, E. J., Yonace, A., Farrington, A. J., Barratt, K. H., & Wakeling, A. (1983). Bulimia nervosa: A placebo-controlled double-blind therapeutic trial of mianserin. *British Journal of Clinical Pharmacology, 15,* Supplement, 195S–202S.

Sheehan, H. L., & Summers, V. K. (1949). The syndrome of hypopituitarism. *Quarterly Journal of Medicine, 18,* 319.

Simmonds, M. (1914). Ueber embolische prozesse in des hypophysis. *Archives of Pathology and Anatomy, 217,* 226–239.

Strober, M., & Yager, J. (1985). A developmental perspective on the treatment of anorexia nervosa in adolescents. In D. M. Garner & P. E. Garfinkle (Eds.), *Handbook of psychotherapy for anorexia nervosa and bulimia* (pp. 363–390). New York: Guilford Press.

Suematsu, H., Ishikawa, H., Kubocki, T., & Ito, T. (1985). Statistical studies on anorexia nervosa in Japan: Detailed clinical data on 1011 patients. *Psychotherapy and Psychosomatics, 43,* 96–103.

Swift, W. J., Andrews, D., & Barklage, N. E. (1986). The relationship between affective disorders and eating disorders. A review of the literature. *American Journal of Psychiatry, 143,* 290–299.

Szmukler, G. I. (1985). The epidemiology of anorexia nervosa and bulimia. *Journal of Psychiatric Research, 19* (2/3), 143–153.

Szmukler, G. I., Eisler, I., Gillis, C., & Hayward, M. E. (1985). The implications of anorexia nervosa in a ballet school. *Journal of Psychiatry, 19,* 177–181.

Szmukler, G. I., McCance, C., McCrone, L., & Hunter, D. (1986). Anorexia nervosa: A psychiatric case register study from Aberdeen. *Psychological Medicine, 16,* 49–58.

Theander, S. (1970). Anorexia nervosa: A psychiatric investigation of 94 female patients. *Acta Psychiatrica Scandinavica,* Supplement, 214.

Theander, S. (1985). Outcome and prognosis in anorexia nervosa and bulimia: Some results of previous investigations compared with those of a Swedish long-term study. *Journal of Psychiatric Research, 19,* 493–508.

Thoma, H. (1967). *Anorexia nervosa.* (G. Brydone, Trans.). New York: International Universities Press.

Tobin-Richards, M. H., Boxer, A. M., & Petersen, A. C. (1983). The psychological significance of pubertal change: Sex differences in perceptions of self during early adolescents. In J. Brooks-Gunn & A. C. Petersen (Eds.), *Girls at puberty* (pp. 127–154). New York: Plenum Press.

Waller, J., Kaufman, M. R., & Deutsch, F. (1940). Anorexia nervosa: A psychosomatic study. *Psychosomatic Medicine, 2,* 3–16.

Walsh, B. T., Steward, J. W., Roose, S. P., Gladis, M., & Glassman, A. H. (1984). Treatment of bulimia with phenelzine: A double-blind, placebo-controlled study. *Archives of General Psychiatry, 41,* 1105–1109.

Willi, J., & Grossman, S. (1983). Epidemiology of anorexia nervosa in a defined region of Switzerland. *American Journal of Psychiatry, 140,* 564–567.

Wilson, G. T., Rossiter, E., Kleifeld, E. I., & Lindholm, L. (1986). Cognitive-behavioral treatment of bulimia nervosa: A controlled evaluation. *Behavior Research and Therapy, 24,* 277–288.

Wolchik, S. A., Weiss, L., & Katzman, M. A. (1986). An empirically validated, short-term psychoeducational group treatment program for bulimia. *International Journal of Eating Disorders, 5,* 21–34.

Wooley, S. C., & Wooley, O. W. (1985). Intensive outpatient and residential treatment for bulimia. In D. M. Garner & P. E. Garfinkle (Eds.), *Handbook of psychotherapy for anorexia nervosa and bulimia* (pp. 391–430). New York: Guilford Press.

III

Special Populations

20

Marital Dysfunction

GARY R. BIRCHLER AND MADELINE GERSHWIN

INTRODUCTION

"They fell in love, got married, and lived happily ever after" is the idealized romantic image ascribed to the institution of marriage in our culture. This notion continues despite the highly publicized prevalence of marital dysfunction and a soaring divorce rate. Although social trends may alter the structure and function of marriage, it would seem that the institution, as a vehicle for legitimizing and formalizing dyadic relationships, will be with us for some time to come. "Marriage counseling" has now become a more accepted form of psychological service. The last decade has seen an explosion of contributions to the marital therapy literature, particularly from the behavioral and family systems perspectives (Gurman, 1981; Jacobson & Gurman, 1986). Social learning theorists have developed improved technologies for treating marital dysfunction that are based on the scrutiny of empirical data. The behavioral therapists' commitment to examine therapy outcome has set the stage for a lively interaction among theorists of opposing points of view (e.g., Gurman & Kniskern, 1978). This chapter examines the historical trends in marriage and marital therapy and focuses on a model of treatment that integrates the behavioral and systems approaches (Birchler & Spinks, 1980). It is the authors' contention that the strictly orthodox approach of either the behavioral or the systems model (or any single therapeutic model) is less effective than a more comprehensive, integrated treatment program.

GARY R. BIRCHLER • University of California School of Medicine, and Psychology Service, VA Medical Center, San Diego, California, 92161. MADELINE GERSHWIN • University of California School of Medicine, San Diego, California 92161.

Trends in Marriage

The traditional marriage with well-defined, gender-determined roles has clearly broken down in our age, when the expectation is that all relational and affective needs will be met in the marriage. Not only are affective needs poorly delineated and conceptually global, but there is little in the education of individuals throughout their lives to prepare them to meet "relationship" needs. Further, society values achievement in the workplace rather than interpersonal competence. An emphasis on "people" skills is somehow suspect. Couples are therefore in the unenviable position of expecting to have ill-defined, little-valued emotional needs met in relationships in which the individuals are unprepared for this challenge. The ground rules were set for a game that has changed.

At a cultural level, the women's movement generated an increase in marital instability beginning in the 1960s when the national consciousness addressed issues of freedom for all oppressed people. Traditionally, marriage has offered more advantages to men than to women (Paolino & McCrady, 1978). Personal growth, professional development, and self-improvement have always been male perquisites within the context of marriage. As women have begun to place a high value on their own independent growth and personal development, there has been a corresponding ambivalence about traditional feminine goals and an increased dissatisfaction with marriage. Not surprisingly, then, as women have gained status and with the corresponding increase in marital instability, husbands have reported increased marital dissatisfaction (Burke & Weir, 1977). The idea of a companionship marriage, which seems a logical outgrowth of shifts in the social norms, remains largely unrealized. Until the society at large places a higher value on interpersonal competence and our social institutions prepare individuals with the behavioral skills required to actualize such an ideal, there will continue to be a wide discrepancy between expectation and reality. In the search for an egalitarian companionship marriage, we have seen the rise of a phenomenon sometimes referred to as *serial monogamy* (Paolino & McCrady, 1978). This pattern may provide an alternative to the traditional lifetime monogamy of marriage. The increased divorce rate may be viewed as an effort to bridge the gap between the expectations of a companionship marriage and the disappointing reality of the present state of the culture.

Trends in Marital Therapy

Historically, couples experiencing marital unhappiness dealt with their problems within the context of the extended family, or they shared their concerns, worries, and fears with a member of the clergy. In the United States, early professional recognition of some need to address marital issues was reflected in the development of the Marriage Consultation Center by Abraham and Hannah Stone in New York in 1929. A few years later, in 1939, Paul Papenoe founded the American Institute of Family Relations. By 1942, pioneers in marital therapy had organized the American Association of Marriage Counselors, which in 1970 became the American Association of Marriage and Family Counselors, reflecting the influence of the fast-growing field of family therapy. The end of World War II saw a dramatic increase in marital instability and a consequent growth in the field of marital therapy.

The technologies for intervention were limited to the predominant psychotherapeutic model of the time, which was essentially psychoanalytic. In 1938, Oberndorf published a classic paper on the psychoanalysis of married couples, and in 1948, Mettleman published a paper on the concurrent analyses of married couples (cf. Paolino & McCrady, 1978). Because the psychoanalytic model is individually and intrapsychically focused, *concurrent* marital therapy (i.e., one therapist seeing each spouse individually) gained in popularity. It remained the most common form of treatment through the psychoanalytic heyday of the 1950s. Today, *conjoint* marital therapy (i.e., both partners seen together) is heavily favored in the treatment of marital conflict. Conjoint treatment focuses on the relationship rather than the individuals and allows the therapist to intervene directly in the interactional process. This modality grew out of the 1960s expansion of new therapeutic technologies and out of the work of the newly emerging field of family therapy, which began in the late 1950s. Behavioral approaches to marital problems were first used in the mid-1960s, having had their original applications in work with individuals. In some respects, the psychoanalytic and behavioral perspectives may be viewed as two sides of a coin. One focuses on the past and the individual's unseen internal processes. The other focuses on the immediate present and the individual's observable behaviors.

In comparison, the family systems point of view focuses concern away from the individuals and emphasizes the interactional process. This paradigm shift in the late 1950s and the 1960s marked a unique contribution to the development of marital therapy. Communication (systems) theorists share with behaviorists an attention to observable data but may have developed a greater appreciation for the subtleties of interpersonal processes than behaviorists (Segraves, 1982).

For most of the 1970s, the three major theoretical schools adopted somewhat adversarial postures, each maintaining an entrenched position regarding the validity of the views and the efficacy of their approaches. However, over the past several years, all three groups have been confronted by the limits of their own models. Psychodynamically oriented clinicians have expanded their clinical repertoires to include behavioral interventions, and behavioral therapists are now examining ways to deal more effectively with the affective issues in therapy. The thrust in all health care nationwide is toward more integrative and holistic approaches. Marital therapists of all persuasions are recognizing the value of a more comprehensive, broadened perspective.

The treatment model proposed in this chapter integrates the major strengths of both social learning theory and family systems theory (Birchler & Spinks, 1980). Moreover, the cross-fertilization provided by the present authors' divergent backgrounds has opened the way more recently to a consideration of psychodynamic factors that impact the interactional process. The behavioral-systems marital therapy (BSMT) model discussed in this chapter follows a basic behavioral format as its strategic approach. However, constant attention is paid to cognitive, affective, and dynamic issues as they influence the interactional process. Additionally, the therapist is sensitive to individual intrapsychic factors, recognizing the clinical reality that internal conflicts are expressed in interpersonal relationships.

The behavioral-systems model (Figure 1) makes several working assumptions about couples presenting for marital treatment. Slightly modified, these assumptions are essentially consistent with those described by Wood and Jacobson (1985):

1. We assume that distressed couples presenting for treatment wish to improve their relationship. Unless evidence gathered during the assessment phase suggests otherwise, this assumption is associated with the belief that couples have already tried to solve their problems on their own.

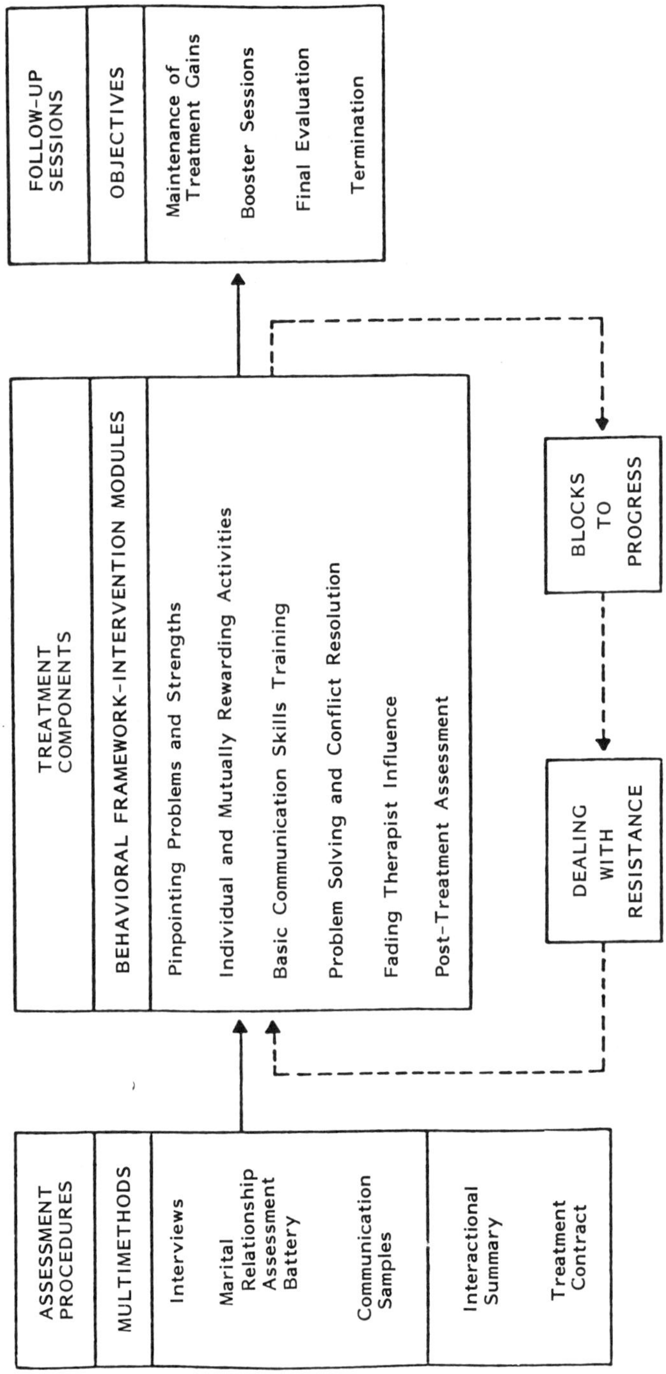

Figure 1. Behavioral-systems marital therapy: Assessment and intervention components.

2. We assume that distressed couples are deficient in basic communication, problem-solving, and conflict-resolution skills. Therefore, conflicts are unresolved and intrapsychic factors often determine the interpretations given by each partner to the experience.

3. Differences in personality and interactional style evolve into sources of frustration and alienation for distressed couples. Previously, these characteristics may have been attractions, and they may still have the potential for strengthening the relationship. This alienation and sense of perceived difference leads to Assumption 4, the lack of a collaborative set.

4. We assume that couples entering treatment deal with the frustration of marital dysfunction by pulling in opposite directions. We believe that, in order for progress to occur, the partners must make noncontingent, bilateral commitments to work on improving the relationship.

5. We assume that successful marital therapy requires more work and energy than can be accomplished in the therapy sessions alone. Therefore, homework is an important part of this model.

6. Progress in therapy rarely moves along an even course. We assume that setbacks and regression to less facilitative behavior will occur during the course of treatment. Preparation for such relapses is essential to maintain therapeutic gains.

7. We assume that distressed couples have little, if any, current experience with positive exchanges in their relationship. The BSMT model includes early attention to increasing the partners' repertoires of positive behaviors. This early intervention is designed to encourage hopefulness and increase motivation.

8. We assume that, in the course of skill training and other behavioral interventions, therapists will have to address certain cognitive, affective, and insight-oriented issues.

This integrative BSMT approach has evolved over the last 12 years and continues to be modified by new developments in theoretical understanding and intervention technology.

SPECIAL DIAGNOSTIC CONSIDERATIONS

The treatment of marital dysfunction is conceptualized in three stages: the *evaluation period, treatment applications,* and *termination.* Throughout all three stages, there may be significant *blocks to progress* (i.e., resistance) to reaching the goals of assessment and treatment. In this section on the evaluation period, multimodal assessment procedures that characterize BSMT approaches are discussed.

Objectives of Assessment

We suggest making an explicit contract with the couple to evaluate their marital relationship before discussing any intention to bring about change or to enter therapy. The first session, preferably and usually with both partners present, is devoted to (1) understanding the nature of the partners' complaints; (2) determining how they came to the decision to seek marital therapy; and (3) finding out what their current intentions and expectations are for improving (or, sometimes, terminating) the relationship. This first meeting is considered successful if the therapist has accomplished the above tasks and has gained a commitment from each spouse to complete the process of marital relationship evaluation. This process is explained as consisting of a series of two or three additional meetings to help the couple learn in detail how their relationship is functioning. After this process, a decision will be made whether to mutually define goals for treatment. Most couples agree to complete this brief evaluation process. Although from a behavioral perspective active treatment does not begin until the evaluation period has been completed, we have found the assessment phase to have a therapeutic effect. Many couples report decreased conflict and increased hopefulness about their relationship.

There are five general considerations for the therapist to keep in mind during the evaluation process. The first is the need to establish a therapeutic alliance with each partner despite the conflict between the partners.

The second consideration is the appropriateness of marital therapy as the treatment for the presenting problems. There appear to be a number of exclusionary criteria that experienced clinicians believe complicate the prospects of a good outcome for conjoint marital treatment. In fact, *individual treatment* may well be required before marital therapy if the presenting complaints include active alcoholism or drug abuse, acute psychosis, moderate to severe paranoid personality disorder, significant affective disorder, borderline personality disorder, moderate to severe character disorders, pathological jealousy, and violence-prone negative interaction cycles. Individual therapy may also be a useful adjunct to marital therapy for individuals suffering from intrapsychic conflicts that have substantial repercussions in their lives.

Marital therapy is generally considered the treatment of choice when one or both partners are dissatisfied with some aspect of the marriage, when both partners are sufficiently committed to the relationship to work for improvement, and when the problems identified have arisen as a function of dyadic interaction. Marital therapy is indicated when solutions to the presenting problems can be conceptualized as resulting from systematic changes in partners' attitudes, beliefs, behaviors, or feelings. *Family therapy* is the treatment of choice if the presenting complaint or the family dynamics are such that a family member outside the marital dyad is the identified patient, manifests significant behavioral or psychiatric symptoms, or otherwise has such a significantly influential impact on the marital or family system that this person must or should be included in the group to be treated.

Third, the therapist must attend to the mix of *awareness of problems, requisite interactional skills,* and *motivation to change* in each partner. Each of these three factors may significantly affect the prospects for successful marital therapy, and each requires somewhat different assessment and treatment interventions.

Fourth, during the assessment process, it is useful to generate hypotheses about the rules, roles, and homeostatic mechanisms that govern the relationship. How are interpersonal messages exchanged? Is affect expressed, and in what manner? What are the implicit and explicit rules about communication? What are the relationship roles, and is there a struggle over roles? What nonfacilitative interpersonal behaviors serve to maintain dysfunction in the system? Last, but not least, what are the strengths in the relationship?

Finally, the fifth consideration during the evaluation period is the assessment of conflict in the relationship from both a content and an interactional-process point of view. We are interested not only in *what* couples disagree about but also in *how* they go about managing and resolving conflict.

Throughout the evaluation process, the therapist considers both the kinds and the priorities of treatment interventions. Information from the five general areas described above provides the basis for these decisions. When appropriate, the rather standardized assessment and treatment model is modified to meet the needs of a given couple. For example, some couples enter treatment in crisis, or they generate crises during the evaluation period. Digression from the standard procedures is therefore indicated to provide supportive or problem-oriented crisis counseling. Also, regarding the standard treatment interventions, the particular order and/or emphasis may differ significantly from one couple to another. For example, some couples enter therapy devoid of positive feelings for one another; others start from a rather good base of affection, humor, and intimacy. Once these differences are determined, treatment plans may be designed to reflect these strengths and weaknesses.

Methods of Assessment

The therapist may use several information-gathering methods to determine what the content- and process-related issues are for a given couple. This diagnostic information is then presented to the couple in such a way that mutually agreed-upon treatment goals are established and pursued. The four diagnostic methods are clinical interviews, self-report instruments, communication samples, and spouse observation in the natural environment.

Clinical Interviews

As discussed above, the first meeting with the couple is typically devoted to a discussion of the spouses' chief complaints, their reasons for initiating therapy, and their past experiences with therapy, and to an invitation to complete two or three more evaluation meetings. It is important to involve both partners in this discussion. Each spouse has both a right and a responsibility to explore and disclose his or her concerns about the relationship. Accordingly, the therapist makes a point of eliciting comparable information from both partners and of reinforcing their sharing by using good listening and validation skills (Gottman, Notarius, Gonso, & Markman, 1976). Even though the spouses may not agree with one another, the therapist demonstrates an understanding of each person's perspective.

At the earliest possible point in the assessment and therapy process, the therapist seeks to establish and reinforce a "collaborative set" (Jacobson & Margolin, 1979) between the partners. This implies that the partners understand that the present status and quality of their relationship is a product of their interaction, and that each person acts, reacts, and otherwise contributes to the existing patterns of interaction that constitute the relationship. Typically, partners enter marital therapy assured that their spouse is to blame for the major problems. Early in the sessions, the therapist asks questions, makes normative statements, administers questionnaires, and uses language that introduces and emphasizes the interactional perspective. Helping couples to understand and believe in this notion is critical to the success of marital therapy.

In the context of gathering information from couples and listening to their complaints, the amount of control the therapist exerts in the session is important. We use the phrase "measured ventilation of feelings" to describe the art of eliciting partners' feelings (sufficiently so that they feel heard and understood) but setting a limit on the amount, the nature, and the intensity of negative affect (to keep control of the session and to minimize destructive comments).

Information relevant to treatment decisions is obtained primarily through the evaluation interviews. Sometimes, one spouse requests an individual interview before or after the initial conjoint meeting. We prefer to do these after the first conjoint meeting if possible, in order to emphasize our bias that the relationship is the treatment unit. Recently, we have found it useful to schedule routinely one individual session with each partner as part of the evaluation process. This session explores family-of-origin information as well as relationship history before the present marriage. These meetings also give the therapist an enhanced perspective on long-standing personality factors that may contribute to the current distress. Other issues that emerge in the individual sessions include one partner's having had an affair, one partner's wanting to end the marriage (but being unable or afraid to confront the spouse), and significant individual problems (e.g., depression, anxiety, suicidal ideation, or severe ambivalence about the marriage). When such significant factors are discovered, a plan is devised for incorporating these issues into the relationship therapy, if appropriate. Occasionally, what is learned in these individual meetings renders conjoint marital therapy inadvisable. For example, one partner may have a private commitment to an ongoing affair or a definite intention to leave the other.

Self-Report Instruments

All of the behavioral and cognitive-behavioral marital-therapy clinical-research programs in the country make extensive use of assessment questionnaires. The purposes of administering these batteries are threefold. First, the data are used for a clinical assessment of the strengths and weaknesses of a given relationship and for treatment planning. By the use of self-assessment inventories, much information is gathered in a cost-effective manner outside the therapy sessions. Second, when the inventories are administered before and after treatment, and at follow-up, the possible effects of the therapeutic intervention are measured. Standardized measures allow for comparisons with other couples and programs. Third, completing the questionnaires introduces the couple to the therapist's perspective regarding the salient dimensions of marital satisfaction and interaction.

Two marriage-assessment inventories commercially available are the Couples Pre-Counseling Inventory (Stuart, 1983) and the Marital Satisfaction Inventory (Snyder & Regts, 1982; Snyder, Wills, & Keiser, 1981). Both of these instruments elicit several kinds of information, including aspects of marital satisfaction, general communication and problem solving, conflict over child rearing, sex and affection, and commitment to the marriage. Most programs use one of two scales to measure the couple's global marital adjustment. Traditionally, the Locke-Wallace Marital Adjustment Scale was used (Locke & Wallace, 1959). More recently, the Dyadic Adjustment Scale (Spanier, 1976) has become popular. These scales are useful for comparing study samples or the pre- and posttherapy levels of the marital satisfaction of each partner.

In our program, the first author has participated in the development of several assessment instruments and has combined them with standard instruments such as the Locke-Wallace Marital Adjustment Scale to comprise a package called the Marital Relationship Assessment Battery (MRAB). The MRAB consists of the following seven self-report inventories, which are completed independently by each spouse. These descriptions indicate the kind of self-report information deemed important in BSMT.

Locke-Wallace Marital Adjustment Scale. General areas of agreement and disagreement on major topics within the relationship are indicated. Empirically derived scale-scores discriminate maritally distressed from nondistressed couples.

Marital Status Inventory. In this scale, prepared by Weiss and Cerreto (1980), 14 true-false questions assess the degree to which each spouse has sought a dissolution of the relationship.

Areas of Change Questionnaire. In this questionnaire, devised by Weiss and others (Weiss & Birchler, 1975; Weiss, Hops, & Patterson, 1973), 34 areas of typical marital conflict are assessed by analyzing couples' requests for behavior change in self and spouse.

Self-Description Inventory. Designed by Wahler (1968), three scales assess individuals' levels of self-esteem, psychological distress, and physical symptoms. The scales indicate individuals' tendencies toward depression, anxiety, denial, and somatic preoccupation.

Responses to Conflict. Birchler (1977) prepared this scale as an index of partners' perceptions of the likelihood that a maladaptive response to marital conflict will occur given the interactional opportunity.

Inventory of Rewarding Activities. Weiss *et al*. (1973) devised and Birchler (1979) modified this questionnaire to assess the types and proportions of recreational activities that each partner has engaged in alone, with the spouse only, with the spouse and other adults, with the family, and with others (excluding the spouse) over the previous 4 weeks. A section on time distribution also indicates what percentage of the previous week was spent working, sleeping, and engaging in rewarding or nonrewarding activities.

Summary of Current Important Issues. To complete the MRAB, each spouse lists, in order of importance, his or her perception of the four most significant relationship, and personal, strengths and weaknesses.

Once the MRAB is completed and scored, a 16-page written summary is given to the clients at the time of the roundtable discussion. This document may be used for assessment and feedback purposes only, or as the basis for the initial therapeutic discussions and homework assignments. For strategic purposes, considerable information is available to emphasize the couple's strengths and weaknesses, or both.

Communication Samples

In our experience, no matter what the couple says or writes about their general communication and problem-solving skills, more, and often different, information is obtained from actual observation of the couple discussing a marital conflict issue. Accordingly, and typically at the beginning of the second evaluation session, the therapist helps the couple to identify a relevant and moderate-intensity marital problem to discuss (i.e., an issue on which they currently disagree). This 10-minute discussion is videotaped while the therapist is out of the room. In situations where videotape is not available, the therapist may stay in the room, disengage from the discussion, and observe the couple's interaction pattern. These displays often provide a unique source of data about dominance and deference, general sending and listening communication skills, problem definition and solution skills, and the type and function of affect generated during the discussion.

Depending on one's objectives, the marital-conflict communication sample may be used for sophisticated research projects, in which each verbal and nonverbal behavior is objectively rated by trained observers using complex behavioral coding systems (e.g., Marital Interaction Coding System—Hops, Wills, Patterson, & Weiss, 1972; Couple's Interaction Scoring System—Gottman, 1979), or the communication sample technique may constitute a purely clinical assessment procedure to facilitate diagnosis and treatment planning. It should be noted that there is a need for an inexpensive, practical clinician's guide to assessing marital interaction in a standardized procedure. Some methods have been proposed (Floyd & Markman, 1984; Thomas, 1977), and a similar project is under development in our program. In any case, a couple's ability to identify, mutually define, and effectively solve marital conflicts is considered a critical requisite for a satisfactory marriage. The observed communication sample provides a method of assessing the basis and the development of this interactional process as often as is appropriate throughout therapy.

Spouse Observation

From the advent of the social learning approach to marital therapy (Stuart, 1969; Weiss *et al.,* 1973) to this day (cf. Weiss & Margolin, 1989), self-reported patterns of spousal interaction observed at home have been integral to the assessment and treatment of marital dysfunction. When this method in particular is used, the distinction between assessment and treatment is blurred. The reason is that most applications of spouse observation are initiated very early in treatment and continue throughout the program, and each week's assessment data become the basis for next week's homework assignment. Such procedures are as simple as "catching your spouse doing something nice" (Liberman, Wheeler, de Visser, Kuehnel, & Kuehnel, 1980) and participating in "caring days" (Stuart, 1980) or "love days" (Weiss & Birchler, 1978), or as sophisticated as having each partner monitor, on a once- or twice-daily basis, over 400 marital interaction behaviors using the Spouse Observation Checklist (cf. Weiss, 1980). By means of this system, the weekly results of spouse-emitted behaviors may be computer-sorted according to a given couple's strengths and deficiencies in 12 important areas of marital interaction.

Developmental Considerations

In addition to the standard assessment considerations applicable to the BSMT model, the authors have been influenced by work done in the area of adult and family development (Carter & McGoldrick, 1980; Colarusso & Nemiroff, 1981; Levinson, Darrow, Klein, Levinson, & McKee, 1978; Sheehy, 1974). Each decade, from the 20s to the 60s, involves a shifting perspective for the individual. Relationships must accommodate to these natural developmental progressions. Additionally, the life cycle of the family consists of a series of periods characterized by states of movement and change or quiescence and stability. The times of developmental change represent an instability in the structure of significant relationships. Developmental milestones for the individual become normative events for the family (e.g., birth, death, launching a career, and retiring). Consequently, in the diagnostic phase of marital therapy, the developmental epochs of family life are important factors because they provide information about universally experienced transitions. Recognizing the developmental tasks considered essential at any given stage enables the therapist to appreciate the realities faced by any given couple. Important implications for treatment may result.

The Treatment Contract

In the typical marital-therapy case, the third or fourth session is devoted to providing the couple feedback based on all the types of assessment data obtained and to agreeing on a treatment plan. We integrate the information obtained into what we call the *interactional summary*. The couple is presented (in terminology that they use and can comprehend) with our understanding of (1) their individual concerns about the marriage, their partner, and their expectations for change; (2) their mutually developed functional and dysfunctional communication and behavioral interaction patterns—in both the instrumental and the affectional domains; (3) their specific efforts and styles of managing conflict—and the positive or negative consequences; and (4) any other information relevant to the current status of and the future prospects for marital satisfaction. During this session, feedback is presented verbally and in writing (concerning the topical and quantitative results of the MRAB) and may include videotaped illustrations of their communication sample. Throughout this presentation, the partners are invited to comment on the impact of this information.

Finally, the goals of the treatment are outlined and typically include work in some particular *content* areas (e.g., sex and affection, household responsibilities, or finances) and in some important *process* areas (e.g., improvement in general communication skills, problem-solving and conflict resolution skills, or sex-role adjustments). In this discussion, the couple is encouraged to endorse or modify the proposed list and to help set priorities for intervention. The therapist then explains how the treatment objectives will be accomplished both at home and through weekly 1- to 1½-hour meetings. Couples are told that the intervention techniques include active discussion, exercise training in general communication and problem-solving skills, behavioral rehearsal, videotape feedback, and a variety of weekly homework assignments. Depending on the number and complexity of the treatment goals, the total number of weekly sessions required is estimated. In practice, the number of sessions (including the evaluation meetings) ranges from about 12 to 40. If a long or complex course of treatment is anticipated, the objectives are broken down into smaller segments, and estimates are given for these (e.g., six weeks to accomplish goals related to marital enrichment and basic communication skills).

FREQUENT CLINICAL PROBLEMS

The major problems encountered by the marital therapist in the outpatient setting may be categorized in three ways: content issues, interactional process issues, and maladaptive cognitions and feelings. Distortions in cognitions and feelings (internal dynamics) may generate a nonfacilitative interactional process, which then leads to specific content-based complaints.

Content issues are a common part of each partner's presenting complaints. These areas of chief complaint have been studied and enumerated in the literature (cf. Birchler, 1979, for several references). Common among these complaints are lack of communication, spouse too moody, spouse demanding and critical, finances, sex and affection difficulties, child management conflicts, and household responsibilities. It becomes apparent during the evaluation process that most content issues are actually a manifestation of dysfunctions in the couple's interactional process.

Interactional process refers here to the *how* of couples' problems. These dysfunctions are typically encountered as deficiencies in communication, problem-solving, and/or conflict-management skills. Distressed couples are notorious for managing the frustration and the inherent negativity associated with marital conflict in one of three styles: escalation of sequences of conflict generation, persistent patterns of conflict avoidance, or some husband–wife or sequential combination of the first two (Gottman, 1979).

Beyond these *faulty behavioral interactions, maladaptive cognitions* and their consequent *affective distortions* play a highly significant role in the etiology of, the maintenance of, and/or the resistance to treatment of marital distress. These cognitions (beliefs) are formed partly in the family of origin and are elaborated in the crucible of life experience. Often, there is great discrepancy between the expectations generated by distorted cognition and the reality of experience in the relationship. The highly structured, rational, nonemotionally focused interventions of behavioral marital therapy may fall short of success when the therapist fails to recognize that there is an internal system of references operating in each partner. The therapist who can address clients' feelings and relate those feelings to misperceptions based on distorted cognitions will experience greater success in dealing with the complexity of couples' presenting problems (Epstein, 1982; Greenberg & Johnson, 1986; Segraves, 1982; Wile, 1981).

TREATMENT APPLICATIONS

Since the mid-1970s, outcome research on the effectiveness of BSMT has been accumulating. The common treatment components in most of the reported studies have been (1) skill training in communication and problem solving and (2) various interventions designed to change spouses' behavior. The results so far, as summarized by Baucom and Hoffman (1986), have indicated that, relative to a wait-list control, BSMT is effective in (1) decreasing partners' negative communication as assessed in observed situations; (2) decreasing self-reported problem areas and behavior change requests; and (3) increasing marital satisfaction ratings. Jacobson, Follette, and Revenstorf (1984) developed some very stringent criteria for determining whether a given BSMT case had improved. They applied these standards to a number of previously completed outcome studies. Overall, approximately half the couples treated improved with BSMT. The available indications were that significant gains in marital satisfaction had been maintained for about half the treated couples at 1-year follow-up (Jacobson & Holtzworth-Munroe, 1986).

This 50% success rate is difficult to interpret. For one thing, few marital therapy programs, other than those behaviorally oriented, have systematically included multimethod, observational outcome measures. Therefore, objective comparisons with alternative approaches are difficult to make. To complicate matters further, one must remember (and this may be critical) that most clinical research projects that have investigated the efficacy of BSMT have typically (1) employed relatively inexperienced graduate students as therapists; (2) conducted relatively brief 10- to 20-treatment sessions; (3) used standardized treatment packages that were not individualized for a given couple; and (4) used small samples of couples that were occasionally suspect as to their level of clinical marital distress. Nevertheless, a 50% success rate maintained for 1 year for significantly distressed couples may be a solid achievement, given that the divorce rate in the general population is also about 50%. That is, helping 50% of the most distressed half of marriages is noteworthy.

Behavioral-Systems Treatment Components

First, referring again to Figure 1, let us review the fundamental treatment components of our behavioral-systems approach. These are (1) pinpointing problems and strengths; (2) establishing individual and mutually rewarding activities; (3) training in basic communication skills; (4) problem solving and conflict resolution; and (5) fading therapist influence (discussed under Termination).

Pinpointing Problems and Strengths

All of the information collected during the multimethod assessment phase is considered in an analysis of both the individuals' and the couple's strengths and weaknesses. Each couple has a unique combination of personality and interactional assets and liabilities. In our experience, treatment planning and the setting of priorities for intervention may be individualized considerably for a given couple within the fundamental framework of the behavioral-systems model.

For example, in one recent case, a dual-career couple presented for therapy. The wife complained primarily about lack of help with household responsibilities and care of the children and about general lack of affection. The husband complained about lack of sex and about the fact that his wife was engaged in so many outside activities that she never seemed to be at home. The husband made an excellent salary but was a hard-driving, obsessive person who demanded perfection in many areas, including household management. The wife was much more easygoing and considerably less organized but was warm and seemed really to care for her husband. The communication sample suggested fair to good communication and problem-solving skills, but other information indicated that the partners spent relatively little time together because of their busy schedules.

Based on an analysis of these factors and the more extensive assessment procedures described above, a treatment plan capitalizing on the couple's strengths and taking into account their weaknesses included (1) using some of their considerable discretionary income to hire a part-time housekeeper to clean the house and to transport the children to enrichment activities after school; (2) having the husband propose a number of mutually rewarding social activities that the wife would then agree to make time for (including some romantically inclined evening and weekend time alone together); and (3) some high-priority weekly ''talk time'' that would allow them to apply their relatively good communication skills to discussing relationship issues and plans for improvement. In this case, little emphasis was placed on remedial communication training, on asking the wife to become more organized to manage the household and the children, or on asking the husband to modify his rather fixed, perfectionistic, and unemotional personality style.

Establishing Individual and Mutually Rewarding Activities

Most couples seeking marital therapy have significant difficulty with independence-dependence-interdependence and intimacy-alienation. Obviously, one's expectations and fears concerning intimate relationships are shaped in previous family and other interpersonal experiences. Ironically, certain partners are interested in an intimate attachment and at the same time may have learned to fear intimacy because of the potential for rejection and abandonment. Frequently, the attitudes and behaviors that an individual adopts to secure intimacy while protecting against rejection are misperceived and misunderstood by the spouse. Consequently, in the absence of open and clear communication, maladaptive, reciprocal patterns of interaction are developed. Early in our treatment program, we use the "individual and mutually rewarding activities" interventions as relatively straightforward procedures for analyzing and addressing these issues. Interventions are targeted at daily, weekly, or project-based time intervals. The well-known, and previously described, caring activities (Birchler, 1983b; Stuart, 1980), love days (Weiss & Birchler, 1975) and consideration interventions (Margolin & Weinstein, 1983) are designed to help couples identify and raise their consciousness regarding daily exchanges of positive instrumental and affectional behaviors. Simple non-problem-area, repetitive behaviors are assigned that demonstrate caring, elicit similar behaviors in response, and are generally incompatible with negative interaction behaviors (e.g., a hug, a favorite meal, or a favor like doing the other's task).

In a larger perspective, the weekly and project-oriented activities of couples are reviewed with the purpose of seeking an effective balance between the partners' personal, independent activities (e.g., hobbies, sports, and clubs) and their mutually rewarding "together" activities (e.g., socializing with friends, going to a show or out to dinner, and vacations and holidays). As mentioned earlier, most distressed couples have significant problems in developing optimal balance in these areas. Education, permission, and specific assignments to develop or to restructure these activities are very helpful. Although the structural assignments appear simple enough, this is often a difficult area in which to make progress. Nevertheless, uncovering and explaining the significant meanings of individually and mutually rewarding activities for each partner are often basic to improvement in the marriage. Here also, the therapist's appreciation of family of origin and long-standing personality issues facilitates this process.

Training in Basic Communication Skills

Communication training (i.e., message-sender and active-listener skills—see Gottman *et al.*, 1976) has traditionally been a central ingredient in most marital enrichment and behaviorally oriented marital-therapy programs (for literature reviews, see Birchler, 1979; Guerney, Guerney, & Cooney, 1985). The efficacy of communication training (CT) *per se* has been difficult to isolate from that of comprehensive treatment programs, which typically combine communication and problem-solving-skill acquisition with other cognitive-behavior-change interventions. Few well-controlled studies have been done. However, as reported in a research review by Baucom and Hoffman (1986), it appears that CT has a greater effect on specific communication-skill variables than it has on marital adjustment overall. The most conservative conclusion at this time is that CT may be an important and constructive treatment component but is neither necessary nor sufficient to account for improvements in marital satisfaction. Our own clinical experience is that CT is often, if not always, an effective organizing and facilitative vehicle for helping couples to identify and modify dysfunctional aspects of their personal beliefs, behaviors, and dyadic interactions. CT also serves to help couples explore, understand, and validate one another's feelings.

In brief, basic CT consists of bibliotherapy, modeling, behavioral rehearsal (in sessions and at home), coaching, and verbal and videotape feedback. Couples are taught how to self-disclose personal messages honestly, openly, concisely, and clearly, and to listen in a way that actively demonstrates interest, support, and understanding (for exemplary CT details, see Birchler, 1983b; Gottman *et al.*, 1976; McKay, Davis, & Fanning, 1983; Strayhorn, 1977).

Although couples rarely enter therapy demonstrating effective communication skills, it is not always clear whether the partners are suffering from skill deficits or performance (i.e., motivational) deficiencies (Margolin & Fernandez, 1985). The assessment process is designed to identify skill deficits as well as related interactional dysfunctions. When indicated, the skill-training process itself may take from two to an indefinite number of weeks (when one half to two thirds of the time in each session is devoted to instruction and practice). Alas, some individuals never seem to progress to the point of being acknowledged, accomplished communicators. In some cases, the other spouse may compensate with gains in communication skills of his or her own. In other cases, the nonspecific effects of the training may still be important, for example, in the development of a collaborative set. In still other cases, the expectations and goals of treatment may have to be modified. In general, however, with considerable practice at home, four to six sessions are devoted to basic communication-skills training.

Problem Solving and Conflict Resolution

Training in problem solving is begun after the partners have achieved and demonstrated a mutual respect for one another and a shared sense of responsibility for their marital distress. In addition, they should have accomplished at least the preliminary objectives of (1) the caring activities; (2) the individual and mutually rewarding activities; and (3) the basic communication-skills training. This problem-solving training procedure is now well developed and fairly straightforward. The process is a product of the problem-solving model described by Goldfried and D'Zurilla (1969) and has been elaborated comprehensively by Jacobson and Margolin (1979) in their problem-solving manual.

Typically, a long list of potential problem areas is derived from all of the major assessment procedures described above. Couples are taught to address these content areas in a progressive manner, going from the relatively easy to the most difficult unresolved problems. The five major steps that we emphasize in problem solving are agenda building, selection of issue(s) for discussion, brainstorming, selection and implementation of the plan for resolution, and subsequent evaluation of the plan (cf. Birchler, 1983b). Initially, the therapist plays a very active instructor role in directing the problem-solving exercises in the sessions. Increasingly, the couple is taught to organize the exercises for themselves and to do more and more of the work at home. In most cases, it is wise to write out the proposed solutions in the form of contracts. This way, the agreed-upon responsibilities and contingencies may be documented and referred to in the future.

The five-step model outlined above is applicable to most but not all marital problems. In our experience the most difficult applications involve basic conflicts concerning commitment to the relationship, trust, jealousy, temper tantrums, predispositions toward anger and hostility, sex and affection (when one or both partners demand spontaneity and passion as the primary characteristic), long-past events that continue to upset one or both partners, and other conflicts that are not in any way amenable to negotiation, compromise, and an experimental approach to resolution. In fact, it is precisely these sorts of problems that present the greatest challenges to marital therapists in general, and to behaviorally oriented marital therapists in particular. The common lack of success with these types of problems also probably explains why many clinicians and clinical researchers are now actively attempting to develop integrated treatment approaches that consider affective, behavioral, cognitive, family systems, and psychodynamic variables. In keeping with this integrative effort, the following section presents some contemporary strategies for dealing with blocks to treatment progress, both before and after they occur.

Dealing with Resistance: Blocks to Progress

We regard as resistance any significant block to progress toward therapeutic goals. Resistance may be a function of behavioral, cognitive, and affective factors affecting any part of the therapeutic system: the individual partners, the therapist, or their interaction (cf. Anderson & Stewart, 1983). One author (Birchler, 1989) discussed the phenomenon of resistance in BMT at length and suggested two management strategies. First, as a normal part of the therapy process, one may *anticipate* various blocks to progress before they occur and take preventive steps. Second, once resistance is recognized in the therapeutic endeavor, remedial action may be taken to remove or modify the threat to progress. Note that any given behavior may or may not represent resistance and must be considered in context as it relates to theoretical orientation and therapeutic progress.

Anticipatory Strategies

To the extent that intermittent resistance to change is expected, good preventive practice dictates designing therapist-intervention options that preclude major problems. In this regard, the first objective for the therapist is to establish his or her credibility as a knowledgeable, competent professional who can facilitate change (Alexander, Barton, Waldron, & Mas, 1983). Such things as good recommendations from referral sources, appropriate office decor and location, therapist dress, and courteous reception are important. A second objective, establishing rapport with the couple, was discussed above. Demonstrations of empathy, warmth, understanding, and control are important in minimizing early blocks to progress. We have found it very helpful to include the partners in the consideration of, and the rationale for, all the various assessment and treatment activities. For example, in-session exercises and homework assignments are made very explicitly, and each partner is personally asked to agree on and commit herself or himself to each significant activity. Any reservations, expressed verbally or nonverbally, are explored at the time of assignment rather than after the fact. Stuart (1980) suggested that the therapist provide *reassurance, redirection,* and *repetition* of the rationale when initial resistance to directives is encountered.

During the treatment phase, five standard therapist interventions serve well to minimize or prevent resistance before it occurs. Some of these interventions have already been mentioned, and all of them may be applied throughout therapy, before or after resistance is encountered.

First, therapists should identify and maximize the clients' *efficacy expectations for change* (Epstein, 1985; Jacobson, 1984; Weiss, 1984). Failure to comply with a treatment regimen may be caused by a deficit in the clients' knowledge of what is appropriate or of what behavior will accomplish the goals, by a skill deficit, or by the presence of both and with the additional presence of fear and doubt (Meichenbaum & Gilmore, 1982). Clients must believe that they, the therapist, and the therapeutic method can be successful.

Providing knowledge and a rationale and maintaining enthusiasm and optimism are facilitative measures that the therapist may take.

Second, the partners' current behavior and functions of behavior may be *reframed* or *relabeled* in positive terms. The objective is to get spouses to alter their dysfunctional or change-inhibiting attributions about the meaning of their partner's behavior, about their distressed marriage, and about prospects for change. Once the basic meaning is challenged, the partners have an opportunity to observe and modify both the functions and the performance of such behaviors. For example, persistent arguments between partners may be relabeled as a relatively positive sign because they demonstrate the partners' investment of energy devoted to the relationship, as opposed to being emotionally divorced.

If relabeling is effective, the spouses may be less intent on blaming each other and more open to adopting the third (and already-discussed) cognitive restructuring: a *collaborative set* (Jacobson & Margolin, 1979). Basically, every opportunity is taken, via the provision of a rationale, bibliotherapy, in-session exercises, and homework assignments, to convince couples that a problem for one of them affects marital satisfaction and is therefore a problem for both of them.

The fourth cognitive intervention designed to minimize blocks to progress is *predicting relapses* during the course of therapy. Here the therapist monitors the therapeutic progress made by the couple and suggests that as part of the normal process of changing, setbacks and reversions to former, familiar styles of interaction are expected to occur. Predicting relapses simultaneously enhances the therapist's credibility and control of the situation and the couple's ability to cope once setbacks occur.

The fifth intervention that may prevent resistance before it occurs is the proper determination, assignment, and follow-up of *homework*. Resistance to BSMT is most often encountered as noncompliance with homework assignments. The skill-acquisition and behavioral-rehearsal aspects of BSMT require compliance both in the sessions and at home during the week. Accordingly, behavioral marital therapists should be experts in assigning homework (for specific guidelines, see Birchler, 1988; Hartman, 1983; Lazarus & Fay, 1982; Martin & Worthington, 1982). The assignment itself must be given in the context of rapport with the clients and relevance to explicit therapeutic goals. The partners should participate in the consideration of what specific assignments, to be done by whom, are appropriate. The assignments should not exceed the partners' competence or motivation levels. Finally, once given, homework assignments must be reviewed, shaped, and modified. The partners' performance must be acknowledged in subsequent sessions. The technology of homework assignments is a deceptively critical aspect of BSMT and its relative success.

Remedial Strategies

Dealing with significant blocks to progress after they occur is an important challenge to any marital therapist. In such cases, the therapist must be prepared to deviate from the straightforward behavioral approach in order to clearly identify and deal with resistance (Spinks & Birchler, 1982). This is an area in which social learning theorists have increasingly and appropriately looked to other contemporary clinicians, orientations, and clinical investigators for innovative therapeutic interventions that can be integrated into the basic cognitive-behavioral approach (e.g., Barton & Alexander, 1981; Birchler & Spinks, 1980; Jacobson & Holtzworth-Munroe, 1986; Margolin & Fernandez, 1985;

Weiss, 1980; 1984). In line with these developments, the following strategies for dealing with resistance include cognitive, behavioral, and affective intervention options, some of which are relatively new to BSMT and expand the theoretical and technical range of the therapeutic interventions available to facilitate change.

Exploring Cognitions, Relabeling, and Cognitive Restructuring

At the earliest sign of a significant pattern or the blatant occurrence of resistance, we suggest that the therapist label the behavior and ask the client or the couple to help explain its meaning. A direct, empathic approach often prompts the client to identify and assert his or her concerns. For example, "I've noticed that you folks have been 10–15 minutes late for our session the past 3 weeks. May we talk about that, and can you help me understand what it might mean?"

It may also help to relabel certain behaviors in a positive light. For example, "You both seem to be upset and discouraged because there has been a significant increase in the number of your arguments over the past 2 weeks. Actually, in the short run, I think that is a positive sign. It demonstrates that you are less willing simply to avoid important issues in the relationship and are more willing to express your feelings. All we have to concentrate on now are effective communication skills so that your discussions will be constructive instead of argumentative."

When resistance has been identified or when dysfunctional cognitions or attributions are suspected, one may use the "search-and-destroy" cognitive-restructuring technique described by Epstein (1985) and Jacobson (1984). Using a one-on-one interviewing technique, the therapist elicits the partners' beliefs about the therapy process and their attributions concerning their spouses. For example, in a case where the wife functionally punishes a newly emitted behavior by the husband (which she formerly requested), the search-and-destroy technique may uncover the wife's attribution, "My partner will never change. He's just doing this because the therapist told him to." The consequence of such a belief may be examined by all, and hopefully, the attribution will be challenged and modified (i.e., destroyed).

In some instances, it may be helpful or necessary to design a hypothesis-testing, cognition-challenging behavioral experiment. For example, clients who believed that feelings of intimacy should precede actions of intimacy have often changed their minds as a function of caring activities assignments. Spouses are asked to behave independently "as if" they especially cared for their partners over a period of several days or weeks. When successful, caring activities demonstrate partners' commitment to the relationship and their willingness to risk and bring about change. Usually, when the partners genuinely participate in these assignments, renewed feelings of respect and caring are experienced.

Identify, Explore, and Express Emotions

With few exceptions, behavioral marital therapists have sought to contain and control partners' emotional expressions, particularly the negative ones. An emphasis has been placed on modifying the spouses' behaviors and cognitions to bring about change in their marital satisfaction (i.e., their subjective feelings). However, when standard BSMT interventions meet with significant blocks to progress, it is possible that helping couples to identify and express their primary feelings, needs, and wants will help them to communicate, to problem-solve better, and to increase the levels of their intimacy (Wile, 1981).

Greenberg and Johnson (1986, p. 262) outlined nine steps of their emotionally focused couples-therapy approach, many of which may well be adapted to dealing with resistance in BSMT. The nine steps are to (1) delineate the conflict issues in the core struggle; (2) identify the negative interaction cycle; (3) access unacknowledged feelings; (4) reframe the problem in terms of underlying feelings; (5) promote identification with disowned needs; (6) promote acceptance of the partner's experiences; (7) facilitate the expression of needs and wants; (8) establish the emergence of new solutions; and (9) consolidate new positions.

Clearly, moving into the area of "core struggles," "underlying feelings," "disowned needs," and "personal vulnerabilities based on past experiences" may take behavioral therapists a long way from objective interactional behavior. However, to the extent that related affect and cognitions mediate behavior change, and that these interventions may be operationalized, they should be investigated systematically. As Jacobson and Holtzworth-Munroe (1986) suggested, the identification of the partners' thoughts and feelings that accompany a mutual escalation of negative affect may be important first steps toward pinpointing the effective behavioral options that each spouse has in these difficult situations.

Interpretive Modeling

Interpretive modeling was developed independently of the Greenberg and Johnson approach, but it is certainly relevant to many of the nine steps of emotionally focused couples-therapy listed above. Interestingly, interpretive modeling is designed specifically to facilitate couples' delineation of core conflicts, to access partners' unacknowledged feelings, to promote their identification with disowned needs, and to facilitate the direct expression of needs and wants (Birchler & Spinks, 1980; Spinks & Birchler, 1982). The procedure incorporates therapists' modeling of good communication skills as they role-play and interpret the assumed attitudes and feelings of the couple. Therefore, interpretive modeling is most dramatic and effective when enacted by cotherapists. However, it is also possible to use it when a single therapist interacts with one of the partners while the other partner observes.

This technique is effective because (1) unspoken issues that are out of the clients' awareness are made explicit and overt; (2) the expression and management of underlying issues are modeled with particular empathic skill, which imparts to the clients a sense of confidence and reduced anxiety; and (3) the clients' catastrophic expectations are diffused as they observe the therapists effectively discussing critical issues. Once the carefully preplanned interpretive-modeling sequence has been displayed, the partners are invited to correct, to modify, and subsequently to continue the discussion on their own. This technique can be a powerful intervention. However, it should be applied cautiously, in an open, hypothesis-testing atmosphere. It is most applicable when the therapists have a good idea of the causes of resistance, after the couple trusts the therapists, and after the partners have acquired basic communication skills so that they can constructively continue the discussion of the uncovered issues on their own.

Antisabotage Procedures

Resistance that is encountered in the form of repeated noncompliance with (otherwise appropriate) homework assignments may often be resolved through the use of antisabotage procedures (Spinks & Birchler, 1982). This intervention consists of four steps: (1) brainstorming with the couple about all the conceivable ways and reasons that there may be noncompliance with the plan; (2) isolating high-probability obstructive attitudes and behaviors for each person; (3) assisting the couple to discuss specifically how the high-risk sabotage behaviors will be countered; and (4) socially reinforcing the couple for anticipating potential problems and solving them in advance of their occurrence. Although the procedure may take half a session to apply, it is a highly effective technique for getting compliance with homework.

Contingency Management

Another standard procedure designed to facilitate compliance with homework assignments is contingency management. This procedure is most relevant in the assessment period and the initial phases of treatment. Given a reasonable amount of rapport with the couple and considerable rationale, the therapist may effectively make further therapy contacts contingent on partners' completion of the agreed-upon homework. It is also possible to use a response-cost paradigm in which certain fees are refunded (or charged) depending on the couple's compliance with various assessment and intervention tasks. Once again, before such contingencies are applied to the couple's performance, consideration should be given to the appropriateness of the assignment in the first place.

Paradoxical Prescriptions

The use of paradoxical prescription in marital therapy (Hare-Mustin, 1976; Soper & L'Abate, 1977) is not incompatible with BSMT (Birchler, 1981). However, in our view, it should be used cautiously and as a last resort when resistance to homework assignments is significant and persistent and the therapist is determined to gain control over the situation. Paradoxical strategies consist of presenting a rationale for prescribing symptoms, or exercises that are designed to put clients in a therapeutic bind. That is, whether they comply with the prescription or resist (i.e., do not comply), constructive movement in the therapeutic process is achieved. The therapist's functional analysis of the symptom or the interactional system must be plausible, and compliance with the assignment must be unacceptable to the clients. For example, prescribing arguing at least three times a day to a constantly arguing couple, because marital conflict represents intimacy to them, probably meets both paradox criteria. If they comply, the therapist gains a measure of compliance and control; if they fail to argue as prescribed, some improvement will have occurred in their interaction.

Individual Contacts

As behaviorally oriented marital therapists have sought effective ways to deal with resistance and, independently, to expand the application of BSMT (e.g., Beach & O'Leary, 1986; Birchler, 1988; Foster, 1986; Hafner, 1986; Jacobson, 1983; O'Farrell, 1986), the once-discouraged meeting with individual spouses outside the conjoint format has emerged as a viable intervention procedure. In most marital therapy cases, we still tend to limit individualized meetings to the assessment phase and to dealing with significant resistance believed to be caused primarily by the partners' personal issues. In individual meetings, the therapist's objectives are to evaluate critically the individual's attitudes, feelings, and behavioral patterns and to identify possible hidden agendas regarding the partners' commitment to change in the relationship. Once obstructive issues are identified, the clients are confronted with the self- or relationship-defeating aspects of their cognitions and behavior. At this point, if appropriate, a plan is made to resolve the problems. Otherwise, it is suggested that relationship therapy be terminated. When used strategically, individual confrontations may be effective because they are a significant departure from the conjoint approach and they therefore "get the attention" of the resistant partner(s).

Termination and Referral

The final option for dealing with intractable resistance to progress is a discussion with the couple about terminating relationship therapy, with or without recommended referrals. Certainly, some couples discover, through their failed attempts at improvement, that the marriage is not viable. Other couples reach a limit in treatment gains that may fall short of the initial goals and expectations, but that nevertheless dictates a break in the weekly therapy sessions. In still other cases, the therapist or the treatment orientation does not work for the given couple, and referral to a different marital therapist is indicated. In any case, we have experienced situations in which the real threat of treatment termination had to be broached before the partners were motivated sufficiently to make significant gains.

Unfortunately, mild to moderate blocks to progress in therapy are the rule rather than the exception, and no one has yet found the formula either for predicting the type of resistance in a given case or for specifying the appropriate remedial intervention once resistance is encountered. This area still represents the art, not the science, of marital therapy.

Fading Therapist Influence

One of the characteristics of cognitive-behavioral-systems approaches to marital therapy that contributes to its relative success in a brief treatment model is the directness and the activity level of the therapist. For example, compared to client-centered and psychodynamically oriented clinicians, we suspect that behaviorally oriented therapists are significantly more active in several respects. Some of the following interventions require that the therapist understand and practice the basic technology developed as part of BSMT over the years; other interventions call on the therapist's natural skills and personality predisposition as the most active ingredient in the brief therapy process. Here is a list of common therapist interventions, many of which occur in most sessions, until substantial progress is made in achieving the goals of treatment. They are ordered randomly:

1. Teaching partners about the nature of functional and dysfunctional relationships.
2. Modeling effective communication and problem-solving skills, including assertiveness, self-disclosure, and empathic listening skills.
3. Structuring and directing interaction exercises (i.e., behavioral rehearsal).
4. Each session, actively setting an agenda and maintaining focus on the goals of treatment.
5. Inducing a "collaborative set" whenever possible by espousing the family-systems interactional-perspective and by encouraging self-change versus other change.

6. Regularly assigning, fostering compliance with, and debriefing homework activities.
7. Whenever appropriate, inducing interaction between partners rather than the therapist talking with the partners individually.
8. Commenting positively on the activities and progress of therapy while maintaining the clients' realistic perspective on the work required to succeed.
9. Encouraging steady progress while anticipating and predicting periodic relapses.
10. Using humor whenever appropriate to keep perspective on the tasks at hand.
11. Specifically identifying, exploring, and modifying partners' cognitions.
12. When indicated, identifying and exploring partners' affective responses.
13. Promoting the generalization and maintenance of treatment gains.
14. Socially reinforcing partners' positive behaviors and attitudes that are extant or emerging.
15. Extinguishing, or explicitly identifying and setting contingencies to modify, negative and destructive behaviors.

Obviously, a therapist who accomplishes many of these things in most sessions is very active indeed. However, approximately two thirds of the way through the treatment, the therapist begins to teach the couple how to take charge of the therapeutic process themselves. Progressively, over the remaining weeks, they are asked to propose the agenda for the sessions, to design the homework assignments, and to trouble-shoot any difficulties that may arise. Near the end of the regular therapy sessions, the therapist serves primarily as a consultant. This is an ideal role to play as the issue of termination is addressed.

TERMINATION

The termination process is the final phase of treatment. For years we have been suggesting that an important part of ending contact is to provide for the long-term generalization and maintenance of treatment gains (Birchler, 1983b; Birchler & Spinks, 1980). One effective way to do this is to phase out the frequency of meetings over several months. A week before the last regular weekly meeting, the couple is asked once again to complete the Marital Relationship Assessment Battery and to provide a 10-minute videotaped communication sample. The MRAB is turned in at the last regular weekly meeting. At this session, detailed plans are made to cover the time interval before the first follow-up meeting. Couples are encouraged to continue to meet weekly at the former therapy hour at home (or out to dinner, etc.) in order to monitor and continue the gains made in therapy. Depending on the likelihood of success in following this plan, most couples are then asked to return in 1 month; some return in 2 or 3 weeks. After the first follow-up visit, a second return visit is scheduled at the same or a longer interval, again depending on stability and progress. These so-called booster sessions are extended in weekly intervals and in number until the gains made in the regular therapy sessions seem to be well maintained or improved on. Even then, couples are encouraged to consider the therapist a consultant on permanent retainer. An annual checkup is suggested, but in any case, at the earliest sign of uncontrolled deterioration in one or both partners' level of marital satisfaction, the couple is encouraged to call the therapist.

SUMMARY

This chapter presents a behavioral-systems model for the outpatient assessment and treatment of marital dysfunction. The approach is similar to that in many standard BSMT programs and features multimodal assessment procedures, behavioral observations, communication and problem-solving-skill training, and related techniques of behavior exchange and modification. In addition, among others, the authors are attempting to expand the range and to improve on the outcome efficacy of the basic social-learning approach by incorporating into the treatment program a variety of family-systems, cognitive-behavioral, affective-behavioral, and, to a lesser extent, psychodynamic interventions. To the degree that these additional interventions have not been empirically validated, they should be considered preliminary and experimental. In the present approach, the relatively nonbehavioral interventions are applied most often either in anticipation or remediation of significant blocks to therapeutic progress following the behavioral format.

This is an exciting era for marital therapy. In the 1980s, the assessment and treatment of marital relationships, as a field in itself, came to fruition (cf. Jacobson & Gurman, 1986). Moreover, expert clinicians who espouse many theoretical orientations are realizing the limitations of narrow perspectives in treating distressed couples. Integrative, innovative approaches are proliferating in the world of clinical practice; research on the relative efficiency and effectiveness of certain interventions and treatment packages is under way across the country. We have seen marital dysfunction addressed by social learning (i.e., behavioral) approaches (Stuart, 1969; Weiss *et al.*, 1973) that have developed into behavioral-systems approaches (Birchler, 1983a; Weiss, 1980), into cognitive-behavioral approaches (Jacobson & Holtzworth-Munroe, 1986; Weiss, 1984), and into a psychodynamic-behavioral approach (Segraves, 1982); its treatment is now also influenced by ego-analytic (Wile, 1981) and affect-oriented psychodynamic approaches (Greenberg & Johnson, 1986). Perhaps enlightened marital therapists will some day fully integrate the field by developing the ultimate "affective-cognitive-behavioral-psychodynamic" approach. It would seem that the complexity of human relationships requires such a broad perspective.

REFERENCES

Alexander, J. F., Barton, C., Waldron, H., & Mas, C. H. (1983). Beyond the technology of family therapy: The anatomy of intervention model. In K. D. Craig & R. J. McMahon (Eds.), *Advances in clinical behavior therapy* (pp. 48–73). New York: Brunner/Mazel.

Anderson, C. M., & Stewart, S. (1983). *Mastering resistance: A practical guide to family therapy.* New York: Guilford Press.

Barton, C., & Alexander, J. F. (1981). Functional family therapy. In A. S. Gurman & D. P. Kniskern (Eds.), *Handbook of family therapy* (pp. 403–443). New York: Brunner/Mazel.

Baucom, D. H., & Hoffman, J. A. (1986). The effectiveness of marital therapy: Current status and application to the clinical setting. In N. S. Jacobson & A. S. Gurman (Eds.) *Clinical handbook of marital therapy* (pp. 597–620). New York: Guilford Press.

Beach, S. R. H., & O'Leary, K. D. (1986). The treatment of depression occurring in the context of marital discord. *Behavior Therapy, 17,* 43–49.

Birchler, G. R. (1977, April). *A multimethod analysis of distressed and nondistressed marital interaction: A social learning approach.* Paper presented at Western Psychological Association Meeting, Seattle.

Birchler, G. R. (1979). *Inventory of rewarding activities.* Unpublished manuscript, University of California Medical School, San Diego.

Birchler, G. R. (1981). Paradox and behavioral marital therapy. *American Journal of Family Therapy, 9,* 92–94.

Birchler, G. R. (1983a). Behavioral-systems marital therapy. In J. P. Vincent (Ed.), *Advances in family intervention, assessment and theory* (Vol. 3). Greenwich, CN: JAI.

Birchler, G. R. (1983b). Marital Dysfunction. In M. Hersen (Ed.), *Outpatient behavior therapy: A clinical guide* (pp. 229–269). New York: Grune & Stratton.

Birchler, G. R. (1988). Handling resistance to change. In I. R. H. Falloon (Ed.), *Handbook of behavioral family therapy* (pp. 128–155). New York: Guilford Press.

Birchler, G. R., & Spinks, S. H. (1980). Behavioral-systems marital and family therapy: Integration and clinical application. *The American Journal of Family Therapy, 8,* 6–28.

Burke, R. J., & Weir, T. (1977). Marital helping relationships: The moderator between stress and well being. *Journal of Psychology, 95,* 121–130.

Carter, E. A., & McGoldrick, M. (1980). The family life cycle and family therapy: An overview. In E. A. Carter & M. McGoldrick (Eds.), *The family life cycle: A framework for family therapy.* New York: Gardner.

Colarusso, C. A., & Nemiroff, R. A. (1981). *Adult development: A new dimension in psychodynamic therapy and practice.* New York: Plenum Press.

Epstein, N. (1982). Cognitive therapy with couples. *American Journal of Family Therapy, 10,* 5–16.

Epstein, N. (1985). Structured approaches to couples' adjustment. In L. L'Abate & M. Milan (Eds.), *Handbook of social skills training and research* (pp. 477–505). New York: Wiley.

Floyd, F. J., & Markman, H. J. (1984). An economical observational measure of couples' communication skill. *Journal of Consulting and Clinical Psychology, 52,* 97–103.

Foster, S. W. (1986). Marital treatment of eating disorders. In N. S. Jacobson & A. S. Gurman (Eds.), *Clinical handbook of marital therapy* (pp. 575–596). New York: Guilford Press.

Goldfried, M. R., & D'Zurilla, T. J. (1969). A behavioral-analytic model for assessment competence. In C. D. Spielberger (Ed.), *Current topics in clinical and community psychology.* New York: Academic Press.

Gottman, J. M. (1979). *Marital interaction: Experimental investigations.* New York: Academic Press.

Gottman, J., Notarius, C., Gonso, J., & Markman, H. (1976). *A couples guide to communication.* Champaign, IL: Research Press.

Greenberg, L. S., & Johnson, S. M. (1986). Emotionally focused couples therapy. In N. S. Jacobson & A. S. Gurman (Eds.), *Clinical handbook of marital therapy* (pp. 253–278). New York: Guilford Press.

Guerney, B. G., Guerney, L., & Cooney, T. (1985). Marital and family problem prevention and enrichment programs. In L. L'Abate (Ed.), *The handbook of family psychology and therapy* (pp. 1179–1217). Homewood, IL: Dorsey.

Gurman, A. S. (1981). Sources of influence in the family therapy field: Publication trends in three major journals. *Journal of Marital and Family Therapy, 7,* 81–87.

Gurman, A. S., & Kniskern, D. P. (1978). Behavioral marriage therapy: 1. A psychodynamic-systems analysis and critique. *Family Process, 17,* 121–138.

Hafner, R. J. (1986). Marital therapy for agoraphobia. In N. S. Jacobson & A. S. Gurman (Eds.), *Clinical handbook of marital therapy* (pp. 471–494). New York: Guilford Press.

Hare-Mustin, R. T. (1976). Paradoxical tasks in family therapy: Who can resist? *Psychotherapy: Theory, Research and Practice, 13,* 128–130.

Hartman, L. M. (1983). Resistance in directive sex therapy: Recognition and management. *Journal of Sex and Marital Therapy, 9,* 283–295.

Hops, H., Wills, T. A., Patterson, G. R., & Weiss, R. L. (1972). *Marital Interaction Coding System.* Unpublished manuscript, University of Oregon.

Jacobson, N. S. (1983). Expanding the range and applicability of marital therapy. *Behavior Therapist, 6,* 189–191.

Jacobson, N. S. (1984). The modification of cognitive processes in behavioral marital therapy: Integrating cognitive and behavioral intervention strategies. In K. Hahlweg & N. S. Jacobson (Eds.), *Marital Interaction: Analysis and modification* (pp. 285–308). New York: Guilford Press.

Jacobson, N. S., & Gurman, A. S. (Eds.). (1986). *Clinical handbook of marital therapy.* New York: Guilford Press.

Jacobson, N. S., & Holtzworth-Munroe, A. (1986). Marital therapy: A social learning-cognitive perspective. In N. S. Jacobson & A. S. Gurman (Eds.), *Clinical handbook of marital therapy* (pp. 29–70). New York: Guilford Press.

Jacobson, N. S., & Margolin, G. (1979). *Marital therapy: Strategies based on social learning and behavior exchange principles.* New York: Brunner/Mazel.

Jacobson, N. S., Follette, W. C., & Revenstorf, D. (1984). Psychotherapy outcome research: Methods for reporting variability and evaluating clinical significance. *Behavior Therapy, 15,* 336–352.

Lazarus, A. A., & Fay, A. (1982). Resistance or rationalization? A cognitive-behavioral perspective. In P. L. Wachtel (Ed.), *Resistance: Psychodynamic and behavioral approaches* (pp. 115–132). New York: Plenum Press.

Levinson, D. J., Darrow, C. N., Klein, E. B., Levinson, M. H., & McKee, B. (1978). *The seasons of a man's life.* New York: Knopf.

Liberman, R. P., Wheeler, E. G., de Visser, L. A., Kuehnel, J., & Kuehnel, T. (1980). *Handbook of marital therapy.* New York: Plenum Press.

Locke, H. J., & Wallace, K. M. (1959). Short-term marital adjustment and prediction tests: Their reliability and validity. *Journal of Marriage and Family Living, 21,* 251–255.

Margolin, G., & Fernandez, V. (1985). Marital dysfunction. In M. Hersen & A. S. Bellack (Eds.), *Handbook of clinical behavior therapy with adults* (pp. 693–728). New York: Plenum Press.

Margolin, G., & Weinstein, C. D. (1983). The role of affect in behavioral marital therapy. In M. L. Aronson & L. R. Wolberg (Eds.), *Group and family therapy 1982: An overview.* New York: Brunner/Mazel.

Martin, G. A., & Worthington, E. L. (1982). Behavioral homework. In M. Hersen, R. M. Eisler, & P. M. Miller (Eds.), *Progress in behavior modification* (Vol. 13) (pp. 197–226). New York: Academic Press.

McKay, M., Davis, M., & Fanning, P. (1983). *Messages: The communication book.* Oakland, CA: New Harbinger.

Meichenbaum, D., & Gilmore, J. B. (1982). Resistance from a cognitive-behavioral perspective. In P. L. Wachtel (Ed.), *Resistance: Psychodynamic and behavioral approaches* (pp. 133–156). New York: Plenum Press.

O'Farrell, T. J. (1986). Marital therapy in the treatment of alcoholism. In N. S. Jacobson & A. S. Gurman (Eds.), *Clinical handbook of marital therapy* (pp. 513–536). New York: Guilford Press.

Paolino, T. J., & McCrady, B. S. (Eds.). (1978). *Marriage and marital therapy.* New York: Brunner/Mazel.

Segraves, R. T. (1982). *Marital therapy: A combined psychodynamic-behavioral approach.* New York: Plenum Press.

Sheehy, G. (1974). *Passages.* New York: Dutton.

Snyder, D. K., & Regts, J. M. (1982). Factor scales for assessing marital disharmony and disaffection. *Journal of Consulting and Clinical Psychology, 50,* 615–623.

Snyder, D. K., Wills, R. M., & Keiser, T. W. (1981). Empirical validation of the Marital Satisfaction Inventory: An actuarial approach. *Journal of Consulting and Clinical Psychology, 49,* 262–268.

Soper, P. H., & L'Abate, L. (1977). Paradox as a therapeutic technique: A review. *International Journal of Family Counseling, 5,* 10–21.

Spanier, G. B. (1976). Measuring dyadic adjustment: New scales for assessing the quality of marriage and similar dyads. *Journal of Marriage and the Family, 38,* 15–28.

Spinks, S. H., & Birchler, G. R. (1982). Behavioral-systems marital therapy: Dealing with resistance. *Family Process, 21,* 169–185.

Strayhorn, J. (1977). *Talking it out.* Champaign, IL: Research Press.

Stuart, R. B. (1969). Operant interpersonal treatment for marital discord. *Journal of Consulting and Clinical Psychology, 33,* 675–682.

Stuart, R. B. (1980). *Helping couples change.* New York: Guilford Press.

Stuart, R. B. (1983). *Couple's Pre-counseling Inventory.* Champaign, IL: Research Press.

Thomas, E. J. (1977). *Marital communication and decision making.* New York: Free Press.

Wahler, H. J. (1968). The Self-description Inventory: Measuring levels of self-evaluative behavior in terms of favorable and unfavorable personality attributes. *Journal of Clinical Psychology, 24,* 40–45.

Weiss, R. L. (1980). Strategic behavioral marital therapy: Toward a model for assessment and intervention. In J. P. Vincent (Ed.), *Advances in family intervention, assessment and theory* (Vol. 1) (pp. 229–271). Greenwich, CN: JAI.

Weiss, R. L. (1984). Cognitive and strategic interventions in behavioral marital therapy. In K. Hahlweg & N. S. Jacobson (Eds.), *Marital interaction: Analysis and modification* (pp. 337–355). New York: Guilford Press.

Weiss, R. L., & Birchler, G. R. (1975). *Areas of change questionnaire.* Unpublished manuscript, University of Oregon, Eugene.

Weiss, R. L., & Birchler, G. R. (1978). Adults with marital dysfunction. In M. Hersen & A. Bellack (Eds.), *Behavior therapy in the psychiatric setting* (pp. 331–364). Baltimore: Wilkins & Wilkins.

Weiss, R. L., & Cerreto, M. (1980). The Marital Status Inventory: Development of a measure of dissolution potential. *American Journal of Family Therapy, 8,* 80–86.

Weiss, R. L., & Margolin, G. (1989). Assessment of conflict and accord: A second look. In A. Ciminero (Ed.), *Handbook of behavioral assessment* (Vol. 2). New York: Wiley.

Weiss, R. L., Hops, H., & Patterson, G. R. (1973). A framework for conceptualizing marital conflict, a technology for altering it, some data for evaluating it. In F. W. Clark & L. A. Hamerlynck (Eds.), *Critical issues in research and practice: Proceedings of the fourth Banff international conference on behavior modification.* Champaign, IL: Research Press.

Wile, D. B. (1981). *Couples therapy: A nontraditional approach.* New York: Wiley.

Wood, L. F., & Jacobson, N. S. (1985). Marital distress. In D. H. Barlow (Ed.), *Clinical handbook of psychological disorders: A step-by-step treatment manual.* New York: Guilford Press.

21

Adolescents and Young Adults

DALE J. HINDMARSH

INTRODUCTION

This chapter reviews the psychotherapeutic treatment of adolescents and young adults with an emphasis on the teenage population. Particular attention is given to the clinical problems presented by child–parent conflicts, school, parental divorce, and suicide in young people. Eating disorders, substance abuse, and depression are important in relation to the adolescent and young adult population but are extensively treated in other chapters of this book. Throughout the clinical and technical sections of the chapter, there is an underlying emphasis on relating the understanding of the case and its management to the developmental level of the teenager.

HISTORICAL INFLUENCES

The psychotherapeutic treatment of adolescents has grown out of specific social needs to manage this age group, and also out of the psychotherapy of children and adults. The four most influential 20th-century movements contributing to adolescent psychotherapy have been the child guidance movement, psychoanalysis, the growth of the medical subspecialty of child psychiatry, and the family therapy movement.

The child guidance movement grew out of the study of juvenile delinquents in the early 1900s. William Healey and his associates established a multidisciplinary evaluation program for juvenile offenders in the Cook County court system in Chicago, and subsequently in the Judge Baker Clinic in Boston. They emphasized the careful collection of historical, medical, and psychiatric data and were among the first to use psychometric

DALE J. HINDMARSH • Western Psychiatric Institute and Clinic, University of Pittsburgh, Pittsburgh, Pennsylvania 15213.

testing as a regular component of their evaluations. Initially, they focused on presenting reports on juvenile offenders to assist the courts in disposition and treatment decisions. They soon determined that an active treatment program was necessary, for without a clinical means of carrying out their treatment recommendations, they found that the teenagers had a high criminal recidivism rate. This need led to the establishment of the child guidance clinics (Healey & Bronner, 1923–1948), which was enthusiastically and financially supported by the then-prominent mental-hygiene movement in adult psychiatry.

The child guidance movement's origins in providing evaluations and treatment for court-referred teenagers established a precedent of public service, compassion, and pragmatism, which have been characteristic of its work over the last 70 years. During this period, the focus of treatment expanded to include emotionally and behaviorally disturbed children and adolescents from a variety of referral sources.

The child guidance movement also influenced the practice of psychotherapy with children and adolescents by establishing new and broader professional roles for mental health personnel. The evaluating functions of the psychiatrist, the testing psychologist, and the social worker were solidified in the "treatment team." At its best, this was a comprehensive multidisciplinary approach to data gathering, case synthesis, and treatment planning. The child guidance movement was also instrumental in the emergence of social workers as psychotherapists. Organizationally, the American Orthopsychiatric Association provided a national forum for furthering the child guidance movement and the professional development of child psychiatrists, social workers, psychologists, and educators.

The second movement that had enormous influence on the psychotherapeutic treatment of adolescents was psychoanalysis. Freud made numerous references to adolescent dynamics and pathology, but the fundamental contributions to the psychoanalytic theories of adolescence and the psychoanalytic treatment of young people came from his followers, a few of whom will be mentioned here.

August Aichhorn, an analytically trained educator working with behaviorally disturbed adolescents, used a liberally pragmatic adaptation of psychoanalytic principles. His writings, especially the book *Wayward Youth* (1925) were very influential. More theoretically bent writers were Anna Freud and Peter Blos, both of whom emphasized the defense mechanisms and the ego development of adolescents (Blos, 1962, 1979; Freud, 1958). These authors also clarified and elaborated on the concept of adolescent turmoil, which is discussed in the next section of this chapter. Another prominent psychoanalyst was the neo-Freudian theoretician Erik Erikson (1958, 1968), whose contributions to adolescent theory are twofold. In his epigenetic stages of development, Erikson described the psychological dilemma and tasks of the eight general ages of life. He described identity formation as the primary psychological task of adolescence, and this formulation has strongly influenced the clinical and popular perception of teenagers over the last quarter century. Erikson's second major contribution was his description of the transformation of adolescent conflicts into lifelong, purposeful working themes in adulthood. In Erikson's views the goal of treatment is not to resolve internal adolescent conflicts but to facilitate the adaptation of neurotic struggles to productive life themes or causes.

A third force in the evolution of the treatment of teenagers was the development of child-psychiatric residency programs, such as those under Leo Kanner at Yale and Loretta Bender at Bellevue Hospital in New York. These programs placed emphasis on advancing the science of child psychiatry and critically examining diagnostic patterns and biological treatments as well as psychotherapy, and their graduates established child psychiatry as a boarded medical subspecialty. The development of departments of child psychiatry and their close relationship to general psychiatric training centers have given the medical community significant influence over the identification of and prescription of treatment for psychologically disturbed teenagers. For example, insurance reimbursement usually requires a standard psychiatric diagnosis by a physician for the approval of payment for psychotherapy.

A fourth, and more recent, influence on the practice of psychotherapy with teenagers is the family therapy movement. The growth of family therapy in the United States has been exponential, and it has a variety of schools and leaders. It is not an exaggeration to describe this movement as a series of treatment models without clear-cut diagnostic criteria, and without the emphasis on scientific study and validation that child psychiatry now appears to strive for. Yet, the influence and popularity of family therapy are undeniable, and its treatment strategies and techniques—opening communications, assigning tasks, practicing specific behaviors, putting time limits on treatments, and viewing the disturbed person as a member of a larger, involved family system—have been very helpful to psychotherapists working with troubled adolescents.

SPECIAL CONSIDERATIONS

There are two emerging concepts in the field of adolescent development and psychopathology that are highly relevant to a therapist's approach to psychotherapy with adolescents. The first is the changing clinical perception of normal adolescence, and the second is the place of adolescent psychiatric disorders in clinical continuums of child, adolescent, and adult psychopathology.

The Concept of Normal Adolescence

By the middle of the 20th century, a theoretical construct of the adolescent psyche was being articulated. This theory, referred to here as the *turmoil hypothesis,* was founded on psychoanalytic principles and was drawn from the clinical experience of analysts working with referred adolescents. It views adolescence as a period of sexual reawakening in which the internal and external relationships of teenagers to their parents undergo fundamental psychodynamic changes, and it posits that these changes are normally experienced as a breakdown of the stable psychological equilibrium of latency. Concerning adolescence, this theory states that there is a necessary disruption of the child's psychological defenses and attachments, resulting in regression and the expression of numerous shifting psychopathological symptoms, all in the service of the ultimate emergence of an independent and competent adult psyche. Accordingly, teenagers experience intense internal turmoil and frequently demonstrate neurotic or psychotic symptomatology. Similarly, alienation from the adult world is seen as prevalent among adolescents, as it functions to assist them in differentiating themselves and emancipating them from their parents. On the other hand, conflict-free stability through the teenage years is considered atypical and a cause for concern to the clinician, in that it implies overdependency and a lack of self-differentiation (Blos, 1962, 1979; Freud, 1958).

The adolescent turmoil hypothesis initially provided a useful model to psychotherapists working with troubled teenagers, as it clinically distinguished these patients from children and adults and attempted to understand adolescent symptoms in a developmental framework. It also encouraged therapists to adapt their techniques as dictated by the psychodevelopmental needs and capacities of their teenage patients, thus allowing much greater treatment flexibility than was traditionally permissible in adult psychoanalysis or psychoanalytic psychotherapy. The turmoil hypothesis was not limited to troubled or disturbed teenagers but was generalized to the overall age group as the normal maturational pathway.

The negative features of the turmoil hypothesis are (1) it blurs normal and pathological adolescent phenomena to the extent that a psychiatric diagnosis is considered of questionable utility for teenagers, and (2) it deemphasizes the continuities between clinical presentations in adolescence with childhood or adulthood (Strober, 1986).

Beginning in the 1950s, and then increasingly over the next quarter century, a number of clinicians and researchers challenged the validity of the turmoil hypothesis. The most influential studies were epidemiological surveys of large adolescent populations that either represented the whole breadth of adolescents in a community or focused on normal adolescents by excluding delinquent and disturbed teenagers. The results of these investigations consistently tend to depathologize the concept of normality in teenagers, as is illustrated below by a review of two of the more influential studies published. The first, by Rutter, Graham, Chadwick, and Yule (1976), is from the United Kingdom, and the second is by Offer and his group working in the American Midwest (Offer, 1986; Offer, Ostrov, & Howard, 1981).

Rutter *et al.* (1976) took a hard look at adolescent alienation and turmoil as part of the Isle of Wight studies. They screened 2,303 14- and 15-year-old adolescents with teacher–parent behavioral questionnaires, and of these, they interviewed 200 randomly selected "general-population" teenagers and 304 "deviant" teenagers as identified by the screening questionnaires. They also interviewed the parents and teachers of the two subgroups. The findings regarding parent–child alienation are striking in that a large majority of the general population teenagers did not feel critical of their parents and very few rejected their parents. The parents of these children similarly reported positive relationships and communications with their children. On the other hand, signs of alienation were much more common between the teenagers and parents when the teenagers had a psychiatric disorder. Furthermore, the alienation appeared to be associated with the disorder rather than being a causal mechanism for the condition. The internal experience of turmoil was also evaluated during the psychiatric interviews. Over 40% of the boys and girls in the general-population sample reported that they sometimes felt miserable or unhappy to the extent that they were tearful or wanted to get away from it all. About 30% endorsed ideas of reference, and about 20% expressed self-depreciation. The feelings of misery contrasted with the incidence of "observed sadness" in the interviews, which was less than 15% for boys and girls in the general-population sample.

Rutter *et al.* concluded from their data (only partially outlined here) that parent–child alienation is not a common feature for adolescents unless the adolescent already has a psychiatric disorder, and that parents continue to have a substantial influence on normal children through adolescence. Feelings of inner turmoil, however, are fairly common and cause appreciable personal suffering but are often unnoticed by adults. The prevalence of diagnosable psychiatric disorders in these adolescents was low (about 13%) and not significantly different from the prevalence of psychiatric conditions in 10-year-olds (about 11%). Thus, adolescents were found to experience some inner turmoil, but its overall effect appeared to be limited, as they maintained good family ties and were generally free of psychiatric conditions. In summary, Rutter *et al.* (1976) stated that "adolescent turmoil is a fact, not a fiction, but its psychiatric importance has probably been overestimated" (p. 55).

Daniel Offer and his group (Offer *et al.*, 1981) conducted large-scale questionnaire studies focusing on the self-perceptions of identified normal adolescents, 13- to 19-year-old middle-class students without social deviancy or overt psychopathology. The questionnaires examined five general areas of "self": psychological self, social self, sexual self, familial self, and coping self. The salient findings in these content areas were strikingly positive. In the area of psychological self, these normal adolescents enjoyed life, tended to be happy with themselves, were usually relaxed, felt healthy, and were proud of their physical development. The social self-perception showed that these normal teenagers derived pleasure from work that was well done, were optimistic about future employment, made friends easily, and believed that they would be successful in their future social and vocational spheres. These adolescents were not afraid of their sexuality and were generally confident in their relationships with members of the opposite sex. In the area of familial self, the findings were consistent with those of Rutter: the predominant feelings between parents and their teenager were mutually positive, and in the vast majority, there was no evidence of a generation gap. Finally, in the area of the coping self, these adolescents believed that they had the skills and confidence to succeed, and they enjoyed novel situations and challenges. They also tended to deny psychiatric symptoms.

Offer (1986) also examined the longitudinal course of a large group of normal male adolescents. He found that the majority fell along three developmental routes. Approximately 23%, the continuous group, had a smooth course of development, essentially free of internal turmoil or external conflict. Another 35%, the surgent group, had alternating periods of "developmental spurts" and periods of turmoil and conflict. A third group, about 21%, demonstrated the prolonged, tumultuous pattern reminiscent of the adolescents described by Anna Freud and other earlier psychoanalytic writers. The remaining 20% of these normal adolescent males could not be assigned to any of the three groups but were described as more similar to the first two groups than to the tumultuous group.

These epidemiological studies delineate a clearer picture of the normal teenage experience, which is less tortured, less alienated, and broader in scope than that described by the turmoil hypothesis. Adolescence is seen as a period of personal development that does not necessarily display regression or conflict. In general, family values and relationships are maintained while the social world expands. Academic and vocational achievement is regarded positively, and the future is optimistically embraced. A significant minority of normal teenagers do appear to suffer through a tumultuous course, and many adolescents describe feelings of misery and unhappiness—but although this is an important facet of life for some, it is not the prevailing experience of the age group. The implication for the therapist is that normal adolescents tend to appear normal, whereas psychiatric symptoms and family alienation are more likely to be associated with real psychopathology.

Continuums of Adolescent Psychopathology

When nonclinical teenage populations are studied, their normal life experience is found to be less symptomatic and more healthy than was previously believed. A careful study of disturbed adolescents, with the use of rigorous standardized evaluations, demonstrates that the majority of cases may be assigned psychiatric diagnoses, and that the diagnoses are reliable and replicable as long as defined symptom criteria are used (Rutter, & Graham, 1968; Strober, Green, & Carlson, 1981). This finding partially contradicts another tenet of the turmoil hypothesis, that diagnosis in adolescents is of little clinical utility because of the fluctuating and frequent symptomatology in both normal and disturbed teenagers.

Many disorders in adolescence are continuations of childhood problems. Rutter *et al.* (1976) found that just under half their psychiatrically disturbed 14-year-olds had disorders persisting from childhood, and that slightly more than half had new psychiatric disorders (p. 47). Behavior problems such as aggressive conduct disorders (Loeber & Stouthamer-Loeber, 1987) and attention deficit disorders with hyperactivity (Cantwell, 1986a; Gittleman, Mannuzza, Shenker, & Bonagura, 1985; Hechtman, Weiss, & Perlman, 1984) are known to continue from childhood into adolescence. Adolescent reactions to childhood language and learning disorders are frequently expressed in disturbances of behavior or as gradually established depressive conditions (Cantwell, 1986b, refers to a type of gradual reactive depressive syndrome in these children as a demoralization syndrome), and childhood affective disorders, especially chronic dysthymic conditions, often continue into adolescence. Kovacs, Feinberg, Crouse-Novak, Paulauskas, and Finkelstein (1984a,b) found a prolonged natural course of several years for childhood dysthymic disorder and a risk of 80% that these children would eventually develop major depressions. Emotional reactions to parental divorce that occurs in childhood are known to continue to trouble some children into and through their teenage years (Wallerstein, 1985), and childhood victims of physical and sexual abuse may suffer long-term sequelae (Steele, 1986). The major childhood psychoses, autism and childhood schizophrenia, are by nature lifelong disorders and thus afflict a percentage of teenagers. Therefore, as a number of childhood psychiatric conditions continue to affect their victims into the teenage years, it is incumbent on the therapist not only to consider a disorder in adolescence in the developmental context of the adolescent period but to determine whether the disorder is of recent or childhood onset.

The distress and functional impairment that are caused by mental disorders provide the therapist sufficient impetus to treat the teenager, but if further justification were necessary, it would be found in the long-term consequences of adolescent disorders. Therefore, let us now consider the continuums of adolescent and adult psychopathology. Longitudinal perspective studies of adolescent psychopathology offer the most persuasive evidence that disturbances of mental health in teenagers increase the risk of similar or related problems in adulthood. Kandel and Davies (1986) reported on the adult sequelae of adolescent depressive symptoms. They resurveyed about 1,000 young adults (average age 24.7 years) who had taken part in a school survey 9 years earlier, and they found that teenage depressive affect for both boys and girls predicted depressed mood in adulthood. Also, it increased the risk of psychiatric hospitalization in women by their mid-20s. In addition, depressed mood over time was associated with impaired intimate interpersonal relationships; dysphoric teenagers had a more distant relationship with their parents, which seemed to express itself in adulthood as an impaired ability to form an intimate and close relationships with their partner or spouse, although the ability to make friends was not noticeably affected.

Other adolescent psychiatric disturbances frequently continue into adulthood as chronic or recurrent disorders: alcohol and substance abuse, antisocial behavior, anorexia nervosa, bulimia, anxiety disorders, obsessive-compulsive syndromes, and various psychopathological symptoms of personality disorders.

Less well appreciated, and more difficult to assess, are the long-term consequences of disruptions of normal growth and development caused by the specific timing of psychiatric disturbances. For example, a high school senior referred to our program developed a suicidal depression that responded well to a combination of hospitalization, antidepressants, and individual psychotherapy. Equally important for this young man from a poor inner-city family was that the timing of the disorder threatened his acquisition of an athletic scholarship, without which he could probably not go on to college. Thus, once his suicidal impulses were under check, the timing of the disorder posed a greater threat to his future than the severity of his symptoms. Adolescence and young adulthood are periods of heightened risk for the impact of mental disorders, as they are times of rapid personal and social development and of choices in life direction, and the functional impairment of even a relatively time-limited disorder may result in lost opportunities with long-term ramifications.

COMMON CLINICAL PROBLEMS

Teen–Parent Problems

The psychotherapist who works with teenagers encounters many whose primary reasons for referral are conflicts between them and their parents. Normal teen–parent disagreements are common, most frequently over such things as standards of dress, haircuts, or going out, and they do not cause serious or lasting disruptions of family relationships (Rutter *et al.,* 1976). These types of disputes are developmental phenomena and are derivatives (1) of teenagers increased peer identification coupled with a heightened self-consciousness of how their peers judge them; (2) of attempts to think and act independently; and (3) of an expanding cognitive capacity for more effective argument and debate.

More serious teen–parent conflicts may arise that exceed the family's capacity for tolerance, at which point a referral to a therapist is appropriate. The adolescent is most frequently presented as the identified patient or client, and typical areas of conflict are rebelliousness against parental authority and values, school problems, sexual promiscuity, illicit drug and alcohol use, antisocial behavior, running away, and suicide threats. The task of the therapist is to evaluate the entire situation (i.e., the nature of the problem, the adolescent, the parents, and the family circumstances), and to determine what type of therapeutic intervention is indicated.

A careful chronological history of the problem will allow the therapist to view the situation in its longitudinal context, as well as to assess its current impact on the adolescent and the family. The longitudinal perspective identifies problems that are chronic in course, and it may indicate either underlying psychopathology in the adolescent, parental deviance, or ongoing dysfunctional patterns of family adaptation. When the history determines that the conflict is of recent origin and is a significant departure from the previous quality of the parent–child relationship, the focus of attention shifts to the recent past and the current situation, and the therapist is impelled to wonder, "Why now?" An illustration of a chronic versus a recent-onset problem is seen in two girls who were both referred for runaway behavior.

Cindy, age 15, had a history of extended runaways back to 9 years of age. She had been adopted at age 3 by court order into a wealthy family that had recently adopted her twin brother. On interview, she was self-assured, articulate, and street-wise. She was a popular and self-centered girl who was remarkably unperturbed by the distress her repeated runs had caused her family. A detailed history revealed that the conflicts between her and her parents had long preceded her first runaway, and that there was strong ambivalence on both sides of the parent–daughter relationship. The courts had insisted on the adoption of Cindy in order to keep her with her twin brother, a decision that the parents would not have made on their own. The recurrent runaways, which her brother did not participate in, reflected the incomplete bonding between Cindy and her parents, as well as her overly autonomous character pathology. This case required long-term individual psychotherapy coupled with family meetings.

Sharon, also 15, was brought to the clinic after her first brief runaway. There had been no serious previous problems between her and her parents, but they were concerned, as they knew that several of Sharon's friends had also run away over the past year. Further evaluation of the parents' concern revealed that they were intimately knowledgeable about the recent community runaways, as Sharon usually informed the parents of her runaway friends' whereabouts. The father had even managed to secretly house a few of the runaway adolescents in the family's basement while he attempted his own brand of crisis intervention. In a large sense, Sharon's runaway was an angry reaction to her father's intense and solicitous involvement with her friends. The girl and her family were otherwise free of serious psychopathology, and the problem was addressed with brief family therapy.

As the above cases demonstrate, qualitatively different levels of adolescent and parent pathology may be expressed through similar teen–parent problems. Part of the evaluation of the problem is also to rule out the presence of more serious psychiatric conditions, such as major depressive disorder, manic-depressive illness, schizophrenia, or neurological impairments, which would further alter the priorities and choice of treatment.

Parent–adolescent conflicts, without complicating major psychiatric disorders, may be approached with a variety of psychotherapeutic strategies. The trends in treatment are (1) not to treat the teenager in isolation but to actively involve the parents and perhaps other nuclear- or extended-family members; (2) to develop a treatment plan or contract that specifies the goals and modalities of intervention; and (3) to limit the time course of the therapy.

Robin, Koepke, and Nayar (1986), at Wayne State University, developed a specific family treatment program for parent–adolescent conflicts that is based on an integration of cognitive therapy, communications theory, and family systems theory. In the initial evaluation period, the therapist looks for deficits in the family's problem-solving and communication skills, for cognitive distortions (unrealistic beliefs and absolutist positions), and for difficulties inherent in the family structure or function—any of which may serve to promote parent–adolescent conflicts. The therapist then outlines the findings to the family and develops a treatment contract. Active treatment involves teaching the family new skills for problem solving and communication, and challenging maladaptive cognitive distortions. The sessions are structured and interactive, and they push the family to explore new alternatives in the perception and management of their conflicts. Homework assignments with feedback sessions encourage the family members to actively try out less conflictual interactive styles, at first addressing minor areas of disagreement and then progressing to more intense or complex problems. The therapist gradually becomes less active in order to facilitate a natural termination of treatment. This psychotherapy model is better suited to motivated families that have a general tolerance of self-examination and that have family roles that are not so rigid as to preclude change.

School Problems

Rutter (1985) asserted that, after symptom reduction, the second essential goal of the treatment of children and adolescents is the promotion of normal development; this assertion is especially apropos when one is treating a teenager with school problems. Even in severely psychiatrically disturbed and functionally impaired adolescents, a primary therapeutic task is to help the teenager to continue his or her education in the most normal and productive fashion possible. In society, the school is the hub of the adolescent's intellectual and social development, and the successes and failures experienced there have major import for both the teenager's present and his or her future. Every therapist encounters exceptions, but the guiding principle when working with adolescents is that a successful school experience fosters normal development, which in turn fosters mental health. Consequently, those problems that threaten a successful school experience deserve careful inspection and prompt intervention.

With this principle in mind, it is reasonable to ask what are the attributes or skills that are most helpful to students in the secondary schools. Zigmond and Kerr and their coworkers investigated this question in a large metropolitan school system (Zigmond & Kerr, 1986; Zigmond, Kerr, Brown, & Harris, 1984). Surveys collected in three large city high schools from the principals, school administrators, teachers, and school personnel, as well as from over 4,000 students, identified a consensus on the skills and problems that affect a high school student's success. The five school survival skills most often rated "very important" were (1) goes to school every day; (2) shows an interest in grades; (3) turns in work on time; (4) arrives at school on time; and (5) plans steps to reach a goal. The five "most serious" problems were (1) makes poor grades; (2) cannot read directions; (3) does not bring pencils, paper, or books to class; (4) gives backtalk to teachers; and (5) fails to finish work. It was also found that both successful and less successful students rated school survival skills similarly, but that the less successful students consistently failed to apply this knowledge. Another notable finding was that educators and students rated personality and social adjustment items as far less important than attendance, class participation, and timely completion of work. It may be that the educational system is not sensitive enough to emotional and interpersonal matters. But the import of these studies is that the professional seeking to counsel or advise teenagers and families about school problems would do well to examine the adolescent's school survival skills in the evaluation and to similarly address these issues when formulating a treatment plan.

The evaluation of school problems is an orderly, comprehensive look at the biological-developmental, psychological, familial, and educational components of the adolescent's difficulty. When gathering a history, it is important to review the adolescent's development for early medical problems (e.g., premature birth, serious illnesses, head injuries, or seizure disorders), maturational abnormalities, and emotional or behavioral traits (e.g., separation anxiety or hyperactivity), which may have contributed to later school difficulties. A detailed school history, beginning with preschool adjustment and progressing chronologically to the present, is mandatory and is greatly aided by attendance records, report cards, and testing results. Standard psychometric and educational tests are quite helpful in the evaluation, unless the student is clearly bright and achieving good marks. The family history and circumstances are important. The parents' educational experience and their expectations of their children may contribute to their child's own school problems, and the value that the parents place on various aspects of school life—academics, popularity, sports, extracurricular activities, attendance, and so on—may indicate their motivation in sending their child for treatment and what types of intervention strategies are apt to garner parental support. Changes in the family circumstance, such as parental separations, recent moves, unemployment, or deaths in the family, should be investigated as potential etiological factors, especially when the school problems are new or have recently intensified. The mental status examination of the adolescent looks first for psychiatric disorders or psychopathological traits that are detrimental to school adjustment and then looks for psychological strengths in the teenager that can be positively used or enhanced in treatment.

School problems may be divided into problems of academic performance, behavioral problems, problems of social acceptance, and problems of attendance. It is beyond the scope of this chapter to discuss these comprehensively, but some salient features in each category are addressed.

Problems of Academic Performance

Problems of academic performance are common in junior and senior high schools, and they are not always an indication for psychotherapy. If the therapist determines that the educational placement seems appropriate, if there is no previously undiagnosed learning disability, and if there are no significant psychopathological symptoms, then the problem is one of capacity, interest, or study habits. Nonretarded, limited intellectual capacity is not a disorder by itself, but it may be associated with one by reaction. An example is a student of low average potential who has the misfortune to have highly motivated parents of superior intellect who cannot accept the C's and D's their child struggles to attain. The treatment here first focuses on the mismatch of family expectations and the adolescent's innate abilities, and then on the student's damaged self-esteem.

Poor study habits *per se* do not require psychotherapy; nonetheless, they frequently arise as issues in treatment. The therapist should be able to counsel teenage clients about more effective study techniques, and to work with the teenager, the parents, and the school, if necessary, to closely monitor the student's progress. The school survival skills mentioned above serve as a useful model for developing a treatment plan.

Primary reading retardation and other learning disabilities are a serious set of disorders that directly affect the school performance of children and adolescents. Their prevalence is estimated at 10%–16% of the population and is even higher in urban and lower-SES populations (Yule & Rutter, 1985). The disorders are heterogeneous and are thought to be due to developmental impairments, perhaps genetically determined, that are related to abnormal neurological maturation. The most common and thoroughly studied is primary reading retardation. It is a chronic and educationally debilitating problem and, by adolescence, is frequently associated with school failure, school conduct problems, and juvenile delinquency (Silver & Hagin, 1985). It can be diagnosed from (1) delays in reading achievement at least two years below age expectations and (2) characteristic verbal-performance discrepancies of twenty or more points on the WISC-R. The treatment of choice is remedial instruction given by special educators. Psychotherapy is not a treatment for learning disabilities, but it may be an appropriate treatment for the learning-disabled adolescent who has concomitant behavioral or emotional problems.

Problems in academic performance may be symptoms of various emotional disturbances. Parental separation and divorce frequently result in a reactive deterioration of school performance in adolescents. Depression may interfere with schoolwork through loss of concentration, fatigue, apathy, and preoccupation. Schizophrenia and other adolescent-onset psychoses severely disrupt the perceptual and cognitive integration that are required in the classroom, and the teenager may also be distracted by hallucinations and delusional thoughts. In each of these examples, treatment of the underlying disorder and (if necessary) special educational assistance are the appropriate interventions.

Behavior Problems in School

The teenager with behavior problems in school is generally referred to the clinic or the therapist by concerned and exasperated school officials. The etiologies of school misconduct are legion, and the therapist faced with a sullen, angry teenager and indignant parents encounters a formidable challenge to his or her evaluation skills. Corroborating sources, such as school principals or counselors, are valuable in the collection and verification of the initial data, and the subsequent treatment may well be a joint project between the adolescent, the therapist, the parents, and the school. Therefore, it is best to obtain permission to contact the school at the outset.

Specific diagnostic considerations in school behavior problems are childhood histories of attention deficit disorder with hyperactivity or learning disabilities. Both groups have conditions whose symptoms persist into adolescence. Adolescents with a history of hyperactive attention-deficit disorders often retain patterns of short attention span and behavioral and cognitive impulsivity. Learning disabilities are also chronic. Both groups have a significant incidence of conduct disorder and juvenile delinquency. Attention deficit disorder is underdiagnosed in teenagers, in that, until recently, the clinical lore was that it disappeared after puberty. Other diagnostic considerations in school misconduct are irritable, depressed states, manic states, personality disorders, and behavioral reactions in school to physical or sexual abuse at home.

The treatment of school misconduct requires, for the best results, an alliance of the therapist with the teenager and the family, a willingness of the school and the family to work together, and good communication channels all around. Close attention to attendance and tardiness, improvement in study skills, self-monitoring of prosocial and antisocial behavior, and regular reports from the school to the home or the therapist may all come into play. Underlying personal concerns may move the treatment into an individual psychotherapy model, or the focus may shift from the school to a parent–adolescent conflict model as described earlier. The therapist needs to be flexible enough to choose a conceptual model and a treatment strategy that fit the unfolding clinical situation, as behavior problems in school are like fevers from an infection; there are multiple possible causal agents, not all responsive to penicillin.

Problems of Social Acceptance

Another type of school problem referral is the teenager who is a social outcast or misfit. These students are either scapegoated or ignored, and they are perceived as peculiar, repugnant, different, or too withdrawn. They usually have depressive symptoms and are keenly aware of their lack of status. They may be highly disturbed or abnormal, but in some cases, and especially in schools with strong clique identifications, they may be essentially normal teens who have not yet found their social network. Some diagnostic considerations are in the affective disorders; chronic dysthymic states and major depressions may hamper an adolescent's social adjustment through isolation, lack of spontaneity, irritability, inability to feel pleasure, and psychomotor inhibition. Another diagnostic consideration is schizophrenia: chronic social isolation whose hallmark is a markedly peculiar personality is one of the risk factors for schizophrenia (Rutter & Garmezy, 1983). Organic personality syndromes related to brain damage may also cause unusual personality features that result in social ostracism.

The treatment for the social outcast, once a psychotic condition or brain damage is ruled out, requires warmth, understanding, and a sense of strategy. The therapeutic relationship in which the adolescent feels liked and valued lays a foundation for more pragmatic interventions. It does not take much to get by in society, and even small changes in appearance and style may appreciably destigmatize an adolescent and improve his or her social adjustment: How do you dress and groom yourself? How do you handle a conversation with a classmate? Through social skills therapy, the therapist and the adolescent address the adolescent's socialization deficits and improve on them in a series of steps designed each time to maximize the chances of success.

Problems of Attendance

School refusal, which is based on anxiety about leaving home or attending school, is a potentially serious problem and is clinically differentiated from truancy (Hersov, 1985). The clinical picture starts with a reluctance to go to school or vague complaints about it, which progress to a total refusal to attend school despite parental entreaties or threats. Some afflicted students profess a desire to go to school but, in the morning, are slow to rise and dress; they become increasingly anxious and unwilling as the time to leave approaches, and the result is another day's absence. The anxiety typically abates once the family acquiesces and allows the adolescent to remain home. There is usually an accompanying withdrawal from peers and outside activities, although some adolescents suffer little impairment in after-school activities that are out of the home. School refusal is an emotional disorder and is generally a manifestation of separation anxiety, a phobia, a depressive disorder, or a combination of these.

Adolescents who refuse to go to school have a less favorable prognosis for treatment success than younger children with the same condition, and the therapy requires firmness and persistence. In evaluation, affective and anxiety symptoms should be carefully ascertained, and teenagers with depression or panic attacks may be considered candidates for adjunct treatment with antidepressants. If school phobia itself is the primary problem, systematic desensitization via gradual increases in the amount of time spent each day at school is sometimes successful. If the adolescent demonstrates a picture of separation anxiety (fears of separation from the parents, persistent fears of harm befalling the parents when the teenager is at school, an inability to sleep at a friend's home, and an anxious desire always to be close to the parents), then the therapist should look for childhood antecedents of separation problems, precipitating events such as recent deaths or illness in the family, or contributory family psychopathology. The following is a typical case example:

Tony, age 14, had begun to refuse school totally in late September and was brought to the clinic in November. He was the youngest of a sibship of four and the only boy. He denied any reason to fear school and each evening vowed to go the next morning. At breakfast, he would start to feel anxious, and the anxiety would increase dramatically as he approached the front door, culminating in a tearful and desperate insistence on staying home. There was a history of reluctance to attend school in the elementary grades, but this had not reached a serious level. None of his sisters had school attendance or separation problems. The evaluation revealed that the family history was positive for serious medical problems; Tony's father had been forced into retirement by two heart attacks and now spent much of the day as a volunteer in a hospital. Tony's mother was even more severely debilitated by a presenile Alzheimer's disease and was essentially homebound. Although Tony denied being concerned about his mother and minimized her deterioration, his school refusal appeared to be a protective move. In a family meeting, one of Tony's sisters upbraided him, saying he might as well go to school because he did not help out at home anyway. Tony angrily retorted, "You don't know what I do for her!"

In this case, clarifying the clinical situation for the family helped them to deal more openly with the mother's Alzheimer's disease. They were able to procure assistance in monitoring her during the day from members of the extended family, and shortly thereafter, Tony returned voluntarily to an alternative education classroom in another part of the school system. He maintained, interestingly, a phobic avoidance of his original school.

Our approach is to identify the prompt return to school as a necessary component of successful treatment, and to work closely with the adolescent, the family, and the school officials to accomplish it. We avoid advising homebound instruction, as it serves to legitimize the student's absence from school. Once the adolescent is back in school, individual psychotherapy addresses the underlying issues, and family sessions are used to provide support to the parents and to implement interventions at the family level. Special attention should be paid to high-risk periods for a reemergence of school absenteeism, for example, the resumption of school following vacations and returning to school after a bona fide illness. Finally, if psychiatric illness in one or both parents is an etiological factor in the student's school refusal, the chances of therapeutic success are significantly less if the parent does not also receive treatment for his or her own disorder.

The Effect of Divorce on Adolescents and Young Adults

The growth of the divorce rate is a major phenomenon in modern industrialized societies, and in the United States, it is estimated that 40% of marriages end in divorce (Wolkind & Rutter, 1985). The rate in mental-health-clinic populations is even higher. The impact of divorce on families is enormous and long-term, causing a loss of family stability; changes in family relationships; changes of residence, often with significant lowering of the family socioeconomic status; and acute and chronic psychological effects on both parents and children. Divorce may precipitate psychopathological reactions in teenagers, resulting in a referral for psychotherapy, or it may be an important component of a larger clinical picture. Common symptoms arising in adolescents following a marital breakup are depressive syndromes, anger at one or both parents, school failure, emotional and social withdrawal, and conduct disturbances, including delinquent behaviors, sexual acting out, and substance abuse.

As divorce is so common, it is worthwhile to look for risk factors and protective factors affecting the eventual adjustment of children and adolescents following marital breakups. The major consistently identified risk factor relates to family discord. Wolkind and Rutter (1985) identified family discord preceding and following a divorce as correlating with a poor adjustment. Similarly, Chess, Thomas, Korn, Mittelman, and Cohen

(1984) found the level of continued conflict and parental hostility to be the major negative factor determining the successfulness of the child's adjustment after a divorce. On the other hand, several protective influences have been identified: more amicable parental separations, the availability of sibling relationships, positive relationships for the parents outside the marriage, and the reestablishment of new intimate relationships for the parents all tend to support normal child and adolescent postdivorce adjustments (Wallerstein, 1984).

In the California Children of Divorce Project, Wallerstein (1984, 1985) and Kelly (1980) longitudinally studied 131 nonclinic children and adolescents from 60 divorced families. The initial interviews were 1–13 months after the divorce, and the follow-up interviews were at 5 and 10 years. Several sets of findings that specifically address the reactions and course of adjustment of the older children and adolescents in the original cohort have been reported. One clinically notable finding was that, in late childhood and early adolescence, there is a strong tendency for the children to identify one of the parents as responsible for the divorce, to choose sides in parental conflicts, and to be intensely angry at one or both parents. Also, older children and adolescents are acutely aware of the dating and sexual activities of their parents.

At 5-year follow-up, a group of the original cohort who were 13–18 at the time of divorce were reevaluated, with a focus on the quality of their young-adult heterosexual relationships (Kelly, 1980). They tended to separate into two general groups. The first group was well adjusted, but its members appeared reluctant to allow themselves to be seriously involved with someone of the opposite sex. They dated, but the relationships were short-lived and the terminations were initiated by the study subjects. The second group was smaller in number. The members of this group had serious and chronic psychological difficulties and were functioning "at a barely adequate level." These young men and women were found to have low self-esteem, depression, and a history of poor school performance following the divorce. Their heterosexual relationships seemed "uniformly impoverished, immature, and ungratifying" but tended to be long term, with the subjects holding onto them in a desperate fashion. At this 5-year follow-up, two thirds of the interviewed subjects did not view marriage as desirable, and this was especially true of the well-adjusted group.

Wallerstein (1985) published a preliminary report on the 10-year follow-up of 40 of the original 131 study subjects. These 40 young men and women had all been in late childhood or adolescence when their parents divorced, and the findings reaffirmed the intensity and chronicity of their reactions. A decade later, the memories of the initial separation were strikingly vivid and affectively laden, and the subjects viewed their childhood and teenage years as being burdened by the divorce. Regardless of the quality of their subsequent adjustment, the subjects shared a sense of deprivation that they related to missing the experience of an intact family, although 30% had also experienced the divorce as a relief from a tyrannical parent. Anger, but not necessarily criticism, toward their parents had diminished. The decrease in anger tended to occur in adolescence and was coupled with a conclusion that the divorce had been inevitable and for the best.

In contrast to previous follow-ups, most of the young adults were now interested in commitments to love and marriage; they also had a strong desire to avoid a divorce for the sake of their own children. A subgroup of the young women in the cohort seemed to have fared less well; they were described as drifting through various jobs and men, frequently pairing up with older men, and they seemed worried, fearful, and despairing. Wallerstein was particularly impressed by the willingness, thoughtfulness, and eloquence that the subjects brought to their 10-year interviews. They seemed to welcome an opportunity to discuss topics that brought back intensely painful memories and feelings, and it was concluded that, for most, the divorce "continued to hold a moderately or highly central position in their psychological functioning" (p. 550).

Psychotherapy can be of assistance both for acute reactions to a divorce and for chronic or residual effects. In the period around the divorce, the therapist can provide support and objectivity, can identify and treat depressive reactions, and can help the adolescent contain angry and/or self-destructive impulses. When adolescents and young adults are still encumbered by a divorce in their childhood, the therapist can encourage them to reexamine their memories and the associated emotions, but now to approach the divorce with a degree of detachment and understanding that were beyond their capabilities as children. Both Blos (1962) and Wallerstein (1985) have commented on the opportunity that adolescent psychological development offers to teenagers to resolve this kind of childhood emotional trauma.

Wallerstein (1984) outlined a series of psychological tasks that face children and adolescents whose parents divorce; these provide a useful framework in psychotherapy: (1) Initially there is the task of acknowledging the marital disruption and then (2) the need to regain a sense of direction and to reassume customary activities, (3) dealing with loss and feelings of rejection, (4) forgiving the parent held responsible by the child for the breakup, (5) accepting the permanence of the divorce (as differentiated from recognizing its actuality), and (6) resolving issues in relationships and acquiring an enduring ability to love and be loved. These tasks require time to accomplish and are in part tied to normal maturational phenomena as well as to the psychological health of the individual. To the therapist, they offer guideposts for assessing the young person's progress in treatment.

Suicide in Adolescents and Young Adults

A subject of enormous concern is the increase in suicides among teenagers and young adults. In the United States in 1981, the reported suicide rate among 15- to 19-year-olds had risen 142% over the same age group in 1960. The rates of recorded completed suicide in males of this age had gone from 5.6 per 100,000 in 1960 to 13.6 per 100,000 in 1981. The rate for 15- to 19-year-old females was lower but had also increased from 1.6 to 3.6 per 100,000. Young adults (age 20–24 years) have an even higher rate of suicide completion, and their rate increase between 1960 and 1981 was comparable to that of teenagers. Young adult male suicides went from 13.7 per 100,000 in 1960 to 25.6 per 100,000 in 1981, and in young adult females, it rose from 2.9 to 5.6 suicides per 100,000. These trends appear to be continuing through this decade (Hawton, 1986).

Although the causes of this "epidemic" have not been proved, there are speculations that it may be related to the breakdown of nuclear- and extended-family ties throughout our culture. The dramatic increase of the divorce rate and the loss of extended-family systems may increase the prevalence of psychopathology among young people while coincidentally depriving them of the traditional support systems. There is also evidence that media coverage of teenage suicides and the dramatic portrayal of adolescent suicide on television result in at least temporary rises in suicidal behavior among young people (Gould & Shaffer, 1986; Phillips & Carstensen, 1986). Corresponding to the increase in suicide rates is a growth in the incidence of suicide attempts, both serious and gestural. The sex ratios of attempts are reversed; estimates of the ratio of female to male attempted suicides ranging from 3:1 to 9:1.

There are a few additional suicide statistics worth noting. Suicide rates are higher among white than among black young people, and the rates are particularly high in American Indian youths (but there is great variation between individual reservation populations). Married teenagers are at higher risk than single teenagers, a phenomenon that is the opposite of the protective effect of marriage in adults. Finally, preadolescents and early adolescents (10–14 years) have demonstrated only a slight rise in suicide rate since the late 1970s; and in 1978, their incidence of suicide was 0.8 per 100,000, one ninth of the rate among 15- to 19-year-olds (Hawton, 1986). Therefore, the problem of suicide in young people, by epidemiological standards, occurs from mid-adolescence through young adulthood.

When a teenager or a young adult complains of suicidal thoughts, a careful assessment of the circumstances and the person's psychological state are warranted. What is the historical context of the suicidal ideation? What led up to it, and when did it begin? Were there clear precipitants, such as boyfriend or girlfriend problems, anticipated punishments, severe stresses, or disappointments? What is the content of the suicidal ideation? Is it vague, such as "I wish I were dead or gone," or has the person considered a specific means? The therapist should inquire into evidence of preparatory planning or activities before a suicidal act. One 16-year-old who had made a serious hanging attempt told his therapist that he was having a recurrence of depressive symptoms and suicidal feelings. Only after patient, detailed questioning and encouragement did he disclose that he had recently procured a rope and had hidden it near a suitable tree in an isolated wooded area. The fantasies and the affect associated with the suicidal ideation should be explored: What will suicide accomplish and how does the person view its impact on family and friends? Are the suicidal impulses related to feelings of anger, rage, sadness, despair, or perhaps relief? Feelings of hopelessness are indications of heightened risk, especially when accompanied by low self-esteem.

If the client has performed a suicidal act, the details of the event should be evaluated for the lethality of the suicidal behavior and the seriousness of the intent. Occasionally, young people make serious suicide attempts with what are, in fact, nonlethal or innocuous means. In these cases, the intent of the act, however inept, is the crucial point, for a subsequent attempt may be more effectively executed. The behavior and feelings after the act are also important clues to its seriousness. Did the young person warn anyone of the attempt or seek help, and how does he or she feel about surviving?

In the psychiatric history, one should look for previous suicide attempts, past or current depression, dysthymic states, evidence of past manic or hypomanic behavior, and substance abuse. Brent (1987) and his colleagues have studied a series of completed adolescent suicides and found bipolar disorders disproportionately represented. They also identified the combination of teenage alcohol abuse and the availability of firearms in the home as significant risk factors for suicidal teenagers. The therapist should also look for evidence of psychosis, such as paranoia or hallucinations.

Family risk factors are a history of suicide and/or suicide attempts in the family, recent losses, and psychiatric disorders among family members. An interesting example of the impact of family psychiatric disorders can be found in Shaffer's review (1974, 1985) of 30 completed suicides in children and adolescents under 15 years of age. Of the deceased children, 55% had family members who had sought psychiatric treatment. Two of the suicides appeared to be directly related to the imminent discharge of a parent from a psychiatric institution.

After gathering the necessary information, a management plan is made. If the risk of suicide is felt to be high, then hospitalization is indicated. In the case of all teenagers and young adults, the family should be involved if at all possible. If the case is judged manageable on an outpatient basis, then a specific plan for communications and emergencies is required. An available, trusted support should be identified and apprised of the situation. For the period of risk, more frequent therapeutic contacts may be arranged, and the therapist should closely monitor clinical changes for improvement or worsening. Medications should be parsimoniously prescribed, and the therapist and the family may need to take special precautions in medication management, such as pill counts and supervision of medication ingestion. It is best to clear the house of guns when a young person is suicidal.

There are a few clinical conditions in which suicide management is particularly difficult. The first is refractory depression with chronic hopelessness and suicidal thoughts and impulses, especially when there is a family history of suicide. Some young people with these symptoms appear, over time, to incorporate suicide as an egosyntonic facet of their self-image and are at perpetual risk of self-destruction. A combination of aggressive antidepressant medication and intensive psychotherapy is indicated. Unstable or rapidly cycling bipolar patients with suicidal thoughts or delusions are another high-risk group. They require expert medication management and a good therapeutic alliance to weather their numerous mood swings and crises.

A third group is made up of female adolescents with histories of extensive and traumatic sexual abuse and exploitation. These girls and young women suffer from a chronic posttraumatic stress syndrome. They are usually dysthymic and prone to serious depressive episodes, and they have great difficulty engaging in positive interpersonal relationships. Their sense of self-worth is severely impoverished, and their perception of the world is fearful and bleak. Their personalities are unstable and immature and often meet the criteria for a diagnosis of borderline personality disorder. The suicidal thoughts and impulses that these young women have are both chronic and polymorphous: suicidal ideation and gestures, self-mutilation, and actual suicide attempts. Again, long-term psychotherapy is probably necessary to gradually provide stability and a sense of self-worth. Antidepressants and low-dose antipsychotics are the medications most commonly useful in these cases and may help to contain their impulses in the early phases of psychotherapy.

The final subgroup we have encountered is made up of adolescent boys and young men with narcissistic and antisocial personality disorders who use potentially lethal suicidal behavior in a way that is partly manipulative and apparently self-gratifying. One narcissistic and dysthymic college student declared that his near-fatal wrist slashing was "the only act of self-affirmation I ever made," and he clearly found satisfaction in the inability of the concerned hospital staff to convince him of the value of living. The sense of control and power that these young men derive from their threats is bolstered by the clinician's appreciation of their aggressive impulsivity and poor judgment. An underlying affective disorder should also be ruled out. In psychotherapy, one endeavors not to challenge their threats and bravado, but to shift their focus to problem solving and to allow them other avenues of narcissistic gratification.

MODIFICATIONS IN TREATMENT APPROACHES FOR TEENAGERS

The fundamental differences between psychotherapy for adults and adolescents lie in the developmental characteristics of teenagers as they influence the context and the techniques of the psychotherapy. There also are trends in psychotherapy for adolescents that are derivatives of larger trends and advances in the diagnosis, understanding, and treatment of psychiatric disorders, both adolescent and adult.

A basic premise of psychotherapy for adolescents is that they are not treated in isolation. At the levels of referral and evaluation, the therapist looks for the contribution of parents, school personnel, and sometimes other adults; these same resources are useful informants on the progress of the teenager's treatment. The question is not whether to include parents and other sources, but to what degree. There are several ready examples. Teenagers with antisocial behavior problems are unreliable reporters, so the therapist requires corroborating sources to help monitor the case. In affective disorders in young people, the symptoms are sometimes less apparent to the teenager than to his or her family, especially in the early phases of an initial episode or a relapse; again, outside reporting is helpful. Treatment for teenagers with social skill deficits is similarly helped by parent observations. School problems, as previously noted, are another example of the usefulness of communications between parents, school personnel, and the psychotherapist, so that the progress of a case may be followed. In practice, it is only with mature older adolescents with emotional disorders that the treatment may be handled with the type of privacy afforded to most adult outpatients.

The counterbalancing factor when sharing information with parents and other sources is the issue of confidentiality. Confidentiality is not as secure when one is working with adolescents as when one is working with adults. Parents have a right to some feedback, and schools may need advice for management and placement. The dilemma for the therapist is to share the necessary information and still sufficiently engage the trust of the teenager to build a therapeutic alliance. Also, confidentiality varies with the selection of the therapeutic modality. In individual therapy, the therapist and the adolescent may agree mutually on an arena of confidentiality and may designate the specific circumstances in which it will not hold; in group and family therapy, the boundaries are looser. When the issue of confidentiality arises, the best tactic is to address it in a straightforward, open fashion. Teenagers do not have complete privacy and consequently do not expect it, but they are concerned that their thoughts and feelings be treated with respect, and they appreciate knowing the boundaries separating confidential and nonconfidential information.

Another trend in the treatment of teenagers, paralleling the same movement throughout the field of mental health, is the increased specification of treatment goals and strategies. This is partly a natural outcome of improvement in the diagnosis of psychiatric disorders, and partly an accommodation to the pressures of cost containment. When funds are limited, so is treatment duration, forcing the therapist to identify the goals and therapeutic modalities that are sensible in the context of brief treatment.

The use of psychopharmacology is an increasingly important trend in adolescent psychotherapy, as a number of disorders in teenagers are under evaluation for their responsiveness to a growing armamentarium of psychoactive medications. Psychopharmacology need not be viewed as a threat to psychotherapy, but it does imply that non-medical therapists will need to collaborate, in many instances, with a psychiatrist or other physician who can prescribe and manage medication. Also, adolescents are not necessarily comparable to adults in medication responsivity; for example, unlike older adults, depressed adolescents have not yet been convincingly shown, in a controlled study, to respond any better to antidepressants than to placebo (Ryan, Puig-Antich, Cooper, Rabinovich, Ambrosini, Davies, King, Torres, & Fried, 1986). Therefore, psychotherapy is still the best treatment available for many depressed adolescents.

Another study addressing medication and psychotherapy for children and adolescents examined the treatment of hyperactive children. It showed that, when hyperactive children have a planned psychotherapeutic regimen in addition to stimulant medication, they have a much lower outcome of juvenile delinquency than hyperactive children treated with stimulants alone (Satterfield, Satterfield, & Schell, 1987). Thus, medications will probably not supplant psychotherapy, and the combination of drugs and therapy is likely to become increasingly prevalent for the more serious disorders. Several specific diagnoses where this trend is recently apparent are adolescent panic disorders, attention deficit disorders, obsessive-compulsive disorders, and some cases of adolescent depression.

Common Problems in Psychotherapy for Early Adolescents

Problems in psychotherapy arise that are specifically related to the maturational level of the adolescent, particularly in early adolescence. A number of clinicians have commented on the difficulties of engaging young teenagers in psychotherapy, and then maintaining them through the course of treatment (Kessler, 1979; Slaff, 1979; Wilson & Hersov, 1985). These teenagers, generally 13–15 years old, are just moving away from childhood and are experimenting with more independent relationships with their families. When they come to treatment, it is almost always at the request of their parents or other adult authorities, and accordingly, they are reluctant participants. Sitting and talking about emotional problems and participating in self-examination are both foreign to and uncomfortable for this age group, and as they tend at this age to discharge tension through action, the less verbally inclined find therapy sessions agonizingly long and awkward. Also, young adolescents are cognitively immature and are often incapable of viewing their problems with detachment or within an abstract conceptual framework. On the other hand, they may find play therapy demeaning and childish.

Another problem, which Kessler (1979) and Wilson and Hersov (1985) have commented on, is the intolerance that young adolescents have for feelings of dependency. Thus, at the point where the therapist begins to work effectively with teenagers, they reexperience the type of dependent feelings that they had toward their parents, and they recapitulate the strivings for independence by becoming less involved in therapy or suddenly fleeing it altogether. Other characteristics of young teenagers that interfere with establishing a therapeutic alliance are their tendency to avoid assuming responsibility for their own difficulties and the use of the immature defenses of denial and externalization. One 15-year-old related an episode of stealing from his mother's boyfriend as follows: "I was walking through his apartment, and my right hand reached out on its own and picked up his radio."

In summary, during early adolescence, the immaturity of the teenagers' defenses and conceptualizations, their intolerance of feelings of dependency, their self-consciousness and fear of disclosure, and their preference for physical action—all work against the communications of individual psychotherapy. The therapist may overcome many of these handicaps by being more interactive and by demonstrating respect for the teenager's integrity and sensitivities. Kessler (1979) found group therapy especially useful for early adolescents, as it diffuses the issues of dependency and takes advantage of the teenager's normal proclivity for peer relationships. Kessler stated:

> The more nearly a youngster has progressed in his development to preadolescence, the more useful phase-appropriate, valued peer relationships can be in therapeutic intervention. Where individual therapy may be actively rejected, group therapy can dilute the dangers of transference and offer peer support, along with alternative solutions to current conflicts. (pp. 153–171)

Art therapy, which allows the indirect and more projective elucidation of themes and emotions, is another approach useful for many adolescents. Its nonverbal component reduces the threat of a therapy session for anxious teenagers, and the creative activity of constructing an artwork is satisfying and often therapeutic in itself.

Treatment Goals

As noted previously, the trend in psychotherapy is to specify more clearly the goals of treatment, which reflect the primary symptoms presented by the teenager and the family, and the disorders, deficits, and other problems identified in the evaluation. The treatment goals should be understandable and sensible to the adolescent and the parents, thus promoting their engagement and sense of participation in the treatment. Rutter (1985) outlined a useful guideline for setting treatment goals, in which he categorized the areas of desired improvement. The first general treatment goal is symptom reduction. The second is the overall promotion of normal development. Third, the therapist fosters the child's sense of autonomy and self-reliance. The fourth goal in treatment is the generalization of behavioral gains beyond the treatment setting itself. The fifth is ensuring the persistence of improvement over time (and, by implication, well after the completion of the treatment), and finally, the sixth goal is environmental changes that will promote the health of the child.

Contraindications to Psychotherapy

Wilson and Hersov (1985) identified certain conditions for which psychotherapy is contraindicated as the treatment of choice: severe disturbances secondary to organic brain disorders, autism, developmental disabilities, and schizophrenia. These disorders require multidisciplinary planning (often emphasizing specific, structured educational environments), the enhancement of family understanding and support systems, and sometimes medication. Psychotherapy for these conditions is usually an adjunctive treatment for secondary reactions to the disorder. Similarly, the following clinical features were identified by these authors as poor prognostic indicators for psychotherapy: poor reality testing, a severe lack of impulse control, a persistent denial of personal problems, psychotic states, and severe conduct disorders (Wilson & Hersov, 1985).

Therapist Attributes

The first qualities essential for successful work with teenagers is liking young people of this age group and finding a challenge in the complications inherent in the adolescent period. Without this attraction and interest to buoy one up, the frequent frustrations that adolescents and their families present will eventually make clinical work with them dissatisfying. The second quality that is important in the therapist is good common sense. This ingredient is not easily defined but denotes an intellectual flexibility in relating the abstract concepts of diagnoses and treatment models to the facts of the young person's life, coupled with an ability to communicate these ideas clearly and without professional jargon. There is evidence that an extroverted, assertive, and open style is helpful with adolescents (Wilson & Hersov, 1985), and in general, the therapist does well to avoid the role of the blank screen. Kessler (1979) further cautioned that a nonjudgmental nondirective therapeutic stance is developmentally inappropriate for many adolescents, who may misinterpret the therapist's neutrality as sanctioning impulses to act out. Finally, a therapist should have the capacity to listen sympathetically to the complaints of a teenager without overendorsing their legitimacy and without obviously taking sides against the parents. An open line of communication between the parents and the therapist will help keep the complaints of the adolescent in perspective.

In summary, successful therapist attributes have a great deal in common with the qualities that are found in good teachers, in good youth-group leaders and coaches, and, for that matter, in good parents. They are adults who demonstrate an evident interest in and enjoyment of teenagers, and who respect and understand their thoughts and feelings but are also able to actively provide direction and positive role-modeling. They are also willing to set limits when appropriate. The differentiating qualities of the psychotherapist are his or her expertise in psychopathology and its treatments and a knowledge of adolescent psychological development.

SUMMARY

Psychotherapy for teenagers is an important component of the management of many of the emotional and behavioral disturbances found in this population. The practice of psychotherapy with teenagers is demanding, as it requires a knowledge of psychopathology, normal development, and the developmental influences of adolescence on the presentation of psychopathology. It also calls for a facility in working with reluctant clients and for communicating effectively with both the adolescent and his or her family, as well as a willingness on the therapist's part to seek out and use outside resources. It is difficult but frequently rewarding work than can effectively reduce the discomfort of disturbed young people and help maximize their recovery and promote their growth and development as they prepare to enter adulthood.

REFERENCES

Aichorn, A. (1925). *Wayward Youth.* New York: Viking.

Alexander, F., & Selesnick, S. (1966). Development in child psychiatry. *History of psychiatry* (pp. 373–387). New York: Harper & Row.

Blos, P. (1962). *On adolescence—A psychoanalytic interpretation.* New York: Free Press. London: Collier-Macmillan.

Blos, P. (1979). *The adolescent passage.* New York: International Universities Press.

Brent, D. (1987). Personal communication on unpublished data.

Cantwell, D. P. (1986a). Attention deficit disorder in adolescents. *Clinical Psychology Review, 6,* 237–247.

Cantwell, D. P. (1986b). *Behavioral disorders.* Presentation at the Annual Review of Child Psychiatry, Chicago.

Chess, S., Thomas, A., Korn, S., Mittelman, M., & Cohen, J. (1984). Early parental attitudes, divorce and separation, and young adult outcome: Findings of a longitudinal study. In S. Chess & A. Thomas (Eds.), *Annual progress in child psychiatry and child development* (pp. 281–289). New York: Brunner/Mazel.

Erikson, E. (1958). *Young man Luther.* New York: W. W. Norton.

Erikson, E. (1968). The life cycle: Epigenesis of identity. In E. Erikson (Ed.), *Identity, yough and crisis* (pp. 91–141). New York: W. W. Norton.

Freud, A. (1958). Adolescence. *The psychoanalytic study of the child, 13,* 255–278.

Freud, A. (1966). *The ego and the mechanisms of defense.* New York: International Universities Press.

Gittleman, R., Mannuzza, S., Shenker, R., & Bonagura, N. (1985). Hyperactive boys almost grown up. *Archives of General Psychiatry, 37,* 937–947.

Gould, M., & Shaffer, D. (1986). The impact of suicide in television movies, evidence of imitation. *New England Journal of Medicine, 315,* 690–694.

Hawton, K. (1986b). Suicide in adolescence. In S. Roy (Ed.), *Suicide,* (pp. 135–150). Baltimore: Williams & Wilkins.

Healy, W., & Bronner, A., (1923–1948). The child guidance clinic: Birth and growth of an idea. In L. Lowrey (Ed.), *Orthopsychiatry* (pp. 14–49). New York: American Orthopsychiatric Association.

Hechtman, L., Weiss, G., & Perlman, T. (1984). Young adult outcome of hyperactive children who received long-term stimulant treatment. *Journal of the American Academy of Child Psychiatry, 23,* 261–269.

Hersov, L. (1985). School refusal. In M. Rutter, & L. Hersov (Eds.), *Child and adolescent psychiatry, modern approaches* (pp. 382–399). Oxford: Blackwell Scientific Publications.

Kandel, D. B., & Davies, M. (1986). Adult sequelae of adolescent depressive symptoms. *Archives of General Psychiatry, 43,* 255–262.

Kelly, J. B. (1980). Observations on adolescent relationships five years after divorce. In S. C. Feinstein, J. C. Looney, A. Z. Schwartzberg, & A. D. Sorosky (Eds.), *Adolescent psychiatry: Developmental and clinical studies* (pp. 133–141). Chicago: University of Chicago Press.

Kessler, E. S. (1979). Individual psychotherapy with adolescents. In J. Novello (Ed.), *The short course in adolescent psychiatry* (pp. 153–171). New York: Brunner/Mazel.

Kovacs, M., Feinberg, T. L., Crouse-Novak, M. A., Paulauskas, S. L., & Finkelstein, R. (1984a). Depressive disorders in childhood. *Archives of General Psychiatry, 41,* 229–237.

Kovacs, M., Feinberg, T. L., Crouse-Novak, M. A., Paulauskas, S. L., & Finkelstein, R. (1984b). Depressive disorders in childhood. *Archives of General Psychiatry, 41,* 643–649.

Loeber, R., & Stouthamer-Loeber, M. (1987). The prediction of delinquency. In H. C. Quay (Ed.), *Handbook of juvenile delinquency.* New York: Wiley.

Offer, D. (1986). Adolescent development: A normative perspective. *American Psychiatric Association Annual Review, 5,* 404–419.

Offer, D., Ostrov, E., & Howard, K. I. (1981). *The adolescent: A psychological self portrait.* New York: Basic Books.

Offer, D. (1986). Adolescent development: A normative perspective. *American Psychiatric Association Annual Review, 5,* 404–419.

Phillips, D. P., & Carstensen, L. L. (1986). Clustering of teenage suicides after television news stories about suicide. *New England Journal of Medicine, 315,* 685–689.

Robin, A. L., Koepke, T., & Nayar, M. (1986). Conceptualizing, assessing, and treating parent-adolescent conflict. In B. B. Lahey, & A. E. Kazdin (Eds.), *Advances in clinical child psychology* (Vol. 9) (pp. 87–124). New York: Plenum Press.

Rutter, M. (1985). Psychological therapies in child psychiatry: Issues and prospects. In M. Rutter & L. Hersov (Eds.), *Child and adolescent psychiatry, modern approaches* (pp. 927–940). Oxford: Blackwell.

Rutter, M., & Garmezy, N. (1983). Developmental psychopathology. In P. Mussen (Ed.), *Handbook of child psychology.* New York: Wiley.

Rutter, M., & Graham, P. (1968). The reliability and validity of the psychiatric assessment of the child: 1. Interview with the child. *British Journal of Psychiatry, 114,* 563–579.

Rutter, M., Graham, P., Chadwick, O. F. D., & Yule, W. (1976). Adolescent turmoil: Fact of fiction. *Journal of Child Psychology and Psychiatry, 17,* 35–56.

Ryan, N. D., Puig-Antich, J., Cooper, T., Rabinovich, H., Ambrosini, P., Davies, M., King, J., Torres, D., & Fried, J. (1986). Imipramine in adolescent major depression: Plasma level and clinical response. *Acta Psychiatrica Scandinavia, 73,* 275–288.

Satterfield, J. H., Satterfield, B. T., & Schell, A. M. (1987). Therapeutic interventions to prevent delinquency in hyperactive boys. *Journal of the American Academy of Child and Adolescent Psychiatry, 26,* 56–64.

Shaffer, D. (1974). Suicide in childhood and early adolescence. *Journal of Child Psychology and Psychiatry, 45,* 406–451.

Shaffer, D. (1985). Depression, mania and suicidal acts. In M. Rutter & L. Hersov (Eds.), *Child and adolescent psychiatry, modern approaches* (pp. 698–719). Oxford: Blackwell.

Silver, A. A., & Hagin, R. A. (1985). Outcomes of learning disabilities in adolescence. In S. Feinstein, M. Sugar, A. Esman, J. Looney, A. Schwartzberg, & A. Sorosky (Eds.), *Adolescent psychiatry* (Vol. 12) (pp. 197–213). Chicago: University of Chicago Press.

Slaff, B. (1979). Adolescents. In S. Harrison (Ed.), *Basic handbook of child psychiatry* (pp. 504–518). New York: Basic Books.

Steele, B. F. (1986). Notes on the lasting effects of early child abuse throughout the life cycle. *Child Abuse and Neglect, 10,* 283–291.

Strober, M. (1986). Psychopathology in adolescence revisited. *Clinical Psychology Review, 6,* 199–209.

Strober, M., Carlson, G. A., & Green, J. (1981). Reliability of psychiatric diagnosis in hospitalized adolescents: Interrater agreement using DSM-III. *Archives of General Psychiatry, 38,* 141–145.

Wallerstein, J. S. (1984). Children of divorce: The psychological tasks of the child. In S. Chess & A. Thomas (Eds.), *Annual progress in child psychiatry and child development* (pp. 263–280). New York: Brunner/Mazel.

Wallerstein, J. S. (1985). Children of divorce: Preliminary report of a ten-year follow-up of older children and adolescents. *Journal of the American Academy of Child Psychiatry, 24,* 545–553.

Wilson, P., & Hersov, L. (1985). Individual and group psychotherapy. In M. Rutter & L. Hersov (Eds.), *Child and adolescent psychiatry, movern approaches* (pp. 826–838). Oxford: Blackwell.

Wolkind, S., & Rutter, M. (1985). Separation, loss and family relationship. In M. Rutter, & L. Hersov (Eds.), *Child and adolescent psychiatry, modern approaches* (pp. 34–57). Oxford: Blackwell.

Yule, W., & Rutter, M. (1985). Reading and other learning disabilities. In M. Rutter & L. Hersov (Eds.), *Child and adolescent psychiatry, modern approaches* (pp. 444–464). Oxford: Blackwell.

Zigmond, N., & Kerr, M. M. (1986). What do high school teachers want? A study of expectations and standards. *Education and Treatment of Children, 9,* 239–249.

Zigmond, N., Kerr, M., Brown, G., & Harris, A. (1984, April). *School survival skills in secondary school age special education students.* Paper presented before the American Educational Research Association, New Orleans.

22

Geriatric Populations

ROBERT S. MARIN

INTRODUCTION

Psychiatric care for the elderly challenges clinicians to orchestrate a broad array of psychosocial and medical skills in dealing with complex clinical and existential problems. Although the elements of assessment and treatment are essentially the same as in other adult areas, the approach to care is altered by the distinctive array of psychological, biological, and social problems one sees in elderly patients. This chapter is intended to acquaint the reader with some of these problems and with the principles of assessment and treatment that apply to their management.

After presenting a few highlights of the field's history, a number of illustrative developmental issues are discussed. This material provides the rationale for the assessment process, which is described in the next section. In the section on frequently encountered clinical problems, the management of the two most commonly encountered clinical syndromes, depression and dementia, is described. Recommendations regarding the use of psychotropic drugs for dementia and depression are included in this section, and psychotherapy is treated separately in the section on the adaptation of treatment approaches to the elderly.

HISTORY

Interest in psychiatric care for the elderly has grown in concert with a variety of societal factors including demographic projections of the elderly population (U. S. Department of Health and Human Services, 1985–1986); epidemiological estimates of the

---

ROBERT S. MARIN • Western Psychiatric Institute and Clinic, University of Pittsburgh, Pittsburgh, Pennsylvania 15213.

psychiatric needs of the elderly (Butler & Lewis, 1982); and service delivery studies showing deficiencies in the availability and utilization of mental health services by the elderly (Cohen, 1980). Simultaneously, we are witnessing a reconstruction or, at least, a reconsideration of our society's values about aging: myths and stereotypes are being examined (Ford & Sbordone, 1980); existential concerns about death and dying are being exposed to ethical scrutiny (Jahnigen & Schrier, 1986); and family and cultural loyalty to the aging is being recognized (Brody, 1977).

The historical roots of these developments may be traced back over centuries. Francis Bacon has been credited with initiating the modern scientific inquiry into geriatric illness in his *History of Life and Death,* published in 1645 (Rowe & Minaker, 1985). Esquirol, in the mid-19th century, described the major mental changes in late life, including early senility and the late-life onset of mania. In the last decade of the 19th century, neuropathological studies by Pick, Binswanger, Alzheimer, and others differentiated cerebral arteriosclerosis, neurosyphilis, and senile dementia. It was also at this time that Emil Kraepelin accomplished the enduring differentiation of dementia praecox and manic-depressive illness (Robinson, 1972).

Despite these contributions, a distinction between functional and organic psychopathology in the elderly had not yet been established. The prevailing view was that "the commonest cause of persistent affective and paranoid symptoms among the aged was cerebral disease" (Roth & Kay, 1962; p. 74). Conversely, a clear relationship between the neuropathology of brain disease and its psychological concomitants was unproved (Robinson, 1972).

Studies from England contributed to progress on these fronts. Measuring cognitive capacities in life and then, after death, quantifying the number of neurofibrillary tangles or the volume of cerebral tissue infarcted by stroke, Blessed, Tomlinson, and Roth (1968) demonstrated quantitative correlations between the severity of mental impairment and the extent of neuropathological changes in patients who had died of stroke or Alzheimer's disease (AD). At the same time, Roth (1955) asserted the separability of functional and organic disturbances in late life and subdivided the area of functional disorders through his descriptions of affective disorders and paranoid illness in the elderly.

Since the 1950s, we have seen enormous changes in our approach to the process and pathology of aging. The biopsychosocial model (Engel, 1977), derived from systems theory, provides a framework that is eminently useful in caring for patients with multiple interacting problems. In virtually every discipline, from the chemistry of free radicals to the social psychology of residential environments, the parameters of normal aging and late-life mental disorders are being addressed. The biopsychosocial model also structures clinical assessment and treatment and defines the rationale for multidisciplinary team functioning, a needed alternative to the traditional, physician-centered approach to care.

SPECIAL DEVELOPMENTAL AND DIAGNOSTIC CONSIDERATIONS

Developmental Issues

Geropsychiatry is a developmental field, that is, a clinical area defined by a phase of the human life cycle. Its foundation in the study of normal aging, gerontology, is built in terms of the varied psychological, social, and biological changes that affect people as a function of time. Knowledge of the problems that may be created by these changes is helpful in the assessment process. Few such problems are unique to late life. Death, disease, disability, and dependency may occur at any age. It is rather their salience and certainty in the lives of the elderly that are distinctive. Awareness of the prominence they may have for individual patients will guide professionals to respond empathically and to discern their presence when patients or their families are unable to articulate their concerns in psychological terms.

Individual Psychology of Normal Aging

Personality. The literature on personality and aging offers a number of concepts to guide professionals in conceptualizing normal development. Perhaps the most important contribution from the empirical literature is the extensive evidence that, contrary to popular belief, continuity and consistency are characteristic of personality traits in later life (McCrae & Costa, 1984; Newton, Lazarus, & Weinberg, 1984). Erikson (1982) depicted the developmental challenge of late life as a crossroad between the sense of integrity and despair. Jung (1923) viewed adulthood and late life as a time when the unconscious parts of the self may be integrated into conscious functioning. Neugarten (1968) proposed that there is an increase, with time, of "interiority," the quality of relying on and strengthening one's sense of self. Social scientists have looked at well-being, life satisfaction, and morale as concepts that may be used to describe the quality of aging (Schulz, 1985).

Cognition. Contrary to myth, the cognitive changes of late life are not specific to the elderly; rather they develop gradually during the middle adult years. Many people are sensitive to the changes in cognitive capacity that characterize normal aging. For example, memory complaints are a state-related aspect of depression (Popkin, Gallagher, Thompson, & Moore, 1982). Normal adults accrue measurable losses in short-term memory, visuospatial skills, language abilities, and problem-solving capacities. Studies on the nature and mechanism of such changes attempt to disentangle cohort and longitudinal effects and to distinguish slowing and fatigability from qualitative changes in specific cognitive capacities.

Biology of Normal Aging

Aging processes may be studied at all levels of biological organization. The structural and functional changes associated with later life begin in the third and fourth decades. Although such changes occur in many organs and systems, the impression of invariant deterioration has proved inaccurate. Some measures (e.g., of hematocrit) show no change in healthy elderly (Rowe & Minaker, 1985). A decrease in resting cardiac output and other cardiac indices in healthy adults may reflect occult cardiac disease (Lakatta, 1985). Such normal processes interact with pathological ones in creating vulnerability to the diseases and dysfunction that many mistakenly regard as typifying late life (Rowe & Minaker, 1985). Age and medication use contribute independently to the higher incidence of medication side effects seen in elderly patients. Physiological changes seen in elderly patients that are of particular importance in psychotropic drug use include (Salzman, 1984):

- Absorption: A decreased gastric pH, splanchnic circulation, and gastric motility.
- Distribution: A decrease in cardiac output, serum albumin, lean body mass, and total body water.

- Metabolism: A decrease in hepatic size, enzyme activity, and blood flow.
- Excretion: A decrease in blood flow, tubular secretion, and glomerular filtration of the kidneys.

Adaptation to Loss and Opportunity

The tension between loss and continued opportunity is a hallmark of aging (Atchley, 1983). The losses that concern the elderly may be symbolic or concrete, psychosocial or biomedical, a matter of fact or of fantasy. They often seem familiar and, at the same time, have unique meanings to patients and their families. Assessment aims to elucidate patients' losses as well as their resources and opportunities and, thereby, to better portray the patient as both a case of particular type and, at the same time, an individual of unique experience and capacities.

The prospect of loss is felt most poignantly through the immediacy of death and dying. It is through the deaths of others that we become acquainted with death and build a framework for dealing with the inevitability of our own death. Inquiries regarding these experiences, patients' fantasies about their own deaths, and the tangible plans they have made for death—through wills, funeral preferences, or discussions with a spouse about how the survivor will conduct his or her life—are always germane to the assessment process.

Bereavement, the state of grieving the loss of a loved one, may be thought of as an instance of the more general developmental challenge of aging: adaptation to loss. Mourning is the process by which humans adapt to loss. Depending on the loss and the individual in question, the mourning period may last minutes, months, or years. For bereavement, the acute period of mourning has been said to last a period of months. Although attenuation occurs throughout the first year, many features of grief persist for years (Zisook & Shuchter, 1985). For other losses, the acute period is generally shorter, depending on the meaning of the particular loss and its functional consequences. In bereavement, there is first an initial period of a few days or weeks when psychological symptoms, insomnia, and appetite loss may be marked. Later, there are periods of increasing length during which the bereaved person feels relatively well. For bereavement, as well as other losses, preoccupation with thoughts and images of the lost object diminish as these images and memories are integrated with associated affects. Initial disturbances in daily activities are corrected, and gradually, the individual engages in new roles and relationships, frequently acquiring new skills and responsibilities in the process.

New Roles

It is practical to define many of the stressors of late life in terms of the disruption of old roles and the need to adapt to new ones. Throughout the adult years, work functions as an organizer of our lives. In varying degrees, it is a vehicle for attaining a sense of independence, competence, control, and social value through one's daily activities. The inability to work, whether at formal employment or as a homemaker, may bring changes in all aspects of life. Marriages may be strengthened by the opportunity for husbands and wives to be together without major external constraint. On the other hand, time together may burden a relationship that depended on external demands to limit intimacy.

Illness and death inevitably cause dramatic role disturbance, and even their possibility is disabling to some. Those who have taken pride in their self-sufficiency may find it impossible to adjust to disability and dependency. Those who have been dependent on others may be incapacitated by the incompetence they feel at having to function on their own. Learning to grieve and to comfort those who are grieving is a life task that comes to the fore in late life. The simple process of expressing condolences to a bereaved relative or friend is a new role in itself, as expressed by a patient who reported, "I pride myself on being able to write a nice condolence note."

Grandparenthood offers enormous opportunities for renewed pleasure but requires parents and children to renegotiate the bounds of interpersonal involvement. The relationships between parents and children may also call for redefinition to deal with parents' becoming dependent on their children. The intangible values of life are brought to the fore by the infirmities of aging because concrete achievements may no longer be feasible. Late life *per se* may be perceived as a personal role in which the prospect of illness and disability and the certainty of death challenge us to commit ourselves to projects knowing, more than ever, that there is uncertainty about whether there will be an opportunity to complete them (Erikson, 1983).

Diagnostic Considerations

This section is an overview of the rationale and content of assessment in geropsychiatry. General principles and organization of care are first discussed. Suggestions regarding the interview of older patients are followed by comments regarding major areas of assessment: medical and neurological evaluation; cognitive assessment; and functional assessment. Discussion of family and community resources is deferred to the discussion of dementia. Although examples are chosen with regard to dementia and depression, the material is recommended as having a general applicability to the care of older psychiatric patients.

General Principles

Ideally, the outcome of geropsychiatric assessment is a holistic understanding of the older person that integrates information from the biological, psychological, and social spheres. Comprehensive assessment, which is our best approximation of this ideal, is best accomplished through the multidisciplinary team process, as no one professional has the time or the skills to address all aspects of this process. For the office-based practitioner, a multidisciplinary assessment may be particularly difficult because the professionals comprising the team may be located elsewhere in the community. In such situations, it is important that one professional assume the role of a case coordinator who will monitor, coordinate, and help patients to integrate the results of the assessment procedures.

Interviewing Technique

The interview technique for older patients is individualized, based on initial and ongoing appraisals of the patients' strengths and limitations. Many older patients who are having difficulty in adapting to late-life stressors have few, if any, significant impairments, and therefore require little or no change in approach. The conventional priority given to respect, genuine interest, empathy, confidentiality, and privacy go most of the way to insuring effective communication. Changing one's approach in such instances may have the unwitting effect of making the patient feel that he or she is seen as "old," impaired, or incompetent.

When objective obstacles to communication are evident, a number of adjustments may be helpful. Hearing-impaired patients are aided by minimizing environmental noise, sitting closer to the patient, making use of whichever ear has better hearing, and lowering the voice pitch. Thus, information from facial expression and vocal intonation may be used more readily. One is cautioned against engaging in the proverbial error of the American in France who tries to make himself or herself understood by talking louder. On the other hand, slowing the rate of speech and pausing between words momentarily may make a dramatic difference.

For the patient with cognitive impairment, simplifying syntax and vocabulary will often make noticeable improvements. Not all response failures should be attributed to amnesia. For example, an anomic demented patient who says she "can't remember" when asked to describe her deceased husband may do better when asked, "What color were his eyes?"

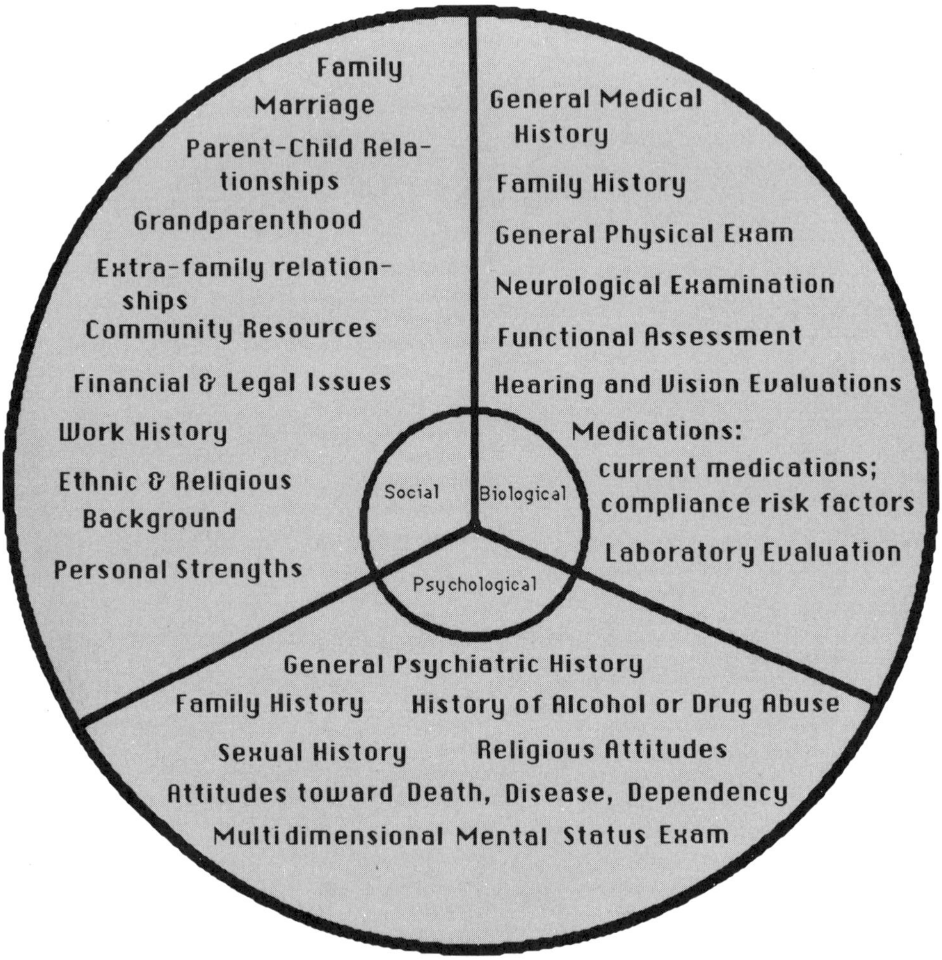
Family
Marriage
Parent-Child Relationships
Grandparenthood
Extra-family relationships
Community Resources
Financial & Legal Issues
Work History
Ethnic & Religious Background
Personal Strengths
General Medical History
Family History
General Physical Exam
Neurological Examination
Functional Assessment
Hearing and Vision Evaluations
Medications: current medications; compliance risk factors
Laboratory Evaluation
Social
Biological
Psychological
General Psychiatric History
Family History
History of Alcohol or Drug Abuse
Sexual History
Religious Attitudes
Attitudes toward Death, Disease, Dependency
Multidimensional Mental Status Exam

Figure 1. Overview of geropsychiatric comprehensive assessment.

Medical Evaluation. Figure 1 outlines the content of a comprehensive, multidisciplinary assessment. Certain basic information should be obtained about virtually all of these areas, although the time for doing so will depend on the patient's current status. Seeking history from family members or professionals is obviously important for cognitively impaired patients. In virtually every new case, a thorough medical evaluation is called for. The importance of hearing and vision assessment cannot be overemphasized, as impairments may contribute to the false impression that the patient has dementia or depression. Neurological evaluation requires a thorough history and neurological examination, whereas the indications for a brain imaging procedure, electroencephalograms, a lumbar puncture, and an erythrocyte sedimentation rate are considered for each new case.

The laboratory evaluation (Table 1) carried out in evaluating elderly patients for secondary causes of depression, dementia, anxiety, paranoia, personality change, and other syndromes is quite similar because there is considerable overlap in the differential diagnosis of these syndromes (Table 2).

Strengths Assessment. It is a liability of the medical model to attend only to patient's problems and pathology. Patients' strengths need also to be identified in the assessment process. Such strengths may be found in the past in terms of patients' accomplishments or memories, in the present in terms of their activities or personal relationships, or in the future in terms of their goals and potentials. Awareness of such strengths can be used directly in the treatment process to help affirm patients' awareness of themselves as competent individuals.

Cognitive Assessment. Cognitive capacity should be evaluated in every older patient. Although the history and the interview process often yield important clues, there is no substitute for carrying out a structured assessment of cognitive capacity. Otherwise, impairments are frequently overlooked (McCartney & Palmateer, 1985). Although the

Table 1. Suggested Initial Laboratory Evaluation for Frequently Encountered Psychiatric Syndromes in the Elderly

Complete blood count
Erythrocyte sedimentation rate
Liver function tests
Renal function, tests, including estimate of creatinine clearance
Serum electrolytes, including calcium and phosphorous
Serum glucose
Serum folate and vitamin B_{12} level
Syphilis screening test
Thyroid function tests
Electrocardiogram
X ray of chest
As indicated:
Heavy-metal and drug-screen procedures
Electroencephalogram
Lumbar puncture
Brain-imaging procedure

Mental Status Questionnaire and related instruments have substantial validity (Gurland, 1980), the Mini-mental State Examination and other instruments that rate multiple cognitive capacities have greater sensitivity (Klein, Roca, McArthur, Vogelsang, Klein, Kirby, & Folstein, 1985), even though they, too, may fail to detect mild cases of dementia, particularly in highly intelligent patients.

Cognitive assessment is used not simply to document the presence or course of impairments. It is also helpful in diagnosis, localization of dysfunction, and management of functional problems.

When there is uncertainty about the explanation for functional or emotional difficulties, cognitive assessment serves a *diagnostic* purpose. Neuropsychological test results are also an aid in differential diagnosis. For example, memory impairments of patients with AD, Korsakoff's syndrome, and Huntington's disease may be distinguished according to the differential effects of encoding instructions, proactive interference, and other test conditions (Moss, Albert, Butters, & Payne, 1986).

Table 2. Some Medical Conditions Frequently Associated with Depression, Dementia, and Other Psychiatric Syndromes in the Elderly

Cardiopulmonary
Hypoxia and/or hypercarbia (e.g., congestive heart failure, chronic obstructive pulmonary disease)
Endocrine
Hypo- and hyperthyroidism
Addison's disease and Cushing's syndrome
Diabetes mellitus
Hypo- and hyperparathyroidism
Hepatic or renal failure
Infection
Syphilis
Tuberculosis
Urinary tract infection
Malignancy
Primary or metastatic CNS tumor
Remote effects of carcinoma (e.g., bronchial, pancreatic carcinoma)
Medication side effects
Anticholinergic drugs
Antihypertensive drugs
Antineoplastic drugs
Psychotropic drugs
Neurological
Degenerative diseases (e.g., Alzheimer's disease, Parkinson's disease)
Cerebrovascular diseases
Trauma (e.g., subdural hematoma)
Hydrocephalic dementia
Vasculitis
Temporal arteritis
Systemic lupus erythematosus
Toxic states
Industrial agents and heavy metals
Vitamin deficiencies
Folate
Niacin
Thiamine
Vitamin B_{12}

Localization is a separate function of neuropsychological testing. For example, it has been proposed (Benson, 1983) that patterns of neuropsychological findings can be used to distinguish between dementias affecting primarily the cerebral cortex (e.g., AD) or subcortical structures (e.g., Parkinson's disease, Huntington's disease, progressive supranuclear palsy, and Wilson's disease).

The demonstration of problems with multiple-step commands, word finding, memory, left–right orientation, and so on, may make *functional* problems comprehensible to the family and, more important, may provide clues to how patients may be helped. For example, confused patients who find difficulty in following multiple-step commands may suddenly seem less confused if family members are shown that the ability to complete requests is much improved by the use of single-step commands.

Functional Assessment. The capacity to function competently is central to a number of important issues in geriatrics. Functional impairment has been found to be a significant correlate of depression in the elderly (Gurland, Wilder, Golden, Teresi, Gurland, & Copeland, 1988) and to have a systematic and specific diagnositc relationship to the stage of illness in AD (Reisberg, 1985). Although 14% of the elderly are considerably disabled, disability rises to over 20% in those over 75.

In view of these facts, ascertaining the areas of a person's current functioning that are intact or compromised is an important component of evaluation. Instruments used commonly for carrying out this assessment are the Activities of Daily Living (Katz, Ford, Moscowitz, Jackson, & Jaffe, 1963) and the Instrumental Activities of Daily Living (Lawton & Brody, 1969). Similar functional information is gathered by multidimensional evaluation instruments such as the Older Americans Resources and Services (OARS, Duke University, 1978) and the Comprehensive and Referral Evaluation (CARE, Gurland, Kuriansky, Sharpe, Simon, Stiller, & Birkett, 1977).

FREQUENT CLINICAL PROBLEMS

Differential Diagnosis

Differential diagnosis in the elderly entails many of the same principles that are applicable to general adult populations. The added difficulties result from the fact that elderly patients are more likely to present with multiple problems and that these problems are more likely to present in unusual ways. The following two sections deal with these issues in connection with depression and dementia, two of the most common problems in geropsychiatry. Both introduce a broad range of diagnostic possibilities and, at the same time, call for the integration of psychosocial and biomedical treatments. Paranoid disorders, which are also seen frequently in the elderly (Roth, 1962), are dealt with in a separate chapter.

Depression

The treatment of depression is one of the most important and fruitful in geropsychiatry. In community studies, elevated levels of depressive symptoms are found in at least 15% of those over 65, bearing out the general impression of the widespread problem of significant dysphoria in the elderly. On the other hand, community studies indicate that, at any one time, 1-3% of elderly will meet the diagnostic criteria for affective disorder (Blazer, Hughes, & George, 1987). Depression interacts with a variety of other problems faced by the elderly. The social withdrawal of depression may lead to an unnecessary burden on spouses or children. The presence of depression increases the morbidity associated with medical disease, and conversely, its treatment has a beneficial effect on the outcome of medical interventions. Depression, along with such associated factors as hypochondriasis, isolation, loneliness, and physical illness (Blazer, 1982), contributes to the fact that the elderly account for 25% of all suicides (Blazer & Williams, 1980; Gallagher & Thompson, 1982a; Gurland, 1976).

Diagnosis of Depression in the Elderly

In the absence of biological or other markers of diagnosis, the criteria for the diagnosis of major depression in the elderly are the same as those for other age groups. Therefore, the foundation of diagnosis continues to be serial diagnostic interviews, including information from reliable informants. Sleep electroencephalography has considerable utility in diagnosing major depression (Reynolds & Kupfer, 1987) and in evaluating patients with mixed symptoms of depression and dementia. However, at present, it remains primarily a research tool. A clear place for the dexamethasone suppression test in diagnosis remains to be demonstrated (Georgotas, Stokes, Krakowski, Fanelli, & Cooper, 1984). The diagnosis of depression in medically ill elderly people is particularly difficult and often relies on evaluating the psychological and vegetative features of depression after optimal medical treatment has been provided (Rodin & Voshart, 1986).

The field continues to grapple with the question: Do elderly patients with a diagnosis of depression present differently from younger patients? Investigations (Blazer, 1982) have provided support for the impression that sadness, guilt, and low self-esteem are less frequent among the elderly depressed than among their younger counterparts. In contrast, feelings of uselessness, pessimism, apathy, and somatic complaints are more common. The variance of these symptoms in elderly depressives makes it difficult to use such differences for individual cases, however. Better suited to individual cases may be a characterization based on the different types of clinical presentation that depression may have in the elderly.

Psychological Presentation. There are many elderly depressives who present little difficulty in diagnosis. Depressed mood, hopelessness, loss of interest, diminished self-esteem, anxiety, guilt, suicidal ideation or death wishes, and social withdrawal dominate the clinical picture, constituting what may be called a psychological presentation of depression. Loss of emotional reactivity and associated physiological changes—sleep disturbance, loss of appetite and libido, weight loss, and diurnal mood change—will be acknowledged.

Somatic Presentations. Although somatic complaints are a common element in such psychological presentations, there are some patients in whom they dominate the clinical picture. Such somatic presentations may be subdivided. Some patients present multiple symptoms deriving from multiple systems. In others, the complaints are referable to a single system (e.g., cardiac complaints). Differential diagnosis is particularly difficult when such symptoms occur in association with an identified medical problem of that system.

The management of such patients warrants close collaboration with an internist. Reliable medical information indicating that the patients' symptoms have persisted despite optimal assessment and treatment should be taken as supporting the possibility of an affective disorder. Specific inquiry regarding the psychological and physiological symptoms of depression often supports the diagnosis of affective disorder, although treatment for depression is frequently indicated nonetheless once appropriate medical treatment limits have been reached.

Physiological Presentations. Whereas the somatic presentations are defined by patients' symptoms, physiological presentations are a function of objective changes. These presentations are characterized by such problems as sleep disturbance, weight loss, diminished food intake, dehydration, mutism, or incontinence. In such cases, physicians properly give first consideration to the existence of medical disease. Dehydration and metabolic problems may have developed as complications of depression but may require emergency treatment. It is important that the possibility of an affective disorder be considered once the medical status is optimized. Even problems such as incontinence or mutism, which are generally considered features of neuromedical disorders, may be seen in patients with major depression. It is a matter of judgment how far to pursue medical diagnosis and treatment. It is critical, however, that the full assessment for depression be carried out and that a course of treatment for depression be considered.

Cognitive Presentations. Elderly patients complaining about problems with memory or other intellectual capacities may be expressing an awareness of actual cognitive problems or concern about the *possibility* of becoming intellectually impaired. A diagnosis of depression should be entertained in either case (Plotkin, Mintz, & Jorvik, 1985). However, to the extent that the complaints are subjective (i.e., unassociated with objective impairment), such problems suggest difficulty in adapting psychologically to aging and they may have a variety of personal meanings. For example, they may express our culture's self-deprecatory stereotypes of aging or the individual's fantasies about what it would mean to be impaired or dependent. Psychosocial interventions are strongly indicated in such cases, and the need for medications should be carefully considered.

When the cognitive complaints correspond to objective difficulties, there are three possibilities:

1. *Normal aging.* The patient is having difficulty adapting to the cognitive changes of normal aging. Formal neuropsychological testing will aid in the evaluation of such relatively mild impairments.

2. *Dementing illness.* The patient has a medical or neurological disease causing cognitive impairment and, associates with this, a depression that may represent either a psychological reaction to or a physiological consequence of this disease. Depending on the primary illness and the severity of the cognitive impairment, the diagnosis in such cases may be organic affective disorder, mixed organic brain syndrome, primary degenerative dementia with depression, or multi-infarct dementia with depression.

3. *Dementia syndrome of depression.* The patient has a major depression in which cognitive problems are prominent enough so that the patient appears to have dementia (i.e., a dementia syndrome of depression).

The term *pseudodementia* has been used, without adequate clarification, to refer to each of these possibilities, creating ambiguities in its clinical implications (Reifler, 1986). Systematic clinical evaluation indicates, contrary to the connotation of *pseudo,* that, among patients with subjective and/or objective cognitive difficulties, one can usually find characteristic psychological and physiological features of depression that can be used to make valid diagnoses (Rabins, Merchant, & Nestadt, 1984). In addition, when objective cognitive impairment is found, a diagnosis of major depression is suggested by a relatively abrupt and recent onset; a history of affective disorder; or cognitive performance failure attributable to poor effort. Scores on the Mini-Mental State Examination in the range of 18–25, which represent mild to moderate impairment, have been associated with improvement on antidepressant treatment (Folstein, Folstein, & McHugh, 1975).

Assessment and Treatment

Only a few points need to be added here to the general assessment principles presented earlier. First, it should be underscored that one must be vigilant in teasing out and developing integrated treatment plans for the many combinations of psychological, social, and medical problems presented by the depressed elderly. For some patients, a single modality of treatment may be indicated, be it psychotherapy, adaptive environmental interventions, medication, or another approach. Most, however, warrant a combination of treatments.

The second point is that errors of omission are probably the major source of error in the management of affective disorders in the elderly. Underdiagnosis may occur either because of an incorrect interpretation of the sometimes unusual presentations of depressive disorders or because the symptoms of depression may be ascribed mistakenly to normal aging or the effects of medical disease or medications.

Undertreatment may occur even when a diagnosis is appropriately made. When patients' subjective distress is ''understandable'' in terms of stress or loss, treatment may be inappropriately withheld. In extreme instances, the elderly may be seen as untreatable simply because they are ''too old.'' Alternatively, some patients receive subtherapeutic antidepressant medication trials because the practioner mistakenly applies to the individual case the general principle that the elderly, as a group, are more at risk for medication side effects.

Thus, when the alternative to treatment for depression is, simply, no treatment, the direction in which to err is almost always in favor of a treatment trial. This principle holds for each of the clinical presentations discussed above. It is important not to equate the presence of cognitive impairment *per se* with the diagnosis of a dementing disease and to look carefully for associated symptoms and history to make the diagnosis of major depression. When there is reasonable concern that a depressive disorder is responsible for or is contributing to dementia, unremitting physical symptoms, hypochondriasis, or personality change, a trial of psychosocial and medication treatment for depression should be carried out, once the secondary causes of such syndromes have been appropriately pursued.

With these principles in mind, the following guidelines are generally applicable to the management of patients with affective disorders. Patients being treated in an outpatient setting for acute depression are generally followed on a weekly basis. At each visit, one assesses:

- The progress of the depressive syndrome
- The personal and social aspects of the patient's functional status
- Psychological, social, and environmental complications
- Compliance with treatment recommendations
- Medical status: weight; blood pressure, including orthostatic change and symptoms; and fluid and nutritional status

- Suicide risk indicators
- Adverse drug effects
- Indications for changes in treatment

Psychotherapeutic interventions are integrated with these monitoring functions. As improvement occurs, the treatment and the frequency of visits are adjusted. Patients who have been suicidal are monitored more closely during the initial period of improvement. It is frequently suggested that geriatric depressions last longer and are less treatment-responsive, although this idea has been questioned (Small & Jarvik, 1982).

Indications for Antidepressant Medication. A trial of at least one antidepressant medication is indicated in major depression and in some cases of dysthymic disorder. More specifically, indications for a medication trial included persistence of the syndrome for at least 2 weeks in the absence of secondary causes of depression (e.g., alcohol use, which can be treated directly); the presence of endogenous features (distinctive dysphoria, diurnal mood change, sleep and appetite disturbance, weight loss, and lack of emotional reactivity); a previous history of improvement with medication; and unresponsiveness to psychosocial and environmental interventions.

Selection of Medications. In the older patient without complicating medical illness, desipramine and nortriptyline are often considered the drugs of choice (Salzman, 1984). Desipramine has the advantage of being the least anticholinergic of the first-generation tricycle antidepressants (TCAs). Nortriptyline has been found to cause relatively little orthostatic hypotension. Both are available in 10-mg tablets, permitting very low initial dosages. With both drugs, one can adjust the dose according to data on therapeutic serum drug concentrations, an important point vis-à-vis trazodone or other newer drugs whose side-effect profiles offer some advantages for some patients. For patients in whom sedation is preferred, nortriptyline has some advantage over desipramine.

Administration. Antidepressant drugs are given initially in small, divided doses in order to minimize side effects. Doses may be increased at intervals of 4–7 days, generally by increments of 30%–50%. Usually, a dose of 25–75 mg per day of these drugs is appropriate, although the range of therapeutic doses varies from 20 to 100 mg per day and, for desipramine, higher. For patients who do not show significant improvement after 3–6 weeks, serum drug levels should be considered. Once patients have responded, medication is maintained for 4–12 months, depending on the nature of the episode. For patients with recurrent depression, longer periods are considered.

Conditions Complicating the Use of Antidepressant Medications. A variety of medical conditions and clinical circumstances dictate the use of other drugs and approaches to treatment. Some of these are briefly discussed here.

1. *Vulnerability to anticholinergic agents.* Patients with narrow-angle glaucoma, dementia due to neurological disease, symptoms of prostate enlargement, or intolerance of other anticholinergic side effects may be offered antidepressants with minimum anticholinergic potency. Monoamine oxidase (MAO) inhibitors, such as phenelzine and trazodone, may be considered for this purpose if desipramine is not tolerated.

2. *Cardiac disease.* Antidepressant therapy is often feasible in patients with cardiovascular disease. The treatment of patients with cardiac disease should not be based only on electrocardiographic findings, but on a total assessment of cardiovascular and general medical status. This assessment is usually best accomplished in collaboration with

an internist or a cardiologist. In either case, the presence of conduction or rhythm abnormalities should not be regarded as an absolute contraindication to antidepressant medications.

Ventricular arrhythmias. From a cardiac standpoint, tricyclic antidepressants are Type I antiarrhythmics (Giardina, Bigger, Glassman, Perel, & Cantor, 1979; Stoudemure & Atkinson, 1988). Thus, the presence of ventricular premature contractions may be an indication, rather than a contraindication, for the use of tricyclics. Because they have antiarrhythmic and conduction effects similar to those of quinidine and procainamide, the use of the latter may have to be decreased or stopped when tricyclic antidepressants are given. Concern about TCA-induced arrhythmias is primarily a feature of acute overdosage and toxic serum levels (Giardina *et al.*, 1979). MAO inhibitors have not been reported to produce arrhythmias. Trazodone, on the other hand, sometimes produces ventricular arrhythmias, particularly in patients with cardiac disease (Pellettier & Bartolucci, 1984).

Conduction abnormalities. The tricyclic (Roose, Glassman, Giardina, Walsh, Woodring & Bigger, 1987), as well as other cyclic antidepressants (Stoudemire and Atkinson, 1988), are not strictly contraindicated in patients with uncomplicated first degree heart block, left bundle branch block, or right bundle branch block. If used in such situations, special precautions including hospitalization should be considered. MAO inhibitors have negligible effects on conduction at usual doses and, therefore, may be preferable. For patients with second degree heart block, AV junctional, bifasciular and trifasciular blocks, cyclic antidrepressants should probably not be used unless a pacemaker has been provided. For the management of these and other cardiac problems, consultation with a cardiologist should be considered.

3. *Cognitive impairment.* Physicians should not be discouraged from treating depression associated with cognitive impairment, whether the cognitive impairment is thought to be secondary to a dementing disease or to an affective disorder. On the other hand, it is advisable to assume that patients with dementing disease are more at risk of developing delirium or other behavioral disturbances as a result of psychoactive drugs. This concern dictates the following modifications in the treatment of depressive symptoms associated with dementing disease, such as primary degenerative dementia or multi-infarct dementia:

- Use drugs with smaller degrees of anticholinergic potency. Desipramine, trazodone, and MAO inhibitors each have advantages in individual circumstances, although nortriptyline is often effective.
- Initiate treatment with minimal doses.
- Make dose increases less frequently.
- Be sure that the drug regimens have been simplified and that drug-free observation has been tried as much as possible.
- Consider MAO inhibitors (Jenike, 1985) as well as ECT for persistent disturbances. Both have been reported to be effective in such patients.

4. *Failure to respond to initial treatment.* Several alternatives are possible if patients are not significantly improved after 3–5 weeks of therapeutic doses of medication. From a biomedical standpoint, these alternatives include further dose adjustment based on a knowledge of serum drug concentrations; the addition of tri-iodothyronine, lithium, or ritalin; a trial on an MAO inhibitor (MAOI) or other cyclic antidepressant; and a combination therapy of cyclic and MAOI antidepressant. Such alterations are made after reevaluating the patient for unrecognized causes of secondary depression, compliance problems, or

diagnostic errors. For patients who remain depressed after vigorous trials with psychotherapies and medication, consideration should be given to in-hospital care and electroconvulsive therapy.

Dementia

The pervasive impact of dementia makes it a paradigm for the application of the comprehensive assessment scheme presented earlier. The care of patients with dementia is rewarding, not only because it is gratifying to discover reversible illness in patients who fear they have an irreversible brain disease, but because of the enormous value that accrues to patients and their families when they find relief from some of the perplexity and helplessness that they confront with diseases that primarily affect the mind.

Differential Diagnosis

The diagnosis of dementia implies the presence of an acquired syndrome of cognitive impairment that is known or presumed, after appropriate testing, to be due to a specified organic cause. The content of such testing was described earlier. Although the differential diagnosis of dementia is extensive, systematic evaluation permits specific diagnosis in almost all cases (Seltzer & Sherwin, 1978). Therefore, the practice of using the general term *organic brain syndrome* as a diagnosis seems difficult to justify. Even in the instance of AD, which is treated by the DSM-III as a diagnosis of exclusion, positive clinical criteria are emerging for making the diagnosis. Thus, rating scales developed for characterizing the severity and the functional status of patients with AD (Reisberg, Ferris, de Leon, & Crook, 1982; Reisberg, Gordon, McCarthy, & Ferris, 1985) have been reported to be of use in discriminating normals and abnormals and in differential diagnosis. With the use of computerized tomography, 83% of a sample of AD victims and normal controls were correctly classified by focusing on the temporal lobe areas, where pathological changes are concentrated. This percentage contrasted to 65% correct when linear indices of sulcal and ventricular enlargement were used (LeMay, Stafford, Sandor, Albert, Haykal, & Zamani, 1986). Similarly, systematic neuropsychological testing indicates that distinctive patterns of memory impairment, language disturbances, apraxia, and visuospatial problems reliably differentiate AD patients from normals and from subjects with other dementias (Benson, 1983; Cummings & Benson, 1983; Moss, 1986). Candidates for biochemical markers of diagnosis continue to be actively pursued (Katzman, 1987).

Unfortunately, most patients with dementia have AD and/or multi-infarct dementia (Cummings & Benson, 1983). However, depending on the population studied, 5%–25% of cases have a medical illness, medication side effects, affective disorders, or other neurological diseases. Many of these conditions are reversible. For a geropsychiatric population, the decision tree in Figure 2 provides a useful approach to diagnosis. Because of the priority that is appropriately given to the psychiatric consequences of medical illness and drug side effects, assessment first asks if features of delirium are present. Recent onset, disturbed attention, short-term memory loss, visual hallucinations, and fluctuations in affect, wakefulness, or cognitive capacity are generally considered diagnostic features. If cognitive change is not occurring in the context of delirium, affective disorders are considered next. If cognitive impairment is present it may be related to normal aging, a dementia syndrome of depression, or a dementing illness in which depression occurs as a consequence of, or as a reaction to, the cognitive impairment.

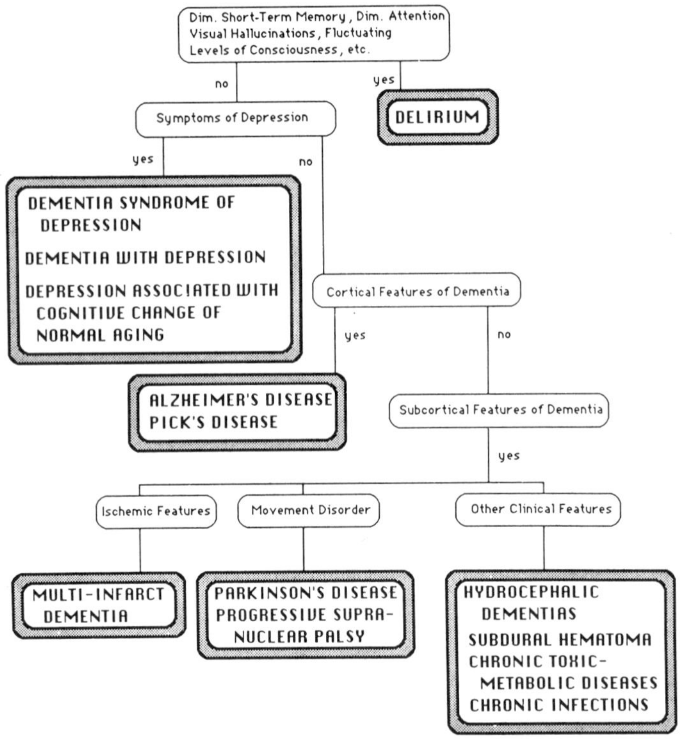

Figure 2. Decision tree for cognitive impairment.

The distinction between cortical and subcortical patterns of dementia, discussed earlier, provides a useful approach at this point. According to Benson (1983), patients with AD and Pick's disease tend to appear alert and to show normal rates of speech and movement, as well as normal posture, but have amnesia, visuospatial deficit, anomia and other language problems, and lack of awareness of their condition. Subcortical lesions, in contrast, tend to produce slowing of speech and movement, movement disorder, slurred speech, and cognitive changes marked by a distinctive type of forgetfulness and "dilapidated" cognition. The cortical-subcortical dichotomy is currently the object of discussion and must be applied with discretion. For example, the impairments produced by brain tumor, stroke, and other vascular disease (e.g., syphilitic or connective tissue vasculitides) produce different syndromes, depending on the brain regions affected. The nosological status of chronic metabolic encephalopathies (e.g., uremia) is uncertain, although it has been suggested that they show features of subcortical dementia (Benson, 1983; Cummings & Benson, 1983).

Treatment

At any stage of illness, interventions may be divided as follows:

Psychological and Behavioral Problems. In the early stages of the illness, when patients have subjective concerns about their cognitive abilities, management focuses on whether objective neuropsychological and functional problems are present. To the extent that a patient's concerns about cognitive impairment are disproportionate to the actual impairments, anxiety, affective, and adjustment disorders should be considered.

When objective impairments are mild, there is generally uncertainty regarding the diagnosis and the prognosis. Patients and families should be carefully evaluated for the understandable anxiety, depression, and helplessness evoked at this point. Vocational and other role changes may need to be considered for the afflicted individual. Plans for reevaluation should be made, as the progression of impairment is often an important diagnostic finding in such circumstances. Interventions focus on ensuring that there will be a full understanding of the current problems and that the ominous possibilities will not compromise current living unduly. It may be helpful at this early stage of the illness to point out that 80%–95% of the elderly showing such minimal objective changes remain unchanged on 4-year follow-up (Reisberg, Shulman, Ferris, de Leon, & Geibel, 1983).

If impairments progress, functional consequences are avoidable, and patients and families enter into the difficult period of having to make changes in their lives and in their plans for the future. This phase, which corresponds for AD patients to the confusional and the early and middle dementia phases of the illness (Reisberg *et al.*, 1982), is in many ways the most stressful because established adult roles and responsibilities are so dramatically changed. Denial, depression, demoralization, and apathy may develop (Reisberg *et al.*, 1985). Persistent or incapacitating depressive symptoms, if unresponsive to social and environmental interventions, may be treated with antidepressant medications. Ergoloid mesylates (hydergine) and methylphenidate may benefit demented patients, particularly those who show apathy, anergia, or mild depression.

Throughout the course of the illness, patients' activities should be structured to maximize the use of their retained capacities. Careful functional and neuropsychological assessment may be helpful in identifying such remaining strengths. For example, patients who value cultural activities may lose the ability to read, yet may be able to enjoy talking books or music. Encouraging activity and the structured use of all competencies becomes increasingly important as initiative and independence become compromised over the years.

Delusions, agitation, and wandering are associated with more severe cognitive impairment. Each may be disruptive to patients and caregivers. Effective interventions require similar combinations of environmental adaptations, social supports, and medications. Environmental adaptations are particularly important for wandering, which responds least well to medication. For example, minimizing the use of restraints or bed rails and maximizing the areas for unimpeded walking, such as a fenced-in yard, may be quite useful (Winograd & Jarvik, 1986). Neuroleptic medications may be used for each of these problems, although wandering is not likely to be helped by medication. Depending on the associated problems, low- and high-potency neuroleptic medications, used in divided doses, may be considered (e.g., thioridazine, 10–100 mg/day; haloperidol, 0.5–3 mg/day). Shorter acting benzodiazepines without active metabolites (e.g., lorazepam, 0.25–0.5 mg; oxazepam, 10–20 mg) are also used, although they may cause increased confusion, memory loss, gait instability, depression, and, paradoxically, agitation. When using such medications with demented patients, several precautions are necessary:

- Be sure that the new onset of such problems does not reflect superimposed medical problems or side effects of other medications.
- Reevaluate the use of such medications frequently (e.g., at 1- to 2- week intervals).

- Dose reduction or drug discontinuation is often possible; behavioral symptoms may be transient even though the disease is permanent.
- Side effects produced by psychotropic drugs are easily overlooked or attributed to the ''natural course'' of the disease. Therefore, vigilance is called for in evaluating new problems that develop while medication is being given.

Social problems. Family and other care providers play a critical and distinctive role in the care of elderly patient with dementia. Contrary to popular myth, it is the rule rather than the exception for the family to be actively involved in the care of the elderly patient (Morycz, 1985). Although they often petition professionals for help, families often do not regard themselves as being in the role of patients. Rather, because they deliver so much of the care to the identified patient, they frequently and appropriately see themselves as care providers. Therefore, helping caregivers balance the responsibilities of these roles is a guiding principle of family treatment.

The specific objectives of family interventions are dictated by a complex interplay between the characteristics of the patient, the family, and the wider social and physical environment of the patient (Morycz, 1985). For patients with minimal impairments, the process of providing families information regarding the rationale of assessment and the significance of diagnosis may suffice. Some caregivers turn to psychodynamic explanations of behavior, often attributing unmistakable signs of brain disease to enduring personality traits or conflicts in their relationship with the patient. Others displace blame to medications, physicians, or themselves. Some families, wanting to leave no stone unturned in their search for a cure, are eager to undertake experimental medication trials. At present, there is relatively little to offer them, although there are some hopeful signs on the horizon. Although the use of experimental drugs is obviously a potentially adaptive approach to their helplessness, it is important, given their low yield at present, that professionals balance their eagerness to support such trials against the potential benefits of helping caregivers confront the feelings of helplessness, fear, or anger that may motivate them to pursue such drug trials. Of the drugs that have been tested under double-blind conditions, only ergoloid mesylates (hydergine), given in doses of 0.5–2 mg/day, have been found with some consistency to provide significant, although modest (and temporary), benefits, possibly secondary to their ability to increase energy or motivation.

Ultimately, for families of patients with progressive dementia, the goal of treatment is to facilitate acceptance of their powerlessness to cause or halt the progression of the illness and, at the same time, to empower them to see the enormous value that their own efforts may have in coping with the disease. The grieving and psychosocial adjustment involved is an ongoing process. Gradually, the focus of therapy shifts to adaptive interventions, that is, to deliberate changes in the social and physical environment of the patient that will facilitate the optimal use of the retained capacities. Over the long haul, caregivers need to realize that providing themselves with a semblance of personal satisfaction will enhance their ability to care for the patient. Providing counsel to this end may help caregivers to overcome their resistances to accepting help, and bringing other family members into the caregiving process may be helpful. Caregivers disabled by physical impairments or depression should be referred for specific treatment.

As this process of maximizing support for the caregiver continues, the resources of the community become relevant. The appropriateness of day-care and respite-care programs, the feasibility of outings with and without the patient, and the desirability of in-home services from nurses, homemaker aids, meal delivery programs, and so on should all be considered. At the earliest appropriate time, patients and caregivers should be encouraged to undertake the weighty process of making decisions that anticipate the later stages of the illness when the patient may no longer be competent. Living wills and other advanced directives may be considered at this time (Jahnigen & Schrier, 1986).

Finally, professionals should not forget themselves in this long process. There is a psychological adaptation called for here. When our patients die, the years of providing professional care necessitate a mourning process for ourselves, as well. For family members and other caregivers, the efforts and burdens experienced for so many years may give way to their own special meanings in the months after the dementia victim's death. This is a phase of the illness about which we know very little. Family members may experience relief, guilt, or depression, among other reactions. The depth of these experiences was suggested by a patient's wife, whose husband had died a few months earlier of AD. Reflecting on her singleminded and singlehanded devotion to her husband's care over the 9-year course of his illness, she commented, "I feel so close to God."

MODIFICATION OF TREATMENT APPROACHES

Psychotherapy for the Elderly

Interest in psychotherapy with the elderly has developed in many directions in recent years. Case reports of fruitful psychoanalyses of older individuals have been presented (Kahana, 1978), and studies comparing the efficacy of different psychotherapeutic approaches have been undertaken (Gallagher & Thompson, 1982b; Steuer, Mintz, Hammen, Hill, Jarvik, McCarley, Motoike, & Rosen, 1984). On the other hand, we still lack the information to choose knowledgeably between different forms of therapy or to address the relative efficacy of psychotherapies and medications for selected problems (Gallagher & Thompson, 1982a).

Supportive and Exploratory Approaches

Although some older patients are candidates for exploratory or insight-oriented approaches, others present a variety of clinical and existential problems for which supportive approaches are preferred (Yesavage & Karasu, 1982). In choosing between these approaches, it is helpful to distinguish between objective and subjective stressors. To the extent that objective stressors and losses dominate the person's life, supportive approaches (i.e., approaches that reduce distress and optimize current functioning), usually dominate the clinical approach. Such stressors include illness, death, material or social loss, role change, loss of functional capacity, and cognitive impairment. To the extent that subjective or anticipated concerns dominate the clinical picture, exploratory or insight-oriented approaches are indicated. Such concerns may include anticipating the conclusion of one's professional career; dealing with stress in marriage or in relationships with children; and facing the prospect of death or disability due to an existing or imagined illness.

The optimal balance point between supportive and exploratory strategies may be modified according to the emotional status and the current stressors of the patient and according to the course of each case. The division between subjective and objective problems is sometimes artificial. Also, it represents only a general guideline. Such traits as intelligence, curiosity, education, and insight increase the extent to which characterological and developmental issues and, therefore, exploratory strategies may be incorporated into treatment. In most patients, a combination of such subjective and objective problems is found.

In most older psychotherapy patients, a number of technical modifications are generally applicable. To the extent that patients are socially isolated or are coping with irreversible, objective loss, it is often appropriate for them to perceive their therapists as real participants in their social support system. To this end, it is common to express a more personal interest in the patient and to share a degree of information about oneself. Touching patients to express such genuine concern or personal relatedness may often be appropriate with older patients. Similarly, the termination of the treatment is often a qualified termination. Therapists usually make explicit their willingness to be contacted again should a problem arise. It is not uncommon to combine psychotherapy with the administration of antidepressant medications.

Cultural stereotypes depict the elderly as self-centered, irritable, hypochondriacal, dependent, hopeless, or, simply, negative. These stereotypes undoubtedly contribute to the frequent impression that elderly patients are less ideal patients and have poorer prognoses than younger patients (Ford & Sbordone, 1980). Although these are inaccurate depictions of the elderly in general, such characteristics are found in some patients, so that it may be difficult for some therapists to build a therapeutic alliance. Thus, these characteristics may contribute to the impression that elderly patients cannot be engaged effectively in psychotherapy. Strategies for dealing with them are clearly called for. To this end, the following sections describe several approaches to psychotherapy with older patients.

Competency Motivation and the Functional Viewpoint

The capacity to function competently is a central theme in the care of elderly patients. Elderly patients usually see themselves as having functioned competently throughout their lives. They have a sense of competency about themselves—a capacity and a desire to see themselves as self-sufficient, responsible, and able to fulfill their roles as spouses, workers, parents, friends, or siblings. Most have lived their lives, fulfilled their social roles, and realized their personal goals with considerable success. To the extent that they have not done so, they have usually adjusted gradually to these disappointments.

This functional viewpoint, which may be seen as a derivative of competence motivation (White, 1959), has a variety of applications to treatment. The functional viewpoint is a valuable tool in alliance building with patients who do not view their problems in psychological terms or who seem mystified or incapacitated by their emotional state. For example, hypochondriacal patients often plead with therapists for medical intervention and seem quite resistant to dynamic interpretations of their emotional status. Often, however, they readily accept the interpretation that they are having emotional difficulty about being unable to function competently any longer. Similarly, patients who seem dependent, apathetic, or depleted (Cath, 1966) may seem like poor candidates for psychotherapeutic interaction. Their lack of initiative is often mistaken for evidence of negativism or lack of motivation. Actually, they are generally quite desirous of being able to function again but feel that their efforts are doomed by the enormity of the problems they face (e.g., death, disease, dependency, and disappointments of various sorts). Here, too, making explicit their motivation to function competently is often a critical step in helping them harness their unimpaired or remaining resources.

Adaptation to Aging: Loss and Opportunity

Psychotherapy with elderly patients may be past-, present-, or future-oriented, depending on the particular combinations of life experiences, the personal circumstances, and the personality of the patient. Elderly patients seen for psychotherapy are often concerned about adapting what they experience as relatively successful and satisfying lives to changing social and environmental circumstances. Of equal importance is their concern about adapting to the shifting combination of their strengths and their declining capacities. In each instance, patients are called on to adapt psychologically to the circumstances of their lives. Not being able to do so with a sense of well-being, satisfaction, acceptance, or integrity is a common concern among older patients. Recognizing that patients are trying to accomplish this adaptation often makes it possible to respond helpfully to their concerns:

Case example: A couple in their 60s entered therapy because of marital conflict. After initial psychotherapy yielded improvement in this regard, they continued to want to visit to talk about their gay manic-depressive son, who was having interpersonal and vocational difficulties. They would talk in detail about his problems, but since neither they nor the therapist could identify a purpose for or benefit from the sessions, the frequency of visits was reduced. At a later time, more frequent visits were resumed when the therapist framed the meetings as part of their ongoing need to accept the disappointment they felt because their son was manic-depressive and because of the helplessness they felt at being unable, now that he was an adult, to care for him as they once had.

The following variety of psychotherapeutic techniques may be viewed as contributing to this process of adaptation:

Cognitive and Behavioral Approaches

Older patients are responsive to behavioral and cognitive therapies (Gallagher & Thompson, 1982b). Gallagher and Thompson (1982b) found that brief (time-limited) behavioral, cognitive, and insight-oriented relational therapy all provided comparable improvement in depression over a 16-week period. However, relapse rates after 1 year were significantly higher for the patients treated with the insight-oriented approach. The advantages of cognitive and behavioral approaches may have been due to their inclusion of specific rationale and skills, a structured treatment approach and the patient's active participation. Cognitive approaches have also been used in the rehabilitation of patients with memory impairments (Yesavage & Karasu, 1982).

Therapy for Bereavement and Other Losses

With respect to treatment, therapy for the bereaved provides a model for other losses. Whether one is adapting to the loss of a spouse or a job, to the change in one's income, or a disappointment in a relationship with a child, the principles of therapy are fundamentally the same:

Identification of the Problem and Its Manifestations. At an early point in treatment, one attempts to indicate explicitly and empathically a recognition of the issues that motivate the desire for treatment. When there has been a discrete loss, such as a death or an amputation, there is little difficulty in identifying the cause of a patient's symptoms. In other instances, these may not be so clear, either because of marked denial or because the problem is an abstract one (e.g., the above couple's need to reconcile themselves to the fact that their son would not have the life they had envisioned for him).

Validating and Facilitating Emotional Response. A host of emotions—sadness, abandonment, rage, guilt, and humiliation, for example—may be aroused by loss. The normal mourning process is impeded when these emotions are the source of anxiety, shame, or embarrassment. In these instances, the therapist must facilitate the expression of these emotions. By doing so nonjudgmentally, one conveys that such feelings are expectable and normal, not reasons for further distress. Generally, the process of facilitating an emotional response entails supporting patients' spontaneous associations and, thereby, the affect connected with them. When this facilitation is not productive, one may prompt patients specifically to talk either about memories connected with the lost object (e.g., vacations together) or about the way in which the loss will affect their lives (e.g., having no one to help take care of the household or needing to accept help as a result of paralysis or memory difficulties). Techniques of reminiscence therapy, described below, may be used.

Emotional and Realistic Acknowledgment of Powerlessness. A critical point in the process of adapting to loss is to come to grips—emotionally and functionally—with the fact that a loss is irretrievable. When abreaction and reminiscence do not seem to contribute to improved emotional or social functioning, it may be helpful to address explicitly the patient's unwillingness to separate from the lost object. Sometimes, the maintenance of the attachment may be seen in terms of internalized representations (e.g., fantasies and memories). Sometimes, it is most evident in daily activities (e.g., a widower's retaining his wife's full wardrobe in their bedroom closet). These and other behaviors symbolize the patients' not having accepted their powerlessness to restore their old reality. Confronting their powerlessness facilitates an expression of the emotions that maintain the attachment. Although there is a point in the mourning process at which the eternal nature of attachments should be affirmed and valued, this point generally comes after such powerlessness has been acknowledged.

Adapting to the new reality. As the loss becomes a psychological reality, patients usually become motivated to make the adjustments in their daily roles, responsibilities, and activities that are necessary to establish optimal functioning. Not infrequently, however, the personal or social resources needed to do so are inaccessible. The loss of a spouse calls for the survivor to find ways to accomplish household tasks that may be unfamiliar or intimidating. Marshaling the resolve to use a prosthesis or to manage legal and financial responsibilities may call for finding and making use of unfamiliar resources in oneself or one's community. In all of these instances, patients may benefit from psychological support to assist them in overcoming their reluctance to make such changes. Simultaneously, clinicians have a responsibility to ensure that the needed skills and community resources can be readily identified and used.

Although life review techniques may be used in the therapy for loss, they have a more general application in facilitating adaptation to aging. Butler (1964) described the life review as a universal psychological process in which people undertake a reevaluation of their successes and disappointments in life. The life review is seen as occurring spontaneously and as operating both consciously and unconsciously. Through the life review, one diminishes the distress associated with personal disappointments, neurotic conflicts, and unattained goals in life. As a result, the balance between one's sense of accomplishment and one's sense of failure in life becomes more positive. The life review is, then, a sort of spontaneous psychotherapy. It is applied to formal treatment when patients' problems are construed in terms of a life review process that has been halted. It is, then, the therapists' role to reactivate it. This reactivation is accomplished by encouraging patients, and sometimes their families, to recall events, ideas, or feelings that have been important to them. Many devices may be used to facilitate this process (e.g., examining photographs or family artifacts; talking with old friends and family; making pilgrimages; or constructing family trees). In some patients, reminiscence may be directly recommended as a process to be engaged in self-consciously. In other patients, one recognizes through these patients' spontaneous thoughts or word choices that they are actively involved in a life review process and simply need help to move ahead with it. For example, some patients need to be encouraged when they cut off their own thoughts saying, "I know I shouldn't dwell in the past."

Self-Psychology and Normal Aging

A central issue in aging is the tension between the continuity and growth of the self, on the one hand, and the prospect of its gradual deterioration and dissolution, on the other. The theory of self-psychology, as developed by Kohut (1971), may be usefully applied to understanding this process, as Kohut's concept of the self provides a theoretical construct through which the stressors of late life may be seen to operate (Lazarus, 1980). Within the theory of self-psychology, stressors and loss threaten the lifelong view of oneself as competent and whole, that is, the cohesiveness of the self. The manifestations of the loss of cohesiveness or the fragmentation of the self, as described by Kohut, coincide strikingly with many of the signs and symptoms presented by elderly patients, for example, defensive self-centeredness; grandiosity; suspiciousness; an empty or anergic sense of depression; a tendency to belittle oneself or feel humiliated; and dependency on others for validation of the self through approval or assistance in basic needs. To the extent that such symptoms represent acute responses to stress, rather than features of adult personality or characterological problems, they should be interpreted as defenses against narcissistic threat or loss, rather than as evidence of narcissistic personality disorder. To illustrate, an elderly woman may be heard to say to an acquaintance as one of a series of woes, "It's hard to remember anything now. My memory used to be the best thing about me." Although her words may suggest self-centeredness as a personality feature, this formulation emphasizes the reactive or regressive nature of these narcissistic features.

Similar interpretations may be applied to transference and countertransference phenomena (Lazarus, 1980). In general, when therapists feel slighted, humiliated, exploited, or unappreciated by their elderly patients, these experiences may be constructively viewed as countertransference reactions evoked by their patients' own narcissistic concerns. By responding to idiosyncratic or problem behaviors as evidence of narcissistic injury, grandiosity and aloofness are less likely to be mistaken for hostility (Lazarus, 1980), dependency is less likely to be responded to as manipulation, and egocentrism is less likely to be responded to as ingratitude.

Clinicians are advised in such instances to resist confronting patients with the defensiveness of their statements, the weaknesses in their personalities, or the deficiencies in their current efforts or social functioning. Because it is precisely the perceptions of themselves in these ways that is proving difficult for them to adapt to, such confrontations tend to provoke either more rigid defenses or less effective functioning. On the other hand, by empathically addressing and supporting patients' sense of narcissistic vulnerability, it is often possible to help them gradually to experience their narcissistic resources as replenished. To this end, empathic understanding is the critical quality in the therapist's verbal and nonverbal communications, in keeping with the critical place given to empathic interpretation in the therapeutic approach to patients with narcissistic disorders (Kohut, 1971). Once such empathic understanding is established, additional supportive measures may be recommended, such as increased activity, initiative, and social interaction.

SUMMARY

There is little question that, even in our current state of knowledge, the major psychiatric disorders seen in the elderly are eminently responsive to treatment. A San Francisco study of outpatient intervention indicated that outpatient treatment could produce a significant reduction in the rate of institutionalization (Simon, Lowenthal, & Epstein, 1970). The information presented in this chapter should be understood within broader basic science, clinical, and sociopolitical perspectives, however. Knowledge about brain function, for example, is likely to produce important shifts in the options available to the seriously impaired elderly patient (e.g., diagnostic contributions from brain-imaging technology or the pharmacotherapeutic implications of neurotransmitter disturbances). Undoubtedly, such scientific knowledge will contribute substantially to clinical progress. At the same time, the potential benefit of our present or future ability to treat such problems will continue to be constrained by a host of financial and administrative problems, which are often, at their heart, matters of social attitude and value. A recent study of mental health care in a primary-medical-care setting (Goldstrum, Burns, Kessler, Feuerberg, Larson, Miller, & Crober, 1987) confirmed the previous findings that elderly patients with mental disorders are significantly less likely to be seen by mental health professionals than younger adults. Cohort-specific characteristics may ameliorate some of these differences, for example, if the elderly of the year 2030 feel less stigmatized by psychiatric problems than their grandparents do today. However, innovations in the delivery and the organization of services (Cohen, 1980; Gurland, Bennett, & Wilder, 1981) and a rational apportionment of financial resources to meet human needs are likely to prove of the greatest importance.

REFERENCES

Atchley, R. C. (1983). *Aging: Continuity and change*. Belmont, CA: Wadsworth.

Benson, D. F. (1983). Subcortical dementia: A clinical approach. In R. Mayeux & W. G. Rosen (Eds.), *The dementias* (pp. 185–194). New York: Raven Press.

Blazer, D. G. (1982). *Depression in late life.* St. Louis: C. V. Mosby.

Blazer, D. G., & Williams, C. D. (1980). Epidemiology of dysphoria and depression in an elderly population. *American Journal of Psychiatry, 137,* 439–444.

Blazer, D., Hughes, D. C., & George, L. K. (1987). The epidemiology of depression in an elderly community population. *The Gerontologist, 27,* 281–287.

Blessed, G., Tomlinson, B. E., & Roth, M. (1968). The association between quantitative measures of dementia and of senile change in the cerebral grey matter of elderly subjects. *British Journal of Psychiatry, 114,* 797–811.

Brody, E. M. (1977). *Long-term care of older people: A practical guide.* New York: Human Sciences Press.

Butler, R. N. (1964). The life review: An interpretation of reminiscence in the aged. In R. Kastenbaum (Ed.), *New thoughts on old age.* (pp. 269–280). New York: Springer.

Butler, R. N., & Lewis, M. I. (1982). *Aging and mental health.* St. Louis: C. V. Mosby.

Cath, S. (1966). Beyond depression—The depleted state: A study in ego psychology in the aged. *Canadian Psychiatric Association Journal Special Supplement, 11,* 239.

Cohen, G. D. (1980). Prospects for mental health and aging. In J. E. Birren & R. B. Sloane (Eds.), *Handbook of mental health and aging* (pp. 971–993). Englewood Cliffs, NJ: Prentice-Hall.

Cummings, J. L., & Benson, D. F. (1983). *Dementia, a clinical approach.* Stoneham, MA: Butterworth.

Duke University Center for the Study of Aging and Human Development. (1978). *Multidimensional Functional Assessment: The OARS Methodology.* Durham, NC: Duke University.

Engel, G. L. (1977). The need for a new medical model: A challenge for biomedicine. *Science, 196,* 129–136.

Erikson, E. H. (1982). *The life cycle completed.* New York: W. W. Norton.

Erikson, J. M. (1983). *Images of aging: Music and musing.* Presidential Symposium for the Arts and Humanities Annual Meeting of the Gerontological Society of America, November 19.

Folstein, M. F., Folstein, S. E., & McHugh, P. R. (1975). Mini-Mental State: A practical method for grading the cognitive state of patients for the clinician. *Journal of Psychiatric Research, 12,* 189–198.

Ford, C. V., & Sbordone, R. J. (1980). Attitudes of psychiatrists toward elderly patients. *American Journal of Psychiatry, 137,* 571–575.

Gallagher, D., & Thompson, L. W. (1982a). Depression. In P. M. Lewinsohn & L. Teri (Eds.), *Clinical geropsychology* (pp. 7–37). New York: Pergamon Press.

Gallagher, D. E., & Thompson, L. W. (1982b). Treatment of major depressive disorder in older adult outpatients with brief psychotherapies. *Psychotherapy: Theory, Research and Practice, 19,* 482–490.

Galenberg, A. (1985). Trazodone-induced conduction delay. *Biological Therapies in Psychiatry, 8,* 7.

Georgotas, A., Stokes, P. E., Krakowski, M., Fanelli, C., & Cooper, T. (1984). Hypothalamic-pituitary-adrenocortical function in geriatric depression: Diagnostic and treatment implications. *Biological Psychiatry, 19,* 685–693.

Giardina, E. G. V., Bigger, J. T., Glassman, A. H., Perel, J. M., & Kantnor, S. L. (1979). The electrocardiographic and antiarrhythmic effects of imipramine hydrochloride at therapeutic plasma concentrations. *Circulation, 60,* 1045–1052.

Goldstrom, I. D., Burns, B. J., Kessler, L. G., Feuerberg, M. A., Larson, D. B., Miller, N. E., & Cromer, W. J. (1987). Mental health services use by elderly adults in a primary care setting. *Journal of Gerontology, 42,* 147–153.

Gurland, B. J. (1976). The comparative frequency of depression in various adult age groups. *Journal of Gerontology, 31,* 283–292.

Gurland, B. J. (1980). The assessment of the mental health status of older adults. In J. E. Birren & R. B. Sloane (Eds.), *Handbook of mental health and aging* (pp. 671–700). Englewood Cliffs, NJ: Prentice-Hall.

Gurland, B., Kuriansky, J., Sharpe, L., Simon, R., Stiller, P., & Birkett, P. (1977). The comprehensive assessment and referral evaluation (CARE)—rationale, development and reliability. *International Journal of Aging and Human Development, 8,* 9–42.

Gurland, B., Bennett, R., & Wilder, D. (1981). Reevaluating the place of evaluation in planning for alternatives to institutional care for the elderly. *Journal of Social Issues, 37,* 51–70.

Gurland, B. J., Wilder, D. E., Golden, R., Teresi, J. A., Gurland, R., & Copeland, J. R. M. (1988). The relationship between depression and disability in the elderly: Data from the Comprehensive Assessment and Referral Evaluation (CARE). In J. P. Wattis & I. Hindmarsh (Eds.)., *Psychological assessment of the elderly.* London: Churchill Livingston.

Jahnigen, D. W., & Schrier, R. W. (Eds.). (1986). *Clinics in geriatric medicine, ethical issues in the care of the elderly.* Philadelphia: W. B. Saunders.

Jenike, M. A. (1985). Monoamine oxidase inhibitors as treatment for depressed patients with primary degenerative dementia (Alzheimer's disease). *American Journal of Psychiatry, 142,* 763–764.

Jung, C. G. (1923). *Psychological types*. London: Routledge & Kegan Paul.

Kahana, R. J. (1978). Discussion of psychoanalysis in later life. *Journal of Geriatric Psychiatry, 11,* 37.

Katz, S., Ford, A. B., Moskowitz, R. W., Jackson, B. A., & Jaffe, M. W. (1963). Studies of illness in the aged. The index of ADL: A standardized measure of biological and psychosocial function. *Journal of the American Medical Association, 185,* 914–919.

Katzman, R. (1987). Alzheimer's disease: Advances and opportunities. *Journal of the American Geriatrics Society, 35,* 69–73.

Klein, L. E., Roca, R. P., McArthur, J., Vogelsang, G., Klein, G. B., Kirby, S. M., & Folstein, M. (1985). Diagnosing dementia: Univariate and multivariate analyses of the mental status examination. *Journal of The American Geriatrics Society, 33,* 483–488.

Kohut, H. (1971). *The analysis of the self.* New York: International Universities Press.

Lakatta, E. G. (1985). Heart and circulation. In C. E. Finch & E. L. Schneider (Eds.), *Handbook of the biology of aging* (2nd Ed.) (pp. 377–413). New York: Van Nostrand Reinhold.

Lawton, M. P., & Brody, E. M. (1969). Assessment of older people: Self-maintaining and instrumental activities of daily living. *Gerontologist, 9,* 179–186.

Lazarus, L. W. (1980). Self psychology and psychotherapy with the elderly: Theory and practice. *Journal of Geriatric Psychiatary, 13,* 69–88.

LeMay, M., Stafford, J. L., Sandor, T., Albert, M., Haykal, H., & Zamani, A. (1986). Statistical assessment of perceptual CT scan ratings in patients with Alzheimer type dementia. *Journal of Computer Assisted Tomography, 10,* 802–809.

McCartney, J. R., & Palmateer, L. M. (1985). Assessment of cognitive deficit in geriatric patients: A study of physician behavior. *Journal of The American Geriatrics Society, 33,* 467–471.

McCrae, R. R., & Costa, P. T. (1984). *Emerging lives, enduring dispositions.* Boston: Little, Brown.

Morycz, R. K. (1985). Caregiving strain and the desire to intitutionalize family members with Alzheimer's Disease. *Research on Aging, 7,* 329–361.

Moss, M. B., Albert, M. S., Butters, N., & Payne, M. (1986). Differential patterns of memory loss among patients with Alzheimer's disease, Huntington's disease, and alcoholic Korsakoff's syndrome. *Archives of Neurology, 43,* 239–246.

Neugarten, B. L. (Ed.). (1968). *Middle age and aging.* Chicago: University of Chicago Press.

Newton, N. A., Lazarus, L. W., & Weinberg, J. (1984). Aging: Biopsychosocial perspectives. In D. Offer & M. Sabshin (Eds.), *Normality and the lifecycle* (pp. 230–285). New York: Basic Books.

Pellettier, J. R., & Bartolucci, G. (1984). Trazodone and cardiovascular side effects (letters to ed). *Journal of Clinical Psychopharmacology, 4,* 119.

Plotkin, D. A., Mintz, J., & Jarvik, L. (1985). Subjective memory complaints in geriatric depression. *American Journal of Psychiatry, 142,* 1103–1105.

Popkin, S. J., Gallagher, D., Thompson, L. W., & Moore, M. (1982). Memory complaint and performance in normal and depressed older adults. *Experimental Aging Research, 8,* 141–145.

Rabins, P. V., Merchant, A., & Nestadt, G. (1984). Criteria for diagnosing reversible dementia caused by depression: Validation by 2-year follow-up. *British Journal of Psychiatry, 144,* 488–492.

Reifler, B. V. (1986). Mixed cognitive-affective disturbances in the elderly: A new classification. *Journal of Clinical Psychiatry, 47,* 354–356.

Reisberg, B. (1985). Alzheimer's disease update. *Psychiatric Annals, 15,* 319–322.

Reisberg, B., Ferris, S. H., de Leon, M. J., & Crook, T. (1982). The global deterioration scale for assessment of primary degenerative dementia. *American Journal of Psychiatry, 139,* 1136–1139.

Reisberg, B., Shulman, E., Ferris, S. H., de Leon, M. J., & Geibel, V. (1983). Clinical assessments of age-associated cognitive decline and primary degenerative dementia: Prognostic concomitants. *Psychopharmacology Bulletin, 19,* 734–739.

Reisberg, B., Gordon, B., McCarthy, M., & Ferris, S. H. (1985). Clinical symptoms accompanying progressive cognitive decline and Alzheimer's disease. In V. L. Melnick & N. N. Dubler (Eds.), *Alzheimer's dementia: Dilemmas in clinical research* (pp. 19–39). Clifton, NJ: Humana.

Reynolds, C. F., & Kupfer, D. J. (1987). Neuropsychiatric aspects of sleep disorders. In R. E. Hales & S. C. Yudofsky (Eds.), *Textbook of neuropsychiatry* (pp. 241–256). Washington, DC: American Psychiatric Press.

Robinson, R. A. (1972). The evolution of geriatric psychiatry. *The Scottish Society of the History of Medicine, 16,* 184–193.

Rodin, G., & Voshart, K. (1986). Depression in the medically ill: An overview. *American Journal of Psychiatry, 143,* 696–705.

Roose, S. P., Glassman, A. H., Giardina, E. G. V., Walsh, T. B., Woodring, S., & Bigger, T. (1987). Tricyclic antidepressants in depressed patients with cardiac conduction disease. *Archives of General Psychiatry, 44,* 273–275.

Roth, M. (1955). The natural history of mental disorder in old age. *Journal of Mental Science, 101,* 281–301.

Roth, M., & Kay, D. W. K. (1962). Psychoses among the aged. In H. T. Blumenthal (Ed.), *Medical and clinical aspects of aging* (pp. 74–96). New York: Columbia University Press.

Rowe, J. W., & Minaker, K. L. (1985). Geriatric medicine. In C. E. Finch & E. L. Schneider (Eds.), *Handbook of the biology of aging* (2nd ed.) (pp. 932–959). New York: Van Nostrand Reinhold.

Salzman, C. (1984). *Clinical geriatric psycho-pharmacology.* New York: McGraw-Hill.

Schulz, R. (1985). Emotion and affect. In J. E. Birren & K. W. Schaie (Eds.), *Handbook of the psychology of aging* (pp. 531–543). New York: Van Nostrand Reinhold.

Seltzer, B., & Sherwin, I. (1978). "Organic brain syndromes": An empirical study and critical review. *American Journal of Psychiatry, 135,* 13–21.

Simon, A., Lowenthal, M. G., & Epstein, L. J. (1970). *Crisis and intervention: The fate of the elderly mental patient.* San Francisco: Jossey-Bass.

Small, G. W., & Jarvik, L. F. (1982). Depression in the aged. *Psychiatric Clinics of North America, 5,* 45–48.

Steuer, J. L., Mintz, J., Hammen, C. L., Hill, M. A., Jarvik, L. F. McCarley, T., Motoike, P., & Rosen, R. (1984). Cognitive-behavioral and psychodynamic group psychotherapy in treatment of geriatric depression. *Journal of Consulting and Clinical Psychology, 52,* 180–189.

Stoudemire, A., & Atkinson, P. (1988). Use of cyclic antidepressants in patients with cardiac conduction disturbances. *General and Hospital Psychiatry, 10,* 389–397.

U.S. Department of Health and Human Services. (1985–1986). Aging America: Trends and projections.

White, R. W (1959). Motivation reconsidered: The concept of competence. *Psychological Review, 66,* 297–333.

Winograd, C. H., & Jarvik, L. F. (1986). Physician management of the demented patient. *Journal of the American Geriatrics Society, 34,* 295–208.

Yesavage, J. A., & Karasu, T. B. (1982). Psychotherapy with elderly patients.*American Journal of Psychotherapy, 36,* 41–55.

Zisook, S., & Shuchter, S. R. (1985). Time course of spousal bereavement. *General Hospital Psychiatry, 7,* 95–100.

23

The Vietnam Veteran

BENJAMIN BURSTEN

INTRODUCTION

Vietnam veterans must be distinguished from Vietnam era veterans. Vietnam era veterans are those who served in the armed forces of the United States during the period of the Vietnam conflict. Although this group includes those who served in Vietnam itself, it also includes those who never left the United States or who served in other geographical areas. Like any unselected group of veterans from any era, this group can suffer a wide variety of psychiatric illnesses, from the anxieties and somatoform disorders to the personality disorders to the mood and thought disorders. Hearst, Newman, and Helley (1986) reported that having served in the armed forces during the Vietnam era increases the likelihood of suicide by 65% and the likelihood of dying in a motor vehicle accident by 49%.

Vietnam veterans comprise a more restricted group within the class of Vietnam era veterans. These are people who saw service in Vietnam itself. They were all in a combat area. In Vietnam, there were no noncombat areas (Van Devanter, 1985). This was a guerrilla conflict that could erupt anywhere at any time.

Vietnam veterans are not immune from anxieties, somatoform disorders, personality disorders, mood and thought disorders, and so on. In that respect, they may not be much different from other Vietnam era veterans. However, the diagnostic condition that concerns us in this chapter is posttraumatic stress disorder (PTSD); this condition sets Vietnam veterans as a group aside from other Vietnam era veterans (Figley, 1978b; Kadushin, Boulanger, & Martin, 1981). Although the study of suicides and motor vehicle accidents cited above did not distinguish between Vietnam veterans and Vietnam era veterans, the

BENJAMIN BURSTEN • 103 Garnet Lane, Oak Ridge, Tennessee 37830.

relationship of postservice stress symptoms to exposure to combat (Figley, 1978b; Foy, Sippreele, Rueger, & Carroll, 1984; Kadushin *et al.*, 1981) and the nature of PTSD as described below make it highly likely that Vietnam veterans comprised a large proportion of the cases reported.

JUSTIFICATION FOR THE GROUP

Is the Vietnam veteran any different from veterans of other combat situations? PTSD—whether called *war neurosis, combat fatigue,* or *shell shock*—has been documented following other wars, and many of the characteristics have been similar (Archibald & Tuddenham, 1965; Futterman, & Pumpian-Mindlin, 1951). Nonetheless, there were some differences between this conflict and others in which our country engaged (Figley, 1978a; Shatan, 1978). The Vietnamese were portrayed as nonhuman, and atrocities were committed under tacit sanction in situations where the line between Vietnamese friend and foe was often impossible to draw. Soldiers arrived and left individually, rather than in cohesive groups. Many found the conflict absurd because the goals were more poorly defined than those of other conflicts and the support of the citizens at home was ambiguous at best. Massive use of drugs and alcohol relieved the tension of trying to survive a guerrilla war until one's tour of duty was up. Homecoming was seldom heroic because the conflict was so unpopular. Often, the veteran was treated with contempt, called a baby-killer, and sometimes even spat on by war protesters. Flemming (1985), while de-emphasizing the uniqueness of the Vietnam conflict, stressed some unusual sociological features of the era: the adolescent soldier was brought up in a period of high expectations, and when he or she returned from the war, our society was in disarray and the system had little to offer. The veteran, having had the normal period for identity consolidation interrupted by Vietnam (Laufer, 1985), returned to an unstable society.

It is not clear that these conditions produced a different type of PTSD from that which has followed other military activities. It does seem likely that these conditions produced a greater incidence of PTSD, and as we shall see below, these conditions found their way into the unique content of the problems expressed by Vietnam veterans.

Why should the Vietnam veteran merit a chapter in this book? If I am talking about PTSD (which I am), why should I not write a chapter about the disorder—the diagnostic category—rather than about a particular group of people who have the disorder? Partly, the answer lies in the fact that there are some differences between Vietnam veterans PTSD and other PTSDs, as I shall discuss in the next section. Partly, the answer lies in the fact that there are powerful forces in both the veteran and the diagnostician that, in contrast to other PTSDs, make it all too easy to overlook the diagnosis. These forces, too, will be discussed in the next section.

Perhaps the strongest reason to devote a chapter to the group of people with this diagnosis is to heighten the diagnostician's index of suspicion. Kolb (1986) advised that all men and women aged 35–45 should be asked about military service in Vietnam. One can draw an analogy with people suffering the effects of industrial toxins. Place of employment is not a diagnosis; however, without a work history, the diagnostician is likely to overlook the diagnosis. The Vietnam veteran is at risk; adequate history-taking will help rule PTSD in or out.

PTSD was formally recognized as a psychiatric disorder by the American Psychiatric Association in 1980, in the third edition of its *Diagnostic and Statistical Manual* (DSM-III). There are four sets of criteria for the disorder:

1. There must be a recognizable stressor of significant magnitude. It is of interest to note that PTSD is one of the few DSM-III disorders that are dependent not solely on the phenomenology of the signs and symptoms, but also on the etiology: the stressor (Green, Lindy, & Grace, 1985).

2. The stressful situation (trauma) must be reexperienced. This reexperiencing may occur through dreams (often nightmares), daytime intrusive recollections of the trauma, or sudden feeling that the trauma is actually recurring.

3. There is numbing or diminished involvement with the external world. There may be a withdrawal of interest from one or from many activities. There may be a feeling of detachment or alienation from others. There may be a blunting or constriction of affect.

4. There must be at least two or a set of assorted other symptoms: hyperalertness and startle, sleep disturbance, guilt about surviving or about activities that were necessary for survival, memory or concentration difficulty, avoidance of situations that are reminiscent of the trauma, and intensification of symptoms when reminded of the trauma by events that have a real or symbolic similarity to the trauma.

Listed as associated features are depression, anxiety, increased irritability and aggressive behavior, impulsive trips or changes in lifestyle and residence, emotional and autonomic lability, headache, and vertigo.

The symptoms of PTSD may appear immediately following the traumatic event or may have an onset that is delayed for months or even years. These characteristics are indeed found in Vietnam veterans with PTSD. Factor-analytic studies of 405 Vietnam veterans seeking counseling gave "substantial empirical support . . . for the symptoms that comprise DSM-III's description of Post Traumatic Stress Disorder" (Silver & Iacono, 1984). Wilson and Krauss (1985) reported similar findings.

The severe stressors, of course, encompass the events of combat. They include loss of buddies; immersion in death and destruction (DeFazio, 1978); witnessing dismemberment and mutilation; constant uncertainty about when or where the next attack would come, where the next booby trap would be, or which Vietnamese were friends and which were enemies; and participation in guilt-provoking atrocities against soldiers and civilians—even against children. The fact that the tour of duty was circumscribed (12–13 months), and that the membership of the fighting group changed frequently because of death or staggered rotation schedules, led to a "a survival mentality" (Wilson & Krauss, 1985), rather than an allegiance to a cause. The mounting stress of combat in Vietnam was interspersed with frequent periods of relative safety—often a time for immersion in drugs and alcohol. Horowitz and Solomon (1978) suggested that this peculiar pattern of stressor and relief alternation promoted the defenses of denial and numbing.

It seems reasonable to include the conditions of homecoming as part of the stressor. It is well established that one of the factors inducing PTSD is the attempt to make sense of the trauma (Gleser, Green, & Winget, 1981; Lifton, 1967). Generally, in wartime, a sense of heroism and patriotism and a clear idea of the purpose of the conflict give a framework of meaning to the hardships. Such factors were often lacking, not only during the veterans' stay in Vietnam, but also in the sometimes hostile receptions they received once back in the United States.

The stressor in Vietnam PTSD is not always readily recognizable. Often, the PTSD is of the delayed variety, first making its appearance months or even years after return from overseas (Horowitz & Solomon, 1978; Shatan, 1978). Actually, it is difficult to ascertain just when the symptoms begin. In the first place, for a variety of reasons to be discussed below, the veteran may not talk about his or her symptoms, and there are many obstacles standing in the way of accurate diagnosis. In the second place, if the initial symptoms are numbing and withdrawal, even the veteran may not clearly recognize that anything is wrong. For example, on close questioning, the diagnostician may discover that there has been a change in the veteran's lifestyle that may not be attributed to Vietnam (Scurfield, 1985). We do know that there may be a considerable delay between the stressor and the perception on the part of the veteran or others that help is needed; however, the condition may have been present much earlier. For these reasons, the category of delayed PTSD will probably be omitted in the next revision of the nomenclature (Boulanger, 1985).

Although the role of the trauma is well established as a precipitant of the PTSD seen in Vietnam veterans, the veteran's previous history and personality are also relevant. They affected the way he or she was able to cope with the experiences in Vietnam (Figley, 1978b; Worthington, 1978) and colored the meaning the individual gave to the trauma (Hendin, Haas, Singer, Gold, & Trigos, 1983). Further, certain personality attributes, such as antisocial, paranoid, and narcissistic traits, were frequently aggravated and enhanced by the Vietnam experience (Wilson & Krauss, 1985). Perhaps the best way to conceptualize this interplay of personality and stressor is to look at the conceptualization in tort law. It is commonly accepted in law that "you take the plaintiff as you find him or her." If you hit an individual who happens to have very brittle bones that fracture easily, you are still liable, even if a more healthy person would have tolerated the blow better. The law says that "but for" the blow, he or she would not be in this crippled position. Whatever might have befallen the person with the vulnerable personality without the stressor of Vietnam, "but for" Vietnam it would not have happened at this time in this way. Further, no study has claimed that all Vietnam veterans who suffer PTSD were unusually vulnerable because of their past history or personality, and there is some statistical evidence showing that previous personality, although related, is not the dominant factor in PTSD (Foy *et al.*, 1984; Wilson & Krauss, 1985). From a diagnostic point of view, the preexistence of a severe personality disorder does not rule out PTSD.

Reexperiencing may take several forms. There may be intrusive thoughts and unwelcome memories. Illusions, such as loud noises momentarily misperceived as mortar fire, occur frequently (Mellman & Davis, 1985). Nightmares are common. Occasionally, there are dissociative states with amnesia afterwards.

Perhaps the type of reexperience receiving the most publicity is the flashback. In the flashback, the veteran briefly imagines himself or herself to be back in the combat situation. The frank brief hallucinations of parts of the combat experience may lead to the incorrect diagnosis of schizophrenia. Hallucinations may be visual, auditory, tactile and pain, or even olfactory with the smell of the jungle or of recent death. The intensity of the flashback is so great that the individual is unaware of where he or she really is and behaves in a manner appropriate to the combat situation (Panzarella, Mantell, & Bridenbaugh, 1978). During the flashback, the veteran frequently exhibits dyspnea, palpitations, diaphoresis, and all the other autonomic signs and symptoms that characterize panic attacks (Mellman & Davis, 1985).

Flashbacks may be triggered by sights, sounds, and even smells that are reminiscent of the combat situation either directly or symbolically. They may also be triggered by a state of arousal heightened by other factors, such as interpersonal stress or drug use or withdrawal before the flashback. In addition, I have encountered flashback situations that seemed to have a cognitive or affective prodrome. In one case, the veteran was a man who had gone camping frequently without flashback. Generally, he wore contemporary leisure clothes. However, on one occasion, ''for some reason,'' he dug out an old uniform that he had not worn for years. During this camping trip, he had a brief flashback in which the woods became the jungle in the combat situation. This prodromal period, which was without misperception or arousal, probably represented the beginnings of the reexperience, which had not yet reached consciousness. Indeed, as Blank (1985b) pointed out, one can even have unconscious flashbacks—in which the behavior subtly indicates the reexperiencing, although the veteran is not aware of the flashback. I have also seen a situation in which the flashback seemed to wax and wane, with alternating periods of flashback and reality orientation. Awareness of these possibilities is important diagnostically; we should not discount the authenticity of a flashback report merely because the veteran appears to have made some ''preparation'' beforehand or knows where he or she is intermittently.

Although public attention has been captured by the aggressive behavior some veterans have exhibited during the flashback, these actions appear to be in the minority. Aggressive posturing (without action) or defensive actions (cringing, hiding, and flight) are frequently observed.

Psychic numbing, with its withdrawal of interest, its feelings of detachment, and its constriction of affect, may alternate with reexperiencing or may predominate. The veteran is not only emotionally dull but often actively resistant to intimate relationships or participation in activities that formerly gave him or her pleasure. The numbing of emphatic responses fosters alienation and detachment from others (Shatan, 1973). Not infrequently, this numbing is promoted by self-medication with alcohol and drugs, although numbing exists in the absence of these substances and cannot be considered an exogenous chemical effect. Many of the activities (or inactivities) of numbing have led to the misdiagnosis of personality disorder. Only careful questioning about the other symptoms of PTSD (particularly the stressor and reexperiencing) can clarify the diagnosis.

Horowitz (1976) provided a useful conceptualization of the relationship between reexperiencing and numbing. Reexperiencing appears to be an attempt to assimilate the trauma into the individual's predominant way of understanding things. The numbing is a defensive attempt to avoid this intrusive and disturbing reexperiencing. The ''Fuck it, it don't mean nothin' '' attitude developed as a way of dealing with the intensity of the experience while in Vietnam is carried over into civilian life. It is sometimes felt as a malaise or a feeling that ''something'' is wrong with the veteran's life. She or he tends to blame others for this unease (Egendorf, Farley, & Remez, 1981).

The remaining symptoms have been reported in numerous studies of the Vietnam veteran with PTSD. Hyperalertness tends to merge with the illusions of reexperiencing. The startle response to unexpected noises or even unexpected touching gives evidence of the veteran's readiness to react. In addition to the specific stimuli that remind the person of Vietnam, the ''survival mentality,'' mentioned above, fosters hyperalertness. It is also related to the pan-suspiciousness seen in many Vietnam veterans (Parson, 1984b); this is not only a lack of trust but also a readiness to react in a dangerous world (Brende, 1981).

Sleep disturbance may be of several varieties, including initial, middle, or terminal insomnia; avoidance or delay in going to sleep; and nightmares. Intermittent interruptions during the night are not uncommon. The existence of nightmares and other reexperiencing phenomena help distinguish the sleep disturbance of PTSD from that of major depressive disorder.

Vietnam veterans frequently exhibit guilt in two areas (Haley, 1974; Horowitz & Solomon, 1978; Lifton, 1973; Shatan, 1973). Survivor guilt is not uncommon. Veterans may feel responsible for the loss of a buddy and may try to undo the death in their minds, or they may wonder why they survived and the other person was killed. There is also guilt over having killed the enemy. It is not uncommon for a veteran to say, "I can still see his eyes looking at me." Very powerful guilt feelings are stirred by remembering atrocities committed, the killing of children, the maiming of women, or the wanton destruction (sometimes under orders) of villages. This guilt is quite different from obsessive guilt in that it represents a reaction to actual events rather than to wishes, impulses, and fantasies. The message that we sometimes give to the obsessive person, that the wish is not the deed, has no place here.

Memory impairment and concentration difficulty may be present. They are probably a consequence of the reexperiencing–numbing struggle. Preoccupation with the trauma may also impair concentration.

Vietnam veterans may exhibit both avoidance of activities recalling the trauma and voluntary exposure to them. It is not uncommon to see alternating periods of avoidance of anything reminding the veteran of Vietnam and periods when the veteran watches war movies on television with intense (and often highly critical) interest. Active seeking of Vietnam-like experiences may take the form of provoking authority conflicts or "sensation seeking" (Wilson & Krauss, 1985). For some, there is a need to re-create the exhilarating aspects of combat (Scurfield, 1985), whether they be the thrill of aggression or of sex. For many, the fighting experience itself was tinged with erotic sensations and sometimes with orgasm. The "adrenalin-filled" experience (Wilson & Krauss, 1985) may also play a role in the use of stimulant-drug taking.

Although all the "associated features" described in the DSM-III may be seen in the PTSD of Vietnam veterans, the factor-analytic study of Silver and Iacono (1984) suggests that aggression and depression be considered cardinal rather than associated features in this population. The prominence of these features, Silver and Iacono argued, makes Vietnam veteran PTSD unique and sets it apart from other types of PTSD. Depression and rage reactions are also prominent in the factor-analytic study of Wilson and Krauss (1985), as are somatic complaints. The veterans are often filled with a fear of loss of control, which, although it may reflect guilty recollections of violence in Vietnam, may also reflect the sensation-seeking, pleasurable aspect of loss of control referred to above. Many of these veterans feel betrayed and scapegoated by their government (Shatan, 1973), and they have lost their ability to trust people. Numbing and alienation not infrequently lead to a need for rootlessness; some veterans want to live in solitude in the woods and some need repeatedly to move. The interplay of these factors, together with the reexperiencing and the numbing, frequently leads to repeated cycles of violent and disruptive interpersonal relationships (Rosenheck, 1985) to a much higher degree than is found in other types of PTSD. The prominence of these "associated features" in such a high proportion of Vietnam veterans with PTSD justifies our treating them as a special subgroup.

In addition, PTSD may be accompanied by profound personality change, especially if the trauma has been repeated and prolonged (Parson, 1984b). Many Vietnam veterans suffer characterological changes that make them antisocial or that cause them to function with borderline personality organizations (Parson, 1984a). These features pose particular problems in diagnosis; when they are present, it is necessary to look for additional features of PTSD. People who have antisocial personalities without PTSD often show little guilt and express strong emotions rather than numbing when trying to manipulate others (Bailey, 1985). People who have borderline personalities without PTSD often fear being alone, in contrast to the isolation of those with PTSD (Parson, 1984a). Because personality change may be part of the reaction to the trauma, the treatment of Vietnam veterans with PTSD may present special problems that are found to a much lesser degree in others with PTSD.

The course of PTSD in Vietnam veterans is uneven and fluctuating (Green *et al.*, 1985). There may be periods of quiescence followed by flare-ups. The signs and symptoms may wax and wane independently of each other; at one time, one feature may predominate, and at a later time, a different feature may be dominant. Lipkin, Blank, Parson, and Smith (1982) described four major presentations: primarily the dramatic symptoms, primarily a major life-course alteration, primarily relationship difficulties, and primarily destruction of the meaning of the self and the world.

Before leaving diagnostic considerations, I should point out that there have been many obstacles to the accurate diagnosis of this condition. Some of these obstacles come with the veterans. As noted above, they are generally distrustful, especially of authority. They have tended to view psychiatrists as aligned either with the hated military (Lifton, 1978) or with the equally hated Veterans Administration, which many Vietnam veterans feel betrayed them. They tend not to talk with psychiatrists spontaneously about their Vietnam experiences (Atkinson, Henderson, Sparr, & Deale, 1982). The delayed onset and the intermittent course of the condition often mislead the diagnostician. Intermittent civilian stress may confuse the picture. The fact that PTSD may be falsified may make diagnosis difficult; this falsification cannot even be easily picked up on the Minnesota Multiphasic Personality Inventory (Bailey, 1985). Although checking military records may be of value, it is inconvenient, and the records may not provide an unequivocal account of combat (Atkinson *et al.*, 1982).

Obstacles are also brought to the situation by the diagnostician. Psychiatrists in training receive very little experience in or information about PTSD. Emphasis in training programs is on such conditions as schizophrenia and the affective disorders —disorders that affect large numbers of people and for which reasonable medication regimens are available. There is currently a deemphasis of those disorders that do not have a clear-cut biological base. The tendency to dismiss as "problems in living" psychosocial and interpersonal conditions finds its way into a psychiatry that increasingly champions medication and leaves the psychotherapy to others. Many Vietnam veterans complain that, when they did go to psychiatrists, they were called "schizophrenic" (after all, they did hallucinate) and were put on neuroleptics. Others say that they were handed medications but the doctor never took the time to talk with them. When the veteran is a woman, the possibility of Vietnam PTSD is even further from the diagnostician's mind (Stretch, Vail, & Maloney, 1985).

Shortly after the cessation of hostilities, partly because of the delay in the appearance of PTSD, the Nixon administration reported that the Vietnam conflict had had a remarkably low incidence of psychiatric consequences (Shatan, 1978). This report created a low index of suspicion, and when psychiatric casualties did appear, the anger toward the government that accompanied them made the complaints seem as much political as psychiatric.

Although the condition is much more widely accepted today, there are still some who doubt the "validity" of the diagnosis (Falcon, Ryan, Chamberlain, & Curtis, 1985; Pitts, 1985; Van Putten & Yager, 1984). The similarity of some of the features to panic and generalized anxiety disorder, to depression, and to various personality disorders has led these workers to speculate that PTSD is a heterogeneous group of disorders that are better classified with these other conditions. Blank (1985a) referred to this as the "comorbidity theory," and both he and Atkinson *et al.* (1982) failed to see the logic in fragmenting PTSD into a variety of other disorders. Those who wish to dismiss the diagnosis of PTSD bolster their argument by some evidence that the reexperiencing and its associated autonomic signs and symptoms may be ameliorated by tricyclics and monoamine oxidase inhibitors (MAOIs). This argument is weak; these drugs are not antidepressants, although they are useful in treating depression. Rather, they are extremely broad-spectrum medications that may affect a variety of conditions either by acting at different sites in the brain or by attacking the common attributes of a variety of conditions. Diagnoses cannot be "valid," much less "real" (Falcon *et al.*, 1985); they are merely ways of classifying data, and their ultimate test is their usefulness (Bursten, 1982). At this stage, at least, the diagnosis of PTSD is very useful in that it leads to a therapeutic approach; disregarding the diagnosis has led to misdiagnosis and poor treatment, a fact to which many embittered Vietnam veterans will attest (Scurfield, 1985).

COUNTERTRANSFERENCE PROBLEMS

Not only are there obstacles that the diagnostician must overcome in order to recognize Vietnam PTSD, but there are also serious countertransference issues that may make it difficult to treat these veterans. Some of them spring from attitudes that have already been discussed. If it is difficult to acknowledge PTSD, the veteran may be seen as having a personality disorder. Unfortunately, many psychiatrists view personality disorders pejoratively and feel that those who carry that diagnosis are merely manipulating others for their own ends. Fortified by some of the popular attitudes mentioned above, the therapist may feel that the veteran is, indeed, a villain or that he or she is merely out for financial compensation (Blank, 1985a; Egendorf, 1978). Therapists who are aware of these attitudes are unlikely to work with Vietnam veterans. However, some therapists may not be aware of these attitudes until the veteran frustrates the treatment enterprise by missing appointments, arriving high or drunk, or resisting treatment within the session. At this time, the attitude may emerge and may influence the course of treatment or the decision to terminate.

The intensity of the veteran's rage and projected sadism may mobilize the therapist's own sadistic impulses. Reports of atrocities may evoke feelings of repugnance, or the excitement and erotism of battle may evoke a prurient interest on the part of the therapist (Haley, 1974). The fear of loss of control, which so often accompanies Vietnam PTSD, may be conveyed to the therapist and may evoke a similar fear. This may be particularly difficult for the therapist to deal with emotionally, because the panic is very real and some of these veterans do lose control. Not infrequently, the veterans have weapons at home; this fact makes the fear of loss of control even more intense for both veteran and therapist (Smith, 1985a).

THE PSYCHOTHERAPEUTIC PROCESSES

Any treatment occurs within a psychotherapeutic context, which includes not only formal psychotherapies but also medication, biofeedback, cognitive restructuring, and so on. It even includes mail-order prayer, although we do not ordinarily refer to this type of interaction as psychotherapy. Treatment occurs within any relationship in which the help seeker relates to a help giver (or to a group of other help seekers who, collectively, are seen as a help giver).

In the case of Vietnam veterans with PTSD, the initial psychotherapeutic context is strongly defined by the help seeker. Many factors obstruct the development of a working alliance. The features of the disorder itself cause difficulty.

The sense of betrayal, the rage, and the fear of intimacy make it exceedingly difficult for many to develop the trust necessary for a working alliance. Where the therapist is identified as part of the government, there is often a serious barrier. To help counteract this barrier, the Viet Nam Veterans Outreach and Counseling Centers (Vet Centers) have been set up to deemphasize that they are part of the Veterans Administration medical program by being away from hospitals and clinics, requiring minimum paperwork, and having an air of casualness and informality. Although this atmosphere helps, veterans are still wary, and it often takes quite some time before they venture in. Being generally suspicious of authority, the veteran cannot tolerate rules that he or she may feel are arbitrary. Whether in a Vet enter or elsewhere, the therapist must tolerate missed sessions, substance abuse, reticence, and acting out. An authoritarian approach on the part of the therapist is generally counterproductive (Parson, 1984b; Shatan, 1973). In many rap-group settings, the help giver does not call himself or herself a therapist; often, first names are used, and there is more of a sense of equivalence (Parson, 1984b; Shatan, 1978). The therapist is advised to take an active role in the process. He or she will be tested for honesty and reliability; there must be a readiness to share feelings and opinions honestly with the veterans (Lifton, 1973). The passive, expectant approach that, in other contexts, may be useful for allowing the transference to develop may be interpreted by the veteran as lack of interest or may encourage the development of paranoid feelings (Walker & Nash, 1981).

Vietnam veterans believe that only another combat veteran can possibly understand what they have been through. Although it is certainly helpful for the help giver to be a Vietnam veteran, it is not absolutely essential, provided that the therapist is sensitive, empathetic, and knowledgeable (Parson, 1984b). It is important that this knowledge include not only therapeutic techniques but also a knowledge of the conditions in Vietnam and the post-Vietnam experiences the veteran is likely to have had. The noncombat veteran or nonveteran who wishes to be a help giver must be willing to learn by reading and by listening (Brende, 1981; Egendorf, 1978). And as I have discussed earlier, the trust process will start with the diagnostic evaluation. The veteran will not always volunteer her or his PTSD symptoms; the help giver must think of the diagnostic possibility and ask about military service and PTSD symptoms.

Parson (1984b) pointed out that, when the therapist is a combat veteran, the trust process tends to be different from when he or she is not. If the veteran can get past the authority problem, he or she tends to band together with the fellow-veteran leader. The noncombat therapist soon undergoes a period of testing, opposition, and disparagement. Any attempt to "pull rank" or to deceive the veteran can be fatal to the relationship. The therapist should not defend his or her "right" to be the help giver. This defense will lead only to contentiousness. An attitude of "Well, it's true, I wasn't there, and there is much I'll have to learn from you, but here I am anyway, and I'm willing to try my best" honestly portrays the situation. The noncombat therapist must not be afraid to ask about events with which he or she is not familiar, but in a manner that conveys a genuine attempt to learn and to understand.

I was one of three coleaders in a Vet Center group. I was older than everyone else, I am not a Vietnam era veteran, and I am a psychiatrist—three strikes against me. Coming directly from a clinic in another city, I wore my usual working attire; I was the only one in the room without jeans. As the testing began in the early sessions, my coleaders phoned me and suggested that it might be easier if I wore jeans. I chose not to do this, but I brought up their suggestion in the next session. I informed the group that this was how I usually dressed when I worked at the clinic. I could, of course, change into jeans, but it would be like ducking into a telephone booth and slipping into my Superman outfit: "I might impress you all, but it wouldn't be me." I continued dressing in my usual manner and was ultimately accepted.

Although the lack of trust is predicated partly on the veteran's experiences, it also has its transference aspects. The arrogance, suspiciousness, disdain, and grandiosity are defenses against involvement and commitment, which, in the veteran's mind, would only lead to further pain (Walker & Nash, 1981). Rage is projected to the therapist (Parson, 1984b), who may be endowed with all kinds of malevolent qualities. However, it is not advisable to interpret the transference early in the treatment. The veteran with PTSD often lacks the psychological stability to tolerate the interpretation, much less to make good use of it. The interpretation is likely to be seen as another instance in which the veteran is misunderstood (Walker & Nash, 1981); the emphasis on his or her personal dynamics is seen as the therapist's attempt to minimize the stresses of war and homecoming (Egendorf, 1978; Shapiro, 1984).

Likewise, because the working alliance is so difficult to cultivate and maintain, interpretations of resistances should be given sparingly, if at all. The reluctance of some veterans to talk about their experiences must be handled carefully. It is best to invite the veteran to talk, again and again if necessary, but the therapist must be willing to take no for an answer. (Egendorf, 1978). Sometimes, education about the process and about PTSD is helpful (Scurfield, 1985), but the therapist must be careful not to let the education become a lecture and then become nagging. Clarification of feelings also helps: "It may be too uncomfortable to talk right now."

On the other side, the veterans, either individually or in groups, may regale the therapist or each other with war story after war story. Although the recounting of experiences is useful (indeed, it may actually be the bond uniting the group; Parson, 1984b), there may come a point where it becomes an end in itself. The war stories continue and the discussion goes nowhere; although it is a way of handling anxiety, it is also a resistance. Egendorf (1978) suggested that, instead of interpreting the resistance, the therapist should ask the veteran for his or her personal feelings about the events reported. This approach moves the discussion off dead center without arousing inordinate anxiety.

The anxiety is most often related to the experiences that the veteran is trying to forget. Reexperiencing is painful and may be associated with loss of reality and panic when a flashback occurs. Even without a clear-cut flashback, the veteran may experience panic when reminded of the stressors. In addition to the anxiety, there is a fear of loss of control (Smith, 1985a; Walker & Nash, 1981). This fear is made more vivid for some because they have lost control and have become violent in combat or in their personal relationships after coming home (Horowitz & Solomon, 1978). Whereas in many therapeutic settings, the aim is to remove inhibitions and to relax controls, such a course may be dangerous in this particular setting. There must be a constant titration between reclaiming the experiences and helping the veteran exercise controls. The therapist must be a "barometer" of the veteran's anxiety (McKinnon, 1984).

There are several methods of dealing with the anxiety of reexperiencing. By not attacking the character defenses directly, the therapist allows the veteran to continue his or her own control measures (Parson, 1984b; Walker & Nash, 1981). A gradual approach to the alleviation of numbing (which will be discussed below) helps to keep the pressure low. Education about PTSD, naming the phenomenon and explaining it, and the encouraging of intellectualization are useful cognitive tools (Horowitz & Solomon, 1978).

Rituals may ease the anxiety. Walker and Nash (1981) suggested giving a 10-minute warning before the end of the session to give the veteran time to get feelings under control before leaving. Ending on time and with a ritual is also helpful. When the patient expresses mounting panic, it is sometimes helpful for the therapist to admit fears of the veteran's loss of control, "but we will learn to control the fear."

Practical measures for dealing with the fear that weapons will be used were suggested by Smith (1985a). He suggested that discussions that may lead to the veteran's leaving the weapons with a friend or on some neutral ground may be helpful.

In addition to the cognitive tools referred to above, other behavioral measures for reducing the anxiety and the danger of loss of control have been reported. Horowitz and Solomon (1978) suggested giving "hierarchical routes of behavior." The veteran is asked to name his or her worst impulse (e.g., to hurt someone). The next task is to think of some action almost, but not quite, as harmful. It might be to slam his or her fist into the wall. Next down the list might be to swear, and so on. A scale is constructed. The veteran is then asked to practice going down the scale and to try to substitute ever lower actions for higher ones.

Imaginal flooding has been used to attack the anxiety-generating experience itself (Fairbank & Keane, 1982; Keane & Kaloupek, 1982). The veteran is asked to imagine the painful experience as long as possible or until the anxiety subsides. The procedure is repeated with each experience in each meaning context. Relaxation, reduction of anxiety, and reduction of flashbacks and nightmares have been reported, but in only very small numbers of veterans.

Relaxation and other stress-reduction exercises must be undertaken with care and caution (Smith, 1985a). Veterans with PTSD have erected rigid control systems, and they often feel the need to be constantly on the alert. Relaxation may be very threatening to them and may precipitate a panic attack.

The whole gamut of medications has been tried in an attempt to control the disturbing symptoms of Vietnam PTSD. Birkheimer, Lindsay, and Muniz (1985) conducted a retrospective review of charts that included the use of antipsychotics, tricyclics, MAOIs, benzodiazepines, and propranolol. They concluded that none of these medications were adequate to ameliorate the symptoms. However, Walker (1982), although acknowledging that no well-controlled studies had been done, suggested that MAOIs may reduce flashbacks and nightmares, that tricyclics are useful for secondary depressions, that brief trials of antipsychotics may help control flashbacks, and that propranolol may help control the autonomic symptoms. In his opinion, benzodiazepines are counterindicated. We must remember the potential for substance abuse in these veterans as well as the tolerance of the benzodiazepines with continued use. The more recent review by Ettedgui and Bridges (1985) tends to support these suggestions.

Perhaps the most intriguing reports are those that suggest the efficacy of MAOIs in reducing and sometimes eliminating flashbacks and nightmares (Cornfield, 1984; Hogben & Cornfeld, 1981; Milanes, Mack, Dennison & Slater, 1984). Although the studies have been preliminary and uncontrolled, the cases reported have shown rapid amelioration of these symptoms. General adjustment has improved, perhaps as a direct effect of the medication or as a consequence of the symptom relief. Cornfeld (1984) suggested that flashbacks represent a REM state during the awake period. This connection with the sleep–waking cycle and the fact that MAOIs are REM inhibitors may provide a mechanism of action if the reported efficacy holds up under further controlled trials. Of course, the use of MAOIs in a group of people with a high incidence of alcohol abuse and self-destructive potential calls for extreme caution.

Control of the anxiety associated with reexperiencing is often regulated by the veteran through the defense of numbing, as I have said above. This numbing itself must be carefully attacked so that the veteran may be reacquainted with his or her feelings. The therapist must constantly be alert to opportunities to direct the veteran's attention to feelings. At the same time, acknowledgement that the feelings may be hard to handle and inquiry about what makes the feelings so difficult are useful therapeutic techniques (Egendorf, 1978). Gestalt techniques, especially role playing, may have a place here, but the therapist must be sensitive to the limits of the veteran's anxiety tolerance. The therapist must remember that the numbing serves a purpose; one must be careful not to go too far too fast (Horowitz & Solomon, 1978). "Going to the Wall" (visiting the Vietnam Memorial in Washington, DC) is a powerful experience that is often avoided for some time. The veteran should be encouraged, but not forced, to go. Seeing the names of buddies evokes strong memories and emotions.

One technique, used at the Vet Center in Knoxville, Tennessee, is particularly evocative. After a few introductory sessions, the group of veterans takes the "airplane trip." The room is darkened, the chairs are arranged in two side-by-side columns, and the veterans (and group leaders) are told that they are on a plane taking them to Vietnam. They are asked to recall and describe their feelings. Some of the reports are quite vivid. In later sessions, useful reference can be made to the feelings expressed on the airplane. (The fact that some veterans may have gone over by boat seems to make little difference.)

Hypnosis may also be helpful when the numbing is too powerful to yield to other techniques. It is useful to help uncover unconscious feelings and repressed painful memories, to provide emotional release, and, in a hypnotherapeutic context, to help the veteran work through the experience and integrate it and its meaning with the rest of his or her personality (Brende, 1985; Spiegel, 1981). Sodium pentothal and amytal interviews may also be helpful (Kolb, 1985; Walker, 1982), particularly when dealing with a dissociative state or affective numbing. Kolb exposes the veteran to the sounds of combat during the drugged state and videotapes his or her reaction. The videotape is then shown to the veteran in the awake state, and the reaction is discussed.

According to Silver and Kelly (1985), hypnosis has several advantages over narcosynthesis: it does not require an anesthesiologist, it can bring back experiences that are more remote in time, and the therapist has finer control over the amount and intensity of the reexperiencing. All authors have stressed the importance of titrating the release of repressed material against the anxiety that such release produces; the therapist must remember that he or she is dealing with a potentially volatile person for whom the numbing is protective.

Special mention should be made of the feelings of guilt. As I stated earlier, many of the guilt feelings differ from those encountered in the usual psychotherapeutic practice. Here, the guilt is not over fantasies but over actual deeds (and sometimes over the joy and excitement experienced while the deeds were being done). To interpret this guilt in terms of unconscious fantasies would only cause the veteran to "realize" that his or her moral dilemma over actual deeds is not being understood. Horowitz and Solomon (1978) suggested what amounts to a cognitive approach. The first task is to clarify the difference between today and the combat situation. It is necessary also to understand the differences between individual and collective responsibility. Then, the question of how much atonement and penance are necessary must be confronted. Finally, one might suggest symbolic retribution in the form of doing something that is "life-affirming" or productive. Haley (1974) encourages the patient to understand the factors that made him or her act at the time in a way that is usually repugnant. The group setting also helps dispel the guilt in other ways. The realization that the veteran is not alone in his or her "misdeeds" and that the group can accept such a "morally bad" person is supportive.

Some veterans express little or no guilt because they are unaware of it (Schwartz, 1984). In other cases, the veteran may express guilt over one incident and seems unable to overcome it. The incident offered for discussion may be the lesser of two "evils"; there may be a far more powerful incident that the veteran is concealing or repressing. In still other cases, persistent somatic complaints and references to agent orange may serve to hide the guilt. Persistent references to others, particularly the therapist, as persecutor may function as a projection of the veteran's own sadism, which helps him or her avoid the guilt. If this situation proves intractable and if a working relationship can be established, interpretation of the transference may be necessary. Schwartz (1984) described this within the context of individual psychotherapy. It should be emphasized, however, that this is not the method of first choice; the dangers of early transference interpretation have been discussed above.

As the numbing subsides and the feelings and painful memories emerge, with the therapist's assistance, the veteran can become aware that "it did mean something" after all and that he or she cared very much. However, a reacquaintance with the lost feelings is not always sufficient. Working through must come in the context of personal meanings (Hendin *et al.*, 1983; McKinnon, 1984). Here, clarifications of the meanings of the experiences, as well as interpretations linking these meanings to other meaningful events before Vietnam, may be helpful. Even though combat stress meets the criterion of the "but for" experience described earlier in this chapter, each veteran has put his or her own personal stamp on the experience as well. For example, one veteran may have grown up in a military family and felt he had to prove his worth and his masculinity, but the conditions of the Vietnam situation did not provide him the scenarios that his father had described from previous wars. Another may have come from an intensely religious and patriotic family, and he or she may have lost God in the chaos of Vietnam. Or the veteran may have had sexual experiences or sexual harassment that engendered strong conflicts with the way he or she had been brought up.

An essential part of the treatment process may be psychosocial rehabilitation (Berman, Price, & Gusman, 1982). When the intensity of the symptoms lightens sufficiently, the veteran should be aided in his or her effort to reenter the community. This aid may involve education, job skill training, and even social skills training.

THE THERAPEUTIC SETTINGS

Probably the original and most widely used setting is the rap group (Lifton, 1973; Shatan, 1973; Smith, 1985b). Started by the Vietnam Veterans against the War (VVAW), they consisted of informal groups of disaffected veterans, many of whom had PTSD. Professionals were invited in to help, but they had tried to maintain a nonauthoritarian manner and to relate to the veterans as equals. The early rap groups were a "counter-VA" movement. It was felt that the public protest helped to give the veterans a sense of purpose and meaning. Far from being neutral, the professionals championed the cause of VVAW in a "shared commitment" with the veterans (Lifton, 1978). Flemming (1985) questioned the usefulness of this advocacy. He felt that it may have goaded the veterans to increased dissatisfaction, which, rather than giving purpose, may have become counterproductive by perpetuating an inclination not to assume responsibility for the veteran's own actions. Needless to say, a similar view was held by the government, which found the rap groups politically embarrassing (Shatan, 1973). After the early beginnings, however, Vietnam PTSD was legitimized, and the efficacy of the informal rap groups was accepted. The Veterans Administration has set up a system of Vet Centers, in which rap groups are a commonly used setting (Blank, 1982).

Parson (1984b) gave an excellent analysis of the rap group processes, many of which have been discussed in the previous section. It is an "oblique technical approach" that avoids transference analysis. The group and the leaders coalesce around the common experiences. The group is supportive and nurturant, and characterological defenses are supported. In this way, splitting, projection, and annihilation anxiety may be contained. Within this context, most rap groups use the various control and antinumbing techniques described above. Parson suggested that Vietnam veterans who are motivated not only to alleviate symptoms but also to change are particularly good candidates; antisocial persons who will manipulate the group, paranoid people who will promote pan-suspiciousness, and schizophrenic veterans who will be disruptive to the group process should be excluded. Parsons saw the following goals for the rap group: management of symptoms, tolerance of closeness and connectedness, some working through of guilt and of preoccupation with death, bolstered self-esteem, the acquisition of meaning of the Vietnam experience, and (in his model) the laying of groundwork for future group work. Probably, the majority of veterans who achieve these results in rap groups do not go on to other types of group work.

Smith (1985b) described different levels of rap groups. After a brief introductory group, the veteran goes into a 10- to 14-week initial working rap group. Those who do well in this group may proceed to a long-term rap group run primarily by the veterans themselves. Others may "recycle" the initial working rap group or participate in other forms of treatment.

Other group settings are more traditionally organized. Walker and Nash (1981) advocated a group psychotherapy in which there are clear lines between therapist and veteran. However, they use many of the techniques mentioned above. They do not feel that the political aspects of the rap groups are relevant any longer. Nonetheless, the veterans will bring up political concerns, having to do both with the Vietnam conflict and with current political trends; in my opinion, at least early in the group experience, these concerns must be addressed and in an honest manner.

In actual practice, group approaches probably run the gamut from the original-style rap groups to more traditional group therapies. Parson (1984b) uses a unique series of groups with which to treat Vietnam veterans. Called the *multiple-group model,* it consists of a series of three differently structured groups through which the veteran may progress. The first group is a traditional rap group, the techniques and goals of which have been described above. After a year or more, those who have done well in the rap group enter a second phase. In essence, the group continues, but its style changes. This "'rap' psychotherapy group" has added to its membership two or three Vietnam era veterans who have served elsewhere. Whereas the emphasis in the first phase is on cohesiveness promoted by a feeling that all members are similar, the second-phase group focuses on the diversity of the members and promotes their differentiation from each other. The leadership role is more pronounced. The goals are to diversify and to shift from the symbiotic sharing of the previous group to greater autonomy and interpersonal relatedness, to deepen trust, to promote an awareness of feelings and how they affect other people, to begin to explore the facade shown to others, and to lay the groundwork for the third phase. The third phase is a psychoanalytically oriented group. The selection of members is made from those in the second-phase group whose dramatic symptoms have disappeared and who are sufficiently integrated to tolerate deep exploration. In addition, a few nonveterans are added. The goals are to achieve characterological change by exploring unconscious mental processes and to work through person-specific meanings of the Vietnam experiences.

Vietnam veterans are seen also in dyadic settings of all types, from counseling (Blank, 1982) to more formal and traditional psychotherapy (McKinnon, 1984; Smith, 1985a). The gamut of techniques discussed above may be used. McKinnon described a brief, focal psychotherapy. In his selection process, because numbing is part of the presenting picture, he does not require the veteran to have the capacity to experience feelings. However, he does look for those who have motivation to rid themselves of the symptoms (having a compensation claim does not disqualify them) and who have a focal problem centering on combat stress whose personal meaning is available to the veteran. Treatment is centered on this focal problem.

Individual and group treatment are not mutually exclusive; in fact, they may be complementary (Blank, 1982; Brende, 1981). Both are used in many Vet Centers.

The veteran with PTSD has a strong interaction with significant others in his or her environment, whether they be close friends or spouses and children (Haley, 1974; Williams & Williams, 1985). Those close to the veteran are exposed to all the behaviors that he or she exhibits. These behaviors may take the form of frightening or physically abusive episodes, isolation and "unwillingness" to work, noncommunicativeness, and so on. Not only do these behaviors make the lives of significant others difficult, but they may also evoke responses that are not helpful to the veteran. Treatment for the family and significant others may be very important, and it is offered by many Vet Centers.

Vietnam veterans who are hospitalized in some general VA hospitals may comprise about 20% of the census; they may comprise 40% or more of the psychiatry service in such hospitals (Starkey & Ashlock, 1984). For this reason, some hospitals have set up special units in which to treat Vietnam PTSD. Some of the programs are brief and serve mainly as a way of inducting the veterans into treatment that is to be continued at a Vet

Center. Others are more ambitious. Sax (1985) reported a program that uses virtually all the modalities discussed above. In addition, there is a ward structure with community meetings chaired by an elected member. A variety of educational classes are also available. The milieu of the peer group on a continuous basis is felt to be helpful. Although Sax reported success with many PTSD patients, even those who were substance abusers and were potentially self-destructive, he felt that those who are preoccupied with revenge and who focus on blaming others are poor candidates for this kind of program.

Berman *et al.* (1982) described a three-phase inpatient program. Using a Vietnam-veteran subculture with a gamut of therapeutic activities, the first phase deals with the crisis; flashbacks and other dramatic symptoms are attended to. This period (30–45 days) is also used to develop trust in the program. During this time, the veteran's outside social situation is also "cleaned up" (e.g., bills are paid). During the second phase, which is of the same length, the veteran is encouraged to develop a sense of personal responsibility. Finally, in the third phase, the veteran attends to rehabilitation through education and entering the job market.

It is not clear what characteristics distinguish inpatients in some hospitals from outpatients, other than geographical circumstances and the availability of beds. Arnold (1985) suggested two sets of criteria: If there is no available outpatient treatment center, inpatient treatment may be justified. If outpatient treatment is available, but the veteran has a poor support system or is likely to have severe outbursts, inpatient treatment is preferable. Many Vietnam veterans who are treated as outpatients in Vet Centers present with frightening symptoms and impulses and could clearly meet a "danger-to-self-or-others" criterion for hospitalization. I suspect that many Vet Center staff members would be more comfortable if there were a greater availability of beds in inpatient programs, for certainly, treating some of these severely troubled veterans as outpatients must sometimes feel like playing Russian roulette.

SUMMARY

The peculiar conditions of the Vietnam conflict have fostered the development of varieties of posttraumatic stress disorders (PTSDs), which have both similarities and differences from other types of PTSD. Because the combat veteran has often been reluctant to discuss his or her experiences, and there has been a long delay before the signs and symptoms have become obvious, the diagnosis is frequently overlooked. Numbing, isolation, and sleep disturbance may be misdiagnosed as depression; hallucinations and flashbacks as schizophrenia or panic disorder; and antagonisms, alienation, and substance abuse as antisocial personality.

Although there are some promising leads, treatment of these types of PTSD with chemotherapy has not yielded consistently positive results. Many veterans have resented those psychiatrists who seemed more interested in their chemistry than in their plight. Psychotherapy, both individual and group, although widespread, is beset with difficulties. Countertransference reactions of anger, fear, and disgust may interfere with the process. The veteran's anxieties, stimulated by the tendency to relive frightening experiences, cause him or her to attempt to avoid issues that need to be addressed. Such numbing and fear of personal commitment often make the veteran a difficult psychotherapeutic candidate. The therapist must constantly walk the tightrope between helping the veteran deal with frightening memories and emotions and keeping their intensity within tolerable limits. Unique problems, such as guilt over atrocities, require special techniques. This difficult therapeutic process may take place in conventional or nontraditional settings.

REFERENCES

American Psychiatric Association. (1980). *Diagnostic and statistical manual of mental disorders* (3rd ed.; DSM-III). Washington, DC: Author.

Archibald, H. C., & Tuddenham, R. D. (1965). Persistent stress reactions after combat: A 20 year follow-up. *Archives of General Psychiatry, 12,* 475–481.

Arnold. A. L. (1985). Inpatient treatment of Viet Nam veterans with post-traumatic stress disorder. In S. M. Sonnenberg, A. S. Blank, & J. Talbott (Eds.), *The trauma of war: Stress and recovery in Viet Nam veterans* (pp. 239–262). Washington, DC: American Psychiatric Press.

Atkinson, R. M., Henderson, R. G., Sparr, L. F., & Deale, S. (1982). Assessment of Viet Nam veterans for posttraumatic stress disorder in Veterans Administration disability claims. *American Journal of Psychiatry, 139,* 1118–1121.

Bailey, J. E. (1985). Differential diagnosis of posttraumatic stress and antisocial personality disorders. *Hospital and Community Psychiatry, 36,* 881–883.

Berman, S., Price, S., & Gusman, F. (1982). An inpatient program for Vietnam combat veterans in a Veterans Administration Hospital. *Hospital and Community Psychiatry, 33,* 919–922.

Birkheimer, L. J., Lindsay, D., & Muniz, C. E. (1985). Posttraumatic stress disorder: Characteristics and pharmacological response in the veteran population. *Comprehensive Psychiatry, 26,* 304–310.

Blank, A. S. (1982). Apocalypse terminable and interminable: Operation outreach for Vietnam veterans. *Hospital and Community Psychiatry, 33,* 913–918.

Blank, A. S. (1985a). Irrational reactions to post-traumatic stress disorder in Viet Nam veterans. In S. M. Sonnenberg, A. Blank, & J. Talbott (Eds.), *The trauma of war: Stress and recovery in Viet Nam veterans* (pp. 69–98). Washington, DC: American Psychiatric Press.

Blank, A. S. (1985b). The unconscious flashback to the war in Viet Nam veterans: Clinical mystery, legal defense, and community problem. In S. M. Sonnenberg, A. S. Blank, & J. Talbott (Eds.), *The trauma of war: Stress and recovery in Viet Nam veterans* (pp. 293–308). Washington, DC: American Psychiatric Press.

Boulangar, G. (1985). Post-traumatic stress disorder: an old problem with a new name. In S. M. Sonnenberg, A. S. Blank, & J. Talbott (Eds.), *The trauma of war: Stress and recovery in Viet Nam veterans* (pp. 13–30). Washington, DC: American Psychiatric Press.

Brende, J. O. (1981). Combined individual and group therapy for Vietnam veterans. *International Journal of Group Psychotherapy, 31,* 367–378.

Brende, J. O. (1985). The use of hypnosis in post-traumatic conditions. In W. E. Kelly (Ed.), *Post-traumatic stress disorder and the war veteran patient* (pp. 193–210). New York: Brunner/Mazel.

Bursten, B. (1982). Narcissistic personalities in DSM-III. *Comprehensive Psychiatry, 23,* 409–420.

Cornfield, R. B. (1984). Traumatic war neurosis: Some pharmacologic and psychophysiologic observations. In H. J. Schwartz, (Ed.), *Psychotherapy of the combat veteran* (pp. 221–252). New York: SP Medical and Scientific Books.

DeFazio, V. J. (1978). Dynamic perspectives on the nature and effects of combat stress. In C. R. Figley (Ed.), *Stress disorders among Vietnam veterans: Theory, research and treatment* (pp. 23–42). New York: Brunner/Mazel.

Egendorf, A. (1978). Psychotherapy with Vietnam veterans: Observations and suggestions. In C. R. Figley (Ed.), *Stress disorders among Vietnam veterans* (pp. 231–253). New York: Brunner/Mazel.

Egendorf, A., Farley, J., & Remez, A. (1981). *Legacies of Vietnam: Vol. 5. Dealing with the war.* Washington, DC: U.S. Government Printing Office.

Ettedgui, E., & Bridges, M. (1985). Posttraumatic stress disorder. *Psychiatric Clinics of North America, 8,* 89–103.

Fairbank, J. A., & Keane, T. M. (1982). Flooding for combat-related stress disorders; assessment of anxiety reduction across traumatic memories. *Behavior Therapy, 13,* 499–510.

Falcon, S., Ryan, C., Chamberlain, K., & Curtis, G. (1985). Tricyclics: Possible treatment for posttraumatic stress disorder. *Journal of Clinical Psychiatry, 46,* 385–388.

Figley, C. R. (1978a). Introduction. In C. R. Figley (Ed.), *Stress disorders among Vietnam veterans: Theory, research and treatment* (pp. xii–xxvi). New York: Brunner/Mazel.

Figley, C. R. (1978b). Psychosocial adjustment among Vietnam veterans: An overview of the research. In C. R. Figley (Ed.), *Stress disorders among Vietnam veterans: Theory, research and treatment* (pp. 57–71). New York: Brunner/Mazel.

Flemming, R. H. (1985). Post Vietnam syndrome: Neurosis or sociosis? *Psychiatry, 48,* 122–139.

Foy, D. W., Sipprelle, R. C., Rueger, D. B., & Carroll, E. M. (1984). Etiology of posttraumatic stress disorders in Vietnam veterans: Analysis of premilitary, military, and combat exposure influences. *Journal of Consulting and Clinical Psychology, 52,* 79–87.

Futterman, S., & Pumpian-Mindlin, E. (1951). Traumatic war neurosis five years later. *American Journal of Psychiatry, 108,* 401–408.

Gleser, G., Green, B. L., & Winget, C. (1981). *Buffalo Creek Revisited: Prolonged psychological effects of disaster.* New York: Simon & Schuster.

Green, B. L., Lindy, J. D., & Grace, M. C. (1985). Posttraumatic stress disorder: Toward DSM-IV. *Journal of Nervous and Mental Disease, 173,* 406–411.

Haley, S. A. (1974). When the patient reports atrocities; specific treatment considerations of the Vietnam veteran. *Archives of General Psychiatry, 30,* 191–196.

Hearst, N., Newman, T. B., & Helley, S. B. (1986). Delayed effects of the military draft on mortality: A randomized natural experiment. *New England Journal of Medicine, 314,* 620–624.

Hendin, H., Haas, A. P., Singer, P., Gold F., & Trigos, G. (1983). The influence of precombat personality on posttraumatic stress disorder. *Comprehensive Psychiatry, 24,* 530–534.

Hogben, G. L., & Cornfield, R. B. (1981). Treatment of traumatic war neurosis with phenelzine. *Archives of General Psychiatry, 38,* 440–445.

Horowitz, M. J. (1976). *Stress response syndrome.* New York: Aronson.

Horowitz, M. J., & Solomon, G. F. (1978). Delayed stress response syndromes in Vietnam veterans. In C. R. Figley (Ed.), *Stress disorders among Vietnam veterans: Theory, research and treatment* (pp. 268–280). New York: Brunner/Mazel.

Kadushin, C., Boulanger, G., & Martin, J. (1981). *Legacies of Vietnam: Vol. 4. Long term stress reactions.* Washington, DC: U.S. Government Printing Office.

Keane, T. M., & Kaloupek, D. G. (1982). Imaginal flooding in the treatment of post-traumatic stress disorder. *Journal of Consulting and Clinical Psychology, 50,* 138–140.

Kolb, L. C. (1985). The place of narcosynthesis in the treatment of chronic and delayed stress reactions of war. In S. M. Sonnenberg, A. S. Blank, & J. A. Talbott (Eds.), *The trauma of war: Stress and recovery in Viet Nam veterans* (pp. 211–227). Washington, DC: American Psychiatric Press.

Kolb, L. C. (1986). Post-traumatic stress disorder in Vietnam veterans. *New England Journal of Medicine, 314,* 641–642.

Laufer, R. S. (1985). War trauma and human development: The Viet Nam experience. In S. M. Sonnenberg, A. S. Blank, & J. A. Talbott (Eds.), *The trauma of war: Stress and recovery in Viet Nam veterans* (pp. 31–57). Washington, DC: American Psychiatric Press.

Lifton, R. J. (1967). *Death in life: Survivors of Hiroshima.* New York: Simon & Schuster.

Lifton, R. J. (1973). *Home from the war.* New York: Simon & Shuster.

Lifton, R. J. (1978). Advocacy and corruption in the healing process. In C. R. Figley (Ed.), *Stress disorders among Vietnam veterans: Theory, research and treatment* (pp. 209–231). New York: Brunner/Mazel.

Lipkin, J. O., Blank, A. S., Parson, E. R., & Smith, J. (1982). Vietnam veterans and posttraumatic stress disorder. *Hospital and Community Psychiatry, 33,* 908–912.

McKinnon, J. A. (1984). Brief psychotherapy of the Vietnam combat neuroses. In H. J. Schwartz (Ed.), *Psychotherapy of the combat veteran* (pp. 125–152). New York: SP Medical and Scientific Books.

Mellman, T. A., & Davis, G. G. (1985). Combat-related flashbacks in posttraumatic stress disorder: Phenomenology and similarity to panic attack. *Journal of Clinical Psychiatry, 46,* 379–382.

Milanes, F. J., Mack, C. N., Dennison, J., & Slater, V. L. (1984, December). Phenelzine treatment of post-Vietnam stress syndrome. *VA Practitioner,* 40–49.

Panzarella, R. F., Mantell, D. M., & Bridenbaugh, R. H. (1978). Psychiatric syndromes, self-concepts, and Vietnam veterans. In C. R. Figley (Ed.), *Stress disorders among Vietnam veterans: Theory, research and treatment* (pp. 148–172). New York: Brunner/Mazel.

Parson, E. R. (1984a). The reparation of the self: Clinical and theoretical dimensions in the treatment of Vietnam combat veterans. *Journal of Contemporary Psychiatry, 14,* 4–56.

Parson, E. R. (1984b). The role of psychodynamic group therapy in the treatment of the combat veteran. In H. J. Schwartz (Ed.), *Psychotherapy of the combat veteran* (pp. 153–220). New York: SP Medical and Scientific Books.

Pitts, F. N. (1985). Editorial. *Journal of Clinical Psychiatry, 46,* 373.

Rosenheck, R. L. (1985). Malignant post-Vietnam stress syndrome. *American Journal of Orthopsychiatry, 55,* 166–176.

Sax, W. P. (1985). Establishing a post-traumatic stress disorder inpatient program. In W. E. Kelly (Ed.), *Post-traumatic stress disorder and the war veteran patient* (pp. 234–248). New York: Brunner/Mazel.

Schwartz, H. J. (1984). Unconscious guilt: Its origin, manifestations, and treatment in combat veteran. In H. J. Schwartz (Ed.), *Psychotherapy of the combat veteran* (pp. 47–84). New York: SP Medical and Scientific Books.

Scurfield, R. M. (1985). Post-trauma stress assessment and treatment: Overview and formulations. In C. R. Figley (Ed.), *Trauma and its wake: The study and treatment of post-traumatic stress disorder* (pp. 219–256). New York: Brunner/Mazel.

Shapiro, R. B. (1984). Transference, countertransference, and the Vietnam veteran. In H. J. Schwartz (Ed.), *Psychotherapy of the combat veteran* (pp. 85–102). New York: SP Medical and Scientific Books.

Shatan, C. F. (1973). The grief of soldiers: Vietnam combat veterans' self-help movement. *American Journal of Orthopsychiatry, 43,* 640–653.

Shatan, C. F. (1978). Stress disorders among Vietnam veterans: The emotional content of combat veterans. In C. R. Figley (Ed.), *Stress disorders among Vietnam veterans* (pp. 43–56). New York: Brunner/Mazel.

Silver, S. M., & Iacono, C. U. (1984). Factor-analytic support for DSM-III's post-traumatic stress disorder for Vietnam veterans. *Journal of Clinical Psychology, 40,* 5–14.

Silver, S. M., & Kelly, W. E. (1985). Hypnotherapy of post-traumatic conditions. In W. E. Kelly (Ed.), *Post-traumatic stress disorder and the war veteran patient* (pp. 211–233). New York: Brunner/Mazel.

Smith, J. R. (1985a). Individual psychotherapy with Vietnam veterans. In S. M. Sonnenberg, A. S. Blank, & J. A. Talbott (Eds.), *The trauma of war: Stress and recovery in Vietnam veterans* (pp. 125–164). Washington, DC: American Psychiatric Press.

Smith, J. R. (1985b). Rap groups and group therapy for Vietnam veterans. In S. M. Sonnenberg, A. S. Blank, & J. A. Talbott (Eds.), *The trauma of war: Stress and recovery in Vietnam veterans* (pp. 165–192). Washington, DC: American Psychiatric Press.

Spiegel, D. (1981). Vietnam grief work using hypnosis. *American Journal of Clinical Hypnosis, 24,* 33–40.

Starkey, T. W., & Ashlock, L. (1984, December). Inpatient treatment of PTSD: An interim report of the Miami model. *VA Practioner,* 37–40.

Stretch, R. H., Vail, J. D., & Maloney, J. P. (1985). Post-traumatic stress disorder among Army Nurse Corps Vietnam veterans. *Journal of Consulting and Clinical Psychology, 53,* 704–708.

Van Devanter, L. M. (1985). The unknown warriors: Implications of the experiences of women in Vietnam. In W. E. Kelly (Ed.), *Post-traumatic stress disorder and the war veteran patient* (pp. 148–169). New York: Brunner/Mazel.

Van Putten, T., & Yager, J. (1984). Post-traumatic stress disorder: Emerging from the rhetoric. *Archives of General Psychiatry, 41,* 411–413.

Walker, J. I. (1982). Chemotherapy of traumatic war stress. *Military Medicine, 147,* 1029–1033.

Walker, J. I., & Nash, J. L. (1981). Group therapy in the treatment of Vietnam combat veterans. *International Journal of Group Psychotherapy, 31,* 376–389.

Williams, C. M., & Williams, T. (1985). Family therapy for Vietnam veterans. In S. M. Sonnenberg, A. S. Blank, & J. A. Talbott (Eds.), *The trauma of war: Stress and recovery in Vietnam veterans* (pp. 193–210). Washington, DC: American Psychiatric Press.

Wilson, J. P., & Krauss, G. E. (1985). Practicing post-traumatic stress disorders among Vietnam veterans. In W. E. Kelly (Ed.), *Post-traumatic stress disorder and the war veteran patient* (pp. 102–147). New York: Brunner/Mazel.

Worthington, E. R. (1978). Demographic and pre-service variables as predictors of post-military service adjustment. In C. R. Figley (Ed.), *Stress disorders among Vietnam veterans: Theory, research and treatment* (pp. 173–187). New York: Brunner/Mazel.

24

Mentally Retarded Adults

Dennis H. Reid and Jeffrey R. Fitzgerald

INTRODUCTION

Mental retardation is one of the most prevalent types of handicapping conditions among the human populace. Although reports of the incidence of mental retardation vary, estimates generally indicate that 3% of the population of the United States is mentally retarded (Beck, 1983). The disability of mental retardation affects afflicted individuals throughout their lifespan, including adulthood—which is the chronological period of concern of this chapter. However, despite the widespread prevalence of mental retardation, mentally retarded adults have historically received relatively little attention from an outpatient treatment perspective. Reasons for the lack of attention as well as recent events that have caused increased professional interest in this area of service provision will be discussed later.

The purpose of this chapter is to discuss the outpatient treatment of mentally retarded adults. In order to elucidate the importance and the existing technology within this component of human services, this chapter begins by presenting a (brief) historical overview of outpatient treatment services for adults who are mentally retarded. Following the organizational format used in other chapters, the historical overview is followed by (1) a summary of the special diagnostic considerations involved in providing outpatient treatment to mentally retarded adults; (2) a synopsis of frequent clinical problems faced by outpatient treatment specialists working with this population; (3) an overview of the modifications often required in this particular area of service provision; and finally, (4) a summary of the progress to date as well as developing (and needed) trends in the area.

Although mental retardation is frequently considered a single entity as a handicapping condition, the mentally retarded population actually represents a very heterogeneous

DENNIS H. REID and JEFFREY R. FITZGERALD • Western Carolina Center, Morganton, North Carolina 28655.

group of people who often have highly divergent treatment needs. Nevertheless, for organizational purposes as well as clarity of presentation, some categorization of subgroups of mentally retarded individuals is warranted. Throughout this chapter, subgroupings are referred to in terms of the *severity* of their mental retardation. The severity or degree of retardation is used for descriptive purposes because, for the most part, the treatment needs of mentally retarded persons vary in accordance with the severity of their retardation. Generally, Grossman's categorization (1983) of the severity of retardation—although by no means perfect—seems to be the most widely recognized. Consequently, Grossman's system is used here; it describes the severity of mental retardation (from least to most severe) with the descriptors *mild, moderate, severe,* and *profound.*

HISTORICAL OVERVIEW

Attempting to summarize the general history of the treatment of mentally retarded individuals—and specifically the outpatient treatment of mentally retarded adults—is difficult. The difficulty is due in large part to the fact that service provision to mentally retarded persons has varied considerably over time based on a wide rage of variables. Treatment services for severely and profoundly mentally retarded individuals, for example, have taken a different course, in many ways, from treatment services for mildly and moderately mentally retarded persons. The availability and variety of treatment services have also differed in recent history for mentally retarded senior citizens and for mentally retarded young adults and children. Nevertheless, there have been some major trends in treatment services in the United States—particularly since the 1960s—that have impacted the mentally retarded population in general as well as the subpopulation of mentally retarded adults. This section describes the most important of the recent trends in service provision, with a special focus on how each trend has affected the outpatient treatment of mentally retarded adults.

Normalization

Probably the most pervasive change in service provision for the mentally retarded in recent history in the United States is the change in the fundamental philosophy underlying the design and implementation of treatment services. Before the mid-1960s, mentally retarded individuals (and especially the most seriously retarded) were viewed as requiring specialized care and treatment in essentially all aspects of their lives. Hence, living arrangements and treatment services were established to be very different and separate from those for the normal populace. The most striking representation of this basic philosophy of service provision was the large, 1,000-plus-bed institution in which mentally retarded persons often lived and, basically, spent their entire existence. Life in the large institutions was, for the most part, very unlike life in the normal communities in which the vast majority of the (nonhandicapped) population lived, worked, and played.

In the 1960s, a change in the philosophy of service provision for mentally retarded persons began in the United States. Based on the service models in the Scandinavian countries and the work of Wolfensberger (e.g., Wolfensberger, 1976), a trend began toward the *normalization* of service provision. In essence, the principle of normalization stressed that mentally retarded persons should be allowed to live their lives as closely as possible to the manner in which the mainstream of society lives. The impact of the normalization principle on services for the mentally retarded has been quite significant and pervasive (see Maloney & Ward, 1979, Chapter 2, for a summary), including major effects on the outpatient treatment of mentally retarded adults. In particular, because of the focus on the living patterns of the nonretarded populace—and because outpatient treatment is a common treatment model for nonretarded persons—outpatient treatment became more accepted (and expected) as an appropriate service model for mentally retarded persons. Actually, however, the impact of normalization on outpatient treatment for adults who are mentally retarded has really been due more to an offshoot of the normalization movement (deinstitutionalization) than to normalization *per se*.

Deinstitutionalization

As just noted, one of the most apparent aspects of service delivery that stood in conflict with the principle of normalization was the predominance of large institutions as a place of residence for mentally retarded persons in the United States. As a result of this conflict, once the principle of normalization began to be adopted, a movement toward *deinstitutionalization* began. The deinstitutionalization trend was represented in three general sets of events. First, mentally retarded persons began to be transferred out of large public residential facilities into smaller and more normal living arrangements. Second, a decrease occurred in the number of individuals who were admitted to large institutions. Third, reforms began to take place within the institutions in an attempt to make institutional living conditions more normal.

The impact of the deinstitutionalization movement has been dramatic and widespread, although not entirely positive (Payne, 1976). From the point of view of the outpatient treatment of mentally retarded adults, the first two facets of the movement just mentioned have been especially influential. The large increase in the number of mentally retarded persons who either stayed in the community without ever being admitted to an institution or were discharged from institutions to the community resulted in a rather tremendous increase in the need for outpatient treatment. That is, all treatment services were no longer congregated within an inpatient model in the institutions; mentally retarded persons, as well as their caregivers and/or advocates, were required to seek (outpatient) services within local communities. Unfortunately, effective community-based services have not always been readily available to mentally retarded persons—a factor that has played a role in some of the failures of the deinstitutionalization movement (see Stacy, Doleys, & Bruno, 1983, for a critical review of community programs).

Right to Treatment

As the normalization and deinstitutionalization movements were beginning to affect services for the mentally retarded, another related trend was developing: *right to treatment*. The thrust of the right-to-treatment movement was the view that handicapped persons have a basic right to receive habilitative services and that, in many cases around the United States, mentally retarded persons were being denied that right. More seriously retarded individuals (e.g., the severely and profoundly mentally retarded) were especially being denied access to treatment services, or such services simply did not exist. The unavailability of habilitative programs (due to prohibited access or to nonexistence) for seriously retarded persons was perhaps most pronounced for persons residing in institutions, but it also represented a serious problem in many community settings.

Probably the best example of the focus and impact of the right-to-treatment movement was the passage of the Education for All Handicapped Children Act (P.L. 94-142) in 1975. Before P.L. 94-142, public school programs reserved the right to determine whether or not a given child or adolescent was, in essence, *too handicapped* to receive services from a school system. As a result, a large number of severely and profoundly mentally retarded persons were denied access to educational services. P.L. 94-142 legally outlawed such denial of services, and consequently, school programs for seriously disabled youth were developed and/or expanded in essentially every geographic region of the United States (see Green, Reid, McCarn, Schepis, Phillips, & Parsons, 1986).

The impact of the right-to-treatment movement in regard specifically to the outpatient treatment of mentally retarded adults was unique. On the one hand, the focus on the treatment rights of handicapped persons led to an increased awareness of, and concern about, adult mentally retarded persons' right to (outpatient) treatment. On the other hand, however, the pervasive and intense impact of the Education for All Handicapped Children Act had a rather inadvertent effect on treatment services for mentally retarded adults. So much energy and so many resources were directed toward developing educational programs for seriously handicapped children and adolescents that relatively little attention and few resources were directed toward services for seriously mentally retarded adults. Consequently, whereas literally thousands of severely and profoundly mentally retarded youth were enrolled in school programs for the first time in the late 1970s and the early 1980s because of P.L. 94-142, many of those same persons were suddenly faced with *no* habilitative services—be they inpatient or outpatient—once they legally aged out of eligibility for public education programs (i.e., when they turned 18 or 21 years old, depending on various state regulations regarding legal school age).

As parents, advocates, and service providers were faced with the sudden lack of treatment services when their sons, daughters, and/or clients became too old for school, the gross lack of services—including outpatient services—for mentally retarded adults became apparent. Subsequently, more resources began to be directed to treatment services for mentally retarded adults. However, to date, the increase in educational and habilitative opportunities that occurred as a result of the right-to-treatment movement has still had considerably more impact on mentally retarded children and adolescents than on adults.

Behavior Modification and Therapy

Whereas the impact of the trends just discussed resulted in increased awareness of the need for outpatient treatment of mentally retarded adults, as well as increased treatment services, the last trend in the service provision of concern here impacted the *content* of treatment regimes. Specifically, since the 1960s, tremendous progress has occurred regarding the development and refinement of behavioral treatment strategies that can be effective with mentally retarded adults. In many ways, the development of behavior-modification and behavior-therapy treatment programs brought new optimism regarding the habilitative potential of mentally retarded persons. To describe the growth in the behavioral treatment procedures that have proved effective with mentally retarded adults would be far beyond the scope of this chapter, and the interested reader is referred to other sources for an overview (e.g., Scibak, 1983; Whitman, Scibak, & Reid, 1983). Suffice it to say at this point that, from a treatment perspective, the wide-scale availability of behavioral procedures has probably had the most significant impact on the potential *efficacy* of outpatient treatment procedures for mentally retarded adults relative to the other developments in service provision over the last several decades. The utility of behavioral treatment procedures—as well as existing shortcomings—is elaborated on later in this chapter.

SPECIAL DIAGNOSTIC CONSIDERATIONS

There are a number of somewhat special diagnostic considerations in regard to providing effective outpatient treatment for mentally retarded adults. Probably the most important concerns in this regard relate to a skill deficit of essentially all adults who are mentally retarded: delayed communicative skills. Difficulties in communicating that are experienced by mentally retarded persons range from articulation problems among individuals who have basic conversational skills to a total lack of any intelligible communicative behaviors.

Because of the pervasive communicative difficulties among mentally retarded adults, many outpatient diagnostic procedures used with other clinical populations that require clients to express themselves are not possible with the mentally retarded (Gualtieri, 1982). Projective techniques and clinical interviews, for example, which require considerable skill in verbal expression, are generally disallowed. Relatedly, many diagnostic instruments that may not require verbal expressive skills *per se* on the part of clients are nevertheless also of little value because of their limited *receptive* language skills, which prohibit clients from understanding a clinician's assessment intent.

The difficulties in using traditional (verbal) diagnostic procedures that arise with mentally retarded adults generally become more pronounced as the severity of retardation increases. To illustrate, whereas certain clinical interview techniques may result in some useful diagnostic information for a clinician working with a mildly mentally retarded individual, such procedures are of considerably less value, if of any value, with a profoundly mentally retarded person. However, even in the former situation, the deficient intellectual capacity of mentally retarded adults compounds the difficulties in using diagnostic strategies that rely heavily on communicative skills (e.g., deficits in memory often prohibit a client's accurate description of significant past events).

One result of the communicative disabilities of mentally retarded adults in regard to diagnostic procedures is that, frequently, caregivers of mentally retarded clients (e.g., parents and group-home staff) must be more involved in the diagnostic process. In particular, the relatively pervasive use of adaptive and maladaptive behavior checklists (see Beck, 1983, for an overview) in diagnostic evaluations of mentally retarded individuals requires a heavy reliance on the caregiver's description of a client's functioning. Reliance on caregiver information frequently results in a somewhat different task for a clinician or diagnostician relative to obtaining diagnostic information directly from a client. In the former case, there is less opportunity for the clinical probing and information seeking that can occur when a skilled diagnostician interacts directly with a client. Additionally, a diagnostician has to be concerned about the accuracy of caregiver information about a client—information that can be intentionally somewhat biased (e.g., if a caregiver perceives that a client must be presented in a certain light in order to receive certain services) or unintentionally distorted (e.g., from a family member who is very emotionally involved with, and/or protective of, a given client).

Partly because of the (potential) inaccuracy that results from relying on caregiver description to obtain diagnostic information about mentally retarded clients, a modification in traditional diagnostic processes that is often needed by outpatient clinicians with this client population is environmental observation (Beck, 1983). In many ways, the most useful means of obtaining relevant and accurate diagnostic information is for a clinician to observe a client in his or her normal living, working, and recreational environments. Unfortunately, such a process can be somewhat costly in terms of a clinician's time (e.g., he or she must travel to various locales). Such a process also requires the consent of a number of individuals in addition to the usual client (or guardian) consent, such as employers and group-home operators, in order to enter various settings for observational purposes. Nevertheless, direct observational methods can be very helpful—and at times essential—in designing and implementing effective outpatient treatment regimes for mentally retarded adults.

FREQUENT CLINICAL PROBLEMS

Summarizing the most frequent types of clinical problems exhibited by mentally retarded adults that are addressed on an outpatient basis is difficult. The difficulty is due to the very large variety of problems that occur across the subpopulations of mentally retarded adults (e.g., mildly, moderately, severely, and profoundly mentally retarded individuals). The clinical problems that a clinician may be faced with on an outpatient basis can range, for example, from low-frequency, dangerously injurious aggressive outbursts by a severely mentally retarded man in a sheltered workshop to the maladaptive eating practices and related obesity of a mildly mentally retarded woman in a supervised apartment-living complex. Nevertheless, certain problems do tend to arise more frequently than other problems among mentally retarded adults and because of their severity and/or widespread detrimental effects in an individual's physical or social environment, these are generally referred more often for outpatient treatment. This chapter section provides examples of some of the most frequent types of clinical problems along with a brief summary of the recommended treatment strategies. Although the treatment approaches to be discussed are tailored as much as possible to the specific types of clinical problems of clients, invariably each client requires some idiosyncratic variations in the general therapy approach. The particular variations depend in large part on the characteristics of the client's social and physical environments, which, as noted earlier, often require direct observation of the client in his or her routine environment by the responsible outpatient clinician. Relatedly, as alluded to in the preceding section, the degree of the severity of retardation of a given client also affects the format of treatment.

Because of the number and variety of reasons for which mentally retarded adults are frequently referred for outpatient treatment, a thorough discussion of recommended treatment strategies for each clinical problem is not possible here because of space limitations. Consequently, only a brief overview is provided, and the interested reader is referred to other sources for elaboration.

Noncompliance

Noncompliance refers to a client's lack of appropriate response to relevant requests or instructions from significant persons (e.g., caregivers and employers) in the client's environment. Noncompliance may be represented by a generalized lack of responding to a variety of instructions across a client's typical day or in relatively restricted situations involving only one or a small number of specific requests. The former type of noncompliance is reflected, for example, in referrals for outpatient treatment for mentally retarded adults who refuse to cooperate with their parents' requests in the home environment in regard to performing the necessary self-care tasks, housekeeping chores, and so on. Examples of the latter type of noncompliance are mentally retarded clients' refusal to go to work or to take prescribed medication.

The recommended treatment strategies involve the same general format for both types of noncompliance in that motivational systems usually need to be established to reinforce compliance with targeted requests (Budd & Fabry, 1986; Kazdin, 1977). Motivational systems involve the systematic provision of desired objects, events, or personal attention when clients do comply with specified requests and/or the withholding of such consequences when clients do not comply. In addition, in the case of generalized noncompliance, caregivers often require training in methods of instructing clients when (and only when) the caregivers can actually *require* compliance by, for example, providing successively more intrusive prompting procedures if a client does not initially comply (see Reid & Schepis, 1986, for elaboration). Caregiver training in this regard is often needed to structure a client's social environment to promote compliant behavior and perhaps, more importantly, to prevent the inadvertent development of client noncompliance by ineffective instruction by caregivers (Reid & Schepis, 1986).

Tantrumming

Tantrumming is typically intense, socially undesirable behavior characterized by one or more of the following: crying, screaming, aggression, self-injury, and property destruction. Such behavior often has very serious consequences for mentally retarded adults in that bodily injury and/or embarrassment to themselves or others results, community agencies or employers discontinue their services to the individuals, and/or costly harm is caused to the physical environment.

The recommended treatment for tantrumming generally takes one of two forms, depending on the presumed causal factors of the outbursts. To illustrate, one relatively common cause of tantrumming is to escape from certain situations: an individual will tantrum to avoid doing something that she or he does not want to do (e.g., a self-care task) or to terminate an unpleasant event (e.g., a work task). Consequently, the recommended treatment approach involves ensuring that the client will be required to fulfill the demands of the situation (e.g., complete a self-care or work task) regardless of tantrumming, so that tantrumming loses its functional (escape) utility for the client. Another treatment strategy is to teach individuals appropriate ways to communicate that they would like to terminate a task (Carr & Durand, 1985). A second common cause of tantrumming is related to physical or social environments that provide relatively minimal stimulation for mentally retarded persons. In the latter case, an individual may tantrum in order to increase social attention (i.e., stimulation) from peers or caregivers. Effective treatment of the latter type of tantrums generally involves teaching caregivers to ignore the tantrum in order to ensure that increased attention will not be provided, or removing a client from an environment that (inadvertently) does provide increased attention via a time-out procedure (Rolider & Van Houten, 1985). Additionally, increased positive attention and stimulation should be provided when a client is engaging in socially desirable behavior and is not tantrumming.

Aggression

Aggressive physical behavior represents a problem among mentally retarded adults that frequently results in a referral for outpatient services because of the ramifications for the individual who is aggressive *and* because of the impact on other individuals in his or her environment. Aggressive behavior, be it a form of mild hand slaps against another person or a full-blown physical assault on someone, is a relatively frequent reason that clients are excluded or expelled from community programs and are referred for institutionalization. Unfortunately, the causes of aggression among mentally retarded adults vary considerably, and hence, there are a variety of recommended treatment strategies—too many to discuss here. However, overall, the treatment for aggression should be based on the identified, or at least presumed, precipitating and/or reinforcing factors associated with aggressive episodes (Carr & Durand, 1985). For example, aggressive behavior that is due to an individual client's wanting to escape from an unpleasant demand situation would be treated differently from aggressive behavior that is independent of demand situations (see the earlier discussion on therapy approaches for tantrumming). Descriptions of treatment approaches for aggressive behavior that vary based on differing causal factors are provided elsewhere (Carr & Durand, 1985).

Property Destruction

In many ways, the impact of maladaptive property destruction by mentally retarded adults is very similar to that of aggressive behavior and, consequently, warrants serious treatment attention. As with aggression, there are a variety of causes of the intentional destruction of property. However, in contrast to aggression, there are two general treatment approaches that can be recommended for working with mentally retarded adults who destroy property, depending in large part on the skill level of the client. With mildly and moderately mentally retarded individuals, a motivation system to positively reinforce appropriate (nondestructive) behavior, similar to that discussed earlier in connection with noncompliance, often represents the treatment of choice. With lower skilled individuals, such as the profoundly mentally retarded, restitution and overcorrection can frequently be quite helpful; the client is required to repair the physical damage that she or he has caused to the environment, and to practice engaging in behavior that is incompatible with property destruction by practicing the appropriate use of the property many times over (see Ferretti & Cavalier, 1983, for a review).

Inappropriate Sexual Behavior

One of the most difficult problems facing clinicians who work with outpatient mentally retarded adults is inappropriate sexual behavior. Sexual activities that result in referrals for outpatient services include masturbating in public, inappropriate touching or fondling of others, and sexual intercourse. The difficulty in treating these types of cases on an outpatient basis is that, not only does a clinician have to determine effective and socially acceptable means of altering the maladaptive practices of a particular client, but the clinician must also remain thoroughly aware of community norms for sexual conduct and ensure that such norms will not be violated. At times, what may seem to be in the best interest of a mentally retarded adult—such as the opportunity to engage in sexual exchange with a consenting partner—may conflict with a given community's standards regarding the sexual behavior of mentally retarded persons.

As with other outpatient clinical problems, the treatment alternatives for inappropriate sexual behavior vary according to the functioning level of the client. Treatment strategies for less seriously retarded persons typically involve an educational process to teach socially appropriate social and dating skills. In addition, more basic sex education is often necessary in terms of teaching an understanding of acceptable physical interactions as well as safe and hygienic sexual practices. For lower skilled mentally retarded persons, these types of instructional practices are generally not very useful, and more direct intervention by caregivers is usually required when inappropriate sexual activity occurs. For example, in treating cases in group-home living arrangements, in which a client may engage in masturbation in the living room or kitchen with other clients present, a caregiver often needs to intervene and redirect the client to his or her bedroom or bathroom—and continue to intervene and redirect over time to successfully teach the client appropriate situations for engaging in various types of sexually related behaviors.

Increasing Production within a Day-Treatment Setting

The clinical problems discussed to this point have focused on discontinuing or decreasing some type of maladaptive activity. There are also problems that are frequently referred on an outpatient basis that require a clinician to find a means of helping a client to *increase* his or her frequency of a given type of activity. Probably the most common example of this kind of outpatient referral is a request to assist a client in increasing his or her productivity within a day-treatment setting. The setting may be one in which clients are performing work, such as a sheltered workshop, or it may be a nonpaid situation, such as a type of adult day-activity program (e.g., an adult education program).

In some ways, insufficient production in a day-treatment setting may seem like a relatively insignificant problem when one considers the ramifications of the other types of outpatient problems noted earlier, such as aggression or deviant sexual behavior. However, insufficient production is a problem that occurs frequently in regard to requests for outpatient treatment assistance. Basically, lack of production can result in a client's being discontinued from a day-service system, which in turn causes other problems because a client is then left with no consistent, constructive activity during the day. This situation often results in the development of maladaptive behaviors as well as a difficult logistical situation for caregivers, who must find a means of providing supervision for a client during the day.

There is a wide variety of procedures that staff in day-treatment settings can use through appropriate clinical consultation to assist clients in increasing their production. Almost all of these procedures involve some type of staff-controlled motivation program and/or an overt and systematic feedback system (e.g., Martin, Pallotta-Cornick, Johnstone, & Goyos, 1980). However, a clinician frequently faces a more systemic problem than finding a way to intervene with a given client to increase production: the day-treatment services offered to clients are provided in a manner that makes it likely that clients will *not* participate and produce at an acceptable rate. The services provided in a day-activity center that does not involve remunerative work, for example, often do not consist of any really *purposeful* things for a client to do (see the following section on treatment modification for elaboration). There is also a frequent lack of any explicit feedback or reward system to encourage sufficient production on the part of clients. Relatedly, if a feedback and reward system is in place, it often is not individualized sufficiently to benefit each client in the setting. In environments where these types of situations exist, the recommended treatment strategy for a clinician who is attempting to assist a mentally retarded adult to improve his or her day-treatment productivity is to work both with the client and with the treatment setting's management to alter its program systems (again, see the section on treatment modification for elaboration).

MODIFICATION AND ADAPTATION OF TREATMENT APPROACHES

As with other special populations discussed in this text, effective outpatient treatment for mentally retarded adults differs along several important dimensions from other types of services for the mentally retarded (i.e., inpatient services and children's services). Perhaps the most useful way to look at the modifications in outpatient treatment services that are needed specifically for mentally retarded adults is to do so in light of the major trends in service provision that were discussed earlier. In this regard, the normalization and deinstitutionalization movements clearly increased the need for more outpatient services for adults, and the right-to-treatment movement helped to heighten professional awareness of the need for more services. In essence, these movements set the stage for the development of a greater number and a wider range of outpatient treatment services for mentally retarded adults than had been provided in the United States before. However, because of the focus of the right-to-treatment movement on mentally retarded children in contrast to mentally retarded adults, the *content* of treatment services has, for the most part, been based on the needs of children and not of mentally retarded adults. Although there is certainly overlap among the treatment needs of mentally retarded children and adults, there are also some serious differences, so that the content of treatment services warrants modification for the latter population. Similarly, although the advent of behavioral treatment approaches undoubtedly resulted in very significant improvements in the efficacy of service provision, there has been a need to alter behavioral strategies specifically for mentally retarded adults who are outpatients. This section discusses these two types of modifications in treatment services.

Modifications in Treatment Content

By the nature of mental retardation, many mentally retarded individuals are in need of special treatment services throughout their life span. During adulthood, a primary focus of treatment services is assistance in acquiring and maintaining some type of remunerative employment. In certain cases, treatment services are used to assist mentally retarded adults to function in the competitive work world with the nonhandicapped populace. However, in many situations, the severity of retardation essentially prohibits a client from truly competing with the nonhandicapped work force. In such cases, treatment services are more frequently directed at assisting mentally retarded adults in succeeding at some type of sheltered employment (Whitman *et al.*, 1983, Chapter 6). In addition, there is a large subpopulation of mentally retarded adults whose mental disabilities and/or accompanying physical handicaps are so severe that even sheltered employment is not likely to be a realistic work goal. This population is typically provided with treatment services that are intended to assist in acquiring more basic adaptive skills that may or may not be related to possibly obtaining some sheltered employment in the future.

The pervasive need for treatment services for mentally retarded adults has resulted in the development of some modifications in traditional outpatient services. In particular, a major modification that has occurred, or that has at least been initiated, pertains to treatment services for lower functioning mentally retarded persons who do not display the skills necessary to allow successful employment on a competitive or sheltered basis. In this case, the modification has been in regard to the *content* of (nonwork) day-treatment services. Specifically, day-treatment programs for very seriously retarded adults have recently been heavily criticized for providing services that offer very little, if any, therapeutic benefit (Green *et al.,* 1986). That is, day treatment services (e.g., services provided in adult day-activity programs and educational programs for adults) have been criticized for focusing on client activities and teaching tasks that offer no assistance to the clients once they leave the day-treatment classroom; the tasks are nonfunctional in terms of assisting the clients to function in their routine living, work and recreational environments (Bates, Renzaglia, & Wehman, 1981; Brown, Pumpian, Baumgart, Vanderventer, Ford, Nisbet, Schroeder, & Gruenewald, 1981).

The difficulty that day-treatment programs experience in providing functional or purposeful teaching to low-skilled retarded clients stems primarily from the developmental model on which these programs are based (Reid, Green, McCarn, Parsons, & Schepis, 1986). The skills to be taught to clients are sequenced according to normal human development—beginning with very simple behaviors, which are sequentially expanded and refined into the complex skills required in normal living experiences. Hence, before a profoundly mentally retarded man is taught to buckle his belt, for example, he might first be taught to establish eye contact in order to develop attending skills, then to put a four-piece puzzle together to develop instruction-following skills, and then to stack toy blocks to develop more refined motor skills. The main problem with this approach for a seriously disabled client is that, even if he acquires the eye contact and the puzzle and block-stacking skills, he still cannot buckle his belt. The former are simply too different from the latter to be of much assistance (Reid *et al.,* 1986).

The developmental strategy just noted, which is typically used in educational programs with mentally retarded *children,* is particularly troublesome when one is working with older adults. Usually, as the difference between a client's chronological age and her or his mental age increases, the developmental goals selected become increasingly irrelevant to assisting the client to function in everyday living (Brown, Branston, Hamre-Nietupski, Pumpian, Certo, & Gruenewald, 1979). In short, traditional readiness-type skills, such as putting pegs in pegboards and stringing toy beads—which are common activities in many day-treatment programs for adults (Green *et al.,* 1986)—may be helpful to children who will have more time and opportunity to progress to more useful tasks but are of questionable value, at best, to seriously retarded adults who have not yet learned the basics of daily living, such as putting on a coat or washing their hands (Reid *et al.,* 1986).

Recognition of the rather pervasive reliance on essentially nonpurposeful activities in day-treatment services for lower functioning mentally retarded adults has led to some significant modifications in the content of those services. Based on a number of suggestions and discussions in the professional literature (Bates *et al.,* 1981; Brown *et al.,* 1979), as well as in recent applied research (Dyer, Schwartz, & Luce, 1984; Reid,

Parsons, McCarn, Green, Phillips, & Schepis, 1985), methods for providing *purposeful* day-treatment services for this population have been developed, and awareness of the importance of providing meaningful services seems to be increasing gradually around the country. Nevertheless, observations of many, if not most, existing day-treatment programs for severely and profoundly mentally retarded adults would most likely reveal a continued predominance of nonpurposeful, "busy-work" activities rather than meaningful teaching tasks.

Modifications in Behavioral Treatment Approaches

As indicated earlier, the development of behavioral treatment strategies—behavior modification and behavior therapy—has had a very significant impact on the effectiveness of the outpatient treatment of mentally retarded adults. However, several key modifications have been needed in the way behavioral treatment strategies are typically implemented with mentally retarded adults relative to other clinical outpatient populations. First, because of the primary impact of the disability of mental retardation (subnormal intellectual functioning), those behavioral treatment strategies that were developed for adults of normal (or above-average) intelligence often have to be modified or abandoned. To illustrate, behavioral contracting, which may be used in behavioral marriage counseling (Knox, 1972), requires a client to understand and agree that if he or she engages in a particular act in the future with his or her spouse, there will be a certain consequence. Such an understanding of the relationship between an action and the resulting consequence may be beyond the capacity of many mentally retarded persons (although certainly not all retarded persons, depending primarily on the severity of retardation). Hence, treatment approaches that required the cognitive ability to relate a cause to effect, as well as similar types of mental reasoning, are contraindicated for many mentally retarded clients.

A second modification in treatment approaches that is often needed pertains to the reason that clients seek outpatient services. Most nonretarded individuals seek outpatient clinical services of their own volition. Because of a variety of factors, it is usually the *caregivers* of mentally retarded adults who seek outpatient services for them. Consequently, the motivation to make a change in one's life may be different for a mentally retarded person. For example, there is a large population of nonhandicapped adults who are willing to voluntarily seek outpatient assistance to reduce or eliminate smoking. Smoking and other forms of tobacco consumption are also a problem among many mentally retarded adults. However, rarely do they express the desire or seek assistance to stop smoking. A large part of the lack of a desire to stop smoking is most likely due to a lack of awareness among mentally retarded adults of the health risks associated with tobacco use.

In essence, the modifications in behavioral treatment strategies that are often needed with mentally retarded adults are really an offshoot of a primary characteristic of many mentally retarded individuals: they remain at least somewhat dependent on caregivers to function successfully in living and work experiences. Of course, the more serious the mental retardation, the more the individuals are dependent on others for survival. Because of this dependence, a modification in treatment provision is required that is more significant than the modifications just discussed. That is, just as many diagnostic procedures must involve the caregivers of mentally retarded adults, the focus of many outpatient *treatment interventions* also has to be the caregivers. Hence, outpatient treatment services are often directed to family members, group-home staff, sheltered-workshop staff, and so on. This type of environmental therapy approach (i.e., environmental in terms of altering the social and interpersonal environment of a client in order to help the client) is one reason that a behavioral focus has been a predominant therapy strategy with mentally retarded adults. Behavioral clinical interventions are generally well suited to altering environmental factors such as the caregiver-controlled antecedent and consequent events that are often needed to change specific client behaviors.

SUMMARY AND FUTURE TRENDS

Although outpatient treatment services for mentally retarded adults has received increased attention in the human service sector during the last decade, much more attention must be given to the expansion and improvement of services that will better meet the treatment needs of this population. The results of the deinstitutionalization and the right-to-treatment movements noted earlier appear to be, in large part, permanent—at least for the foreseeable future. Consequently, there will continue to be a large population of mentally retarded adults in need of outpatient treatment services. In addition, the wide range of clinical problems experienced by this population will require a rather wide range of specific treatment strategies.

As more professional attention is directed to the outpatient treatment needs of mentally retarded adults, it is likely that the human service field will become more aware of serious gaps in the traditional provision of services to this clientele. One such gap that has recently begun to receive professional attention is psychopathology among mentally retarded populations. Historically, psychopathological conditions involving, for example, emotional problems and affective disorders have been a low priority for clinical treatment and research with the mentally retarded (Gualtieri, 1982). The lack of professional attention to these and other psychiatrically related disabilities has been highlighted by the recognition that the incidence of psychopathology among the mentally retarded population is quite high (Matson & Barrett, 1982a). Much more professional attention and study are needed to determine effective means of treating mentally retarded persons who have psychiatric disabilities. Fortunately, this traditional gap in service provision is beginning to receive increased professional attention, and beneficial developments in this area are likely to be forthcoming (see Matson & Barrett, 1982b, for an overview).

Another gap in service provision is treatment services for *elderly* mentally retarded persons. As noted earlier, the thrust of the right-to-treatment movement for mentally retarded individuals has primarily affected children and adolescents. As also noted previously, the focus and content of treatment programs for mentally retarded children and adolescents are often quite irrelevant to mentally retarded adults. When considering the needs of *elderly* mentally retarded persons, the content of treatment programs (e.g., habilitative and educational programs) that have long been used with younger persons is likely to be even more irrelevant. However, all things considered, very little is known about the treatment needs of (and related human services for) the elderly retarded. Considerable research is needed to determine those needs and both the outpatient and inpatient services that will be required. Professional ingenuity will undoubtedly be needed in this area of research because many treatment issues are very complex. For example, although it is accepted that many mentally retarded persons remain dependent to varying degrees on caregivers during their senior years, it is not so clear that the mentally retarded must receive *habilitative or training* services throughout their lives. The question of whether a mentally retarded adult can ''retire'' from certain (or all non-life-sustaining) treatment services must be addressed. If there is a point in a mentally retarded person's life at which treatment or habilitative services should be discontinued, what is that point, and who makes the determination? Relatedly, what should the focus be for the caregivers of dependent mentally retarded adults who are ''in retirement''?

Questions such as these must be answered if all of the treatment needs of mentally retarded adults are to be satisfactorily addressed. Although there is much work still to be done to determine how to effectively meet the many and varied outpatient treatment needs of mentally retarded adults—as well as to ensure that, as treatment knowledge increases, the improved technology will actually be applied to day-to-day service provision—currently, there is good reason for optimism. During the last two decades, tremendous advances have occurred in the development and provision of therapeutic services for mentally retarded persons. If the attention given to this population continues, it is quite likely that very significant improvements will occur. As a result, our ability to provide effective outpatient treatment services to mentally retarded adults should improve dramatically.

REFERENCES

Bates, P., Renzaglia, A., & Wehman, P. (1981). Characteristics of an appropriate education for severely and profoundly handicapped students. *Education and Training of the Mentally Retarded, 16,* 142–149.

Beck, S. (1983). Overview of methods. In J. L. Matson & S. E. Breuning (Eds.), *Assessing the mentally retarded* (pp. 3–26). New York: Grune & Stratton.

Brown, L., Branston, M. B., Hamre-Nietupski, S., Pumpian, I., Certo, N., & Gruenewald, L. (1979). A strategy for developing chronological-age-appropriate and functional curricular content for severely handicapped adolescents and young adults. *Journal of Special Education, 13,* 81–90.

Brown, L., Pumpian, I., Baumgart, D., Vanderventer, P., Ford, A., Nisbet, J., Schroeder, J., & Gruenewald, L. (1981). Longitudinal transition plans in programs for severely handicapped students. *Exceptional Children, 47,* 624–630.

Budd, K. S., & Fabry, P. L. (1986). Parent and family planning. In R. P. Barrett (Ed.), *Severe behavior disorders in the mentally retarded* (pp. 235–271). New York: Plenum Press.

Carr, E. G., & Durand, V. M. (1985). Reducing behavior problems through functional communication training. *Journal of Applied Behavior Analysis, 18,* 111–126.

Dyer, K., Schwartz, I. S., & Luce, S. C. (1984). A supervision program for increasing functional activities for severely handicapped students in a residential setting. *Journal of Applied Behavior Analysis, 17,* 249–259.

Ferretti, R. P., & Cavalier, A. R. (1983). A critical assessment of overcorrection procedures with mentally retarded persons. In J. L. Matson & F. Andrasik (Eds.), *Treatment issues and innovations in mental retardation* (pp. 241–301). New York: Plenum Press.

Green, C. W., Reid, D. H., McCarn, J. M., Schepis, M. M., Phillips, J. F., & Parsons, M. B. (1986). Naturalistic observations of classrooms serving severely handicapped persons: Establishing evaluative norms. *Applied Research in Mental Retardation, 7,* 37–50.

Grossman, H. J. (Ed.). (1983). *Classification in mental retardation.* Washington, DC: American Association on Mental Deficiency.

Gualtieri, C. T. (1982). Forward. In J. L. Matson & R. P. Barrett (Eds.), *Psychopathology in the mentally retarded* (pp. ix–xi). New York: Grune & Stratton.

Kazdin, A. E. (1977). The token economy: A review and evaluation. New York: Plenum Press.

Knox, D. (1972). *A behavioral approach to marriage happiness counseling.* Champaign, IL: Research Press.

Maloney, M. P., & Ward, M. P. (1979). *Mental retardation and modern society.* New York: Oxford University Press.

Martin, G., Pallotta-Cornick, A., Johnstone, G., & Goyos, A. C. (1980). A supervisory strategy to improve work performance for lower functioning retarded clients in a sheltered workshop. *Journal of Applied Behavior Analysis, 13,* 183–190.

Matson, J. L., & Barrett, R. P. (1982a). Preface. In J. L. Matson & R. P. Barrett (Eds.), *Psychopathology in the mentally retarded* (pp. xiii–xiv). New York: Grune & Stratton.

Matson, J. L., & Barrett, R. P. (1982b). *Psychopathology in the mentally retarded.* New York: Grune & Stratton.

Payne, J. E. (1976). The deinstitutionalization backlash. *Mental Retardation, 14,* 43–45.

Reid, D. H., & Schepis, M. M. (1986). Direct care staff training. In R. P. Barrett (Ed.), *Severe behavior disorders in the mentally retarded: Nondrug approaches to treatment.* New York: Plenum Press.

Reid, D. H., Parsons, M. B., McCarn, J. M., Green, C. W., Phillips, J. F., & Schepis, M. M. (1985). Providing a more appropriate education for severely handicapped persons: Increasing and validating functional classroom tasks. *Journal of Applied Behavior Analysis, 18,* 289–301.

Reid, D. H., Green, C. W., McCarn, J. M., Parsons, M. B., & Schepis, M. M. (1986). *Providing purposeful training for severely handicapped persons: A trainer's guidebook.* Morganton, NC: Western Carolina Center.

Rolider, A., & Van Houten, R. (1985). Movement suppression time-out for undesirable behavior in psychotic and severely developmentally delayed children. *Journal of Applied Behavior Analysis, 18,* 275–288.

Scibak, J. W. (1983). *Behavioral treatment.* In J. L. Matson & J. A. Mulick (Eds.), *Handbook of mental retardation* (pp. 339–350). New York: Pergamon Press.

Stacy, D., Doleys, D. M., & Bruno, J. (1983). Implementing behavioral programs in the community. In J. L. Matson & F. Andrasik (Eds.), *Treatment issues and innovations in mental retardation* (pp. 37–60). New York: Plenum Press.

Whitman, T. L., Scibak, J. W., & Reid, D. H. (1983). *Behavior modification with the severely and profoundly retarded: Research and application.* New York: Academic Press.

Wolfensberger, W. (1976). Will there always be an institution? II. The impact of new service models. In M. Rosen, G. R. Clark, & M. S. Kivitz (Eds.), *The history of mental retardation collected papers* (Vol. 2, pp. 415–432). Baltimore: University Park Press.

25

Mentally Ill Substance Abusers

Bick Wanck

INTRODUCTION

Mentally ill substance abusers have two illnesses. The first is the substance abuse pattern, one that may involve signs of physical dependency including tolerance and withdrawal, and that often creates problems in employment, relationships, and legal areas. Second, this group suffers more severe emotional and cognitive disturbances than those one ordinarily sees in people who abuse substances. The overlap between the two illnesses often leads to diagnostic confusion and complicates treatment strategies.

Differing philosophies from diverse treatment and recovery groups further complicate the development of consistent treatment approaches for mentally ill substance abusers. Because each treatment group has differing perspectives and backgrounds, these groups subject mentally ill substance abusers to differing diagnoses and treatments. Tragically, the result is frequent rejection or inadequate treatment. Substance abusers with concomitant mental illnesses may bounce from one treatment orientation to another and typically receive either no care, interrupted care, or poorly coordinated care. When rejection from treatment occurs, it often stems from a failure to understand the complexities involved in diagnosing and treating mentally ill substance abusers. Psychiatric education, for example, has been particularly deficient on the addictions.

Helping mentally ill addicts engage in abstinence and sobriety is of crucial importance in treatment. Whatever the type of substance abuse, it takes a toll in terms of illness and premature death. Furthermore, persistence in active substance abuse may render efforts to stabilize the mental illness ineffective. In one sense, mental health treatment may be viewed as supportive of the effort of maintaining the substance abuser in a state of sobriety. Conversely, however, patients may be unable to attain sobriety without adequate

BICK WANCK • Saratoga Therapy and Training, Saratoga Springs, New York 12866; and Albany Medical College, Albany, New York 12302.

treatment of their mental illness. Thus, treatment staffs must address both conditions adequately. Triaging and the timing of the treatments are crucial.

TERMINOLOGY

Clinicians and researchers have applied various terms to this group. *Dual diagnosis* is a popular term applied to patients who evidence at least one substance-abuse diagnosis and, in addition, at least one mental-disorder diagnosis. Programs addressing the problem are called *dual diagnosis programs*. One study (Kofoed, Kania, Walsh, & Atkinson, 1986) referred to this group as psychiatrically impaired substance abusers (PISA). This writer prefers the term *mentally ill substance abusers* because substance abuse appears as a diagnostic entity in the third edition of the American Psychiatric Association's *Diagnostic and Statistical Manuel of Mental Disorders* (DSM-III; APA, 1980). Furthermore, *mental illness* is more inclusive a term than *psychiatric illness* and implies a subset of mental disorders that may result from addictions.

The term *mentally ill substance abuser* also highlights the difference between substance abuse and mental illness. *Mental illness* evokes an association of greater than normal emotional distress or cognitive disruption; mental illnesses involve symptoms that generally do not respond to the usual addiction-treatment approaches. Although emotional distress and cognitive disruption frequently accompany substance abuse disorders, the symptoms do not constitute diagnostic categories unless they are unusually severe.

I use the term *substance abuse* appears throughout this chapter to be consonant with the DSM-III. Both chemical abuse and chemical dependency appear under the category of substance abuse. In this chapter, I do not discriminate between psychological addiction and physical addiction; rather, I use the term *substance abuse* to mean severe disruption because of substance use with or without physical tolerance. The term *addiction* also appears in this chapter as a synonym for *substance abuse,* although with the recognition that differing levels of severity and differing patterns of addiction exist.

EPIDEMIOLOGY

Figures on the rates of mentally ill substance abusers, though quite variable, suggest a large population. Kofoed *et al.* (1986) performed a computation on data from the National Institute of Mental Health (NIMH) Epidemiologic Catchment Area Studies (Myers, Weissman, Tischler, Holzer, Leaf, Orvaschel, Anthony, Boyd, Burke, Kramer, & Stoltzman, 1984) and found that 21%–39% of substance abusers also met the criteria for another DSM-III diagnosis at some time during the 6 months preceding their evaluation. Some of the study's coexisting mental-illness diagnoses may not be valid because the researchers failed to control for substance-induced abuse mental disorders which may have mimicked primary mental disorders in some subjects.

In another study, Fischer, Halikas, Baker, and Smith (1976) found that one third of the patients admitted to a general psychiatry hospital for mental illness were also substance abusers. Powell, Penick, Othmer, Bingham, and Rice (1982) reported that almost two thirds of male alcoholics fulfilled the criteria for one or more additional psychiatric syndromes, primarily affective disorders and antisocial personality disorder. Weiss and

Rosenberg (1985) found that 22.6% of alcoholics met the criteria for one or more anxiety disorders. Finally, in a study of a group of 533 opiate addicts in treatment, 70.3% were diagnosed as having an additional mental disorder (Rounsaville, Weissman, Kleber, & Wilber, 1982).

The diagnosis of mental illness in substance abusers is fraught with methodological problems. Reviewing the literature on the prevalence of depression in alcoholics, for example, Keeler, Taylor, and Miller (1979) found rates varying from 3% to 98%. They demonstrated that the use of differing diagnostic techniques threatens the reliability of such studies. Using three different diagnostic instruments to assess recently detoxified alcoholics, they reported that the rates of depression varied from 8.6% to 43%, depending on the instrument.

Another fundamental methodological issue concerns whether one should seek to diagnose mental illness in substance abusers during the course of treatment. Schuckit (1985), endeavoring to diagnose pure major affective disorder in treated alcoholics, assigned the diagnosis only if alcoholic patients had symptoms that met the diagnostic criteria for major affective disorder either (1) before the first major life problem attributable to alcohol or (2) after 3 or more months of abstinence. Using this method, he found that only 2% of the alcoholics he studied had "true" major affective disorder.

Using a similar approach with cocaine addicts, Gawin and Kleber (1986) sought to separate cocaine addicts with primary mental-illness diagnoses from those with secondary mental illness by waiting 10 days before making the diagnosis. They also noted, however, that symptoms such as dysphoria, anxiety, and irritability may accompany cocaine craving for 10 or more weeks after the last dose of cocaine. This finding suggests that their 54% rate of other DSM-III Axis I mental-illness diagnoses would probably have been lower had they waited the 10 weeks it takes for the early-abstinence craving phase to pass.

The wide discrepancies in the reported rates of coexisting mental-illness diagnoses and addiction diagnoses underscore the difficulty faced by clinicians in making accurate diagnoses. Studies to date suggest that roughly one third of all mental patients have substance abuse problems and that at least one third of all substance abusers have mental illness.

HISTORICAL OVERVIEW

Four core concepts about substance abuse have developed throughout history. They have strongly influenced our treatment approaches to mentally ill substance abusers. These concepts also help to explain the divergence in the theories expounded by various groups treating and helping the mentally ill substance abuser today. These differing views help to explain why mentally ill substance abusers frequently "fall between the cracks" of the various treatment and recovery options. These four concepts illustrate the struggle through recent history to try to understand the etiology of substance abuse. The four concepts about addiction, in historical order of development, are

1. The moral weakness concept
2. The psychological disease concept
3. The spiritual impoverishment concept
4. The biological disease concept

Throughout an examination of historical events, the following discussion demonstrates how these concepts have developed and how they influence current treatment, attitudes, and approaches.

Historical evidence shows that people have pondered the relationship between substance abuse and mental illness for some time. In A.D. 1037, the Arabic physician Aurcenna died of an opium overdose (Seixas, 1980). This event served to highlight similar tragedies and to open discussion about the extent and nature of the dangers of opium use. In the early 1800s, Thomas De Quincey wrote a book entitled *Confessions of an English Opium Eater*. In a follow-up article in 1822, he wrote, "was it opium or was it opium in combination with something else that raised these storms?" (Ebin, 1961, p. 52). His "storms" were bouts of emotional chaos and disordered thinking. Rephrased, his question was: How much are these problems caused by the effect of the drug and how much are they caused by other processes? De Quincey's query was perceptive and, at the time, controversial. When he posed his question about the etiology of his illness, addiction was viewed as a moral weakness.

The Moral Weakness Concept of Addiction

During the 1820s and 1830s, the Inebriety Movement gained momentum and became popularized. By the mid-1830s, millions of Americans were registered members of the Inebriety Movement and had chosen not to use alcohol. The movement spread internationally. Those who participated in the Inebriety Movement saw addiction as an evil scourge, and they endeavored to stay free of its influence through a life of abstinence.

Another powerful movement in the 19th century was the Women's Christian Temperance Union (Seixas, 1980). This group viewed alcohol as a tool of the devil. Alcoholism was seen as evidence of moral weakness—the inability to resist the temptation of evil.

Given the limited understanding of the physiology of addiction and the general attitudes at the time, this perspective was an understandable one. Nineteenth-century society viewed alcoholism as a destructive phenomenon of epidemic proportions, causing loss of employment, broken homes, public drunkenness, child abuse, and other forms of violence. The social philosophers could understand this phenomenon only by identifying it as morally abhorrent. If the offending substance was labeled "evil," it could be isolated and avoided. People could then support one another's efforts to abstain from "demon rum" and thus escape the devastative effects of alcoholism. From a public health perspective, the isolation and avoidance of the pathogen (alcohol) may have helped to limit the spread of the disease.

The problem with the moral weakness approach was that it fostered an attitude of hopelessness and a lack of respect for the alcoholic. Just as alcohol was seen as the creation and tool of the devil, alcoholics were seen as the devil's disciples—destined to a lost life and lost morality. Nineteenth-century society viewed alcoholics as morally flawed, lacking the willpower to resist temptation. The moral weakness concept of alcoholism contributed to a sense of despair and shame for alcoholics and their families. This societal attitude, in turn, probably worsened the course of the disease for most alcoholics.

The Psychological Disease Concept of Addiction

The moral weakness concept was the predominant means of understanding addiction by laypeople and health-care workers alike until the 1870s. In 1870, Joseph Parish, a psychiatrist, founded the American Association for the Cure of Inebriates (Jaffe, 1978). This group held the conviction that addiction was not a moral failure but a psychological disease that could be treated medically. This new theory heralded the beginning of the psychological disease concept of addiction, in which addiction was seen as either a symptom or a cause of mental illness. In 1877, an American psychiatrist, John Mitchell, concluded that there was a close relationship between alcohol abuse and insanity (Seixas, 1980). He based his conclusion on 26 years of experience with "lunatics" and also stated that excessive drinking might lead those who were predisposed to insanity to become insane (Jaffe, 1978).

Sigmund Freud unwittingly became involved in the addiction scene with his 1884 paper "On Coca." In it, he proposed that cocaine be used for nonopiate detoxification from morphine addiction (Byck, 1974). Freud found cocaine to have numerous medicinal benefits and was himself an intermittent heavy user. In current conceptualization, Freud was a victim of the first cocaine epidemic, which occurred in the 1880s (Musto, 1986). Given his cocaine abuse and his self-diagnosed neurosis, Freud was one of our most famous mentally ill substance abusers. A tragic footnote is that he ultimately lost his life to cancer of the jaw because of his strongest addiction: tobacco dependence.

In the early 1900s, proponents of the psychological disease concept of addiction persisted in their approach to addiction. An American psychiatrist, Thom Williams, advanced the belief in 1912 that drug users were neurotic and suffered from feelings of inadequacy that led to depression and a desire to alleviate their depression through the use of drugs (Jaffe, 1978). Until 1919 and the advent of Prohibition, mental health workers generally agreed that inebriety was a symptom of mental illness. With the onset of Prohibition, societal attitudes returned to a pervasive sense that addicts were incurable; this time, alcoholics were seen as incurable psychopaths rather than incurable followers of evil (Seixas, 1980).

The 1930s psychoanalytic writing about drug addiction emphasized the "hedonic" aspects of the addict, who was relentlessly driven to a search for "superpleasure." Thus, in social terms, the addict was seen as an irresponsible, pleasure-seeking, incurable psychopath. There was a strong sense of frustration on the part of treaters and despair on the part of addicts. This despair gave rise to a new theory regarding the etiology of addiction and to an innovative and successful treatment for addicts.

The Spiritual Impoverishment Concept of Addiction

The spiritual impoverishment concept of addiction began in the 1930s when a frightened alcoholic realized that without help he would die. Out of desperation, he traveled to Switzerland to meet with Carl Jung. Jung's treatment involved spiritual principles and was successful in helping the man arrest his alcoholism. Exuberant with the results, he returned to the United States and met with Bill Wilson, also an alcoholic, who was disenchanted by the medical approach to treating his disease. Bill Wilson was influenced by the man's work with Carl Jung, by Jung himself, and by the book *The Varieties of Religious Experience: A Study in Human Nature* (1961) by William James. Along with others, Bill Wilson developed the 12 steps and 12 traditions of Alcoholics Anonymous (AA), a lifelong, nondenominational, spiritually based program for recovery (Thomsen, 1975). Remarkably, alcoholics themselves ultimately developed the most successful treatment for the disease.

The thesis that laid the foundation for AA was that alcoholism progressively led to a loss of health, relationships, and values. The founders of AA felt that the alcoholic was spiritually impoverished and in need of support and discipline through fellowship with a group and through belief in a higher power. AA provided hope for the alcoholic, something the medical system had been unable to do. Understandably, a mistrust of the medical system developed along with AA principles.

Meanwhile, psychiatry continued to struggle with the diagnosis and treatment of substance abusers. Because alcoholics had severe lifestyle disruption and often presented with disordered thinking and emotional disturbances, they were frequently misdiagnosed as schizophrenic or manic-depressive. Alcoholics were subjected to treatment with neuroleptics, antidepressants, and electroconvulsive therapy (ECT). Such misdiagnoses and mistreatments served to further polarize AA and the psychiatric treatment field. From the gap between the two approaches, however, a new concept and treatment approach has recently arisen: the biological disease concept of addiction.

The Biological Disease Concept of Addiction

Proponents of the biological concept of addiction see addiction as a medical illness like diabetes. For support, they cite *The Disease Concept of Alcoholism* (1960) by Jellinek, genetic studies by Goodwin (1983), and research on neurotransmitters. By describing addiction as strictly a biological problem, one can erase the issue of culpability, diminish the guilt, and more readily confront the denial. Although it often disregards the importance of the environmental and psychological contributors to addiction, the biological disease approach helped addicts by simplifying their initial perception of their disease and by focusing their efforts on the most important aspects of treatment: abstinence and sobriety.

The biological disease concept became a competing theory with the psychological disease concept. During the 1970s and 1980s, psychoanalytic circles generated a proliferation of papers describing the developmental problems suffered by addicts. Generalizing from specific cases, many of these theorists implied that, by understanding the developmental lags and conflicts in individual addicts, one could decipher the underlying reasons for their drug use. Some writers matched specific personality types with the addictive drugs (Milkman & Frosch, 1973). Using this theoretical concept, for example, Khantzian (1985) suggested that heroin addicts were self-medicating their rage. Ultimately, a rift developed between the proponents of the biological disease concept and those of the psychological disease concept.

In the late 1970s, as the biological and the psychological disease proponents differed, some mental-health researchers began to discriminate between addicts with coexisting mental illness and addicts who did not have mental illness. Fowler, Liskow, and Tanna (1977) reported that addicts had no greater rate of mental illness than nonaddicts. More recently, writers (Gawin & Kleber, 1986; Schucket, 1983) have begun to differentiate between mental illness symptoms caused by substance abuse and mental illnesses having a non-substance-abuse etiology. The four basic theories of the etiology of addiction (the moral weakness, spiritual impoverishment, biological disease, and psychological disease concepts) still draw adherents and often lead to diagnostic and treatment difficulties for the mentally ill substance abuser. Much of society and some treatment staff still see addicts as immoral individuals without the willpower to resist temptation. The psychological disease concept is still popular among clinicians; for example, the DSM-III classifies addictions as mental disorders.

Although different theoretical constructs serve to increase overall understanding, they may also polarize treatment staff, intensify extremist positions, and decrease treatment options. The 1980s, however, ushered in a period of consolidation in which proponents of the various concepts learned from one another and modified their treatment approaches as they incorporated what they had learned. As a result, for the first time, the mentally ill substance abuser received more attention. Such efforts have raised the hope that the mentally ill substance abuser will obtain the best treatment available.

SPECIAL DIAGNOSTIC CONSIDERATIONS

Before determining whether a patient has a true (primary) mental illness or a substance-induced (secondary) mental illness, clinicians must determine two issues. The first is whether a mental illness exists in a substance abuser, and the second is whether a substance abuse pattern exists in a patient with symptoms of mental illness. The diagnosis of substance abuse in a patient with mental illness rests largely on history, which, in turn, may be imperfectly reported by the patient. Because of the problems of denial and minimization, the patient's history is often unreliable, and it may be necessary to corroborate the history by interviewing other people. Family, friends, and employers often provide detailed histories, although they, too, may be influenced by denial. Occasionally, the clinician makes the diagnosis of substance abuse through personal observation, such as signs of intoxication in the session, the smell of alcohol, or variable cognitive and mood states that cannot be explained by the reported information. At other times, evidence may emerge from blood tests, such as abnormal liver enzymes from heavy alcohol use. Laboratory studies should include urine-drug-screen and blood-alcohol-level tests, which the clinician should reorder randomly during the course of treatment if there is a question of active substance abuse. Because of the pervasiveness of denial, a history suggestive of substance abuse generally indicates that it exists.

In order to determine whether mental illness exists in a substance abuser, the clinician needs to take a thorough history for emotional disturbance, a thinking disorder, eating and sexual aberrations, and maladaptive patterns of behavior. The history should also include questions about suicidal thoughts or behavior and assaultiveness. Often, the history requires collaboration by family, friends, or employer. Another sign that mental illness exists occurs within a substance-abuse-treatment population when other patients point out that a given patient does not fit their social culture. Another indication that a substance abuser may have coexisting mental illness is an inability to grasp the meaning of recovery. Because this inability frequently results from denial, the person may need staff confrontation. Persistence in difficulty fitting into an addiction-recovery treatment program often corroborates an initial impression of the presence of a mental illness.

Once the clinician and the treatment staff have established the presence of a mental illness in a substance abuser, they must determine whether it is a primary mental illness or a secondary (substance-induced) mental illness. Several techniques exist to aid the clinician in making this differential diagnosis. Determining the timing of the symptoms is important. If the symptoms existed before the person's substance abuse, the symptoms at that time were not substance-induced. If the mental illness symptoms existed during substance use but before a full substance-use pattern developed, the symptoms are likely to represent a mental illness. If the symptoms of mental illness persist during an active addiction pattern, they may represent a primary mental illness, possibly, but not necessarily, worsened by the substance abuse pattern.

It is interesting that no current research designs include diagnoses of substance-induced organic mental disorders, such as organic affective disorder or organic delusional disorder, as classified in the DSM-III (APA, 1980), perhaps because of the relatively short term and the reversible nature of most substance-induced mental-illness symptoms. In addition, clinicians may view these conditions as such an inextricable part of the addictive illness that they do not merit separate diagnostic labels. Because some symptoms persist past the early detoxification or abstinence phase, there appears to be a diagnostic and treatment reason to use these diagnoses in more severe cases.

Another piece of information that is important in making the differential diagnosis is family history. When a patient presents with substance abuse and symptoms of a thinking disorder, coupled with a family history of schizophrenia, there is a possibility that the symptoms represent a true psychotic illness. However, even with a strong genetic history of psychosis, a psychotic substance abuser may have a time-limited toxic psychosis rather than a true thinking disorder.

The differential diagnosis of primary versus secondary mental illness can be most accurately made retrospectively. Except for dementia, substance-induced mental illnesses are time-limited. One can rule them out by waiting them out. Alcohol-induced depression rarely lasts longer than 3 weeks after the last drink. Cocaine- or amphetamine-induced psychosis rarely persists beyond 6 weeks after the last drug use. If mental illness symptoms persist beyond the time expected for substance-induced symptoms, they generally indicate the presence of a primary mental illness. Although the family history and the timing of the onset of the mental illness are important diagnostic determinants, the most accurate diagnostic test is waiting out possible substance-induced symptoms. The following section outlines the lengths of time within which symptoms of various substance-induced mental illnesses abate.

Thus, an imposing challenge facing clinicians is whether to treat mental illness symptoms during the early period of abstinence. Active treatment during this phase makes the diagnosis more difficult to establish. For example, by treating depressed alcoholics immediately, one cannot determine if their depression symptoms were substance-induced or due to primary mental illness. Generally, clinicians should suspend pharmacotherapy for mental illness symptoms until there is clear indication of a primary mental illness. If the patient urgently needs medication, it may be wise to withdraw it carefully after a few weeks to determine whether the illness is primary or secondary.

SPECIFIC DIAGNOSTIC COMBINATIONS

As the clinician searches to rule out or diagnose primary mental illness in the substance abuser, it is important to remember that any type of substance abuse may coexist with any type of primary mental illness. Moreover, substance abuse may exacerbate the symptoms or course of any mental illness. Paradoxically, however, substance abuse may also cause or induce symptoms of mental illness. Some writers have referred to substance-induced or secondary mental illnesses as "mimicry," emphasizing the temporary and generally fully reversible nature of these conditions, but failing to give full credence to the degree of suffering and incapacitation involved and to the occasional need for treatment intervention. Because substance-induced mental illnesses may have the same symptoms as true mental illnesses, clinicians can easily be led to a misdiagnosis. Misdiagnosis, in turn, may cause excessive or inappropriate treatment and inaccurate labeling. The specific diagnostic combinations in this section illustrate some of the more common examples of substance-induced mental illnesses; those that have been misdiagnosed historically as primary mental illnesses. Other examples of diagnostic combinations illustrate interesting interactions between mental illnesses and substance abuse patterns.

Depression and Alcoholism

Probably the most commonly misdiagnosed combination is alcoholism and depression. Reported rates of concurrent major depression and alcoholism range from 3% to 98% (Keeler *et al.,* 1979). Thus, following the literature, some clinicians rarely treat alcoholics with antidepressants, and others almost always do. The following discussion presents the reason for such a wide discrepancy in the diagnostic rates for depression with alcoholism.

People who are actively alcoholic, who are in alcohol withdrawal, or who have recently ended a heavy drinking bout often experience dysphoria and feelings of worthlessness. They generally evidence insomnia, anorexia, decreased libido, and low energy. Quite often, they feel suicidal and, tragically, may occasionally succeed in their suicide efforts. Because these symptoms are precisely those of major depressive disorders, it is little wonder that these individuals are frequently diagnosed as having depression and are determined to need antidepressant medication.

One group of researchers (Keller, Klerman, Lavori, Coryell, Endicott, & Taylor, 1984) recommended that treatment for depression accompanying alcoholism begin as soon as possible after the onset of depressive symptoms. Other researchers have interpreted depressive symptoms in alcoholics differently. Schuckit (1983) reported that depression in alcoholics is time-limited and usually disappears without active antidepressant treatment after a period that varies in duration from 2 days to 2 weeks of abstinence. In another study (Wiengold, Lachin, Bell, & Coxe, 1968), 70% of 73 alcoholic patients exhibited symptoms consistent with depression. The symptoms of depression remitted spontaneously with abstinence, irrespective of the treatment used. Additional support for the early spontaneous remission of the symptoms of depression in newly abstinent alcoholics stems from a study of the dexamethasone suppression test (DST) in alcoholics (Dackis, Baily, Pottash, Stuckey, Extein, & Gold, 1985). This group studied nondepressed alcoholics and found that abnormal DST results (positive for depression) normalized after 3 weeks of abstinence.

In a detailed description of primary and secondary depression in alcoholics, Schuckit (1986) reported much higher rates of secondary depression than of primary depression. He found that, in one group of alcoholics, about 30% had had an alcohol-induced affective episode during their years of heavy drinking. He found that the "severe depressions occurring during heavy drinking rarely run the course of primary affective episodes" (p. 142). This finding is consistent with another report (Dave & Wanck, 1985) that, in an alcoholic rehabilitation program, only 3 of 400 alcoholics needed treatment with antidepressant medication.

The time-limited secondary depression associated with alcoholism is quite common, whereas primary major depression in alcoholics appears to occur approximately as often as does primary major depression in the general population. The diagnosis of primary major depression can be made only if the symptoms persist longer than 3 weeks after the last drink. Because secondary depression in alcoholics is so time-limited, the differential diagnosis can be made in less than a month, provided the patient has stopped drinking.

Depression and Cocaine Abuse

Like alcoholism, cocaine abuse commonly coexists with depression. Cocaine abusers appear with a variety of mental health symptoms, including, for most, symptoms consistent with depression. The most familiar period of depressive symptomatology in cocaine abusers is known as the post-cocaine-use "crash." The crash in cocaine abuse has been described (Gawin & Kleber, 1986), as has the crash in amphetamine abuse, which causes a similar postuse depression (Kramer, Fischman, & Littlefield, 1967). The symptoms of the crash are generally the same as the symptoms of major depression. In addition to neurovegetative signs, patients experience extreme dysphoria, with sadness, anxiety, and irritability. They also often have temporary but strong suicidal urges. These signs may be accompanied by paranoid feelings that may attain psychotic levels. Virtually everyone who engages in a chronic, severe, repetitive binge pattern of cocaine abuse experiences the crash. It generally starts within an hour after the last dose of cocaine (or amphetamine) and lasts from several hours to 1 week.

A longer phase of post-cocaine-binge depression was described by Gawin and Kleber (1986) as a "withdrawal phase" starting within a few days after the "crash" phase and lasting from 1 to 10 weeks. This "cocaine abstinence depression" is characterized by sadness, anxiety, irritability, and anergia. The hallmark of this phase is a strong craving for cocaine. As in the "crash" phase, the symptoms of the "withdrawal" phase may be confused with primary depression. The way to rule out depression is to wait out the symptoms. One can either avoid treating the depressive symptoms pharmacologically for 10 weeks or discontinue pharmacotherapy on a trial basis at the end of the 10-week withdrawal phase.

Other Combinations of Affective Illness and Substance Abuse

Drugs of abuse are also known as mood-altering chemicals. Pharmacologically, they alter affect both during their use and following the discontinuation of heavy use. Substance abuse in general, because of its disruptive effect on many aspects of people's lives, may lead to feelings of guilt, shame, and worthlessness. Because of its addictive aspects, substance abuse may lead to feelings of hopelessness and helplessness. Conversely, early recovery, because of its epiphonic and liberating effect, may lead to euphoria through the exhilarating "pink-cloud" effect. Finally, substantial mood shifts are quite common during the first year of recovery while neurotransmitters reequilibrate and lifestyle stabilizes.

Specific substances—caffeine and nicotine—may induce affective conditions and thus merit inclusion here. Although clinicians are aware that stimulants, including cocaine, may produce a hypomanic or manic effect, many are unaware that the powerful mood-elevating effect of caffeine may produce dysfunction and significant impairment. Caffeine intoxication and abuse are quite common among addicts in recovery (coffeepots are standard equipment at most AA meetings). Both acute and chronic heavy caffeine use may present exactly as does hypomania or mania. Nicotine, a powerfully addictive stimulant, may produce mood shifts during intoxication; nicotine is also notable for causing extreme mood shifts and confusion during withdrawal. Idiosyncratic manic episodes are also seen occasionally during sedative intoxication and withdrawal. As in other drug-induced mental-illness symptoms, discontinuation of the drug and waiting for the symptom period to pass may reveal the presence or absence of more enduring psychopathology.

Psychosis and Cocaine and Amphetamine Abuse

Heavy cocaine abuse may affect thinking as well as mood. The typical thinking disorder of chronic cocaine intoxication is paranoia. Cocaine-induced paranoid delusions may be quite intense. The delusions often center on fears of being caught by police or confronted by significant others. No matter what the route of administration, chronic heavy cocaine use may cause a previously sane person to hallucinate, to experience delusions, and to talk incessantly and incoherently. This phenomenon is clearly neurochemical in origin, although it may look like a true paranoia, schizophrenia, or nonsubstance-induced atypical psychosis. It generally remits with the cessation of cocaine use.

During early abstinence, however, psychotic delusions may accompany dysphoria and other symptoms of depression. Thus, the condition resembles major depression with psychotic features. In this case, the psychotic symptoms generally recede with the depressive symptoms. Occasionally, patients develop longer term cocaine-induced psychotic symptoms, most frequently of a paranoid delusional type. This condition has also been called a *toxic psychosis*. Ordinarily, this condition runs its course within a few weeks and does not require treatment. Occasionally, it is severe enough to warrant antipsychotic mediation treatments. Trial discontinuation of the medication should be attempted around the 2-month mark to rule out longer lasting psychopathology and to reduce the risk of side effects in those who no longer need the medication. Similar effects occur with amphetamines. Amphetamines are well known for their disorganizing quality at high doses. Postuse psychosis is seen even more frequently with amphetamines than with cocaine. Nevertheless, it, too, is time-limited. Making the proper differential diagnosis between postuse psychosis and schizophrenia depends on waiting to see whether the symptoms remit.

Anxiety States and Sedative Abuse

Clinical evidence indicates that individuals with anxiety diagnoses may abuse sedatives. Sedatives of abuse include alcohol, benzodiazepines, and barbiturates. In addition to their sedating effects, these drugs have an antianxiety effect. They also intensify anxiety when, during chronic use, their effect periodically wears off, producing a withdrawal state. Sedative and anxiety states interact in a number of ways. Primary anxiety states (e.g., generalized anxiety, phobias, and panic states) may coexist with primary sedative abuse. The symptoms of anxiety disorders may be reduced by the sedating effects of drugs but may also be intensified by the withdrawal effects of drugs. Moreover, the shame and guilt of addiction may intensify sociophobia and agoraphobia. Generally, intense sedative-induced anxiety and phobic symptoms pass within 2 months of the last drug or alcohol use. Persistence of the symptoms may indicate a primary anxiety illness.

Anxiety and phobic states in alcoholics have received increased attention in recent years. Mullaney and Trippett (1979), studying inpatient alcoholics, found that one third had debilitating phobias and that another third were borderline phobic. In another study of inpatient alcoholics (Bowen, Cipynyk, D'Arcy, & Keegan, 1984), 25% were diagnosed as phobic, and 44% were diagnosed as having anxiety disorders. Yet another group (Smail, Stockwell, Canter, & Hodgson, 1984) found that over half of the active alcoholics studied had phobias. All of these studies involved either active alcoholics or alcoholics in withdrawal or very early abstinence. There is evidence (Stockwell, Smail, Hodgson, & Canter, 1984) that chronic heavy drinking exacerbates such conditions and that abstinence leads, in many cases, to resolution of the symptoms of those conditions. It appears that chronic alcoholism may exacerbate and induce anxiety and phobic states. Such alcohol-induced states are generally reversible within a few weeks of abstinence.

Determining whether an anxiety or phobic state is alcohol-induced or whether it is a primary illness coexisting with alcoholism remains a diagnostic challenge. Several studies have examined family histories and the timing of the onset of each illness (anxiety versus alcoholism). One study demonstrated that a family history of affective disorder frequently accompanies a primary anxiety illness (Manjack & Moss, 1981). Anxiety disorders have been found to antedate the onset of alcoholism in patients who have symptoms of both disorders (Bowen *et al.*, 1984). The likelihood of an anxiety or phobic disorder's being primary and not alcohol-induced is greater if the anxiety or phobic disorder started before the alcoholic drinking pattern. The likelihood of a primary disorder is even greater if the anxiety or phobic condition persists despite several weeks of abstinence from alcohol.

Dementia and Alcoholism

The one substance-induced mental illness that, in many cases, is irreversible is alcohol-induced dementia. Although alcoholism may produce dementia through head trauma and nutritional deficiencies, such as thiamine deficiency, alcohol itself appears to have a directly damaging effect on brain tissue (Dietrich, 1977). This thesis has been supported by the finding of significant cognitive impairment in abstinent alcoholics who averaged 24 years of heavy drinking (Svanum & Schladenhauffen, 1986). A significant degree of ventricular dilation has been observed in demented alcoholics. In a number of cases, followed for 6 months to 1 year of abstinence, this dilation seems to remit (Carlin, Holgate, Wilkinson, & Rankin, 1978). Thus, in some cases, alcohol-induced dementia may be partially reversible with abstinence. In other cases, it is likely that, with abstinence, there may be a stabilization of the dementia—no worsening but also no improvement.

Alcoholics may become demented from causes other than alcohol. Alzheimer's disease (primary degenerative dementia), multi-infarct dementia, and dementia of other etiologies may afflict alcoholics. Establishing the diagnosis involves the same process that one uses in differentiating other substance-induced versus primary mental illnesses. If the dementia predated the alcoholism, it is likely that a non-alcohol-induced dementia exists. The symptoms of dementia may have been exacerbated by the effect of alcohol, or the primary dementia may even coexist with an alcohol-induced dementia. In the case of alcohol-induced dementia with abstinence, the cognitive losses either remain unchanged or improve, whereas in Alzheimer's disease or multi-infarct dementia, the symptoms worsen.

Personality Disorders and Substance Abuse

Personality disorders appear to account for a large percentage of mentally ill substance abusers. Studies surveying such diagnostic combinations have shown a 50%–90%

rate of personality disorders in narcotic addicts (Khantzian & Treece, 1985) and rates of 20%–49% of antisocial personality disorder in alcoholics (Hasselbrock, Meyer, & Keener, 1985; Powell *et al.*, 1982). The patients in these studies were either actively addicted to substances or had last used drugs or alcohol within a few days or a few weeks of evaluation for personality disorder. Consequently, the rates may be inaccurately high because of the confounding factor of substance-induced symptoms. For example, heavy drug users often resort to antisocial acts in order to pay for their habit. During abstinence, such behavior usually extinguishes and there is no further evidence of a primary antisocial-personality disorder. Similarly, the use of alcohol and other drugs may cause individuals to make poor judgments in interpersonal relationships, thus disrupting those relationships. Alcohol and drug use may also lead to confusion and distorted self-representation, effects that may resemble the symptoms of personality disorders. Anecdotal evidence suggests that some patients require several months of abstinence before clinicians can determine whether a primary personality disorder persists. Patients may need that length of abstinence before confusion clears, self-representation improves, and adequate reparation of damage to relationships occurs.

As in other diagnoses, to determine whether a primary personality disorder exists, one can gain important information from early life events. Emotional, physical, and sexual abuse and emotional and physical neglect are particularly crucial in the development of personality disorders. Although some people emerge from childhood trauma seemingly unscathed, most "survivors" of early familial disruption, abuse, or neglect are left with maladaptive coping skills that persistently recur. Such symptoms of character pathology may be severe enough to warrant a personality disorder diagnosis. In the case of substance abusers, the presence of premorbid (preaddiction) character pathology may help confirm a tentative diagnosis of character pathology coexisting with a substance abuse pattern.

Adult Children of Alcoholics

The term *adult children of alcoholics* (ACoAs) describes a large group that has recently begun to receive a great deal of attention in the counseling field. There are millions of adults in the United States who were raised by alcoholic parents. The term *adult children of alcoholics* has also emerged from the addiction treatment literature as a label for a condition (Woititz, 1983). Descriptions of the characteristics of adult children of alcoholics abound (Cermak & Brown, 1982; Gravitz & Bowen, 1984; Woititz, 1983).

Although the descriptions vary somewhat, there is a general consensus that most adult children of alcoholics have trouble with intimacy, appear to function well although they feel continually stressed, are confused about what they feel and want, experience chronic feelings of inadequacy, have a tendency to respond to others, and experience a need to control their emotions. Along with these characteristics, many adult children of alcoholics experience chronic dysphoria.

The characteristics of adult children of alcoholics are shared by many who do not have alcoholic family backgrounds. Many of those who were raised in abusive, neglectful, or emotionally rigid families share the characteristics described above. Adult children of alcoholics, however, probably represent the largest subset of mentally ill substance abusers. Many appear to have a genetic predisposition toward alcoholism (Bohman, Sigvardsson, & Cloninger, 1981; Cloninger, Bohman, & Sigvardsson, 1981;

Goodwin, 1983). In addition, most adult children of alcoholics, in modeling their parents, have learned to use mood-altering chemicals to deal with strong feelings.

Although adult children of alcoholics do not always meet the criteria of psychiatric diagnoses, they are often burdened with significant character pathology. The character pathology afflicting these substance-abusing adult children of alcoholics often becomes apparent when, despite several years of successful sobriety, they continue to feel dysphoric. This pathology may also become apparent in substance abusers who, despite their best efforts, continue to relapse into their substance-abuse patterns.

Substance Abuse Coexisting with Other Forms of Craving

Eating disorders, paraphilias, and pathological gambling are often considered problems of self-regulation and impulse control. These disorders, however, like substance abuse, involve obsessional craving and compulsive action and involve ambivalent thoughts about a forbidden act. When craving overcomes anxiety, the person carries out the compulsive action. Relief is often followed by guilt. For most people, these behaviors are shrouded in secrecy and are guarded by minimization and rationalization.

In many cases, problems with eating, sex, and gambling are mirror reflections of the severity of the addiction to a substance rather than a primary problem. Poor judgment, loosened inhibitions, and amnestic episodes may account for isolated or intermittent sexual indiscretions. Prostitution, excessive gambling, and frequent petty thefts may represent an addict's solution to the financial burden of supporting the addiction. If the eating disorder, paraphilia, or pathological gambling existed before the substance abuse pattern, or if these problems persist once the person has attained abstinence, they may represent a primary disorder.

Because primary disorders involving eating, sex, and gambling involve craving, they lend themselves well to some of the same treatment principles used for substance abuse. Some treatment programs consider eating disorders, paraphilias, and pathological gambling forms of addiction and use AA self-help recovery concepts. This approach is often helpful to substance abusers who may already have been acculturated to that language. Eating disorders in particular, however, may be so severe as to warrant medical treatment before the substance abuse pattern is fully addressed.

Self-Medication

A tantalizing question that has arisen in recent years is whether mentally ill substance abusers use drugs as a means of treating their mental illnesses. Chronic young-adult patients have severe psychopathology and may become stuck in the "revolving door" of frequent hospitalizations interspersed with frequent outpatient clinic treatments. Because of the move to deinstitutionalization that has taken place in the United States since the 1960s, and because these patients have limited financial resources, they are periodically thrust into an impoverished environment. Emotional pain and social exposure to drug use may thus be contributing but not sufficient factors in drug use, as not all young mental patients develop drug problems.

Although one can come to no firm conclusion about the relationship between primary mental illness and substance abuse, some researchers have presented evidence to support a relationship between drug choice and psychological state, suggesting a self-medication process in these individuals (Khantzian, 1985). Although some substance abusers use any drug available and deny having a preference, most substance abusers have a drug they prefer. This phenomenon has been described as the "drug of choice phenomenon" (Wieder & Kaplan, 1969), the "preferential use of drugs" (Milkman & Frosch, 1973), and the "self-selection process" (Khantzian, 1975).

Although most substance abusers experiment with drugs until they find their favorite one, there are exceptions to this rule. Some substance abusers are fearful of legal reprisals and limit themselves to alcohol. Some substances such as crack (the smokable alkaloid of cocaine) may be so powerfully addicting that users become addicted before discovering their true drug preference. Nonetheless, most substance abusers select a favorite drug. Two categories of substances that illustrate this process are opiates (e.g., heroin) and stimulants (i.e., cocaine and amphetamines).

Several authors have argued that those who use heroin and other opiates select those drugs for their antiaggression and antirage effects (Khantzian, 1985; Milkman & Frosch, 1973). These researchers have described the effectiveness of opiates in counteracting the ego-disorganizing effects of aggression. Not surprisingly, they found that many opiate addicts were exposed to extreme aggression and violence in childhood and had evidenced lifelong difficulties with their own rage (Khantzian, 1985). I have heard many opiate addicts claim that the antirage effect of opiates is unparalleled by any other drug.

Other writers have described the antipsychotic effect of opiates and have suggested that this effect may figure significantly in the selection of opiates by some patients. The antipsychotic action of opiates may involve a decrease in dopamine secondary to an increase in prolactin (Gold, Redmond, Donabedian, Goodwin, & Extein, 1978). Morphine, for example, was deliberately used in the treatment of psychosis in the 19th century (Comfort, 1977), and the use of methadone has been considered by some clinicians for intractable psychosis (Khantzian, 1985). Some schizophrenics do appear to use opiates preferentially, perhaps for their antipsychotic effect. Nicholson and Treece (1981) found that opiate addicts receiving high doses of methadone had significant impairment of object relations, possibly suggesting that they had chosen opiates for an ego-stabilizing effect.

Although considerable work has been done on the antipsychotic effects of opiates, attention has also focused on the antidepressant and other effects of opiates. One group (Rounsaville *et al.,* 1982) demonstrated that depressed addicts used opiates as self-treatment for dysphoria. Another group (Gold *et al.,* 1982), using clinical, neuroanatomical, and biochemical evidence, claimed to elucidate the antimanic, antidepressant, and antipanic effects of opiates. With specific effects ascribed to opiates in so few studies, it is premature to draw conclusions regarding why some substance abusers prefer opiates, although this preliminary evidence encourages further study of the psychodynamics and neurophysiology of opiate addiction and of other substance-abuse illnesses.

In the case of stimulants, including amphetamines and cocaine, researchers have offered numerous suggestions about the effects and reasons for selection. Milkman and Frosch (1973) suggested that amphetamine addicts use amphetamines to support feelings of diminished self-worth. Khantzian (1985) offered two explanations for cocaine selection: cocaine's effect of overcoming the dysphoria and anergia of depression and cocaine's ability to energize those with a frenetic lifestyle. He also suggested that cocaine is selected by individuals with preexisting depression, attention deficit disorder, cyclothymic disorder, and bipolar disorder. Several researchers have suggested that the neurophysiological mechanism of action of cocaine euphoria may involve activation of dopaminergic pathways in the brain (Dackis, Gold, Davis, & Sweeney, 1985–1986; Gawin & Kleber, 1986). Cocaine also causes release of catecholamine neurotransmitters (Gawin & Kleber, 1986).

Amphetamines appear to involve a similar neurophysiological mechanism of action. Although the use of stimulants may result in a short-term improvement in mood, this effect reverses following discontinuation of the stimulant. In the case of cocaine, increased beta-adrenergic, alpha-adrenergic, and dopaminergic receptor binding, along with neurotransmitter depletion, probably leads to craving and the frequent abstinence dysphoria (Gawin & Kleber, 1984). Thus, stimulants may be chosen for their energizing actions, but ironically, for many, continued use produces the opposite effect because of neurotransmitter depletion.

At present, the limited understanding of the psychodynamics of drug use and of the actions of neurotransmitters does not permit definitive conclusions about drug preference, although the fact remains that substance abusers demonstrate drug preferences. Social, legal, and financial factors may contribute to drug selection, but psychodynamic and neurophysiological factors appear to be more significant. By better understanding the psychodynamic and neurophysiological determinants of drug choice, clinicians will be able to address patients' treatment needs more effectively and more clearly differentiate uncomplicated substance abusers from mentally ill substance abusers.

FREQUENT CLINICAL PROBLEMS

The preceding sections addressed establishing the proper mental-illness diagnosis. Once the clinician has made a diagnosis or ruled out mental illness, treatment become paramount. This section presents a discussion of the clinical problems that frequently arise in addiction treatment.

One clinical problem arises when the patient is exposed to conflicting diagnoses and treatment recommendations. The alcoholic patient with manic-depressive illness illustrates this process. A treating psychiatrist or other mental-health worker may not ask about the patient's drinking history, or the patient and clinician may collude in minimizing the extent and consequences of the drinking. The addiction treatment may be sabotaged if the clinician asks the patient to "drink less" or reassures the patient by failing to diagnose substance abuse. Conversely, the addiction counselor may not discuss the manic-depressive illness or may suggest that the symptoms are attributable to the effects of alcohol. Patients may be advised by their addiction counselors and by members of the AA groups not to take lithium. Patients risk rejection by either group by failing to comply with these mutually exclusive proscriptions.

When addiction and mental health professionals and self-help peers understand the problem ares that each addresses, treatment may be powerfully effective. A mental-health professional who understands the concerns of his or her addiction-professional counterpart may help coordinate an effective treatment strategy for the patient with a primary mental illness and for the patient's family that respects the addiction treatment philosophy. If the patient attends an AA meeting opposed to the use of medication, the mental health clinician may instruct the patient not to discuss his or her use of lithium, or to attend meetings that are specifically designed for mentally ill substance abusers, and to select an AA sponsor who will support the patient in his or her recovery from both illnesses.

Another clinical problem arises when mentally ill substance abusers resist attending

AA or NA (Narcotics Anonymous) meetings. The reasons are many: denial of the addictive illness, heavy exposure to the mental health culture, and sometimes, the nature of the mental illness. Such self-help involvement, however, is crucial in most cases to effectively arrest the substance abuse pattern even if the person has stopped drinking or using drugs. Consistent AA and NA involvement significantly reduces the risk of relapse into the substance abuse pattern through confrontation of denial and reinforcement of the principles of sobriety.

Often, mentally ill substance abusers see their mental-health professionals only and have no contact with the addiction recovery community. Other mental-health professionals insist that these patients attend AA or NA but fail to assist them in becoming acculturated to a subculture that has its own language and perceptions and that is based on group involvement. The mental health professional may need to assign these patients to a therapy group whose goal is member involvement in the self-help recovery community. These groups are generally led by a professional who is a recovering alcoholic or addict, and they focus on educating patients about addiction and about recovery group involvement. Peer pressure is helpful in urging them to actively attend AA or NA. Patients "graduate" from the group when they have become effectively involved in recovery groups.

Another clinical problem that frequently arises in outpatient practice is the patient's use of alcohol or drugs while in treatment. Outpatient mentally ill substance abusers should be required to undergo periodic random blood-alcohol-levels tests and urine drug screens. The clinician should clearly state this requirement at the beginning of treatment or when he or she becomes aware that an alcohol or drug problem exists. The clinician should present the necessity of testing as one important component of the effective treatment of a difficult problem. The rationale for prohibition of the use of alcohol and other drugs by substance abusers in treatment is that the vast majority of addicts are unable to use addictive substances without eventual relapse.

If an outpatient continues to use alcohol or drugs, the clinician must decide either to alter the treatment or to refer the patient elsewhere. A substance-abusing patient who uses drugs in treatment indicates that more involvement is needed in addiction treatment efforts. If the alcohol or drug use is not imminently dangerous, the first step may be to refer the patient to outpatient addiction counseling and to advise intensified self-help involvement. At this stage, the patient should attend one AA or NA meeting per day for 90 days and should select an AA or NA sponsor who follows the patient's self-help group attendance. If these measures are ineffective, the next step may involve referral to an intensive day or evening outpatient rehabilitation treatment program. If the patient continues to be addicted or is in danger medically, psychologically, legally, socially, or occupationally, he or she may require referral to an inpatient detoxification or rehabilitation program.

A final and unfortunate clinical problem is that of the iatrogenically addicted patient. At times, iatrogenic addiction is unavoidable, as in terminally ill patients who are in great pain. Sometimes medically created addiction is not wholly necessary but is rationalized as acceptable by the physician because of the condition, for example, that of a patient with chronic pain. Often, however, iatrogenic addiction occurs without the physician's awareness and commonly involves sedatives, particularly benzodiazepines, prescribed for sleep or anxiety. Giving a suspected substance abuser temazepam (Restoril), flurazepam (Dalmane), or triazolam (Halcion) for sleep is ill advised because it may create an addiction. Giving lorazepam (Ativan) or diazepam (Valium) for anxiety or giving alprazolam (Xanax) for agitated depression may result in iatrogenic addiction to the substance. These medications may also result in a relapse to the substance originally abused by the patient. With any patient, it is essential to take a careful history for possible substance abuse and to avoid addicting drugs if possible. The use of benzodiazepines and barbiturates for sleep or anxiety is questionable in the general population and is contraindicated for substance abusers.

Modification of Treatment Approaches

One of the phrases in AA, "first things first," applies well to the treatment of mentally ill substance abusers. Patients at risk of inflicting self-harm during a substance-induced condition, such as cocaine abstinence depression, must be treated for their suicidal feelings before treatment of the addiction begins. Similarly, patients who are acutely psychotic from an amphetamine-induced psychosis must be stabilized before the addiction can be effectively addressed.

Many mental illnesses are less severe but still require uninterrupted treatment. If manic-depressive illness, schizophrenia, and major depression have been effectively stabilized with medication and psychotherapy before the patient presents for treatment of substance abuse, treatment of the mental illness should continue concurrently with the treatment for substance abuse.

A more difficult decision arises concerning the treatment of milder mental illness. Dysthymic disorder, generalized anxiety disorder, cyclothymic disorder, and personality disorders often respond to psychotherapy that incorporates variable aspects of support, confrontation, and uncovering work. These conditions, however, often do not require treatment as urgently as does the substance abuse illness, particularly when the substance abuse pattern produces significant life disruption. Because of the patient's strong tendency to deny his or her addiction, focusing on other problems may lead him or her to minimize the addiction and to avoid treatment for it. The addiction, moreover, may produce mood swings and confusion that may persist for some time, as discussed earlier. Most recovering addicts say they benefited most from concentrating on their addiction in the first year and returning to psychotherapy after they reached the 1-year sobriety mark. This course may not be advisable for substance abusers who never gain a significant period of sobriety because of repeated relapse. Often, dysphoria from personality disorders and mild affective illnesses feel overwhelming and lead to a return to drug use. For such patients, psychotherapy is helpful as long as its aim is to support sobriety.

Substance Abuse Treatment

The most striking defense mechanism of all addicts, including mentally ill substance abusers, is denial. Addicts tend to minimize the amount or impact of their drug and alcohol use, and they rationalize the acceptability of their drug and alcohol use patterns. Consequently, they are almost invariably poor historians. The astute clinician suspects a substance abuse pattern when there is any mention of a drug or alcohol problem by the patient or the patient's family. If a pattern of substance abuse is suspected, the clinician should confront the patient, using care, as confrontation may lead to a flight from therapy. Gently providing the patient with clear evidence of the alcohol or drug abuse pattern and confronting the patient's rationalizations are sometimes effective, especially if the clinician includes a family member or a concerned friend. If this approach fails, the patient may need a specialized form of confrontation called *intervention*. Interventions involve concerned family members, friends, and employers who unexpectedly confront the patient about his or her drug use. The participants are coached in advance to share with the patient how they have been affected by the patient's addiction. Interventions are effective only if it is clear that there are negative consequences if the patient does not agree to treatment. The patient may face the choice of going for treatment or losing his or her job or family.

If the denial is severe enough to warrant an intervention, inpatient treatment is often indicated. In other cases, however, patients do well in outpatient addiction treatment. Day treatment programs generally run for weeks or months and are followed by individual and group addiction-counseling. When the patient is unable to maintain abstinence during the course of outpatient addiction-counseling, he or she may require inpatient rehabilitation, including detoxification if the addiction involves significant tolerance or withdrawal.

Alcohol and drug withdrawal may pose a serious health risk to the patient, although it is less dangerous in mild cases. Combining prescribed detoxification medications with street drugs may be dangerous, and outpatient monitoring may be difficult. Inpatient detoxification usually lasts less than 1 week and includes counseling and self-help group attendance along with medical treatment of the withdrawal. Patients are then referred to counseling and self-help groups.

The two forms of inpatient addiction rehabilitation programs are those associated with psychiatric hospitals (which generally have a psychiatrist coordinating the patient's care) and rehabilitation programs (in which addiction counselors coordinate the patient's treatment program and psychiatrists may be available on a consulting basis). Generally, mentally ill substance abusers with severe or potentially unstable mental illnesses do best in psychiatrically based programs. Patients with less mental-health impairment generally do well in rehabilitation programs in which they quickly become acculturated to the addiction recovery community. Some form of addiction counseling and self-help group involvement should follow inpatient detoxification and rehabilitation hospitalization.

A drug that has seen great recent popularity with a seemingly high rate of addiction is crack, or rock, the smokable alkaloid base of cocaine. Addiction to it tends to accelerate at frightening speed, usually leading to significant life disruption in months or even weeks. Because of the rapidity and severity of this addiction, most patients cannot be initially treated as outpatients.

A final note in this discussion of substance abuse treatment is the importance of the family. Substance abuse has been called a family disease for two reasons. The family may unwittingly support or enable continued addiction by making excuses for intoxicated behavior and by covering up for indiscretions. Paradoxically, the family may also enable continuation of the addictive pattern by nagging or berating the patient to stop drinking. The family can, however, with help, support the patient's recovery efforts by holding to negative consequences for continued drug use and by not interfering with the patient's schedule of counseling and self-help group appointments.

Addiction is also a family disease because emotional involvement with a substance abuser often leads to confusion, anger, disappointment, and self-doubt. The disease affecting family members has been called *codependency,* a term that refers to one's placing greater importance on another person's feelings and behaviors than on one's own (Cermak, 1984). Family members often have their own denial and rationalization of their loved one's substance abuse patterns. They may be either rageful or masochistic; their lives may revolve around worrying about the addicted family member. Their codependency may be more severe if the addicted family member has been neglectful or abusive toward them.

Appropriate treatment of the family includes involvement in Al-Anon (the self-help recovery group for families of alcoholics and other addicts), ACoA (Adult Children of Alcoholics), Alateen (for teenagers with addicted parents), and Alatot (for young children of addicts). In addition to self-help involvement, family members often benefit from individual, group, and family psychotherapy or counseling. In the course of treating the family, it is important to take histories for hidden substance-abuse patterns in the other family members.

Psychotherapy

Another form of treatment that is helpful to many mentally ill substance abusers is the combination of psychotherapy and addiction counseling. In a review of the literature from 1970 to 1983, five out of seven studies demonstrated that opiate-dependent patients treated with psychotherapy and drug counseling showed a better outcome than those treated with drug counseling alone (Woody, Luborsky, McLellan, O'Brien, Beck, Blaine, Herman, & Hole, 1983).

Researchers from the drug-dependence treatment unit associated with the University of Pennsylvania studied 110 methadone-maintenance patients. They treated opiate addicts with either drug counseling alone, drug counseling combined with cognitive-behavioral psychotherapy, or counseling combined with supportive-expressive psychotherapy. They classified these patients as having low, mid, and high severity of psychiatric symptoms. The results demonstrated overall greater benefits for patients receiving either type of psychotherapy combined with drug counseling. Furthermore, it was the patients with the high-severity symptoms receiving psychotherapy plus counseling who showed the most improvement compared to those receiving counseling alone (Woody, McLellan, Luborsky, O'Brien, Blaine, Fox, Herman, & Beck, 1984). Although more studies are needed, these findings suggest that psychotherapy combined with counseling is more helpful than counseling alone for mentally ill substance abusers. Supportive-expressive psychotherapy is probably the form most commonly used with mentally ill substance abusers. It involves an exploration of relationship issues, including transference. Because it is supportive, the psychotherapist is more actively involved in the session than an analytically oriented psychotherapist would be. Mentally ill substance abusers appear to respond best to psychotherapists who establish a positive transference in the beginning of treatment and remain relatively active throughout the course of treatment.

Certain modifications of supportive-expressive psychotherapy should be made when one works with mentally ill substance abusers. Because substance-abusing patients use denial, minimization, and rationalization, the therapist should pursue the issues underlying contradictory statements and elaborate explanations. During the course of treatment, the therapist should minimize the level of anxiety experienced by the patient because abusers have a low tolerance of anxiety, and anxiety-provoking analytic techniques may renew substance abuse or may lead to a flight from therapy. Psychoanalysis, in fact, is contraindicated for substance abusers because of its tendency to provoke greater levels of anxiety than they can tolerate without relapsing into active substance abuse.

Cognitive-behavioral therapy is active, directive, and often time-limited, and it is frequently effective with mentally ill substance abusers. The therapist identifies the patient's negative beliefs and guides the patient to replace them with more realistic ones.

Such an approach may be effective with substance abusers because it is warm and supportive, and it addresses the hopelessness about not being able to achieve sobriety.

A highly effective form of treatment for mentally ill substance abusers is group psychotherapy. Like individual psychotherapy, it should be supportive rather than anxiety-provoking. Group psychotherapy is particularly effective in confronting self-sabotaging behaviors and defenses such as rationalization and intellectualization. As noted in the substance-abuse-treatment section, group psychotherapy may be used to encourage patients to attend Alcoholics Anonymous and Narcotics Anonymous meetings and should not replace those meetings.

Some therapists use the behavioral technique of contingency contracting (Kleber & Gawin, 1984), which involves the patient's agreeing to undergo random blood-alcohol-level measurements (breathalizer) and urine drug screens. The patient and the therapist determine in advance what negative consequence will result from a positive lab finding. This consequence may involve, for example, the therapist's sending a prewritten self-disclosure of the patient's active substance abuse to the patient's employer.

No matter what form of psychotherapy is prescribed, certain ground rules should apply. One is prohibition of substance use during the course of treatment. Many addiction-treatment personnel maintain that continuing to treat an actively substance-abusing patient reinforces continued substance use.

Another ground rule in the treatment of mentally ill substance abusers is that the patient attend self-help recovery-group meetings. As indicated in the substance-abuse-treatment section, patients should be instructed not to discuss the pharmacological treatment of their mental illness in self-help meetings unless they know that the group will be accepting and supportive. They should be encouraged to select an AA or NA sponsor who will support their recovery from both illnesses.

Whenever psychotherapy is provided for a substance abuser, the therapist should be familiar with the natural course of addictive illnesses and with the process of recovery from addiction. If psychotherapy is indicated, it should accompany AA or NA attendance and, whenever possible, addiction counseling. In addition, a unified team approach to treating mental illness and substance abuse simultaneously in one setting has been shown to be superior to treating each disorder in separate settings (Kofoed *et al.*, 1986). Because this approach is frequently not possible, therapists are advised to maintain close contact with their colleagues in addiction counseling in order to provide continuity of care.

Pharmacotherapy

The outpatient pharmacological approaches to mentally ill substance abusers include medical detoxification, the pharmacological treatment of primary mental illnesses, and the pharmacological treatment of substance abuse. Each approach requires a modification of established procedures. In all three approaches, medication should be used sparingly and cautiously; many of the medications in a clinician's armamentarium are drugs of abuse. If prescribed to a substance abuser, they could precipitate a relapse into active substance abuse. The sedating or energizing side effects of some medications may be reminiscent of intoxicated states, and they induce craving. Even nonaddicting medications that are only slightly mood-altering carry the risk of reinforcing the patient's tendency to use substances to alter undesired mental states. When using medication with this group of patients, the clinician must establish a clear need for the use of the medication and should closely monitor the patient's use of it.

Outpatient detoxification is generally inadvisable because of the severity of withdrawal symptoms and because of the difficulty of monitoring the patient's clinical course and use of detoxifying medication. Drug withdrawal conditions may be quite dangerous. Alcohol detoxification is more dangerous than withdrawal from any other drug, including heroin or cocaine. The seizures, convulsions, and delirium—part of the delirium tremens process—are associated with significant mortality among alcoholic patients undergoing detoxification.

Withdrawal from other drugs is less life-threatening, but still serious. The symptoms of withdrawal from sedatives may include seizures and elevated pulse, blood pressure, and temperature. Patients withdrawing from stimulants, including cocaine, frequently feel suicidal. Patients experience an intense craving for drugs during withdrawal and often relapse into substance abuse. It is frequently impossible to monitor withdrawal symptoms adequately on an outpatient basis. For the more severe withdrawal conditions, inpatient detoxification is recommended.

In mild cases of withdrawal, however, the clinician may attempt outpatient detoxification. The clinician should arrange for frequent medical evaluations and for a responsible friend or relative to dispense the medication.

The choice of medication, if one is needed for withdrawal, depends on the drug of abuse. Alcohol withdrawal is most commonly treated with benzodiazepines. Alcoholics with advanced liver disease respond to oxazepam (Serax) because it is not metabolized in the liver. In some countries, alcohol withdrawal is treated on an outpatient basis with carbamazepine (Tegretol), but this treatment remains experimental in the United States.

Benzodiazepine withdrawal is often treated with phenobarbital because it does not produce an intoxicating effect. Mild cases of barbiturate withdrawal similarly respond to phenobarbital. One should note that Valium withdrawal seizures may occur up to 3 weeks after the last dose. Outpatient opiate withdrawal, in most cases, may be effectively treated with clonidine.

Stimulant withdrawal does not ordinarily require medication unless severe abstinence depression occurs. In such cases, the short-term use of antidepressants may be indicated. The clinician may continue the use of antidepressants if it becomes clear that the patient has a coexistent major depression.

Although the diagnosis of mental illness in substance abusers was discussed earlier in this chapter, it is important to discuss the medications frequently used to treat mental illness that are contraindicated in the substance abuser. Clinicians should avoid prescribing amphetamines and benzodiazepines. This prohibition includes alprazolam (Xanax), which is frequently given to anxious-depressed patients. If an antidepressant is indicated, the clinician should choose one with low sedating effects. Amitriptyline (Elavil) is occasionally sold as a street drug for its sedating effect. Thus, although it is not addicting, it may stimulate a craving for sedatives that are addicting. Similarly, one should avoid monoamine oxidase inhibitors, especially for patients who abuse stimulants, because these medications have been abused for their energizing effects. They should be prescribed only if other pharmacotherapy is ineffective.

If an antipsychotic medication is indicated, it is best to use a relatively low-sedating, low-dose, high-potency medication, for example, trifluoperazine (Stelazine) or thiothixene (Navane). Chlorpromazine (Thorazine) and other strongly sedating antipsychotic medications are often abused. Although the medications are not addicting, their mood-altering side effects may stimulate a craving for drugs that are addicting.

Other medications given to mentally ill substance abusers include those used to treat substance abuse. Disulfiram (Antabuse) has been widely prescribed for alcoholism. By blocking the action of alcoholic dehydrogenase, it causes acetaldehyde to accumulate when a person drinks alcohol. This reaction leads to an extremely unpleasant syndrome with symptoms of flushing, palpitation, hyperventilation, nausea, and vomiting. Disulfiram should be used with healthy patients. Its effectiveness is based on aversive conditioning. Because it remains effective as long as 1 week after the last dose, it continues to provide incentive for patients who experience craving so that they can seek support and prevent relapse. Some therapists oppose the use of disulfiram because patients may believe that the disulfiram is sufficient and they need not attend AA meetings. For some alcoholics, this attitude leads ultimately to relapse. For alcoholics who chronically relapse or for mentally ill substance abusers who are receiving acute care for their mental illness, disulfiram may be a rational short-term adjunct to treatment.

Some researchers have warned against the use of disulfiram for patients with schizophrenia or bipolar illness (Liddon & Satran, 1967). Because disulfiram may inhibit dopamine-beta-hydroxylase, it may exacerbate psychotic symptoms by producing a buildup of dopamine. One group (Kofoed *et al.*, 1986), however, used disulfiram effectively with their patients at doses of 250 mg a day and advised stabilizing patients on appropriate psychiatric medication before starting disulfiram.

Some reports have suggested that lithium is helpful in treating alcohol abuse. Early research into the use of lithium (Wren, Kline, Cooper, Varga, & Canal, 1974) demonstrated that depressed alcoholics who received lithium evidenced a slight improvement when compared to those who did not receive lithium. Although some subsequent studies have been more optimistic, the use of lithium for alcoholism is generally not indicated where bipolar or cyclothymic disorders do not exist.

Two medications are currently in common use as treatments for opiate addiction. Methadone, a long-acting opiate, is generally reserved for patients with an opiate addiction that is unresponsive to other forms of treatment. It has the advantage of removing the patient from the street environment and reducing the crime and adverse medical consequences associated with street drug use. But its disadvantage is that it is an addictive drug that, given its long half-life, may be particularly difficult to stop. Methadone for maintenance treatment is available only at designated clinics across the United States. Naltrexone is the second medication used to treat opiate addiction. It is a nonaddictive opiate antagonist that, at a dose of 50 mg per day, blocks the effect of approximately 25 mg of intravenous heroin (Greenstein, Arndt, McLellan, O'Brien, & Evans, 1984). Naltrexone appears to be most effective with addicts who have a strong self-motivation to stop their use of opiates.

Most of the medications used to treat cocaine abuse are ordinarily used to treat psychiatric disorders. Gawin and Kleber (1984) reported a significant improvement in cocaine abusers treated with desipramine; these patients showed a decreased craving for cocaine 2–3 weeks after starting it. This time period coincides with the time course described for receptor changes and positive responses to tricyclic antidepressants in patients with major depression. All the patients in the study experienced less cocaine craving on desipramine, whether or not they had symptoms of affective illness. Gawin and Kleber suggested that desipramine reversed the dopaminergic and beta-adrenergic receptor changes that occur with long-term cocaine use. They pointed out that such a "blocking" effect also appears to operate in amphetamine addiction.

Researchers have also investigated the effect of lithium carbonate on cocaine abuse (Cronson & Flemenbaum, 1978; Gawin, & Kleber, 1984). In their study, Gawin and

Kleber (1984) found lithium carbonate to be effective in reducing cocaine craving only in cyclothymic patients. Other patients continued cocaine use despite lithium treatment. Khantzian (1983) reported effectiveness of methylphenidate (Ritalin) in treating cocaine abuse. It appears that methyphenidate is effective in treating cocaine abusers who have symptoms of attention deficit disorder, residual type. Because of the potentially addictive property of methylphenidate in substance abusers, clinicians should reserve it for severe cases of attention deficit disorder, residual type.

Dackis and colleagues (1985–1986) proposed the use of bromocriptine to reverse the dopamine depletion effects of cocaine. This unproven experimental approach is currently not advised in the routine treatment of cocaine abusers. The results of these studies on the pharmacological treatment of cocaine abuse suggest an approach to the mentally ill cocaine abuser. If the patient has symptoms of major depression, desipramine or imipramine would be the medication to use. If the patient has cyclothymic disorder and difficulty in maintaining abstinence from cocaine, a trial of lithium may be warranted.

Additional Treatment Approaches

Because mentally ill substance abusers have two disruptive illnesses, their treatment needs are often quite diverse. They should have complete physical examinations at the beginning of treatment; because of the debilitating effects of their illnesses, they frequently need ongoing medical treatment. As their conditions often result in legal and social problems, they frequently need the support of social services and should be referred to these services. As a result of educational or occupational disruption, patients often benefit from vocational rehabilitation of remedial education. Because they often have been incapable of competent self-care, they frequently need help in establishing behavioral patterns that include adequate nutrition and exercise. One may need to combine any or all of these approaches with addiction treatment, mental health treatment, and self-help recovery to adequately address the treatment needs of this group.

SUMMARY

Mentally ill substance abusers are frequently exposed to three treatment approaches, from the mental health field, the addition treatment field, and the self-help recovery community of Alcoholics Anonymous or Narcotics Anonymous. Each of these approaches has its own language and its own belief systems. Through their involvement in these systems, mentally ill substance abusers frequently receive conflicting diagnoses and treatment recommendations. The challenge facing clinicians from both the mental health and the addiction treatment fields is understanding each other's philosophy of treatment and opening the lines of communication.

It is frequently difficult to diagnose mental illness in substance abusers. Substance abuse often presents the same symptoms as primary mental illness. At times, symptoms arising from substance abuse are severe enough to warrant a diagnosis of a substance-induced (secondary) mental illness. Substance-induced mental illnesses are, aside from dementia, reversible and remit earlier than primary mental illnesses. In addition to persistence of the symptoms, a family history of mental illness and a pre-substance-abuse history of mental illness support the diagnosis of a primary mental illness.

The treatment of mentally ill substance abusers involves a multifaceted approach.

Some form of substance abuse counseling is indicated in order to confront the denial and rationalization associated with addiction. Self-help recovery-group involvement is important if the patient is to maintain a sober lifestyle. Family treatment is indicated for two reasons: so that the patient gains the support of loved ones, and so that family members address the self-destructive patterns of codependency that develop as a result of their reactions to the substance abuser.

Supportive psychotherapy is indicated for patients with mental illness, whereas strictly analytical psychotherapy is contraindicated because of its anxiety-provoking effect. Group psychotherapy is indicated to confront the denial of addiction and to confront self-destructive characterological behavior patterns that may lead to relapse into substance abuse. Medical treatment and social work involvement are important, along with assistance with legal, social, and occupational problems and counseling on nutrition and exercise.

The outpatient treatment of mentally ill substance abusers, although complicated by numerous approaches, may be effective with the appropriate combination of therapies. At times, persistent substance use during treatment indicates a need for inpatient detoxification or rehabilitation. The occasional intensification of mental illness may indicate a need for psychiatric hospitalization. Such interruptions should represent brief interludes in a patient's overall treatment course, so that mentally ill substance abusers can spend most of their lives out of the hospital. To accomplish this end, they require a well-coordinated, multifaceted treatment approach.

REFERENCES

American Psychiatric Association. (1980). *Diagnostic and statistical manual of mental disorders* (3rd Edition). Washington, DC: Author.

Bohman, M., Sigvardsson, S., & Cloninger, C. W. (1981). Maternal inheritance of alcohol abuse: Cross-fostering analysis of adopted women. *Archives of General Psychiatry, 38,* 965–969.

Bowen, R. C., Cipynyk, D., D'Arcy, C., & Keegan, D. (1984). Alcoholism, anxiety disorders, and agoraphobia. *Alcoholism: Clinical and Experimental Research, 8,* 48–50.

Byck, R. (1974). *Cocaine papers by Sigmund Freud.* New York: New American Library.

Carlin, P. L., Holgate, G. W. R. C., Wilkinson, D. A., & Rankin, J. G. (1978). Reversible cerebral atrophy in recently abstinent chronic alcoholics measured by computed tomography scans. *Science, 200,* 1076–1078.

Cermak, T. (1984). Children of alcoholics and the case for a new diagnostic category of codependency. *Alcohol Health and Research World, Summer,* 38–42.

Cermak, T. L., & Brown, S. (1982). Interactional group therapy with the adult children of alcoholics. *International Journal of Group Psychotherapy, 32,* 375–389.

Cloninger, C. R., Bohman, M., & Sigvardsson, S. (1981). Inheritance of alcohol abuse: Cross-fostering analysis of adopted men. *Archives of General Psychiatry, 38,* 861–868.

Comfort, A. (1977). Morphine as an antipsychotic: Relevance of a 19th century therapeutic fashion. *Lancet, 2,* 448–449.

Cronson, A. J., & Flemenbaum, A. (1978). Antagonism of cocaine highs by lithium. *American Journal of Psychiatry, 135,* 856–857.

Dackis, C. A., Bailey, J., Pottash, A. L. C., Stuckey, R. F., Extein, I. L., & Gold, M. S. (1984). Specificity of the DST and the TRH test for major depression in alcoholics. *American Journal of Psychiatry, 5,* 680–683.

Dackis, C. A., Gold, M. S., Davies, R. K., & Sweeney, D. R. (1985–86). Bromocriptime treatment for cocaine abuse: The dopamine depletion hypothesis. *International Journal of Psychiatry in Medicine, 15,* 125–135.

Dave, M., & Wanck, B. (1985). Depression in alcoholics: Implications for treatment. *Journal of the American Medical Association, 254,* 231.

Dietrich, R. A. (1977). Plasmalogen content of cerebellum samples from alcoholic and nonalcoholic humans. *Alcoholism: Clinical and Experimental Research, 1,* 11–32.

Ebin, D. (1961). *The drug experience; first-person accounts of addicts, writers, scientists and others.* New York: Grove Press.

Fischer, D. E., Halikas, J. A., Baker, J. W., & Smith, R. L. (1976). Frequency and patterns of drug abuse in psychiatric patients. *Diseases of the Nervous System, 36,* 550–553.

Fowler, R. C., Liskow, B. I., & Tanna, V. L. (1977). Psychiatric illness and alcoholism. *Alcoholism, 1,* 125–128.

Gawin, F. H., & Kleber, H. D. (1984). Cocaine abuse treatment: Open pilot trial with desipramine and lithium carbonate. *Archives of General Psychiatry, 41,* 903–909.

Gawin, F. H., & Kleber, H. D. (1986). Abstinance symptomatology and psychiatric diagnosis in cocaine abusers: Clinical observations. *Archives of General Psychiatry, 43,* 107–113.

Gold, M. S., Pottash, A. C., Sweeney, D., Martin, D., & Extein, I. (1982). Antimanic, antidepressant, and antipanic effects of opiates: Clinical, neuroanatomical, and biochemical evidence. *Annals of the New York Academy of Sciences, 398,* 140–150.

Gold, M. S., Redmond, D. E., Donabedian, R. K., Goodwin, F. K., & Extein, I. (1978). Increase in serum prolactin by exogenous and endogenous opiates: Evidence for antidopamine and antipsychotic effects. *American Journal of Psychiatry, 135,* 1415–1416.

Goodwin, D. W. (1983). The genetics of alcoholism. *Hospital and Community Psychiatry, 34,* 1031–1034.

Gravitz, H. L., & Bowden, J. D. (1984). Therapeutic issues of adult children of alcoholics. *Alcohol Health and Research World, Summer,* 25–42.

Greenstein, R. A., Arndt, I. C., McLellan, A. T., O'Brien, C. P., & Evans, B. (1984). Naltrexone: A clinical perspective. *Journal of Clinical Psychiatry, 45*(9, Sec 2), 25–28.

Hesselbrock, M. N., Meyer, R. E., & Keener, J. J. (1985). Psychopathology in hospitalized alcoholics. *Archives of General Psychiatry, 42,* 1050–1055.

Jaffe, A. (1978). Reform in American medical science: The inebriety movement and the origins of the psychological disease theory of addiction, 1870–1920. *British Journal of Addiction, 2,* 139–147.

James, W. (1961). *The varieties of religious experience: A study in human nature.* New York: Collier Books.

Jellinek, E. M. (1960). *The disease concept of alcoholism.* New Haven, CT: College and University Press.

Keeler, M. H., Taylor, C. I., & Miller, W. C. (1979). Are all recently detoxified alcoholics depressed? *American Psychiatric Association, 4,* 586, 588.

Keller, M. B., Klerman, G. L., Lavori, P. W., Coryell, W., Endicott, J., & Taylor, J. (1984). Long term outcome of episodes of major depression. *Journal of the American Medical Association, 252,* 788–792.

Khantzian, E. J. (1975). Self selection and progression in drug dependence. *Psychiatry Digest, 10,* 19–22.

Khantzian, E. J. (1983). An extreme case of cocaine dependence and marked improvement with methylphenidate treatment. *American Journal of Psychiatry, 140,* 784–785.

Khantzian, E. J. (1985). The self-medication hypothesis of addictive disorders: Focus on heroin and cocaine dependence. *American Journal of Psychiatry, 142,* 1259–1264.

Khantzian, E. J., & Treece, C. (1985). DSM-III psychiatric diagnosis of narcotic addicts. *Archives of General Psychiatry, 42,* 1067–1071.

Kleber, H. D., & Gawin, F. H. (1984). The spectrum of cocaine abuse and its treatment. *Journal of Clinical Psychiatry, 45*(12, Sec. 2), 18–23.

Kofoed, L., Kania, J., Walsh, T., & Atkinson, R. (1986). Outpatient treatment of patients with substance abuse and coexisting psychiatric disorders. *American Journal of Psychiatry, 7,* 867–872.

Kramer, J. C., Fischman, V. S., & Littlefield, D. C. (1967). Amphetamine abuse pattern and effects of high doses taken intravenously. *Journal of the American Medical Association, 201,* 305–309.

Liddon, S. C., and Satran, R. (1967). Disulfiram (Antabuse) psychosis. *American Journal of Psychiatry, 123,* 1284–1289.

Milkman, H., & Frosch, W. A. (1973). On the preferential abuse of heroin and amphetamine. *Journal of Nervous and Mental Disease, 156,* 242–248.

Mullaney, J. A., & Trippett, C. (1979). Alcohol dependence and phobias: Clinical description and relevance: *British Journal of Psychiatry, 135,* 563–573.

Munjack, D. J., & Moss, H. B. (1981). Affective disorder and alcoholism in families of agoraphobics. *Archives of General Psychiatry, 38,* 868–871.

Musto, D. (1986, June 11). Lessons of the first cocaine epidemic. *The Wall Street Journal.*

Myers, J. K., Weissman, M. M., Tischler, G. L., Holzer, C. E., III, Leaf, P., Orvaschel, H., Anthony, J. C., Boyd, J. H., Burke, J., Jr., Kramer, M., & Stoltzman, R. (1984). Six-month prevalence of psychiatric disorders in three communities. *Archives of General Psychiatry, 4,* 959–967.

Nicholson, B., & Treece, C. (1981). Object relations and differential treatment response to methadone maintenance. *Journal of Nervous and Mental Diseases, 169,* 424–429.

Powell, B. J., Penick, E. C., Othner, E., Bingham, S. F., & Rice, A. S. (1982). Prevalence of additional psychiatric syndromes among male alcoholics. *Journal of Clinical Psychiatry, 43,* 404–407.

Rounsaville, B. J., Weissman, M. M., Kleber, H., & Wilber, D. (1982). Heterogeneity of psychiatric diagnosis in treated opiate addicts. *Archives of General Psychiatry, 39,* 161–166.

Schuckit, M. (1983). Alcoholic patients with secondary depression. *American Journal of Psychiatry, 6,* 711–714.

Schuckit, M. A. (1985). The clinical implications of primary diagnostic groups among alcoholics. *Archives of General Psychiatry, 11,* 1043–1049.

Schuckit, M. A. (1986). Genetic and clinical implications of alcoholism and affective disorder. *American Journal of Psychiatry, 143,* 140–147.

Seixas, F. A. (1980). A historical perspective of alcoholism. In E. Gottheil, A. T. McLellan, & K. A. Druley (Eds.), *Substance abuse and psychiatric illness: Proceedings of the second annual Coatesville-Jefferson conference on addition* (pp. 76–84). New York: Pergamon Press.

Smail, P., Stockwell, T., Canter, S., & Hodgson, R. (1984). Alcohol dependence and phobic anxiety states: 1. A prevalence study. *British Journal of Psychiatry, 144,* 53–57.

Stockwell, T., Smail, P., Hodgson, R., & Canter, S. (1984). Alcohol dependence and phobic anxiety states: 2. A retrospective study. *British Journal of Psychiatry, 144,* 58–63.

Svanum, S., & Schladenhauffen, J. (1986). Lifetime and recent alcoholic consumption among male alcoholics. *Journal of Nervous and Mental Disease, 4,* 214–220.

Thomsen, R. (1975). *Bill W.* New York: Harper & Row.

Weingold, H. P., Lachin, J. M., Bell, A. H., & Coxe, R. C. (1968). Depression as a symptom of alcoholism: Search for a phenomenon. *Journal of Abnormal Psychology, 73,* 195–197.

Weiss, K. J., & Rosenberg, D. J. (1985). Prevalence of anxiety disorder among alcoholics. *Journal of Clinical Psychiatry, 46,* 3–5.

Wieder, H., & Kaplan, E. H. (1969). Drug use in adolescents: Psychodynamic meaning and pharmacogenic effect. *Psychoanalytic Study of Childhood, 24,* 399–413.

Woititz, J. G. (1983). *Adult children of alcoholics.* Pompano Beach, FL: Health Communications.

Woody, G. E., Luborsky, L., McLellan, A. T., O'Brien, C. P., Beck, A. T., Blaine, J., Herman, I., & Hole, A. (1983). Psychotherapy for opiate addicts: Does it help? *Archives of General Psychiatry, 40,* 639–645.

Woody, G. E., McLellan, A. T., Luborsky, L., O'Brien, C. P., Blaine, J., Fox, S., Herman, I., & Beck, A. T. (1984). Severity of psychiatric symptoms as a predictor of benefits from psychotherapy: The Veterans Administration-Penn study. *American Journal of Psychiatry, 141,* 1172–1177.

Wren, J. C., Kline, N. S., Cooper, T. B., Varga, E., & Canal, O. (1974). Evaluation of lithium therapy in chronic alcoholism. *Clinical Medicine, 81,* 33–36.

IV

Special Topics

26

Ethical and Legal Issues

C. V. HALDIPUR AND ROBERT C. LONG

INTRODUCTION

The development of ethics as a form of professional self-regulation has a history as long as that of medicine itself. The best known example of an early ethical code is the Hippocratic oath, which dates back to the fourth or fifth century B.C. Similar codes were established elsewhere. In ancient India, for instance, the code forbade physicians to treat certain classes of individuals or diseases with a poor prognosis.

Although these oaths contain specific rules that today might seem elitist, sections dealing with decorum and the instruction "to help, or at least do no harm" continue to be relevant. The Hippocratic oath, for one, was modified with the advent of Christianity, and with subsequent modifications, it continues to serve as a model code of conduct for health-related professionals. Because of advances in the sciences and events such as the Nuremberg trials after World War II, the simple rules of conduct that most clinicians learned at the bedside, such as "Primum non nocere" ("First, do no harm") are no longer enough, and professional organizations have established increasingly detailed ethical codes. Most professional organizations in the mental health field now have their own codes, and questions of ethics that were not addressed in the earlier editions of most professional textbooks are now being discussed, sometimes at great length. There are also many articles and monographs devoted exclusively to the topics of law and ethics in the mental health field.

One approach to moral reasoning and the rationality of moral principles—the question of right and wrong—stems from utilitarian thinkers, particularly Mill (1977), who stressed the significance of thinking about consequences. He accepted, as the foundation of morals, utility, or the greatest-happiness principle that "actions are right in proportion

C. V. HALDIPUR • Richard H. Hutchings Psychiatric Center, Syracuse, New York 13210. ROBERT C. LONG • Benjamin Rush Center, Syracuse, New York 13202.

as they tend to promote happiness, wrong as they tend to produce the reverse of happiness'' (p. 80).

Many ethical dilemmas that clinicians face can be phrased in utilitarian terms, such as instances in which the good of an individual patient (a term the authors prefer over *client*) has to be balanced against the consequences to society as a whole. However, it is not always easy to know with certainty, and in all instances, whether an intervention will promote the happiness of an individual. Would the greatest-happiness principle help the clinician deal with a patient who plans suicide as an escape from a miserable socioeconomic existence?

One of the challenges to such utilitarian thinking was made by Ross (1977), who, though not denying the importance of consequences, pointed to ''certain duties of perfect obligation, such as those of fulfilling promises, of paying debts, of telling the truth, which admit no exception whatsoever in favor of duties of imperfect obligations, such as that of relieving distress'' (p. 89). Clinicians' ethical dilemmas may also be viewed as pertaining to obligations and duties in the relationship with the patient. The crux of many ethical and legal situations is the degree of responsibility attributed to each party in the relationship.

Moral disputes are expressed in terms of rights, duties, and values. Analyses of ethical questions and adjudication of ethical disputes in mental health practice may occur through two separate, but not mutually exclusive, modes of reasoning: first in terms of consequences, or through a teleological (Greek *telos,* ''end'') approach; and second, in terms of obligations, or through a deontological (Greek *deon,* ''obligation'') approach (Engelhardt & McCullough, 1981). Jonsen and Hellegers (1977) explained the two theoretical approaches thus:

> Virtue is the inner spirit of morality; action is its outer manifestation. The virtuous physician without skills may be comfort, but cold comfort, to one who seeks cure. Medicine is a practical science: theory and experience evoked in clinical decision and action. Medical ethics, then, must be as concerned about the rightness of acts as about the goodness of the agent. A theory of virtue is a necessary, but not sufficient, part of medical ethics.
>
> Ethics provides a second, complimentary theory, often called the theory of duty, that defines the criteria whereby actions are judged right or wrong. It analyzes the relationship between intentions and consequences, motivations and circumstances. It studies the conditions of freedom and responsibility underlying imputation of guilt and innocence. (p. 132)

We might have substituted *clinician* for *physician* and *clinical* for *medical* in the quotation above, as the perspective on ethics is the same regardless of professional specialty. It is such theoretical bases that constitute current ethics, with its emphasis not simply on consequences (i.e., doing good), but also on duties such as being truthful, informing patients, and confidentiality—in short, respecting patients' autonomy.

The proponents of ''bioethics,'' a relatively new school of ethical thought, dispute the deductive approach to ethics and see concepts such as autonomy as the basis for fallacious ''reformist changes [which] have done considerable harm to patients'' (Sider, 1986, p. 406). Bioethics proposes a system of ''applied clinical ethics'' that is based on respect for individuals, rather than autonomy, and ''on affirmation of life, empathy, and norms of adaptive growth'' (Ciccone & Clements, 1984, p. 399). The bioethicists also make the point that

> The bottom line in all of [these] cases . . . is responsibility. . . . Decisions made by . . . patients or their relatives should also take into account the biological facts in the individual case, and physicians have the responsibility of determining what is good medical practice. (Potter, 1986, p. 401)

Even the strongest proponents of the "egalitarian–consumer model" would agree that a well-informed consumer is a prerequisite, and that bioethics creates a counterbalance to what has been called the *Pontius Pilate syndrome* (Trosko, 1984, cited in Romano, 1986), in which the clinician washes his hands of all responsibility for decisions.

Much of our practice is governed by laws such as those on confidentiality, civil commitment, and informed consent. Every clinician, at one time or another, is likely to be faced with legal questions, and many professional societies now offer legal counsel or advice to their members through attorneys for a fee. Although there is a tendency to view these laws as latter-day nuisances contaminating the sacrosanct therapist–patient relationship, the earliest known attempt to regulate medicine dates from A.D. 1240, when Frederick II decreed, among other things, the minimum qualifications for physicians and enacted the medieval version of our pure-drug laws.

An important question on the connection between laws and morality is: Can laws dictate morality? There are those, like philosopher Hart (1977), who argue that it is rational for society to defend certain basic moral values and that there is often moral reasoning behind what society puts into laws. Indeed, Hart argued that a collection of individuals becomes a society largely due to a "shared or public morality" (Wasserstrom, 1971, p. 51). Whatever the merits of this argument, the debate on various mental-health laws continues.

One of the severest critics of such laws is Thomas Szasz (1974), who has taken a libertarian position on matters such as the insanity defense, civil commitment, and other paternalistic interventions. His works are best read as those of a moral philosopher challenging the very *raison d'être* of psychiatry, the disease concept of insanity, and laws based on this premise, such as the civil commitment statutes, that deprive an individual of civil liberties. Despite the controversial nature of his views and his polemical style, his works are popular and have served to raise many ethical questions relating to psychiatric practice.

Paternalistic behavior is pervasive in clinical practice; treating patients without consent, the use of placebos, and civil involuntary commitment are but a few examples. Dworkin (1977) defined paternalism as "roughly the interference with a liberty of action justified by reasons referring exclusively to the welfare, good, happiness, needs, interests or the values of the person being coerced" (p. 191). Laws mandating the use of seatbelts or helmets, requiring a license to practice certain professions, and, of particular relevance to clinical work, allowing civil commitment procedures based on the welfare of the patient are paternalistic in purpose.

Clinicians, though accustomed to respecting and honoring patients' autonomy and freedom, may in certain situations be required to take extraordinary measures, such as committing a dangerous patient to a hospital. The current commitment laws arose following the well-known 19-century case of Mrs. E. Packard, who was committed to a state hospital under a statute that permitted a woman to be committed by her husband without adequate proof of insanity. In reaction to such abuses, most modern civil commitment statutes now have two theoretical bases: first, the "police power" when an individual is considered dangerous, and second, *parens patriae* power for individuals who are unable to care for themselves, the latter clearly paternalistic in motive. Even Mill (1956), the champion of individual liberty, acknowledged certain exceptions to his principle, but the paternalism embodied in present statutes often goes beyond the protection of society.

There is a common model for much outpatient work: A therapist and a patient enter into a contract, by which one party, the therapist, agrees to help the other, the patient, with a specific problem. One could argue that what goes on between the two is nobody else's business; the two are, after all, consenting adults. However, fees for service are increasingly paid for by third parties—insurance companies or the government—and the laws alluded to earlier are increasingly making the therapist accountable to outside agencies. Patients are increasingly taking their complaints either to the ethics committees of a professional organization that the therapist belongs to or to the courts. Sexual contacts and alleged overcharging are frequent complaints heard by ethics committees. Lawsuits against psychiatrists and psychologists are said to be increasing to "crisis proportions," and case law precedents such as the *Tarasoff* decision, to be discussed later, are dramatically affecting clinical practice.

In this chapter, we cannot possibly examine all of the laws or situations that raise ethical concerns that one is likely to encounter in outpatient practice. Instead, we address some frequently encountered ethical and legal dilemmas, outline relevant aspects of the legal system and some of its reasoning, and then end the chapter with a few words on prevention.

CURRENT ISSUES

One reason for the development of ethical codes for professional self-regulation, from ancient to modern times, is the implicit recognition of the vulnerability of the patient. The very act of seeking help for pain and suffering from another individual takes a modicum of trust in the caregiver and faith in the professional's ability, two elements likely to foster dependency. From their early origins in the temple of Delphi in ancient Greece to modern-day secular society, the health-related professions have had a certain aura about them. The very title *Doctor* often conjures up an image of a kind, gentle, and even omnipotent person. Most who enter the health-related professions are themselves likely to have encountered such a person, real or imagined, in their formative years. The stage is thus set for what is now referred to in psychoanalytic practice as *transference,* conceptualized as the re-creation of a parent–child relationship. Socioeconomic changes have done little to eradicate such imagery; health-related professionals, though no longer thought of as godlike, continue to command respect, if not adulation. The therapist–patient relationship cannot, therefore, be equal. There is always the potential for exploitation.

In the therapist–patient relationship, a dyad, the therapist's first and most important concern must be for the patient. Despite important changes in the socioeconomic climate in the past century, it is a truism to restate that principle. Yet, it is becoming increasingly difficult to perceive the relationship in strict dyadic terms; the traditional entrepreneurial model is rapidly becoming history. Most Western industrialized societies have one form or another of nationalized health care. In the United States, perhaps the only exception, many mental-health professionals work at least part time within an organization, and almost all derive payment from third parties. The amount charged for services is being regulated by insurance companies and more recently diagnostic related groups (DRGs), and peer reviews regulate the duration of treatment. In short, it is not always possible for therapists to tailor treatment to an individual based solely on his or her idea of what is best. What guidance could a therapist receive from a professional ethical code when faced with a mandate to terminate treatment despite her or his clinical judgment to the contrary? It is clear that codes established primarily to assist clinicians with individual patients are increasingly becoming obsolete, and a number of them are being revised in order to keep up with the changing times.

Mental health professionals are being called on to testify in courts and to work for industries, corporations, and other organizations. Here, too, our present ethical codes are often of little assistance. Some of the situations that clinicians are apt to confront could not have been foreseen when the current codes were formulated. Perhaps nothing has quite shaken the conscience of health-related professionals as much as the Nuremberg trials did after World War II. The trials revealed shockingly inhumane acts by physicians in concentration camps. In the past few years, there have also been revelations about the political abuses of psychiatry, particularly in the Soviet Union, and some, not quite so blatant and abhorrent, in the United States (Stone, 1984). Such revelations suggest the need to continue to revise the existing ethical codes. Could such abuses have taken place if the professionals worked for the individual patient rather than for the state? For now, this remains a rhetorical question. It is against the backdrop of the foregoing discussion that we attempt to address some specific contemporary ethical issues.

Informed Consent

In order for most psychiatric interventions to succeed, an atmosphere of mutual trust has to be created. The clinician's adherence to the principles of confidentiality and informed consent complements full disclosure on the part of the patient and is crucial for the desirable outcomes of symptom relief or cure. It is also possible to perceive the aims of all mental-health treatment as an attempt to support the autonomy and free choice of the patient (Szasz, 1974). Informing the patient of the disorder, the treatment and its risks and benefits, and the alternatives enhances the patient's autonomy. Hence, there is teleological and deontological justification for the doctrine of informed consent; it can be said that informed consent "is the basis of all psychiatric interventions and that without it no psychiatric intervention can be justified" (Redlich & Mollica, 1976, p. 125).

In the unequal clinician–patient relationship, it is the clinician's special knowledge that creates the advantage. Thus, informed consent is meant to force the clinician to give the patient the knowledge that will make him or her an equal bargaining partner (Stone, 1979). It is generally defined as the duty of the clinician to explain the procedure to the patient and to warn him or her of any material risks or dangers inherent in or collateral to the therapy, so as to enable the patient to make an intelligent and informed choice about whether to undergo such treatment (Miller, 1980).

Although the ethical commitment of the clinician is a protection for the patient against exploitation, the legal profession has used the doctrine of informed consent to increase the patient's autonomy. Two legal principles are embodied in the current view on informed consent: First, because of the special knowledge of the clinician and the helplessness of the patient, the relationship is "fiduciary" and therefore imposes a duty on the clinician to disclose to the patient all pertinent facts regarding the condition and the treatment. Second, there is the doctrine of self-determination (Miller, 1980). In 1914, Justice Cardozo stated this principle in this way: "Every human being of adult years and sound mind has a right to determine what shall be done with his own body" (cited in Miller, 1980, p. 2100).

The standards for legally sufficient disclosures vary from state to state. Traditionally, the duty was measured by a professional standard: the customary practices of professionals in the area, or what a reasonable professional would disclose in similar circumstances. Since the 1970s, however, a shift has occurred toward "patient-oriented" standards (i.e., what disclosures a patient would require in order to make a reasoned decision). However, clinicians are still expected to disclose only material risks and not all the possible risks of any treatment. One guiding principle for clinicians may well be to disclose risks that would be significant to the patient, which can be assumed to be the most serious and most common adverse effects of treatment. If the patient decides to proceed, knowing both the most serious and the most common risks, it is assumed that the patient would have consented if he or she had also known the less serious or uncommon risks.

There are several questions in outpatient psychiatric practice regarding informed consent. First, there are questions related to emergency treatment, which physicians are especially apt to confront. When a patient is an immediate source of danger to himself or herself or others in that he or she presents a clear threat to life or limb, consent is not required to treat or take other actions, but only to the extent necessary to mitigate the immediate threat. Second, there is the issue of competency to consent. When a patient's judgment is extremely impaired—because of acute psychosis, for example—it may be possible to obtain judicial consent to treat over the patient's objection. Patients whose judgment is sufficiently impaired to warrant this action are usually inpatients, however. Third, there are few specific and known material risks of psychotherapy, and informed consent may well take the form of simply notifying the patient about the alternative forms of treatment that may be available. Fourth, clinicians may be called as consultants in questionable cases to determine if a patient is capable of consenting to medical treatment. The determination of competency is based on whether the patient has the capacity to understand the nature of the disorder, the risks involved in treating it, and the consequences of not treating it.

Questions have been raised about how valid informed consents for surgery or medical treatments are, and mental health practice raises even more serious questions in this regard. Often, clinicians face dilemmas in informing the patient about serious diagnoses such as schizophrenia or latent homosexuality. One's clinical judgment may dictate that such disclosures be carefully timed, but failure to disclose such information may not allow the patient to truly consent to the recommended treatment. And finally, there is the question of minors and those impaired as a result of psychosis and dementia. Parents or legal guardians (the latter, if they are not one and the same) may consent for minors under the age of 18, but the consent must be informed and specific. The general consent to treat minors, which is often obtained at the beginning of treatment, is not regarded as informed as it relates to specific treatments and is therefore invalid. In some states, minors who are married, who are themselves parents, or who are between the ages of 16 and 18 and have been declared legally emancipated may consent for themselves. Although it is often useful and prudent to involve in treatment decisions the family of a psychotic or demented patient, the parent of an adult, a spouse, or an adult child of a patient may not legally consent to treatment over the patient's objection unless they have been empowered to do so by a court of law. In these cases, a judicial intervention may be the only alternative available to clinicians.

Finally, although most outpatient mental-health treatment is entirely voluntary, several states are contemplating statutes that would allow "outpatient commitments" for treatment. In addition, people may be placed on probation or parole following conviction for a criminal offense, and treatment may be mandated as a condition of remaining at large. When psychiatric treatment is mandated, ethical and legal questions may be raised about the validity of informed consent. It is still important to inform patients in these situations, particularly regarding the available alternatives, although their freedom to choose may be quite restricted.

Confidentiality

"The concept of professional confidentiality refers to the obligation of certain professions to respect information revealed in professional activities. Professional secrecy in medicine is mentioned in the Hippocratic Oath" (Redlich & Mollica, 1976, p. 133). Most modern ethical codes and practice standards contain a proscription related to the release of confidential information without the patient's permission. The Standards for Providers of Psychological Services of the American Psychological Association (1977b), for example, provide that

> The psychologist shall not release confidential information, except with the written consent of the user directly involved or his or her legal representative. (Standard 2.3.5, Interpretation)

Despite the long-standing ethic in all mental-health professions related to confidentiality, and the embodiment of the concept in many state and federal statutes, this tenet is rarely respected in legal proceedings. A patient who puts his or her mental status at issue is regarded as having waived his or her legal "privilege" with respect to information related to it. Thus, the patient who pleads insanity, who alleges psychological damages in a lawsuit, who presents "mental cruelty" as grounds for a divorce, or who engages in a child custody battle usually waives the right to confidentiality and subjects all prior mental-health treatment to scrutiny before the court. Even if the patient does not place her or his condition at issue, the courts frequently direct the release of information or the testimony of clinicians on the presentation of an argument that the interests of justice are so served. Similar dilemmas arise with respect to confidentiality and laws that require the reporting of child abuse and, more recently, the reporting of impaired professionals to licensing boards and offices of professional discipline. In each of these instances, the legal system recognizes the need to balance the welfare of the society against the privacy and the best interests of the patient. The American Psychological Association's Standards explicitly acknowledge this situation:

> If directed otherwise by statute or regulations with the force of law or by court order, the psychologist shall seek a resolution to the conflict that is both ethically and legally feasible and appropriate (American Psychological Association, 1977b, 2.3.5 Interpretation)

The standards do not suggest how the psychologist should do so, nor do they address the restoration of a therapeutic relationship after the patient has heard the clinician compelled to testify under oath about his or her often unfavorable opinion of the patient's mental condition. It is for this reason that many professional codes and standards also state that the professional "is responsible for informing the client of the limits of confidentiality" (American Psychological Association, 1977a, 6d). This dictum again raises the difficulty of balancing the establishment of trust with the need for candor regarding the limits of privacy in the therapeutic relationship.

Other issues that arise in the context of confidentiality are based on the patient's understanding of the purpose of the professional contact or the structure of the therapeutic relationship itself. In the course of

> standard clinical observation the patient is subjected to . . . intensive and extensive exploration of his personality and social relations. Even when this is done with the patient's explicit consent,

he is hardly ever aware of the depth and meaning of such explorations. (Redlich & Mollica, 1976, p. 133)

Information may also be obtained from collateral contacts who are unknown to the patient; this information may be damaging if it becomes known to the patient or to third parties. These issues become especially significant if the information is used for research purposes or in the publication of illustrative case summaries, despite the attempts of clinicians to disguise the case. Potentially damaging information that is unknown to the patient imposes an additional responsibility on the clinician when the patient consents to the release of information to another party, as in arranging ancillary services, or when the patient seeks access to his or her own records relating to treatment. It is for this reason that releases of information approved by the patient should be highly specific and limited to the minimum information necessary, and that clinicians must be judicious in their review of the materials to be released either to a third party or to the patient.

Confidentiality is also a significant problem when therapy is not conducted individually (e.g., couples and group therapy). Although these therapies may be justified clinically and economically, patients are under no ethical or legal obligation to maintain the confidences of their fellow patients. The group leader may emphasize the value of confidentiality, but he cannot enforce it outside the group. Besides the seemingly universal human tendency to gossip, there are situations in which patients may have compelling reasons to violate the confidences of their fellows. It is clear that ethical, and not just clinical, considerations may have to be addressed in deciding to forgo individual approaches with certain patients.

One final note on the limits of confidentiality relates to third-party payments. The increase in peer-review reimbursement controls has created a concomitant increase in the amount of information that must often be shared to establish the need for services and therefore to justify reimbursement for them. This is particularly true when the peer review organization (PRO) has questioned or disallowed payment, and the service provider must supply detailed treatment information to sustain an appeal of the adverse determination. Although this issue is of smaller concern when the PRO directly receives and presumably safeguards the information, our cost-conscious age has spawned some employers who self-insure and contract for limited professional-review services. In some of these cases, the employer receives the treatment information directly, and the potential for the misuse of sensitive material is greater.

The Duty to Warn

The issue that may have generated the greatest controversy and consternation within and between the mental health and the legal communities in the late 1970s and the 1980s is the so-called *Tarasoff* decision. Variously referred to as the "duty to warn" and the "duty to protect," the reasoning of *Tarasoff et seq.* touches on many ethical tenets and concerns.

Tarasoff v. Regents of the University of California began with the meeting of Prosenjit Poddar and Tatiana Tarasoff in the fall of 1968. Mr. Poddar became obsessed with Ms. Tarasoff and, in the fall of 1969, stabbed her to death after she rejected his romantic advances. Before the murder, Poddar had been evaluated at a University of California Hospital and was prescribed neuroleptic medication and admitted to weekly outpatient psychotherapy sessions with a psychologist. During the course of the therapy, Poddar revealed fantasies of harming or killing Tarasoff, and the therapist learned through other sources that he was seeking to purchase a gun.

The therapist consulted with the supervising psychiatrist and the psychiatrist who had evaluated Poddar for admission, and it was determined that hospitalization should be carried out. The mental health professionals contacted the campus police where Poddar was a student and asked for their assistance in committing him. The campus police went to Poddar's residence and, after questioning, accepted his denials that he intended any harm and left without taking further action. Poddar dropped out of treatment, and no further action was taken by the mental health professionals to detain him before the murder.

The Tarasoffs sued, alleging negligence in not confining Poddar or warning Tarasoff. The case was initially dismissed on the basis that no "duty" existed, but it was subsequently reinstated when the California Supreme Court ruled in 1974 that a "duty to warn" did exist under the circumstances. In 1976, the case was heard again, and the court broadened its original ruling to a "duty to protect" by determining that the clinicians had options other than warning the victim that would have met their duty to her.

The *Tarasoff* decision is a prime example of the effect of case law on the legal system and on mental health practice. Although technically limited to the jurisdiction of the California court, the *Tarasoff* precedent precipitated a nationwide reaction, as therapists in other jurisdictions feared that similar reasoning would be applied by other courts. At the same time, clinicians in many jurisdictions (New York, for example) faced an absolute statutory prohibition on taking actions consistent with the California court's ruling, such as violating confidentiality by warning a potential victim. In one of the most far-reaching decisions to date, the Vermont Supreme Court may have extended the "duty to protect" to all mental-health professionals, establishing a single standard of care for all levels of clinicians, and including property as well as persons under the protection umbrella (Stone, 1986).

One ethical dilemma created by *Tarasoff* is the conflict between the duty to warn and the constraints of confidentiality. If a therapist is obligated to warn or take other actions relating to the expressed violent or destructive impulses of the patient, is it ethical to permit or encourage the patient's belief that what is said in therapy will be held confidential? Conversely, what will be the effect on the development of trust in the therapeutic relationship if the therapist greeted each new patient with a warning about the limits of confidentiality? Even if patients continued in therapy, they would be likely to avoid any discussion, and therefore resolution, of problems related to violent or destructive impulses.

The *Tarasoff* decision also directly affects the clinician's judgment in conducting therapy. Some clinicians have resorted to avoiding any discussion of violent or destructive impulses as a way of avoiding the *Tarasoff* dilemma. Others have found themselves delving disproportionately into the slightest indication of such impulses in an attempt to ferret out the correct course of action. Regardless of the tack taken, such amendments in the face of *Tarasoff* are clearly distortions of the therapeutic process, with implications for both the outcome and the duration of therapy. In many cases, the clinician's interests in protecting potential victims and himself or herself are in conflict with the patient's interest in resolving the problems that led to therapy in the first place.

In an excellent overview of the *Tarasoff* decision and nearly 20 subsequent cases in various jurisdictions, Beck (1985) noted that there is no unanimity among the courts on the "duty to protect" or, where held, its parameters. Beck also noted that, in 46 States and the District of Columbia, there has been no ruling on the issue.

Legislative redress of the problem has provided little guidance. In New York, for example, the legislature amended the confidentiality statute (33.13 NYS Mental Hygiene Law) to permit *Tarasoff*-type warnings, but it specifically included the statement that this statutory permission to warn does not necessarily impose a duty to do so. Despite the legal ambiguity, the "duty to protect" has, in effect, become a national standard of practice, as therapists have incorporated its provisions into their repertoire, and clinicians are advised to proceed accordingly (Beck, 1985, p. 33).

Predicting the Future

Another dilemma created by the *Tarasoff* decision pertains to the noted unreliability of clinical predictions of future behavior, especially dangerousness. This problem also arises in many courtroom situations when clinicians may be called on to predict a prognosis for rehabilitation or suitability for child rearing. Extensive reviews of the literature have found that two out of three predictions of dangerousness are not borne out within 5 years after the prediction has been made (Monahan, 1981). Similar results may be expected with other, similar types of predictions.

There are many reasons for the poor prediction record of mental health professionals. Clinicians must often base predictions on incomplete information, especially when the patient whose behavior is being predicted stands to gain from concealing unfavorable information, such as when the patient is attempting to avoid commitment. Regardless of the depth of our knowledge of the patient, almost all behavior is situational as well as dispositional. Our recognition of self-defense as a valid excuse for murder is an acknowledgment of the situational nature of such behavior. Both situational and dispositional factors change with time, and the longer into the future a prediction extends, the greater is its uncertainty. There is also a lack of standardized methods and parameters for making such predictions, which contributes to poor reliability between clinicians. And many events that are subject to prediction, including violence, are truly infrequent occurrences; the result is a phenomenon known as the *base-rate problem,* in which even very accurate prediction methods produce significant error rates.

Clinicians are expected and sometimes required to make predictions, however, in both the clinical and the legal arenas. Knowing that such predictions are fallible, the ethical clinician must seek as much information as possible about both the patient and the situations to which the prediction will apply, must limit predictions to the immediate future, must adopt standardized methods that are supported by the literature, must be wary of predicting uncommon events, and must qualify any predictions that are communicated to others, with regard to each of these factors.

Ethics in the Courtroom

When called to testify in a court of law, to whom does the therapist owe his or her allegiance: the patient, the party paying for the testimony, the state, or some vague and personalized notion of justice? Consider an example in which a clinician is asked to examine a creative artist charged with high treason, the sure punishment for which is execution. If the clinician were to testify that the individual is insane (a strictly legal concept), long-term incarceration in a mental hospital rather than death might be meted out. Now, if the person is not truly insane, it may be argued that the truth would, in fact, hurt the patient. It is likely that precisely such a dilemma was faced by mental health professionals when they examined Ezra Pound, the great American poet, who was charged with treason for collaborating with fascists during World War II.

This dilemma has become more common with the incorporation of psychiatric examination into death penalty statutes. In Texas, for example, there is a requirement that the prosecution establish incorrigibility as a condition of imposing the death penalty. One practitioner earned the moniker of "Dr. Death" because of the predictability of his testimony about the future actions of those he examined in capital cases. In another case, a person was found incompetent to proceed after a death sentence had been imposed. The dilemma for the clinicians in the case might have been to choose between effectively treating the patient so that he could be put to death, or failing to treat him so that he would remain psychotic and alive.

Although forensic psychiatry and psychology are increasingly specialized fields, clinicians in nonforensic outpatient practice may occasionally be called on to testify in the courts. As was noted earlier, current ethical codes do not offer much guidance to clinicians, although the issues involved have been the subject of inquiry (Ciccone & Clements, 1984; Stone, 1984). In addition to the questions of agency (Whom does the clinician work for?), confidentiality, and prediction, there are ethical questions related to giving an opinion about patients who are deceased and cannot be examined (such as in a malpractice suit following a suicide), basing opinions on retrospective examinations conducted long after the event in question (such as assessing criminal responsibility), and answering purely hypothetical questions. All of these situations are fairly common in criminal and civil court cases, and those who are frequently involved with forensic matters will find the aforementioned articles particularly helpful.

Others who may be called on to submit an opinion to a court should follow some basic guidelines. First, if possible, the patient should be informed about the purpose of the examination beforehand, including whom the clinician is working for and being paid by. Second, the clinician should be aware of the purpose of the report or testimony. Psychological and psychiatric testimonies are being used for everything from capital punishment to child custody cases. It is prudent to ask the party who solicits or summons the testimony the exact purpose of the professional opinion in the case and the *specific* question to be addressed, as the true reason is not always apparent. Third, the clinician should make every effort to base statements and opinions on strict standards of truth and scientific knowledge. When opinions are based on personal bias or are highly speculative, the clinician should clearly state the qualifications on his or her opinion or, better yet, state that he or she has no *professional* opinion on the question, as one cannot be compelled to have an opinion. The general public is increasingly skeptical of mental health professionals battling in courts with contradictory opinions. When these opinions are not scientifically based, the testimony serves only to confuse the trier of facts, or to provide a convenient pseudoscientific rationalization to justify a previously held conclusion. Clinicians have a responsibility to restrict their courtroom testimony to their areas of competency; by doing so, they will also further the interests of justice.

Sexual Exploitation of Patients

Some years ago, most clinicians listening to an allegation of sexual liaisons between a therapist and a patient would have dismissed it as a manifestation of eroticized transference or wishful thinking. Although it is difficult to obtain hard data on the magnitude of this problem, it is now widely accepted that sexual exploitation does occur and that it is not as infrequent as was once believed. In a recent nationwide survey of U.S. psychiatrists, nearly 7% of the male and 3% of the female respondents acknowledged sexual contact with their patients (Gartrell, Herman, Olarte, Feldstein, & Localio, 1986). Most victims are females who are taken advantage of by their male therapists. Indeed, sexual exploitation is one of the most common complaints heard by professional ethics committees and is the subject of many lawsuits, most resolved in favor of the complainant.

The defense that the liaison was consensual is not accepted, the courts generally holding that the dependency of the therapeutic relationship, and what clinicians would call transference, precludes a truly voluntary decision on the part of the patient. Because it is now clear that a sexual liaison between a therapist and a patient is detrimental to and traumatic for the patient, a defense that the act was part of the therapy is no longer credible. Even in the case of a sexual relationship that develops after the termination of treatment, it is difficult to argue that the clinician did not take advantage of the therapeutic relationship with the patient. Professional organizations do not condone such behavior, and the American Psychiatric Association (1985, Section 2), for one, specifically forbids sexual activity with patients. Clinicians are thus likely to face professional censure as well as litigation, and some insurance carriers now specifically exclude coverage for liability arising out of sexual activity with patients. It is often unclear if this caveat also includes the cost of the legal defense, especially if the allegations are eventually proved to be untrue. In certain states, the clinician may also jeopardize his or her license to practice, though much depends on how closely the licensing authorities work with professional societies.

Finally, there is the issue of what clinicians should do when confronted with revelations by a patient of sexual exploitation by a colleague. Should one hide behind the veil of confidentiality? Regulations may require reporting such allegations to the proper authorities. It is also worth noting that many clinicians who sexually exploit a patient are likely to do so with more than one individual, and a case may therefore be made that the patient should be encouraged to take the complaint to the appropriate agency for investigation. Stone (1984) offered some valuable practical advice to clinicians in this regard:

> The therapist who is convinced that a patient has been victimized can suggest to the patient that they both or that the patient alone discuss the situation with a consultant (the administrator). If the patient agrees, thereafter the consultant would assume responsibility for ensuring a knowing waiver of confidentiality. The patient and consultant can press appropriate ethical and legal remedies, while the therapist and patient can remain in a traditional therapeutic relationship if that seems desirable. (p. 210)

Not all who exploit their patients sexually are the same. Some are impaired themselves and others display flawed character (Stone, 1984). But as Webb (1986) noted:

> In the final analysis the integrity of our profession lies in the integrity of our individual practitioners. We must continually remind ourselves of the power of the doctor-patient relationship. The power that offers the capacity to heal contains the capacity to cloud therapeutic objectivity. In the covenant with our patients we realize our greatest therapeutic potential. Threats to the covenant damage our basic professional integrity. (p. 1150)

LEGAL PROCESS

Hart (1977), to whose work we alluded earlier, suggested that there are primary rules that impose duties and secondary rules that instruct us on how to adjudicate the primary rules. Another way of viewing this distinction is the familiar dichotomy between content and process. There are laws and court rulings that impose a legal duty on clinicians (e.g., the duty to warn, the duty to inform, and the duty to report child abuse). There are also laws that define criminal behavior, and there are contracts. Together, these laws, rulings, and contracts establish legal "content." The "rule of law" is actually a system of hierarchical rules. Federal rules supercede state rules in matters of mutual concern, and in each system, the U.S. Constitution take precedence over statutes, or laws, which take precedence over administrative regulations. Each successive level of rules generally provides greater detail consistent with the principles set forth by the broader codes. The courts interpret the application of all of these rules to a given set of facts in accordance with separate procedural rules and in the context of "case law" (the recorded prior decisions of other, similar court cases) and "common law" (the recognized past practices of society). It is this historical continuity, with principles dating back several centuries, that forms the backdrop for judging current events.

In most noncriminal matters or "torts," a legal term for civil wrong, negligence theories establish the process by which duties (the content) are adjudicated. Simple negligence is "a breach of duty causing injury." All four elements (i.e., duty, a breach of that duty, injury, and a causal link between the two) must be established for a finding of negligence. Professional malpractice is a special case of negligence.

Let us consider, at some length, the four elements that the party bringing suit (the plaintiff) tries to establish in typical malpractice cases. First, the plaintiff tries to establish that there was a duty to the patient. In most cases in which a therapist agrees to see a person for a problem, a duty to the individual is established by virtue of the professional relationship. This duty may vary according to the condition of the patient and the nature of the relationship, and it becomes a fundamental issue if the plaintiff claims abandonment. It is customary for clinicians to see a patient for one or more sessions to determine whether they can continue to work together. The patient, however, may misunderstand the purpose of these visits and may expect more. The clinician may become liable for abandonment if, after several sessions, she or he abruptly terminates therapy without properly informing the patient of the reasons for the termination or making a referral for continued care. When clinicians are referred patients for testing or diagnosis by various agencies, it is prudent to explain to the patient the purpose of these visits. In such cases, the duty is not to treat but to investigate or diagnose. The legal mandate reinforces a good clinical practice of establishing a "therapeutic contract" with a clear understanding about the purpose and frequency of visits, fees, and other conditions of treatment.

The second element of negligence is establishing that a breach of duty occurred. The breach of duty could be an act of commission (such as violating confidentiality), or it could be an act of omission. What is generally at issue is whether the clinician conformed to the standards of care existing in the community. In professional malpractice, expert opinion is relied on to establish a "standard of care" that determines if a duty existed and if it was breached. The "duty" owed in simple negligence cases is the duty to behave as a "reasonable person" would under the circumstances; the "duty" owed in professional malpractice cases is to behave as a "reasonable and qualified professional" would under the same circumstances. Thus, in malpractice cases, the plaintiff's attorney tries to establish, first, the standard of care that existed under the circumstances (the duty owed the plaintiff by the defendant) and, second, that a breach of that duty (a deviation from reasonable professional behavior) occurred.

The standard of care applicable to clinicians is usually limited geographically to the community of practice (the "strict-locality" rule). In other words, due consideration is usually given to the fact that sophisticated skills and tools may not be available to practitioners in various areas, such as a CT scan to a physician practicing in a remote locale. Therefore, the plaintiff's attorney usually draws from the pool of local experts and relies on their stated practices to establish the standard of care in that community. An exception to this rule occurs in a highly specialized practice when there is no one else with expertise in the immediate locality, and a regional or national standard must be applied.

It is also generally assumed that the various professions in the mental health field have differing expertise: a social worker or psychologist would not be expected to have the same ability to diagnose a medical illness as would a psychiatrist, although they may be expected to make an appropriate referral to rule out such an illness. In short, various disciplines are judged by different standards of care specific to each discipline, based on the testimony of qualified professionals from the local community.

It is unclear whether the courts will continue to honor geographic and discipline-specific standards to the same degree as they have to date. With vast improvements in travel and communications, and with increasing specialization, on the one hand, and broader recognition of nonmedical mental health professionals, on the other, it is becoming increasingly difficult for clinicians to claim, other than in extraordinary circumstances, geographic or discipline-specific standards. A recent case in Vermont may have set a precedent for a ''higher standard of care'' that transcends professional boundaries. Stone (1986) concluded, based on this decision, that, ''as far as organized settings are concerned, [the decision] transforms what are arguably different and lower professional standards of care for nonmedical psychotherapists into a single and higher psychiatric professional standard'' (p. 354).

Laws, prior court cases, and guidelines established by professional organizations or institutions establish principles that can all be used to demonstrate a standard of care. Let us consider, as an example, electroconvulsive therapy (ECT). The American Psychiatric Association task force report on ECT (1978) offers certain guidelines about indications, contraindications, and investigations that should be done before the prescription of such treatment. But policies of the institution that the clinician practices in or local ordinances against the uses of ECT, such as in Berkeley, California, may determine the local standards for prescribing ECT in some instances.

The third element in malpractice cases is to establish that harm came to the patient. Suits for emotional injury due to negligent psychotherapy are unlikely to succeed, and indeed, there are virtually no reported cases imposing liability for negligent psychotherapy resulting in purely emotional harm (Klein, Macbeth, & Onek, 1984). Yet, the principle of emotional trauma has long been established in the law (awards for ''pain and suffering'' are cases in point), and mental health professionals have also recognized that psychotherapy may at times be harmful to patients. The problem may well be establishing a causal link between a certain technique in psychotherapy and adverse emotional consequences. On the other hand, clinicians may be held liable for making an erroneous diagnosis of a serious mental disorder and thereby for causing ''pain and suffering'' to the patient. In situations in which alternatives to psychotherapy are available, such as psychotropic drugs, clinicians should advise patients about the risks and benefits of all the available treatment modalities, and the patient should be encouraged and assisted to make an informed choice.

The majority of mental-health-related malpractice cases involve the use of somatic therapies such as psychotropic drugs. In the past few years, lawsuits against psychiatrists over tardive dyskinesia have been increasing. With most drug treatments, side effects, major or minor, are likely to occur. But tardive dyskinesia is often dramatic and irreversible, and in jury trials, awards are likely to be high when the patient is seen to have marked abnormal facial and tongue movements. As was noted earlier, the questions center on the adequacy of the treatment and on conformity with accepted standards. Was the treatment appropriate for the condition? If, for instance, the patient was prescribed medication not clearly indicated by the patient's symptoms, the liability is increased. Appropriate tests should be carried out before instituting certain treatment (e.g., because of potential teratogenic effects, pregnancy tests in sexually active women of child-bearing age before treatment with lithium carbonate, or appropriate investigations to rule out increased intracranial pressure before the use of ECT).

Physicians are expected to keep themselves informed of the current literature and to familiarize themselves with contraindications, dosages, and the side and adverse effects of the medications they prescribe. Nonmedical practitioners who are working with a patient taking psychotropic medications are also expected to be generally familiar with the side and adverse effects of those medications. Nonmedical clinicians should also be familiar with the symptoms of medical diseases that may mimic psychopathology, so that they know when to make a referral to a physician to rule out an organic condition manifesting itself as a psychological disorder (Bockar, 1976). Even if all of the appropriate procedures are followed, failure to obtain the patient's informed consent may increase liability. Because this issue has gained increasing importance in recent years, it was discussed at some length earlier in the chapter.

And finally, the causal link between the breach of duty and harm to the patient needs to be established. There are few cases of harm arising out of totally unexpected and clearly negligent acts on the part of clinicians, the legal term for which is *res ipsa loquitur* ("that speaks for itself"). An example in surgery would be finding a pair of forceps in a patient's abdomen after routine surgery. In mental health practice, though, such instances are rare. Sudden, unexpected, and grave adverse effects can and do occur, such as suicide, or sudden death following treatment with certain neuroleptics. But they cannot always be attributed to negligence on the part of the clinician. One should note in this context that clear and unequivocal proof is not necessary to establish the link between treatment and harm. Consider the example of tardive dyskinesia, which may occur spontaneously in some cases. However, the chances that tardive dyskinesia will occur in patients receiving neuroleptic medication are higher, and the courts are likely to attribute the "proximate cause" of the symptoms to the side effects of neuroleptics and to hold the prescriber liable.

It is estimated that as many as 20% of malpractice cases against psychiatrists may be over patients' successful or attempted suicides (Klein *et al.*, 1984). Although it is generally accepted that suicides are difficult to control on an outpatient basis, the question of liability usually centers on whether the clinician adequately assessed the patient's suicide potential and whether the risks and benefits of different preventive strategies were considered in response to these indicators. The strategies may include hospitalization, a change in the treatment plan, recourse to medication, or obtaining a second opinion. Clinicians may, of course, make erroneous judgments even after following appropriate procedures, such as obtaining a good history, reviewing previous records, and formally assessing suicide potential. But such errors in professional judgment do not constitute negligence if the clinician acted in accordance with professional standards.

One final issue related to malpractice actions is liability for the errors of others. Normally, an individual clinician cannot be held liable for the actions of someone else, but there are three legal principles that are exceptions to the rule. The first, "borrowed servant," pertains to another who is directly under the control of the clinician. One example, again drawn from surgery, is a surgeon directing the actions of a subordinate in an immediate, step-by-step fashion (this situation is very rare in mental health practice). The second area pertains to the more general and more common "supervision" of an allied professional or paraprofessional. Although a supervisor cannot be held liable for the actions of a subordinate or associate, the supervisor *can* be held liable for negligent supervision. Unfortunately, many clinicians are nominally supervising an associate, but they do not, in fact, have a formal supervisory relationship. If someone is practicing "under supervision" and a formal supervisory relationship cannot be shown, the supervisor may also be held liable for negligent acts. The final exception to the rule is the legal principle of "joint and several liability." The target of many of the current calls for tort reform, this principle provides that, in a case where more than one party is determined to have caused an injury, all such parties are responsible for the full amount of the damages. As a result, a clinician may be assigned 10% of the responsibility for an injury but may end up paying 100% of the damages if the other parties found to have been at fault are unable to pay. This situation is not actually liability for the actions of others but disproportionate liability for one's own negligent contribution to the harm.

Although tort law is the most common concern of many clinicians with the legal system, three other areas of law warrant brief mention. Criminal law intrudes on clinical practice in two ways, first, through the use of expert opinion in deciding such matters as criminal competency and culpability and, second, through the criminal prosecution of clinicians. Examples of criminal complaints that have, on occasion, arisen from clinical practice include battery, which is the unlawful touching of another and is also a tort; sexual misconduct or sexual abuse, a specific form of battery; unlawful imprisonment; falsifying records; obstructing governmental administration; and fraud. Although these cases are relatively rare, it should be noted that criminal intent is not always required and that the consent of the victim is no safeguard, as the capability of giving consent is often an issue when psychiatric patients are involved. It should also be noted that many insurance policies or indemnification laws specifically exclude intentional or criminal wrongdoing from their coverage.

Another area of relevance to the clinician is contract law. A contract is defined as an agreement, *written or oral,* between two or more persons, that is enforceable by the courts. There are both express contracts, in which an overt promise is made, and implied contracts, in which the nature of the relationship, actions, or behavior of the parties imposes a binding contract even though there has been no express agreement. Thus, there are legal as well as ethical reasons for ensuring clarity in relationships with patients, and for not making promises that one is not fully prepared to keep.

STRATEGIES FOR CONTEMPORARY OUTPATIENT PRACTICE

Two seemingly contradictory threads of continuity throughout the preceding sections have been (1) the extent of controversy that surrounds most ethical and legal issues in the mental health field and (2) the degree to which good practice, ethical practice, and legally prudent practice coincide. In this section, we turn our attention to the prevention of legal difficulties through the application of strategies that are consistent with avoiding ethical dilemmas and ensuring good clinical practice. We will also apply these same strategies to the resolution of ethical and legal dilemmas, as even the best clinical skills and the most reasoned practice may not preclude all of the complications of modern outpatient practice.

From a legal perspective, the reduction or avoidance of untoward negative incidents in patient care is called *risk management.* Risk management has received a great deal of discussion in recent years, as escalating liability costs have drawn the attention of practitioners, insurers, and accrediting bodies to the need for something more than traditional quality-assurance programs. Risk management is an organized strategy for identifying risks to patients and practitioners and taking positive steps to minimize those risks.

In larger organized settings, risk management assumes a formal, sometimes overly bureaucratic form, often involving several full-time people to collect, analyze, and act on voluminous information. Many small clinics and independent practitioners have correctly felt that such systems are irrelevant to their context, and they have tended to disregard risk management concepts along with the bureaucracy they have spawned. It is, however, a mistake to regard risk management as something that comes in only one size and shape, or that depends on formal programs for its effectiveness. Bennett and Simpson (1984) presented a conceptualization of risk management that is as basic as the ''three R's'': reason, records, and rapport. These concepts may be applied in any clinical setting, and if applied correctly, they contain inherent checks and balances. They are most effective when applied at the level of the individual practitioner, regardless of context, because the individual practitioner has the most control over the interactions with patients. In this regard, many clinicians would do well to remember the famous line of Walt Kelly's Pogo: ''We have met the enemy, and they is us.''

Reason

The first of the three R's is reason. Reason enters into risk management in several ways. First, clinical practice should, of course, be well reasoned. Clinicians are trained to carefully assess a patient's strengths and weaknesses, and to undertake treatment that is tailored to the needs and abilities of the individual. Each course of treatment should be well thought out, and the clinician should carefully apply his or her knowledge, training, experience, and intuition, not only to project the expected course of the treatment, but also to anticipate possible deviations and to address them in a planned way.

Second, reason is embodied in a legal duty to behave as a reasonable and qualified professional would behave under the circumstances. This legal duty introduces the concept of *community standards,* and it is the community standards that provide an ongoing sense of balance to the individual practitioner. It is comparing one's own views with a shared worldview that provides perspective, what in clinical terms is often referred to as *reality testing.* And it is this perspective that permits the accurate assessment of appropriate actions. Inherent in the need to contrast ones own standards with community standards is the need to become aware of what those standards are. Common practices such as continuing education, consultation, second opinions, and simple discussions of clinical issues are not just good risk management, they also lead to good patient care.

Records

The second of the three R's is records; good documentation of the patient's care is the single greatest defense against legal risk. It is also essential to good patient care in any kind of practice involving more than a single clinician. It is the most reliable, and often the only means of detailed communication between multiple professionals involved in the care of a single patient. Finally, good documentation contributes to good care even when only one clinician is caring for the patient. It permits a review of and reflection on past interactions with the patient that are not subject to the vagaries of human memory, and it is the only reasonable way to transmit knowledge about a patient to another practitioner if need be (e.g., if it becomes necessary to temporarily or permanently transfer the care of the patient, or if a consultation is warranted).

Credibility is at the heart of good records. They should be timely; information should be recorded when obtained, not after it has been corrupted by hindsight and weaknesses of memory. They are accurate; they record what actually happened and when it actually happened. And they are thorough; they record all of the relevant information, separating the wheat from the chaff, and they record the *reasoning* used by the clinician throughout the course of treatment, including the reasoning of other professionals. It is important to note that credibility of records is established by the quality of what is written, not the quantity. Just as in informed consent, the key to good record-keeping is to note the most common and most significant information, and then to show how applying professional judgment to this information led to a well-reasoned course of action. Writing everything into the records out of fear that it may someday become significant documents the clinician's apparent inability to identify the significant facts on which to base a judgment. One final note on credibility relates to ''after-the-fact'' entries. A note written after a significant adverse event has occurred has no credibility, as the secondary gain of such a note is so obvious. Unorthodox practices such as ''squeezing in'' a line within a note or inaccurate dating are also quite easy to detect, and they impugn the credibility of the entire record, regardless of when the entry was actually made.

Rapport

The last of the three R's is rapport. Rapport is important from two perspectives: rapport with colleagues and rapport with patients. Throughout the previous sections, we have discussed various situations in which there is an ethical imperative to share information with the patient. Good clinical practice also dictates a good rapport with the patient; there must be trust and good communication for the therapy to proceed. Rapport is especially important when one is treading on thin ice. Risky cases, risky procedures, or difficult situations should stimulate the desire to communicate carefully both with the patient and with professional colleagues.

In some situations where rapport is critical, it also seems counterintuitive: the natural tendency when something has ''gone wrong'' is to become defensive and to avoid sharing information with the patient or significant others. It is in precisely these situations that the wise clinician establishes personal contact with the patient or the family, if appropriate, and offers sympathy, empathy, and an honest discussion of the *facts* of the situation. In many situations, such an approach may minimize the damage, may allow for the resurrection of treatment, and may prevent more formal actions.

The reactions of many clinicians when a legal action is filed against them is strikingly similar to the stages of grief described by Kübler-Ross (1969). Initial denial, characterized by minimizing the seriousness of the situation, quickly gives way to anger directed toward the patient, his or her family, the lawyers, the courts, colleagues, administrators, insurance companies, or others. Both denial and anger are counterproductive, of course, as they tend to alienate those involved and to inhibit the clinician's ability to resolve the situation or even to formulate an effective defense. The clinician may also move through stages of guilt, bargaining, and depression, in which she or he may attempt to "undo" or compensate for the injuries suffered by the plaintiff, regardless of the clinician's responsibility or control over them. These reactions are particularly damaging to the clinician, as this stage often coincides with the "discovery" or trial phases of the legal process, when self-doubt may lead to legally incriminating statements that irreparably harm the defense. Being the target of a legal action is very stressful, and the similarities noted above suggest that, for some individuals, it may be equivalent to the death of a close friend or relative. Under these circumstances, a clinician's rapport with colleagues and significant others is critical, and formalized professional counseling during the active phases of the suit should be considered if for no other reason than the fact that it affords a relatively safe forum in which to discuss the issues raised by the trauma.

SUMMARY

In the collective psyche of mental health professionals, the benign face of the blindfolded symbol of justice has been replaced by a Janus-like figure, a far more grotesque face confronting the practitioner. The average clinician is unfamiliar with and intimidated by forensic issues. The process of entering a courtroom is apt to raise the anxiety of all but a few seasoned forensic specialists. Nationwide calls for tort reform are punctuated with a quotation from Shakespeare: "Kill all the lawyers." Whatever the nature of such reforms, it is clear that ethical and legal considerations have inexorably changed the practice of mental health professionals, and the clock can hardly be turned back.

Ignorance may contribute to some clinicians' fears. Few clinical training programs require any formal courses in ethics and law. Understanding the foundations of law and ethics enables one to make sense of the maze of rules and regulations that govern clinical practice, especially when one realizes that regulations pertaining to such things as confidentiality, informed consent, and record keeping reinforce the need to attain rapport and to have a good rationale for what we do, two basic ingredients of successful therapy. Clinicians do, through their individual and collective morality, shape the rules, and the rules, in turn, shape our moral views. Knowledge of these topics will not totally obviate litigation because we cannot eliminate human error or adverse outcomes, but such knowledge does, in the long run, make us better clinicians and help us to serve our patients better.

REFERENCES

American Psychiatric Association. (1978). *Task force report 14: Electroconvulsive therapy*. Washington, DC: Author.

American Psychiatric Association. (1985). *The principles of medical ethics with annotations especially applicable to psychiatry*. Washington, DC: Author.

American Psychological Association. (1977a). *Ethical standards of psychologists*. Arlington, VA: Author.

American Psychological Association. (1977b). *Standards for providers of psychological services*. Arlington, VA: Author.

Bennett, H. M., & Simpson, H. H. (1984). *Hospital law seminar* Presented in New York, May 7, 8. Nashville: Health Law Institute.

Beck, J. C. (Ed.). (1985). *The potentially violent patient and the Tarasoff decision in psychiatric practice*. Washington, DC: American Psychiatric Press.

Bockar, J. A. (1976). *Primer for the nonmedical psychotherapist.* New York: Spectrum.

Ciccone, J. R., & Clements, C. (1984). Forensic psychiatry and applied clinical ethics: Theory and practice. *American Journal of Psychiatry, 141*(3), 395–399.

Dworkin, G. (1977). Paternalism. In S. J. Reiser, A. J. Dyck, & W. J. Curran (Eds.), *Ethics in medicine: Historical perspectives and contemporary concerns.* Cambridge: Massachusetts Institute of Technology.

Engelhardt, H. T., & McCullough, L. B. (1981). Ethics in psychiatry. In S. Arieti & H. K. Brodie (Eds.), *American handbook of psychiatry* (2nd ed., Vol. 7). New York: Basic Books.

Gartrell, N., Herman, J., Olarte, S., Feldstein, M., & Localio, R. (1986). Psychiatrist-patient sexual contact: Results of a national survey: 1. Prevalence. *American Journal of Psychiatry, 143,* 1126–1131.

Hart, H. L. A. (1977). Laws and morals. In S. J. Reiser, A. J. Dyck, & W. J. Curran (Eds.), *Ethics in medicine: Historical perspectives and contemporary concerns.* Cambridge: Massachusetts Institute of Technology.

Jonsen, A. R., & Hellegers, A. E. (1977). Conceptual foundations for an ethics of medical care. In S. J. Reisner, A. J. Dyke, & W. J. Curran (Eds.), *Ethics in medicine: Historical perspectives and contemporary concerns.* Cambridge: Massachusetts Institute of Technology.

Klein, J. I., Macbeth, J. F., & Onek, J. N. (1984). *Legal issues in the private practice of psychiatry.* Washington, DC: American Psychiatric Press.

Kübler-Ross, E. (1969). *On death and dying.* New York: Macmillan.

Mill, J. S. (1956). *On liberty.* (1859) Indianapolis: Liberal Arts Press.

Mill, J. S. (1977). Utilitarianism (1871). In S. J. Reiser, A. J. Dyck, & W. J. Curran (Eds.), *Ethics in medicine: Historical perspectives and contemporary concerns.* Cambridge: Massachusetts Institute of Technology.

Miller, L. J. (1980). Informed consent: 1. *Journal of the American Medical Association, 244,* 2100–2103.

Monahan, J. (1981). *The clinical prediction of violent behavior.* Rockville, MD: National Institute of Mental Health.

Potter, V. R. (1986). Applied bioethics and the crisis in health care. *Psychiatric Annals, 16,* 399–401.

Redlich, F., & Mollica, R. (1976). Overview: Ethical issues in contemporary psychiatry. *American Journal of Psychiatry, 133,* 125–156.

Romano, J. (1986). A psychiatrist's view of the state of medical ethics: Progress and peril. *Psychiatric Annals, 16,* 390–394.

Ross, W. D. (1977). What makes right acts right? In S. J. Reiser, A. J. Dyck, & W. J. Curran (Eds.), *Ethics in medicine: Historical perspectives and contemporary concerns.* Cambridge: Massachusetts Institute of Technology. (Originally published 1930.)

Sider, R. C. (1986). Moral direction and misdirection for residents in the psychiatric emergency room. *Psychiatric Annals, 16,* 405–407.

Stone, A. A. (1979). Informed consent: Special problems for psychiatry. *Hospital and Community Psychiatry, 30,* 321–327.

Stone, A. A. (1984). *Law, psychiatry and morality.* Washington, DC: American Psychiatric Press.

Stone, A. A. (1986). Vermont adopts *Tarasoff:* A real barn burner. *American Journal of Psychiatry, 143,* 352–355.

Szasz, T. S. (1974). *The myth of mental illness* (rev. ed.). New York: Harper & Row.

Trosko, J. E. (1984). Scientific views of human nature: Implications for the ethics of technological intervention. In D. H. Brock (Ed.), *The culture of biomedicine: Studies in science and culture, Vol. 1.* Cranberry, NJ: University of Delaware Press.

Wasserstrom, R. A. (1971). *Morality and the law.* Belmont, CA: Wadsworth.

Webb, W. L. (1986). Editorial: The doctor-patient covenant and the threat of exploitation. *American Journal of Psychiatry, 143,* 1149–1150.

27

The Suicidal Patient

JEROME A. MOTTO

INTRODUCTION

Suicidal patients occupy a special place in any clinician's practice, largely because of the social, legal, and ethical implications of self-destructive behavior in our culture. As suicide is the most visible cause of mortality in persons with emotional disorders, intense family concern and a sense of professional vulnerability bring a certain urgency to the issues involved. A sound approach to these issues does not always preclude a suicidal outcome, but it can help to minimize preventable deaths, which constitute a tragic human loss and a source of severe stress to therapists and to vulnerable survivors.

Outpatients pose obvious risks related to the limited contact with the therapist and the frequent lack of a consistent support system, as compared with inpatients. However, the high frequency of suicidal states, the clinical import of autonomy, current pressures to use the "least restrictive alternative" as regards treatment, third-party payers' vigorous efforts to minimize the use and duration of inpatient care, the numerous chronically disturbed patients in urban centers, patient resistance to hospitalization, and therapists' reluctance to resort to involuntary measures—all contribute to the very large number of suicidal persons treated as outpatients.

This discussion reviews the background and current status of problem areas relevant to the outpatient treatment of suicidal adults, with suggested approaches to dealing effectively with those areas. Much of the material will be familiar to experienced clinicians, and many of the points will appear obvious. However, when adverse outcomes are reviewed, it is sometimes the obvious that has been overlooked.

JEROME A. MOTTO • University of California, School of Medicine, San Francisco, California 94143.

Etiology of Suicidal States

A wide range of psychological, social, and biological issues are known to contribute to the impulse to end one's life. Every suicidal person can be viewed as representing a unique combination of these issues. They can be grouped in various ways (Shneidman, 1985, pp. 23–40), one of which is the following four basic etiological patterns, which are not mutually exclusive.

Depressive suicide involves intense rage that the person represses but experiences as self-destructive impulses in the context of depressive symptoms. It is usually regarded as a manifestation of a depressive disorder. Though Freud's early exposition (1949) and Menninger's later elaboration (1938) of this concept have generally stood the test of time, in practice Freud's observation, that "any blow to the ego"—not only the loss of a significant person—can generate the underlying rage, is most pertinent to suicide. Although estimates vary widely, about 35% of suicides belong in this group. It includes those variants referred to as a *hidden depression* and *depressive equivalents,* often seen in persons with considerable ego strengths and well-developed obsessive defenses.

A *symbolic suicide* is one in which the self-destructive act achieves a symbolic goal, for example, to sacrifice oneself to redeem humankind, to achieve rebirth, to communicate with a dead relative, to satisfy the demands of a perceived persecutor, or to further a highly valued goal or tradition. About 10% of suicides are in this group, most of them having psychotic disorders. The suicidal act often has a bizarre quality that reflects the presence of the thought disturbance.

Suicide resulting from organic dysfunction is the effect of various organic conditions that compromise brain function, especially toxic and delirious states. In this poorly defined group, the suicidal mechanism is unclear, and the frequency is difficult to determine. The self-destructive impulse appears to represent a primitive pattern that may occur in the course of a delirium, with no recall whatsoever after the sensorium is clear. Persons who abuse alcohol, drugs, or medications are at special risk. About 5% of suicides are in this group.

Suicide for relief of pain involves a level of emotional pain that exceeds the person's tolerance, producing an irresistible need for relief from the pain rather than a desire to die. Persons with a low pain threshold thus constitute a chronic risk for suicide because so many life experiences can cause the threshold to be exceeded. Even persons with a high threshold may experience acute and overwhelming pain levels that precipitate an unexpected suicide. This kind of suicide has been referred to as "panic" suicide. A desperate need for relief from emotional pain is probably the most frequent etiology of self-destruction, accounting for about 50% of completed suicides.

Innumerable variations exist. Current developments such as effective life-support systems, a progressively older population, and potentially fatal disorders such as AIDS are producing more "rational" suicides, which are aimed at precluding future situations foreseen as unbearably painful, rather than termination of a current state.

The major problem associated with etiology is the close and long-standing association of suicide with depression, so that in nondepressed individuals, the potential for suicide tends to be underemphasized. Too often, an unexpected suicide elicits an expression of surprise, such as "I didn't think he or she was depressed." We must remain aware that not only depression but psychotic states, organic cognitive disturbances, and "any blow to the ego" that produces psychic pain should alert us to this possibility.

Recognition and Initial Assessment

The recognition of suicidal states starts with the awareness that any degree of perturbation can generate self-destructive ideas and impulses. These are so often unexpressed that routine inquiry about them is essential in every thorough assessment of a person's emotional state. Although one must be mindful that depression is only a part of the suicide problem, it usually feels natural and comfortable to approach the issue of suicide with a systematic review of the symptoms of a depressive disorder. This stems from the circumstance that the person is being seen because of some stressful experience.

Every clinician should use his or her own interviewing style, but a typical sequence for this inquiry would be: "Do you ever have times when you feel sad or discouraged about the way things are going? How frequently does that occur? How severe does it get? How long does it last? Does it sometimes interfere with things that you would ordinarily have no trouble with, like working, sleeping, eating, or just doing things around the house? Does it make you withdraw from your usual social or other activities? Do you have crying spells? Does the sadness sometimes lead to your being critical of yourself? At times do you feel that your situation is hopeless? Does it ever get so bad that you wonder if life is worth continuing, that you think of suicide? How persistent are such thoughts, how strong have they been, and was much effort required to resist the idea? Have there been any impulses to carry this idea out? Have any plans been made? How detailed have they been? Have any tentative or preliminary actions been taken, such as collecting pills or obtaining a gun? What deterred you? Do you think those feelings can be managed if they recur? Is there anyone you can turn to for help at such times? Would you be able to call me if you felt you couldn't control the impulse?"

The key question is about suicidal thoughts. If the response is negative, and if other sources of information do not contradict this response, it can be assumed that, at least for the present, a potential suicidal crisis is not being overlooked. It is possible for a person to mislead the interviewer, but we have to accept that there is no way to avoid that risk other than by doing all we can to establish a relationship of trust with the person.

If the response regarding suicidal thoughts is affirmative, the focus shifts from recognition to assessment. This is a critical process, as the degree of risk is a major element in planning clinical management.

A potential problem associated with the recognition of a suicidal state is that, when the clinician becomes aware that suicide is an issue, the anxiety that is generated can produce denial and rationalization; for example, "If I ask about suicide, it will make her more upset than she already is. I don't want to push her into it"; "I might put the idea into his mind"; "He won't admit it to me anyway"; and "There's nothing I could do about it". Thus, communication too often breaks down, and suicidal feelings are not openly examined. Of the many difficulties in the field of suicide prevention, anxiety about full and open inquiry seems most widespread. This problem is greater when the patient is a distinguished person or a fellow professional who may join with us in denying the presence of a serious situation.

Clinical Assessment

The brief inquiry detailed above gives us the basis for a preliminary estimate of suicide risk. It assumes that going directly to the heart of the issue is a practical and effective clinical tool, and that patients will provide valid information if an attitude of caring concern is communicated to them.

A more definite estimate of risk is achieved by supplementing the direct inquiry with inferential data that have been recognized as "high-risk factors." These have been derived primarily from descriptive studies of completed suicides, clinical experience, and common sense. The most important and widely recognized of these are the following:

Having a *history of a suicide attempt* is an important clue to the person's resistance to a self-destructive act. A first attempt seems to meet with the most psychological resistance; subsequent attempts require progressively less intensity of motivation to find overt expression. Two or more prior episodes or any serious attempt in the past warrants special concern.

Feelings of hopelessness have been found to be more closely associated with attempted suicide than is intensity of depression (Beck, Steer, Kovacs, & Garrison, 1985). No single high-risk factor is a dependable indicator of risk by itself, but a sense of hopelessness can be considered the most important of these supplemental considerations.

The specificity and degree of detail in a suicidal plan are an indicator of high risk that can be readily assessed. This was initially identified from experience with callers to a suicide prevention center (Litman, 1974).

Termination behavior needs no translation for one to recognize its pertinence to suicide risk. Making or revising a will, checking insurance, giving away valued possessions, or in any way negating the future can convey self-destructive intent with compelling clarity.

The presence of a lethal instrument in the home or at the workplace is clearly relevant. Though one can devise a suicidal act in almost any setting, the ready availability of a weapon in an impulsive moment can greatly increase the risk.

The presence or the threat of an extremely painful emotional experience of any kind is easily recognized as an important consideration in assessing suicidal risk. Especially in the presence of psychosis or when there is a background of drug or alcohol abuse, such circumstances must influence our judgment. In the absence of an objective measure, it is often useful to ask simply, "Do you think you can stand it?" and to give the response considerable weight.

The uncertain significance of specific risk factors in a given case suggests several precautions. First, make no assumptions, even reasonable ones. Second, obtain information from family members or others, if available. Third, keep in mind that "paradoxical findings" frequently appear in empirical studies (Motto, 1985), indicating that the logical interpretation of a given clinical observation may be misleading.

Dynamic Approaches to Risk Assessment

No matter how carefully we inquire about suicidal issues, the special characteristics of each individual remain a critical determinant of risk. In the absence of an established "explanation" for suicide, a number of dynamic approaches have been suggested (Berent, 1981; Furst & Ostow, 1979; Litman, 1975; Ringel, 1976).

The most detailed argument for the role of a dynamic formulation in estimating suicide risk was presented by Buie and Maltsberger (1983). They focused on the crucial role of one's degree of dependency on external sources of emotional support ("self-objects"); the estimate of risk is determined by the clinician's judgment about whether these "self-object resources" are sufficient to sustain the person. The time and training required for such a judgment may not be available in many settings, for example, in emergency rooms or crisis clinics, where decisions must be made without delay. In a stable outpatient setting, however, incorporating a dynamic approach into the process of estimating suicide risk may be not only appropriate, but required for sound clinical practice.

Objective Estimates of Suicide Risk

The use of objective clinical measurements to provide a quantified estimate of risk is still in the developmental stage. None of the well-known psychological tests (e.g., the Rorschach, the Thematic Apperception Test, or the Minnesota Multiphasic Personality Inventory) have proved helpful, and the simple quantification of known risk factors (e.g., Patterson, Dohn, Bird, & Patterson, 1983) adds little to our subjective impression.

Empirically derived suicide-risk scales (Braught & Wilson, 1970; Farberow & MacKinnon, 1974; Motto, Heilbron, & Juster, 1985) have a role in the assessment of psychiatric inpatients, from whom they were derived, though an attempt to apply these scales to a varied population of depressed outpatients did not seem very promising (Clark, Young, Scheftner, Fawcett, & Fogg, 1987). One large prospective study of depressed outpatients has been reported (Fawcett, Scheftner, Clark, Hedeker, Gibbons & Coryell, 1987). A formal suicide-risk scale was not developed, but hopelessness, anhedonia, and mood cycling during the index period differentiated the subjects who eventually became suicides.

Recent attempts to develop biological measures of suicide risk stem from the early recognition of increased levels of biogenic amines in states of internal agitation or turmoil (Bunney & Fawcett, 1965). Though a number of biological compounds have been studied, primarily 5-hydroxyindoleacetic acid (5-HIAA) in the cerebrospinal fluid (e.g., Traskman, Asberg, Bertilsson, & Sjostrand, 1981), these efforts constitute an area of continuing research rather than practical clinical tools. None of them have a clear application to risk assessment at this time (Motto, 1986).

The Problem Inherent in Risk Assessment

The basic problem of risk assessment is the multiplicity of the determinants and the unique set of characteristics possessed by each patient. In the absence of truly objective measures, the final decision about suicide risk is an intuitive judgment. Whatever approach or combination of approaches we use, our perceptions of the data must eventually be synthesized into an informed estimate that is entered into the record and that serves as a guide in treatment and management.

The recognition and assessment of suicide risk are preliminary to and overlap with treatment, which in turn is carried out within the context of management decisions. The importance of management, which should provide optimal conditions for effective treatment, is intensified in the case of a suicidal patient because all other efforts are contingent on the patient's survival. Thus, management decisions have a certain priority in the treatment plan because they are geared to ensuring survival, sometimes at the expense of optimal treatment. Though a sharp distinction is implied here between management and treatment, in practice all interactions with patients have treatment implications, and in some situations, management decisions may have even greater therapeutic impact than formal treatment measures.

The unique characteristics of both patients and therapists requires that treatment guidelines for suicidal persons be put in the most general terms:

1. Treat the patient as best you know how (Murphy, 1972).
2. Maintain an "active relatedness."
3. Take more initiative with a poorly motivated suicidal patient than you might take if the patient were not suicidal.
4. Focus on symptom relief and on the underlying disorder that generates the suicidal impulse.
5. Consider the patient–therapist relationship the patient's primary sustaining force.
6. When the suicidal crisis is over, continue the follow-up for a prolonged period (at least 3–6 months).
7. Collaborate with the patient's own support system (family, work, etc.) as closely as circumstances permit.
8. Be prepared for manifestations of extreme dependency, such as expressions of utter helplessness, and repeated requests that the therapist respond to "What should I do?" A high tolerance for this behavior is necessary to prevent a growing resentment toward such demands. Responses such as "I would trust your judgment on that," "I don't have an answer, but we can work on that at our next session," and "How have you handled that in the past?" can be useful.
9. Do not underestimate the critical importance of sleep and of maintaining a sense of productivity. A frantic effort to find relief from insomnia frequently triggers an overdose of drugs. In depressive states, the side effects of antidepressant medications (e.g., amitriptyline or doxepin) often suffice for sleep but may require supplementation with a benzodiazepine such as flurazepam (Dalmane) or lorazepan (Ativan).
10. Try to maintain an attitude of quiet confidence that the patient's problems can be resolved, even though the means of resolution are not evident. Experienced clinicians can attest to the value of such optimism, based on the observation that very few human conflicts are immutable. The effects of time alone often modify what persistent effort and spontaneous events do not. Helping a person simply to endure a period of severe crisis can thus be a lifesaving procedure that began in a hopeless-looking situation.
11. Be sure to caution your patient that recovery involves some ups and downs. Nothing is more shattering to depressed persons than to experience a ray of hope, only to have it disappear in a subsequent fluctuation that they interpret as

meaning that they are back where they were before. This may contribute to many instances of suicide during a period of improvement, which have marked such periods as being fraught with special risk.

12. Persons with alcoholism present special problems because the alcohol serves as both a defense against pain and a source of new pain. Be especially cautious if the person has stopped drinking because of threats of divorce, jail, and so on, as the relinquishing of the alcoholic defense may push the patient to suicidal behavior.
13. In serious situations do not handle the matter alone. A responsible family member, a minister, or another person in the patient's life should be included in the treatment plans. In many situations, consultation with a psychiatrist or with a nonpsychiatric colleague is indicated as well. Be candid with the patient about such consultations.
14. Finally, remind yourself that you are not God, that responsibility for the person's life is not on your shoulders, and that your role is to offer what assistance you can and that is all. With this in mind, it may be easier for you to relax and deliberately work out a feasible plan.

Management guidelines can be stated more specifically, but some of the problems encountered are best presented in a clinical context. The process of thoroughly and systematically clarifying the emotional state of the patient is in itself the first step in management, as it is conducive to a sense of sharing or "relatedness," of being both understood and accepted, all of which are emotional lifelines to a desire for continued existence. It is essential that this desire be maintained and nurtured. A sense of rejection, belittlement, or unworthiness intensified during a suicidal state is the most common precipitant of suicidal behavior. Even one dependable source of esteem can suffice to sustain the patient through the crisis, and that source is often the therapist. The various considerations involved are discussed in detail by Litman (1966), Mintz (1966), Tabachnick (1970), and Mayer (1971).

Situation 1

A 38-year-old male professional spoke of preoccupation with suicide as "the only thing left." He was extremely tense and agitated, and he chain-smoked. He showed no psychotic manifestations and no crying or despondency, although he revealed numerous signs and symptoms of extreme anxiety. He was very self-critical, belittling himself for his inability to function effectively, to control his feelings, to work at his profession, to concentrate, or even to account for his emotional state. Seeing a therapist was acutely embarrassing for him; it was equated with "wallowing in self-pity." Because the only supportive persons available had exhausted their abilities to cope, the patient was finally persuaded to see the interviewer.

The therapist decided to hospitalize this patient without delay, based on his clinical judgment that the suicide risk was so high that survival outside a protective setting was unlikely. Though the patient had considerable strengths, they were not readily available to him at the time. Some rapport was established, but a firm relationship with the patient could not be accomplished in so short a time. The patient had an adamant resistance to psychiatric hospitalization, so arrangements were made with the patient's internist to admit him to the medical ward of a hospital for a thorough physical evaluation. This was an obvious compromise.

The Management Problem. The first management decision is to determine the treatment setting. Then, the decision has to be reconsidered repeatedly as the intensity of the suicidal state fluctuates. The clearest indication for hospitalization is simply the judgment of whether the person will survive as an outpatient. That judgment is largely intuitive, even when aided by specific criteria as discussed above. At times, high-risk persons with near-psychotic levels of disorganization have been treated as outpatients because in work situations they seemed able to use their defenses, especially obsessive patterns, effectively. Others can be managed at home when home is experienced as a protective environment. When no readily available setting affords relief, a hospital becomes the preferred setting.

The use of "contracts" is pertinent here. To the extent that a relationship of mutual trust and respect is formed, a patient's agreement to continue in treatment, to arrive at appointments, or not to kill himself or herself can be negotiated. Many therapists who do not identify their work with behavioral modification techniques often make an implicit contract with the patient through an inquiry such as "Can I count on seeing you next week?" or "Can you make it till Thursday?" Such agreements require a firm relationship to warrant much reliance. It has been advised that, with adolescents, it is not reasonable to depend on implicit or explicit contracts even when a good relationship exists.

A power struggle with suicidal patients must be avoided if at all possible, as the patient ultimately has the most power. In this case, using a nonpsychiatric inpatient setting was a means of the buying time to set up a stronger support system. If the patient had refused any form of inpatient care, the examiner was prepared to accept the risk of outpatient treatment rather than force the issue by initiating a procedure that the patient could not agree to.

Situation 2

At the request of his internist, the patient was seen several times in the hospital by a psychiatric consultant and was subsequently discharged to resume therapy with that consultant. The night before the first scheduled outpatient session, the patient made a serious suicide attempt, the consultant could not be reached, and the original clinician was again contacted. In spite of numerous protests, the patient voluntarily entered the psychiatric unit of a general hospital after it was made clear that involuntary measures would be used if necessary. It was learned that the patient had agreed to the arrangements for outpatient care in spite of financial obstacles, and when these proved insurmountable, he felt trapped and helpless, and he acted on a strong surge of self-destructive impulses.

The Management Problem. A serious suicide attempt by an outpatient is a clear indication for inpatient care unless there is an overriding counterargument. No such counterargument was recognized here.

The support system needed to be solidified before the resumption of the higher risk of outpatient treatment. In this situation, the examining psychiatrist, who had established a good relationship with the patient, was prepared to insist on psychiatric hospitalization after the suicide attempt even if it meant relinquishing his potential therapeutic role because of the patient's resentment. This is an example of management taking precedence over treatment, of a potentially antitherapeutic step being deliberately taken in order to ensure survival.

If both the patient and the family are firmly opposed to hospitalization, and the family assure the therapist that they will provide the necessary observation and support, the resumption of outpatient care can be considered. The management decision is often a matter of choosing the lesser of two evils, which usually amounts to making thorny clinical judgments.

A special obstacle is introduced when the patient is a professional person. It is important to resist the impulse to rationalize because of the patient's professional role or position in the community. If the therapist is forced into compromising optimal management, the decision should be clearly documented. For example, it should be noted that hospitalization is indicated, recommended, and refused, and that the requirements for involuntary measures are not present, or that, although hospitalization is indicated, the patient's ultimate best interests are served by the acceptance of an alternate plan.

The simplest solution to this kind of dilemma is to inform the patient and the family that, if the recommended measures are not acceptable, the therapist will have to withdraw from the case as soon as another can be found. This is an appropriate action if the therapist is forced into an untenable position, but it tends to be resorted to unnecessarily early by some clinicians, who thus compound the suicide risk by generating feelings of abandonment in a person highly sensitive to rejection.

Situation 3

At the patient's request, the therapist who had first seen him undertook to develop an outpatient treatment plan. After discussions with the patient and his family, it was agreed that, after discharge from the hospital, three outpatient sessions a week would be used. Care was taken to ensure that the financial arrangements would be feasible. The sessions were arranged to minimize interference with the patient's work schedule, though it was necessary for the therapist to modify his own work time to do so. The initial emphasis was on day-to-day stresses and vegetative functions, and whatever time remained was used to obtain a detailed psychiatric history.

The Management Problem. The first weeks and months following discharge from the hospital are a vulnerable time for suicidal patients and call for special supportive measures. Any change in treatment personnel, however temporary, may precipitate a crisis. Even in a stabilized situation, a therapist's absence due to illness or vacation can bring about the interruption of a vital sense of communication or a resurgence of feelings of abandonment, with accompanying suicidal impulses. Suicide-prevention and crisis centers often receive calls from patients in such a situation, and much more persuasive evidence is available from coroners' records. This problem is common in training institutions, as trainees often move in and out of clinical assignments and frequently move away after the completion of their training. A report of four suicides at one such institution reveals that three of them occurred in the context of vacation interruptions (Kolodny, Binder, Bronstein, & Friend, 1979).

To provide maximum support in the situation described above, the patient was instructed how to reach the therapist at any time, day or night, including weekends and holidays. This arrangement included providing a home telephone number and informing the patient when the therapist would be out of town for a day or more and how to reach him during that time. The term *instructed* is used advisedly. It must be conveyed that the therapist *wishes* the patient to call if at any time she or he feels unable to cope. Patients who are oversensitive to appearing dependent or "imposing on the doctor's valuable time" can easily be lost to suicide in an intercurrent crisis, a life crisis arising in the course of treatment. Conveying to such patients simply that, if they must call, their calling will be acceptable to the therapist is not appropriate because it implies only a willingness to tolerate their needs rather than a desire to respond to them. The ready availability of the therapist is rarely abused in these circumstances. As Mayer (1971) pointed out, the suicidal person's need is not so much to have the therapist immediately available as to know that the therapist's concern extends beyond the ordinary conditions of treatment. The same concept applies to the therapist's making special scheduling arrangements. This approach raises questions of a theoretical nature, but it remains a facet of the sound management principle referred to as *active relatedness*.

Situation 4

Amitriptyline, up to 300 mg/day, was used for 4 weeks as a supplement to psychotherapy, but it had no observable benefit and was gradually discontinued. The patient's emotional state stabilized over the ensuing weeks, and after 2 months of psychotherapy, the sessions were reduced to twice weekly. Diazepam was used, 5–10 mg one to three times daily, to reduce tension, especially in the work setting. Six months after treatment began, a series of discouraging personal and work-related developments was associated with a resurgence of intense suicidal impulses. The patient said he had concealed the return of self-destructive impulses over the preceding week as a way of retaining complete control. At one point, a planned suicide attempt, using carbon monoxide from his car exhaust, was interrupted by the unexpected appearance of a neighbor. Erratic sleep and alcohol intake accompanied thoughts of hopelessness about personal goals and discouragement about the outcome of some professional projects. The patient reluctantly agreed to reenter the hospital, but after a 24-hour delay in finding an available bed, he indicated he thought he could manage with office visits. The very decision to use the hospital again seemed to exert a stabilizing influence on the patient and to reassure family members that a backup resource was available. The therapist arranged daily therapy sessions and had scheduled telephone contact on Saturdays and Sundays. Plans were discussed with the family. The sessions dealt primarily with vegetative functions, especially adequate sleep, with the remaining time being focused on dynamic issues. After 2 weeks of daily sessions, the patient's emotional state had returned to baseline, and the prior therapy schedule was resumed.

The Management Problem. The main focus of treatment for suicidal patients should be on the underlying pathology. To the extent that this includes mood, thought, and anxiety disorders, the use of psychotropic medications is indicated. The diagnosis, however, is often unclear, so that, in a given case, the use of medications may be controversial. In the case discussed above, the therapist saw the problem primarily as a characterological one for which no specific medication exists; thus, pharmacological agents were used only for symptom relief such as sleep (Dalmane, 30 mg at bedtime) and anxiety. Despite the patient's reluctance to use anything suggesting dependence, a firm insistence was maintained on the vital importance of sleep. This was the clearest reason to give medication to this patient. In depressed patients, it is common practice to give a therapeutic dose of a tricyclic antidepressant at bedtime to obtain both antidepressant (treatment) and sedative-hypnotic (management) benefits.

The toxicological properties of tricyclic antidepressant and antipsychotic agents dictate that they be used cautiously in high-risk patients. It is difficult to prescribe a therapeutic dose without providing a potentially lethal supply. Giving frequent small prescriptions is generally preferable to asking a family member to dispense the medication, as the latter method expresses clear doubts about the patient's ability to resist suicidal impulses. Each person is unique, however, and the implications of how the medications are handled should be discussed with the patient to ensure compliance. Some experienced clinicians suggest that prescribing small quantities of an antidepressant to reduce suicide risk fosters noncompliance and offers a false sense of security (Ayd, 1987), but each case must be considered individually. Trazadone and fluoxetine are least toxic in overdose.

Continuous monitoring of the suicidal impulse is an accepted aspect of management, but it is clear from the situation above that we cannot always assume we are getting accurate information. The patient realizes that telling the therapist about resurgent suicidal impulses will lead to deterrence, so the therapist must depend in part on the patient's ambivalence toward death to remain informed.

By this point in the therapy, the therapist felt enough confidence in his relationship with the patient to defer hospitalization in spite of the obviously increased risk. The judgment was an intuitive one that defined objective criteria because it was a function of the therapist's anxiety level as well as the clinical situation.

An acute suicidal state requires either prompt hospitalization or massive support for the patient. Psychological interpretation at such a vulnerable time can generate a feeling of distance that can be lethal. This should not preclude the use of dynamic understanding, but such interpretation should be at a level and in a form that reflects acceptance, caring, and concern rather than intellectual explanation.

The therapist should be in contact with the patient's support system—family, close friends, minister, and employer—and should be available to support and advise them in acute situations. Permission to respond to their inquiries or to communicate with them is best obtained from the patient as early in therapy as possible, to preclude awkward dilemmas later about confidentiality.

Situation 5

Fourteen months after beginning treatment, the patient was in a stable emotional state, was doing well on the job, was cautiously optimistic, and was working on long-term issues on a once-a-week schedule. Dalmane (30 mg) was used occasionally to help the patient sleep.

The Management Problem. In this situation, management decisions are dictated by the philosophy and style of the therapist and the patient, rather than by considerations of patient survival.

Special Management Problems

Situation 6

The suicidal patient's support system is weak or nonexistent.

The Management Problem. For impulsive or labile patients who may not be able to reach the therapist at a given moment but can benefit by having an understanding person to talk with, a suicide-prevention and crisis center may be available, providing telephone access to such a person at any hour of the day or night. Some of the trained volunteers in these centers are as skilled—and more experienced—in managing suicidal persons than many professionals. They are trained to support the patient's relationship with a therapist, and they can provide valuable supplemental services. Of course, their effectiveness varies, but a trial use of such a facility is warranted in high-risk patients who have no support system of their own.

In most community settings, there are various programs to provide help for persons with limited resources. Such programs are usually difficult to keep track of, and their effectiveness is often impossible to assess. An emergency-room intake worker usually knows about such programs, and suicide-prevention centers generally have up-to-date information about the available resources in addition to the counseling they offer to callers. When there are no crisis centers or programs available for people in need, a high-risk person may require hospitalization simply because of the lack of resources elsewhere. Despite grumbling from ward staff or utilization review personnel, this is a sound basis for admission until an alternate resource can be found. Although such a situation does not often occur in private practice, it is a common dilemma in public facilities.

Situation 7

The patient is perceived as using the threat of suicide as a means of controlling the therapist or the environment. Common terms are ''if you don't put me in the hospital,'' ''if the doctor doesn't give me something to get rid of this pain,'' ''if my wife doesn't come back,'' or ''if they reduce my disability payments.'' Innumerable variants of this situation are known, the common theme being that someone else's specific action, or lack of it, is identified as being responsible for the patient's suicidal impulse. Less obvious forms involve repeated impulsive or unconscious passive-aggressive demands for demonstrations of caring by others in the patient's world.

The Management Problem. The first consideration is a careful assessment of the patient's goals and the reasonableness of his or her requests. Often, the patient wants something that is justifiable, but because the request is put in the form of an abrasive, threatening demand and is experienced by the therapist or others as ''manipulative,'' resistance is generated, and refusal is rationalized as ''not playing into the patient's dependent needs.'' This can easily lead to a power struggle in which the patient has the ultimate power, and a suicidal act may ensue.

If the patient's demands have merit, it should be acknowledged that they do in spite of the irritation created. The treatment plan should then include discussion with the patient of how much more readily others would respond to his or her needs if they were expressed in a different way.

If the demands do not have merit, the needs that generate them should be identified, if possible, and alternative means should be formulated to meet them. For example, a 42-year-old male draftsman lost his job, spent his resources on alcohol, and was evicted from his hotel room. His demand for hospital admission because of suicidal impulses was seen, after evaluation, as a request for the gratification of legitimate dependent needs. These were identified and validated, and a plan was worked out for providing a nonhospital setting where he would obtain food, shelter, and medical attention. The patient's uncertainty that his needs would be met were expressed by his asking if the examiner wanted to be responsible for the patient's suicide. The examiner responded that the patient would be the one to decide if he would commit suicide, and that the examiner could not prevent that. He did want to help the patient as much as possible, however, and felt that making suitable arrangements for him would give that help. The patient seemed to accept the statement with relief, and he left in good spirits.

Whenever a clinician is challenged as to whether she or he can thwart a patient's suicidal intent, it is generally appropriate to acknowledge that the patient has ultimate control of that decision. Making such an acknowledgment is simply a recognition of reality, though we can exert some short-term control. The therapist must be comfortable with his or her own limitations in order to deal with this reality effectively, and to avoid feelings of frustration, anger, and resentment that can handicap both judgment and therapeutic effectiveness.

A frequent source of such feelings is the management of what are termed *borderline patients,* particularly that subgroup that manifests chronic self-mutilating behavior and suicidal acts. Of special concern are those with malignant narcissism and those whose characteristics include impulsive suicidal gestures, withholding information, alcohol or drug abuse, and emotional aloofness or withdrawal.

Though individual cases vary widely, Kernberg (1983) offered four guidelines for working with such patients:

1. The secondary gains of suicidal behavior have to be diagnosed and controlled. It is important that patients learn that the threat of suicide has no power over the therapist.
2. The therapist should tell the family and all those concerned that the patient is chronically a high suicide risk. The therapist should not give any kind of assurance that his or her treatment will eliminate this risk.
3. With patients who present chronic suicidal and/or self-mutilating potential, that potential must be explored consistently and woven into the exploration of all the patient's interactions with the therapist.
4. It is important that the therapist who treats a borderline patient with chronic suicidal potential in an outpatient setting not accept unrealistic or impossible treatment arrangements that require unusual efforts or heroic measures on his or her part.

One may dispute what constitutes "unusual efforts," which are clinically indicated at times, but the point is clear that the therapist must come to terms with his or her own limitations regarding the prevention of suicide. This implies not only accepting that the therapist cannot always control the patient's behavior, but making that clear to the patient and to interested third parties as well. An important element in this acknowledgment is to accept that the patient is likewise unable to control all aspects of his or her behavior (e.g., repeated late-night calls, suicide threats), some of which can be so stressful to the therapist that intense feelings of frustration and anger toward the patient are generated. These negative feelings can so disrupt the relationship that a suicide is precipitated.

It is customary to attribute these hostile feelings to the characteristics of the patient. On another level, we might view such anger as representing a regressive process on the part of the health-care worker, who is, after all, responding to symptoms of the patient's pathology. Were these symptoms to be controllable, the person would not be a patient in the first place. Such regression is essentially a universal vulnerability, and the task becomes a matter of devising a means of setting our own limits, for example, telling the patient, "If you continue these late-night calls (suicide attempts, drinking episodes, etc.), I will have to stop seeing you." One may set a limit on the duration, frequency, or nature of behavior, but the message is generally the same: If the therapist's tolerance is exceeded, the therapeutic effort will have to be transferred to someone else. When the relationship with the patient is firm, such measures may have a significant stabilizing effect. However, if the frustration tolerance of a therapist is not very high, borderline patients who are chronically suicidal should probably not be in his or her caseload.

Situation 8

The patient has a lethal quantity of medication and refuses to relinquish it to the therapist or a relative.

The Management Problem. The significance of the cache should be explored before deciding on any action. At one pole is the control-oriented person, usually with obsessive defenses, for whom access to a way out is a precondition for sustained psychotherapeutic work. In this situation, it may be best to support the person's sense of control over his or her fate and to direct one's efforts toward the sources of psychic pain. In time, the cache may lose some of its emotional load and may be relinquished spontaneously.

At the other pole is the person who is impulsive and unpredictable, for whom ready access to a lethal weapon is not likely to have a stabilizing influence. If the patient is a child or an adolescent, or if his or her situation involves alcoholism, psychotic elements, organic cortical dysfunction, or emotional lability, the therapist should insist on the removal of any readily accessible lethal instrument. Each situation deserves an evaluation of the issues it presents, with an intuitive judgment about the ultimate best interests of the patient.

GROUP THERAPY

"Outpatient treatment" generally implies individual, office-based psychotherapy, but many persons in depressed and suicidal states can benefit considerably from group treatment as well. Most reported experience is in long-term open-ended groups (Billings, Rosen, Asimos, & Motto, 1974; Farberow, 1972; Motto & Stein, 1973). There is general agreement that group therapy for suicidal persons is best used as a supplement to other therapeutic measures, and not as a substitute for them. Groups formed expressly for depressed and suicidal patients are referred to here, not the inclusion of suicidal persons in other therapy groups. In traditional group therapy, the emergence of a severe suicidal crisis tends to destabilize the group, whereas in a special group for suicidal persons, group cohesion and support are intensified by such crises. Group members also tend to establish supportive relationships outside the group meetings to a far greater extent than in other therapy groups. This holds for adolescents as well as adults (Ross & Motto, 1984). The empirical information about efficacy is sparse, but encouraging (Frey, Motto, & Ritholz, 1983). The results of a large nonrandomized study indicate that suicidal persons in special group therapy have a lower rate of suicide than comparable patients in other treatment settings (Billings, 1974). A serious obstacle to the availability of group resources is that, although many clinicians are glad to have their high-risk patients participate in such groups, too few group therapists are inclined to conduct them. Those who do generally take the well-advised measure of having one or two cotherapists work with them.

INVOLUNTARY HOSPITALIZATION

A special problem is often encountered in which a suicidal outpatient who has been determined to need hospital care refuses, raising the question of involuntary hospitalization. Each state has specific criteria and procedures for involuntary hospitalization, generally a variant of the determination whether, because of mental illness or chronic alcoholism, the person is a danger to herself or himself, a danger to others, or severely disabled (unable to provide for her or his own food, clothing, shelter, or daily needs). Each clinician likewise develops criteria that may be more specific, for example, a high-risk patient who is (1) psychotic; (2) delirious; (3) panicked; (4) depressed or has any severe psychiatric disorder; or (5) threatening to commit suicide in the clinician's presence. In doubtful situations, a consultation is appropriate, and if the clinician is still doubtful, involuntary hospitalization is usually the more conservative course.

This is an aspect of management that deserves close collaboration with family members, who can sometimes persuade the patient to accept hospital care voluntarily. At other times, they are invaluable in helping with practical matters of transportation and physical assistance during the admissions process. The rationale should be discussed with them, and their concurrence should be obtained if possible. If the family are firmly opposed to inpatient care, consider the possibility of their accepting responsibility for the patient's safety at home, which may be preferable to entering into a power struggle with them.

MEDICAL-LEGAL CONSIDERATIONS

Special guidelines are needed to avoid legal vulnerability in treating suicidal persons, an issue that can plague therapists in every health-care discipline. Though put in terms of legal considerations, these measures are facets of optimal professional care and record keeping. Beyond taking appropriate steps to treat the underlying disorder, five procedures deserve special emphasis.

First, document the inquiry regarding the recognition and assessment of the suicide risk, indicating what information was obtained and the estimated degree of risk determined to be present. Include specific vulnerabilities that could influence the severity of risk in changing circumstances.

Second, document the plan devised to deal with the estimated risk, for example, the frequency of sessions, the use of medications, any discussion with family or others, and the arrangements for keeping communication open or responding to emergencies. If hospitalization was considered, include the rationale for outpatient care.

Third, document that the plan was actually carried out, for example, that meetings were scheduled, medications were given, and phone calls were made.

Fourth, as for any complicated clinical problem, if an equivocal situation arises, obtain consultation from an experienced colleague and document the consultation.

Fifth, try to work with the family members as fully as circumstances permit. That is, unless the patient prohibits contact, listen to the family's concerns and questions, support them within the limits of confidentiality, and try to acknowledge both their intimate knowledge of the patient and the severe strain that such a situation can impose on them. If the family know you are seeing the patient, it violates no confidentiality if they contact you and give their perspective as well as respond to your questions. It is, of course, generally desirable to inform the patient of any such contact, even if some discomfort may be associated with it. Document any interactions with family members or others.

If these few measures are adhered to, from the suicide prevention viewpoint the patient will be receiving optimal care, a clinically valuable record will be generated, and the therapist's legal vulnerability will be minimized even if an error in judgment or fate conspires to bring about an adverse outcome. The basis for confidence in this position is that the therapist will have done in good faith essentially everything that one can do in such a situation.

COPING WITH A PATIENT'S SUICIDE

Even when optimal treatment is provided, an outpatient therapist who accepts high-risk patients is likely eventually to lose a patient to suicide. Though one can prepare for this eventuality intellectually, the emotional experience it precipitates may still be very stressful. Understandably, the most vulnerable therapists seem to be those in the early stages of a professional career. Characteristic responses seem to follow a sequence. The initial stage reflects both expressions of acute psychic pain and defenses against it, especially by repression and denial. Words used to describe the feelings encountered include *disbelief, crushed, stunned, panic, exposed, too angry to speak, alarmingly alone, why me?, shame, guilt, embarrassment, inadequacy, helplessness,* and *need for expiation or punishment.* Thoughts turn to fears of legal suits, indignant relatives, professional and public disgrace, embarrassing questions, and the loss of other patients' confidence. Ruminations of self-doubt are common, as are fantasies of insisting that, henceforth, all patients sign an oath not to commit suicide, feelings of being unable to tolerate such an experience again, impulses to refuse ever to treat another high-risk patient, and thoughts of going into radiology.

An overlapping intermediate state follows, predominated by feelings of loss, sadness, grief, soberness, tears, loneliness, dreams about the patient, and an increased sense of closeness to other patients and to family members. Hyperalertness to suicide risk in new patients is noted, with more careful inquiry, greater readiness to hospitalize, and more conservative management and discharge plans.

Many therapists then go through a resolution phase in the form of feeling weathered and initiated. Accompanying this phase is an awareness of increased maturity and tolerance to stress, as well as greater thoughtfulness about the meaning of clinical responsibility. Concepts such as magical expectations and fantasies of therapeutic omnipotence also take on new meaning. Professional limitations seem more acceptable and shortcomings more forgivable. Expressions of "Maybe it's just as well—he suffered a great deal," or "I think I did everything I could—perhaps it was inevitable," are common among therapists at this stage.

More experienced therapists are not immune to this sequence; much depends on their theoretical, philosophical, and clinical background. In general, they experience a greatly condensed version of the initial stage. The extent of the intermediate stage depends primarily on the intensity and duration of the treatment effort and on the characteristics of the patient and his or her family; these can precipitate a full-blown grief reaction. The thoughts of an experienced therapist after a patient's suicide might run as follows:

> Did I do everything that could be done to prevent this suicide? No, I have never done everything that could be done. I took some risks; I denied some risks. I was too exhausted at that critical moment to provide support. I delayed calling, contacting the family, and reassessing self-destructive impulses. I let wishful thinking and rationalization take over when hardheaded action was called for. So I found myself explaining to the family—thank God I'd discussed the risk with them earlier—and to the deputy coroner. The family was surprisingly supportive, even grateful, and appreciative of all the time and effort and patience they had noted but never spoken of. They seemed to include me as a family member to share the loss. The newspaper report played up the

> painful parts—the youth, the brilliance, the promise, and the survivors. I wonder if it would have changed things if I had only . . . if I hadn't only . . . What a relief it would be if I never had to work with a suicidal patient again. I don't have to. Why do I keep going through all this? But if I don't, who will? Are other therapists more competent, tougher, less vulnerable, and more effective than I am? I wonder what Dr. X goes through in this situation—he's been at it as long as I have. If I avoid these tough ones, I'm rejecting the people who most need help, and I have as much experience with this as anyone. There's no real answer to all this. I know I'll feel better about it before long and will go on as before. I didn't do everything that could have been done, but I did what I could, given my limitations. I just wish I hadn't been so exhausted that night. I wish I hadn't been misled by so many earlier false alarms. I wish, I wish. Maybe it wouldn't have changed anything if I'd called back. I wonder. But I certainly know what I'll do if that situation ever arises again.

The therapist's major concern should be to maintain a realistic perspective in regard to the outcome with high-risk patients so that his or her effectiveness is not compromised by the loss of a patient by suicide. This applies to the therapist's emotional well-being and vulnerability to burnout as well as to the impact of the suicide on her or his psychotherapeutic efforts with other patients.

Litman (1965) wrote that a supportive consultation with another professional person after a suicide proved to be of great psychological benefit. If the therapist had discussed the problem with others before the suicide, such a consultation could give support to his or her feeling that he or she had done everything possible.

Another possibly helpful measure described by Litman (1965) is for the therapist to review the case and present it to a group of colleagues with the question, "What can we learn from this?" Such an exercise is more easily carried out in institutional settings than in private practice, and the spirit of mutual support and shared responsibility makes such a project easier to accept and to view objectively.

On another level, a therapist's efforts to assist the family with questions and feelings created by a patient's suicide have also proved beneficial to the therapist. Externalizing the focus, verbalizing the thoughts, and supporting and responding to questions provide the therapist with the reassurance that he or she has a needed and helpful role. Some families also provide direct assurance of their continued esteem for the therapist and their appreciation of the effort expended. Work with family members may also identify the therapist as a grieving fellow survivor; therapists often have an emotional need of such identification that is greater than their need to deal with professional image problems.

On still another level, some therapists can draw on support from their own families and close friends. If high-risk patients are a part of one's caseload, urgent or odd-hour calls can lead to the development of a supplemental relationship between the patient and the therapist's secretary or spouse. If the patient commits suicide, these persons can realistically share the feelings and help with any need to restore self-esteem.

As the intensity of the emotional response to a patient's suicide diminishes, residual feelings may be addressed, and a sense of closure may be achieved by writing up the experience as a scientific report.

The intensity of the feelings surrounding the loss of a patient to suicide can create a barrier of anxiety in some professionals that prompts them to avoid further work with suicidal patients. We applaud those therapists described by Litman (1965), however, who express the view that, having lost a patient to suicide, they would consider the next suicidal patient a special challenge; the experience of their patient's death could increase their understanding and sensitivity as persons and therapists and could improve their professional judgment.

SUMMARY

How a therapist can best handle a specific situation involving suicide risk depends on too many considerations to allow her or him to rely on a set of guidelines derived from others' experience alone. The points discussed in this chapter can provide a starting point, but the final decision is always an intuitive judgment based on the unique circumstances of each patient. The guidelines offered are all derived from clinical practice, and they represent the commonest dilemmas. Most of the suggestions have resulted from painful lessons that it is hoped others can avoid.

The focus has been on the special characteristics of patients, but therapists also have unique qualities. These are manifested in their treatment philosophy, their management style, and their temperament and will necessarily modify how they deal with the problem of suicide. One issue that applies to all clinicians, however, is the need to document the basis for management decisions. Whatever approach is taken, the rationale should be recorded in detail for both clinical and medicolegal reasons. Other considerations important to all suicidal situations include the value of collaboration with the patient's own support system and recognition of the patient–therapist relationship as the most significant element in both management and treatment.

Finally, we need to continue reminding ourselves that our goal is to reduce premature, unnecessary, and tragic deaths to a minimum. This means we will still lose some patients to suicide, and unless we are prepared for that eventuality, we are not fully prepared to treat them. The effort to do so can make this one of the most satisfying of all psychotherapy endeavors, even though we accept the fact that the outcome may be determined to a large extent by forces beyond our control. Sound management and treatment are simply means by which those forces are influenced in the direction of survival and reduced risk.

REFERENCES

Ayd, F. (1987). What quantity of antidepressant to prescribe for outpatients? *International Drug Therapy Newsletter, 22,* 17–18.

Beck, A., Steer, R., Kovacs, M., & Garrison, B. (1985). Hopelessness and eventual suicide. *American Journal of Psychiatry, 142,* 559–563.

Berent, I. (1981). *The algebra of suicide.* New York: Human Sciences Press.

Billings, J. (1974). *The efficacy of group treatment with depressed and suicidal individuals in comparison with other treatment settings as regards the prevention of suicide.* Doctoral dissertation, California School of Professional Psychology, San Francisco.

Billings, J., Rosen, D., Asimos, C., & Motto, J. (1974). On long-term group therapy with suicidal and depressed persons. *Life-Threatening Behavior, 4,* 160–170.

Braught, G., & Wilson, N. (1970). Predictive utility of the revised suicide potential scale. *Journal of Consulting and Clinical Psychology, 34,* 24b.

Buie, D. & Maltsberger, J. (1983). *The practical formulation of suicide risk.* Cambridge, MA: The Firefly Press.

Bunney, W., & Fawcett, J. (1965). Possibilities of a chemical test for suicide potential. *Archives of General Psychiatry, 13,* 232–239.

Clark, D., Young, M., Scheftner, W., Fawcett, J., & Fogg, L. (1987). A field test of Motto's risk estimator for suicide. *American Journal of Psychiatry, 144,* 923–926.

Farberow, N. (1972). Vital process in suicide prevention: Group psychotherapy as a community of concern. *Life-Threatening Behavior, 2,* 239–251.

Farberow, N., & MacKinnon, D. (1974). Prediction of suicide in neuropsychiatric hospital patients. In C.

Neuringer (Ed.), *The Psychological Assessment of Suicide Risk* (pp. 186–224). Springfield, IL: Charles C Thomas.

Fawcett, J., Scheftner, W., Clark, D., Hedeker, D., Gibbons, R., & Coryell, W. (1987). Clinical predictions of suicide in patients with major affective disorder. *American Journal of Psychiatry, 144,* 35–40.

Freud, S. (1949). *Mourrning and melancholia.* In *Collected Papers* (Vol. 4). London: Hogarth Press.

Frey, D., Motto, J., & Ritholz, M. (1983). Group therapy for persons at risk for suicide: An evaluation using the intensive design. *Psychotherapy: Theory, Research and Practice, 22,* 281–292.

Furst, S., & Ostow, M. (1979). The psychodynamics of suicide. In L. Hankoff & B. Einsidler (Eds.), *Suicide: Theory and clinical aspects* (pp. 165–176). Littleton, MA: PSG Publishing.

Kernberg, D. (1983). Clinical management of suicidal potential in borderline patients. In C. Pfeffer & J. Richman (Eds.), *Proceedings, 15th Annual Meeting, American Association of Suicidology* (pp. 43–46). Denver, CO: American Association of Suicidology.

Kolodny, S., Binder, R., Bronstein, A., & Friend, R. (1979). The working through of patients' suicides by four therapists. *Suicide and Life-Threatening Behaviors, 9,* 33–46.

Litman, R. (1965). When patients commit suicide. *American Journal of Psychotherapy, 19,* 570–576.

Litman, R. (1966). Acutely suicidal patients: management in general medical practice. *California Medicine, 14,* 168–174.

Litman, R. (1974). Models for predicting suicide risk. In C. Neuringer (Ed.), *The psychological assessment of suicide risk* (pp. 177–185). Springfield, IL: Charles C Thomas.

Litman, R. (1975). The assessment of suicidality. In R. Pasnau (Ed.), *Consultation-liaison psychiatry* (pp. 229–236). New York: Grune & Stratton.

Mayer, D. (1971). A psychotherapeutic approach to the suicidal patient. *British Journal of Psychiatry, 119,* 629–638.

Menninger, K. (1938). *Man against himself.* New York: Harcourt, Brace & World.

Mintz, R. (1966). Some practical procedures on the management of suicidal persons. *American Journal of Orthopsychiatry, 36,* 896–903.

Motto, J. (1985). Paradoxes of suicide risk assessment. *Hillside Journal of Clinical Psychiatry, 7,* 109–119.

Motto, J. (1986). Clinical considerations of biological correlates of suicide. *Suicide and Life-Threatening Behavior, 16,* 1–20.

Motto, J., & Stein, T. (1973). A group approach to guilt in depressive and suicidal patients. *Journal of Religion and Health, 12,* 378–385.

Motto, J., Heilbron, D., & Juster, R. (1985). Development of a clinical instrument to estimate suicide risk. *American Journal of Psychiatry, 142,* 680–686.

Murphy, G. (1972). Clinical identification of suicidal risk. *Archives of General Psychiatry, 27,* 356–359.

Patterson, W., Dohn, H., Bird, J., & Patterson, G. (1983). Evaluation of suicidal patients: The SAD PERSONS scale. *Psychosomatics, 24,* 343–349.

Ringel, E. (1976). The presuicidal syndrome. *Suicide and Life Threatening Behavior, 6,* 131–149.

Ross, C., & Motto, J. (1984). Group counseling for suicidal adolescents. In H. Sudak, A. Ford, & N. Rushford (Eds.), *Suicide in the young,* (pp. 367–392). Boston: John Wright–PSG.

Shneidman, E. (1985). *Definition of suicide.* New York: Wiley.

Tabachnick, N. (1970). The crisis treatment of suicide. *California Medicine, 112,* 1–8.

Traskman, L., Asberg, M., Bertilsson, L., & Sjostrand, L. (1981). Monamine metabolites in CSF and suicidal behavior. *Archives of General Psychiatry, 38,* 631–636.

28

Office Practice

EDWARD DENGROVE

INTRODUCTION

This chapter is written from the point of view of a board-certified psychiatrist in private practice for some 40 years. Long experience has made it possible to hone and chisel the initial hour interview to a point where sufficient material is elicited to begin treatment before the patient leaves the office. This is a decided advantage. The patient leaves with feelings of hope and some idea of the goals of therapy. Shortcuts in therapy derive from years of trial and have had time to prove their worth, strengthen the patient–therapist relationship, and result in a more comfortable practice.

Although my primary perspective is psychiatric, other professionals can gain from a similar approach to their patients. The difference, of course, lies in the more medical concern of the psychiatrist and the ability to prescribe psychopharmacological agents. Medications have now become an essential part of treatment for many emotional and mental disorders, and it behooves the nonmedical therapist to work closely with a medically trained practitioner who can prescribe them knowledgeably.

HISTORICAL OVERVIEW

In reviewing the 40 years in which I have been in practice, the gains in therapy appear to be immense. In my residencies, psychoanalysis was king. This is no longer so. More brief therapies have displaced the lengthy and insight-oriented psychotherapies with a multitude of shorter and more effective techniques. Psychopharmacology, with its brilliant discoveries in the neurotransmitter field, has revolutionized chemical approaches to aiding the patient. The bromides and barbiturates have given way to the safer ben-

EDWARD DENGROVE • 541 North Edgemere Drive, West Allenhurst, New Jersey 07711.

zodiazepines, the more efficient neuroleptics, and the antidepressants. Cold packs and insulin-shock therapy have been displaced by electric shock therapy, still effective when used appropriately, though more limited in usage. Legal concerns about patients' rights have emptied the mental hospitals, unfortunately not always to the benefit of the patient. Only now is there a gradual return to a more humanitarian concern about the needs rather than the rights of patients.

CURRENT THEORETICAL APPROACHES AND PRINCIPLES AND EMPIRICAL FOUNDATIONS

Movement has taken place in the direction of shortening treatment, with less emphasis on characterological changes and more on symptomatic relief and reeducation toward self-help. Psychodynamic formulations are still useful, but it is recognized increasingly that insight alone may not account for more than 10% of the gain, emotional expression and ventilation perhaps 30%, and "working through," with homework and enhancement of a supportive network of family and friends and job, the remaining 60% of patient benefits. Eclectic methods suited to patients' needs appear to be the trend of the future.

Within the context of the patient–therapist relationship, the first order of business is diagnosis and assessment. The third edition of the American Psychiatric Association's *Diagnostic and Statistical Manual of Mental Disorders* (DSM-III; APA, 1980) must be satisfied if only because so many of one's fees come from those who demand a clear-cut diagnosis. In years past, it was fashionable to leave out the diagnosis and to concentrate instead on the problem and the patient. This no longer holds true, and one must define the findings through the five axes of the DSM-III in addition.

Diagnosis is followed by goal setting with the patient and establishing therapeutic strategies. These may range from short-term, with the emphasis on symptom relief and counseling, to long-term supportive help, particularly if full recovery is not possible but survival without the need for hospitalization is required.

A variety of common features are attributed to the therapist, the therapy procedures, and the patient (Lambert, 1986). These include support factors such as therapist warmth, respect, empathy, acceptance, genuineness, positive relationship, reassurance, identification with the therapist, structure, trust, catharsis, and release of tension; learning factors such as insight, rationale, cognitive learning, changing expectations for personal effectiveness, and self-acceptance; and action factors, such as encouragement to face fears, taking risks, mastery efforts, reality testing, modeling, practice, and working through. These factors would seem to operate more potently at certain times during the process of therapy. Further, one must recognize that spontaneous remission can take place, together with placebo effects, in addition to the more specific benefit of therapies such as hypnosis and systematic desensitization. Virtually all schools of therapy accept the notice that such therapist–patient relationship variables are fundamental in the formation of progress in therapy and a working alliance.

TECHNICAL METHODS AND STRATEGIES

Because diagnosis is important and preferably accomplished in as short a time as possible, a behavioral approach offers advantages. It is important to emphasize that target behaviors involve the identification of "emotional habits" and faulty cognitions. "Symptoms" merely denote the patient's awareness of the reactions that go on within.

Some years ago, I treated a young married woman who worked as a waitress. Her presenting complaints were the usual phobic ones: fear of shopping, fear in church, fear of crowds, and other interpersonal tensions. In addition, she presented three rather unusual features: difficulty with vision in that things seemed small (micropsia), a tendency for her voice to sound far off, and a feeling that she was fading away, all indicative of a need to avoid facing her problems directly. Asked what she could not face, she described her fears again. I proceeded with systematic desensitization. At first, she made excellent progress and returned to her job. Then, she struck a plateau, and I discovered that she was not fully relaxed, though she had so indicated. Simultaneously, she was having problems with her mother, her daughter, and her husband. It took a longer period to relax her sufficiently for further progress to ensue. She then left her job because she did not want to get involved in her employer's personal problems.

She resolved her external problems with her husband, her daughter, and her mother, but in other areas of her life, progress was lacking and she complained bitterly of not feeling well. At this time, she had lost the specific fears that had brought her into treatment initially, and now she addressed herself to the fact that she could not find another job and her fears that she could not keep it even if she had one. I confronted her with her fear of work, and she replied that people at work—and no other place—made her nervous. I was not happy with this answer. She then confessed that it was not concern about the people at her job that made her nervous but the fact that, if she went to work, her family would suffer. If she worked the morning shift, her daughter would have no way of getting to school 2 miles away and her mother, whom she visited daily, would not have her comfort and help in shopping. If she went on the evening shift, her daughter would not have a hot meal; neither would her husband. She felt that she had to do the right, good, and expected thing. On the other hand, she complained that she was not doing what she wanted to do: she wanted to go to work and have time to go out with her girl friends. She feared that her husband would beat her as her first husband had. Although they were not getting along well, this was not true. The therapeutic focus was now far removed from her original fears. A different approach involving marital counseling and assertive techniques seemed strongly indicated.

If this conflict had been disclosed earlier in treatment, much time would have been saved, and the treatment results would have been more certain. How can a therapist determine these events sooner? A simple listing of fears is insufficient for diagnostic purposes. As Joseph Wolpe (personal communication, 1964) remarked, "Without correct identification of the relevant stimulus elements, one may expend a great deal of time and effort without results." One can form conclusions about important hierarchical items through skillful interrogation, the use of fear interrogation, field surveys or other questionnaires and assessment techniques, autobiographical notes, the letter association technique (Dengrove, 1962), and various psychophysiological measurements. Unfortunately, patience and luck still play an important role.

Stevenson and Hain (1967) decried the failure to identify with sufficient precision the exact stimuli of the patient's neurotic responses, declaring that the therapist can waste valuable time by tackling wrong elements in his or her neurotic reactions. They illustrated their point by analyzing the barber shop phobia, and by insisting that one does not merely settle for the general environment in which it occurs (i.e., the barber shop as a whole). There may be a fear of scrutiny by others, a rebelliousness against social customs, impatience with delays, fear of confinement, fear of mutilation, anxiety-arousing experiences with chairs resembling barber chairs, sexual arousal, issues of seniority, and other explanations for the phobia (including a multiplicity of stimuli that touch off the phobic response).

A stutterer whom I had been treating stuttered more while dictating to his stenographers. He changed stenographers without effect, and desensitization to these women produced no reduction in his affliction. Further diagnostic probing indicated that he was not bothered by individual stenographers but by the fact that what he was dictating was being made a matter of public record and he would be held accountable for it. A change to assertiveness techniques helped overcome this complication. Similarly, an agoraphobic who feared walking away from her home was really afraid of encountering dogs, and desensitization to these animals enabled her to walk freely again.

According to Meyer and Crisp (1966), the presence of historically earlier sources of anxiety may complicate recovery. Thus, the presenting symptom may be the result of higher order conditioning or secondary generalization, yet the basic source of the symptoms may still be present, acting on the individual and influencing the course of the presenting complaints. Consequently, it, too, must be ferreted out and dealt with in addition to the secondary complaints. I have not found this to be much of an obstacle, particularly if I use the letter association technique. (Details of this technique are outlined in the section dealing with diagnostic procedures.)

Davis (1958) pointed out that memory images are perceptions, just as are those caused by current people or objects, and that we respond to the stimuli in memories just as we do to those in other perceptions. The recall of a scene once painful can evoke anxiety not as an old, derepressed emotion, but in response to the stimulus for anxiety occurring in the immediate perception. Thus, memory of a cruel mother may stimulate present anxiety rather than release old anxiety.

Clarke (1968) concluded that the permanence of early learning depends not only on the age of the child and the duration and intensity of the experience but, more particularly, on its later reinforcement. Early learning will fade if not reinforced. Similarly, Montenegro (1968) suggested that, rather than concern ourselves with the past history, we should become more involved in the present conditions that are maintaining and reinforcing the patient's symptomatology. Behavior therapy is directed primarily to removing or counteracting the circumstances that are perpetuating the given behavior problem. Yet, it is important to stress the fact that, when treating higher order learning and bypassing the original learning situation, relapse is likely to be the net result.

Lazarus (1966) emphasized the part played by others in the continuance of a symptom. In one instance, he had to call in the husband and the mother and inform them that they were inadvertently reinforcing the patient's dependency by displaying concern and expressing reassurance whenever she complained of minor somatic discomforts. They were requested not to pay attention to these negative statements, but to reward independent responses. Presumably, it is impossible to become an agoraphobic without the aid of others who submit to the inevitable demands imposed on them by the sufferer. These "sufferees" play a vital role in sustaining and maintaining the agoraphobic behavior and in making lasting therapeutic change unlikely unless they are treated concurrently.

One needs to desensitize not only to the act, but to anticipation of the act as a separate hierarchy. Sometimes, the anticipation takes on an obsessive quality, and we must revert to thought-blocking procedures. Furthermore, it is not merely anticipation of the act *per se* that must concern us; there is also general anticipation of the future. As one patient told me, "I can do the little things, like drive around the block; then I think ahead to what will be expected of me, and I fall apart and don't even want to do the little things.'' We must, in some way, convince the patient to look at the scene one portion at a time. Particularization prevents or reduces feelings of overwhelming anticipatory anxiety.

Wolpe (1964) wrote of pervasive aspects of anxiety that may be difficult to ferret out, such as space, time, one's own body, light verticality, and light–shade contrasts. I recall treating a woman who had developed a phobic state after a car had rammed into her home in the dark. She became sensitized to the dark and to outside car noises but was not aware of these specific irritants, complaining only of general nervousness with tension headaches.

Lang (1964) wrote of the pressure of partially digested food against the wall of the intestine, or of a phase of peristalsis itself, as an interoceptive conditioned stimuli for anxiety, such as might follow family arguments during or following a meal. Gantt (1964) noted that the Russians have successfully conducted conditioning experiments using many subtle internal cues such as an increase in bladder tension, thyroid gland secretions, and metabolic changes. He added that it may be very difficult to extinguish these, and that, certainly, the individual person is unaware of what is producing the changes in his or her visceral system.

The emphasis, thus far, has been on the need to distill basic and primary problem areas in endeavoring to diagnose the covert and overt factors responsible for the patient's presenting complaints. Lazarus and Serber (1968) pointed out that, in making a behavioral diagnosis, one should carefully separate deficits from basic anxiety responses. For instance, it is important to keep in mind that a male patient's inability to approach eligible females may be not a function of anxiety about women, but a reflection of inadequate learning, simple naïveté, and poor verbal skills. Phobic complaints may be secondary to a psychotic process requiring antipsychotic medication, and in some phobic reactions, depression may be the predominant illness, requiring antidepressive medication, environmental manipulation, and assertiveness training. Other phobic cases may warrant reeducation and direct instruction, modeling, and practice, plus rational discussions of ethics and morality.

Lazarus (cited in Abramovitz, 1970) further pointed out that one of the chief limitations of behavior therapy as then practiced was the application of specific techniques that ignored values, attitudes, and beliefs, and that failed to define the particular goals of the patient or to orient the therapy toward their attainment. Individual therapy imposes limitations on the person-to-person exploration of these specific behaviors. As Lazarus put it, ''Many facets of a problem which may elude the scrutiny of even the most perspicacious therapist often become clearly delineated during or after an intensive group discussion'' (in Abramovitz, 1970, p. 255). All in all, clinicians should strive to obtain information about their patients from many sources: observation, measurement, inquiry, outside opinion, and, above all, a detailed exploration of stimulus antecedents and behavioral consequences.

PROCEDURES FOR DIAGNOSTIC EXPLORATION

A systematic approach to history taking (Table 1) leads to a practical diagnostic evaluation within the first half-hour of the first session. The latter half of the initial interview can then be devoted to initiating treatment. I like to see the patient leave after the first visit feeling considerably better and more hopeful about the future.

The questions asked in Table 1 cover fairly completely the complaints of most

Table 1. History Taking

How do you feel? What are your complaints?

Headaches—Any other aches or pains?
Ascertain: Where do you feel the pain? Does it stay there or go to any other place? What is it like: aching, pressing, throbbing, etc.? How often do you get it? How long does it last? What brings it on? What relieves it? Do you suffer nausea or vomiting with it, visual difficulty, dizziness? Other accompaniments?

Nervousness: Are you tense, restless, irritable or impatient, jittery or jumpy, readily, tired, shaky?

Appetite and weight loss.

Sleep difficulty: Trouble falling asleep, interrupted sleep, restless sleep, early waking? Do you have nightmares or bad dreams of any kind?

Memory—concentration.

Sweating, hot flashes, faint feelings or fainting spells, dizziness, weakness, noises in the ears.

Trouble with stomach: Indigestion, nausea or vomiting, diarrhea or constipation, pains in abdomen, heartburn, gas.

Trouble with heart: palpitations, double beats or skipped beats, pains in chest.

Trouble with lungs: tightness in chest, shortness of breath, coughing, choking feelings, things sticking in throat, hard to swallow.

Trouble with bladder: difficulty holding or passing water, go too often during day or night, pain in passing urine.

Any fears: Delineate and detail, circumstances, onset, etc.

Depression, crying spells, suicidal thoughts.

Trouble with sexual life: detail.

Trouble with social life: detail, sports involvement.

Smoking habits, drinking habits, drug habits, taking medications at all, prescription or over-the-counter.

Worries of any kind: Health, future, ability to work, finances.

Changes in menstrual periods, menopause.

Past and personal history: Any serious illnesses, operations or injuries in past: details. Any nervousness: detail, previous treatments.

Married or single, children, how get along with spouse, details of marriage relationship.

Family history: Mother and father, siblings, details of how get along, etc.

Work history.

Any police record, juvenile or adult.

Military service: Details, including type of discharge and hospitalizations, exposure to combat.

Education: Schools attended, achievements, grades, problems with authorities, sports involvement.

Hobbies: Other interests.

Religious affiliation: Attendance and involvement.

Group affiliations.

Draw-a-Person production.

Three wishes.

What kind of person are you (self-evaluation)? Do you anger readily, what do you do about it?

Request: Autobiography
List of fears, list of angers, list of pleasures, list of what he or she would like to see different about self.

Optional: Fear survey (Wolpe & Lang, 1964)

Reinforcement survey (Cautela & Kastenbaum, 1967)

Specific questionnaire re alcoholic habits, etc.

Other psychological tests: Maudsley Personality Inventory, MMPI, other tests of assessment

Letter association techniques for pinpointing etiology.

patients. Simultaneously, the patient's mode of dress, speech, and comportment are observed, whether anxious or depressed, restless or apathetic, intelligent, responsive, and the like. First impressions, though fleeting, are valuable. One can tell much of a patient's inner feelings by the facial expression, particularly about the eyes. Telling the patient one's impressions in a conversational and interested voice will put him or her at ease.

The Draw-a-Person production[1] is a favorite addition of mine because of the wealth of information it gives about the patient in a very short time. I offer patients a pad and pencil and ask them to draw a picture of a person from head to toe, not just a head, and not a stick figure. The interpretation of these drawings is beyond the scope of this paper but there is much literature on the subject. There is nothing like experience, however, to give one the feel of the response, particularly when every patient seen and treated is given the test.

I also use the three-wishes test as a matter of routine. One simply asks the patient, "If you had three wishes, what would you wish for?" The information derived assists in helping the patient to establish goals of treatment. The patient's self-evaluation is often helpful and may tend to corroborate or refute the therapist's own evaluation. Sometimes, added data are obtained for hierarchy building.

The patient is requested to bring in a list of fears, as complete as possible, in order to add to the facts and impressions already secured during the first session. It is highly important to "target" the symptoms and to be certain that what the patient claims to fear is truly the target. Detailed interrogation usually supplies the items needed for the setting up of hierarchies, emphasizing the people, places, objects, and situations that engender anxiety.

I ask the patient to prepare an autobiography (Annis, 1967). The length of the manuscript, left to the discretion of the patient, should be at least several pages long. The purpose is to fill in possible gaps in the history obtained at the first session in the hope that further material for therapy will be supplied. The autobiography also has the effect of making the patient participate more actively in therapy.

Requesting patients to list at their leisure those traits they would like to see different about themselves adds to the determination of treatment goals. It is also helpful to add all the things that irritate patients and make them angry, as well as the times they may have wished to be more aggressive but failed to assert themselves.

Useful information may sometimes be obtained from the addition of a Fear Survey Schedule (Bernstein & Allen, 1969; Lanyon & Manosevitz, 1966; Rubin, Katkin, Weiss, & Efran, 1968; Rubin, Lawlis, Tasto, & Namenek, 1969; Scherer & Nakamura, 1968; Wolpe & Lang, 1964), a Reinforcement Survey Schedule (Cautela & Kastenbaum, 1967), and other specific questionnaires or psychological tests and assessments.

The letter association technique (Dengrove, 1962), devised some years ago, has proved most useful in pinpointing targets. It shortens immeasurably the time needed and is used in each treatment session for ongoing diagnosis. In essence, the moods of the patients are set by asking them to close their eyes and to relax as much as possible. They are to think of a particular symptom, to relate it to the last setting or event in which it was felt, and to attempt to relive or reconstruct—to whatever extent is possible—the feeling tones of the complaint. As a rule, only a few seconds are required for this phase.

Then they are asked to give the very first letter that comes to mind—not the second

[1]I recognize the nonbehavioral nature of these procedures but still find them useful as samples of behavior reflecting the patient's inner life.

or third, but the very first one. This specification is necessary because there are times when the patient will toy around with the alphabet.

The letter is noted, and the patient is then asked to give the very next letter that comes to mind. In all, five letters of the alphabet are obtained. If any letter that follows is sequentially related to the one given before it, the patient may be instructed to scatter the next one, that is, to pick it out from any other place in the alphabet. The initial letter, *A*, and difficult letters, such as *Q*, *X*, and *Z*, are most often used to resist the process and may be disregarded.

There are occasions when patients insist that they cannot think of a letter. In this case, one urges them to make some attempt. After all, who does not know the alphabet? Remind the patient that there are only 26 letters. If there is still resistance, one need only point out the letters of the alphabet in written form and ask the patient to look at the list and choose one. I prefer patients to think of all the letters as printed on bits of paper, placed in a hat, and then thrown into the air; they are to choose the one that is grasped as the pack comes down in a shower.

When five letters have been taken—the number is arbitrary and could be only one—they are listed vertically in order. Patients are then allowed to open their eyes and are requested to give the first word—again only the first one—that comes to mind and that begins with each of the letters previously chosen.

In this way, we have five words listed. The patient is asked to make a sentence using each word, or to free-associate with each word (i.e., saying what it brings to mind and how it connects up with the symptom). Almost always, the words form a battery of information related to the original difficulty, and no word is without meaning in relation to the person's difficulty, no matter how far-fetched it may seem at the time. The information so derived is often dramatically related to the patient's difficulties; often, patients themselves see the connection.

Timing is important. Those who delay in giving a letter should be urged to do so as quickly as possible. It is essential to prevent the patient from mulling over the alphabet, particularly during second or subsequent experiences with this method. Thinking about the subject is not desired; the more quickly the letter is pulled out of the air, the more useful it is for our purpose. Tell the patient not to think about it, just to say it. Nor is one to be distracted by a patient's desire to give a full word, as the word may be only a "red herring." One wants only the letter. Associations may be given afterward.

As an example of this approach, a 37-year old housewife presented complaints of "ungodly thoughts going through my head. I sit and cry and cry and cry, and I don't know why." Asked to give five letters, she produced the following and their associations:

F—free—The boat won't let me be free financially.
G—good—It's good for my husband. He enjoys it.
P—poor—It's making us broke.
B—boat—The same thing.
B—Bob—My husband.

This series led into the precipitating event of her depressed state, which had been the purchase of a boat by her husband and the consequent strain on their finances. Further exploration led to her other conflicts and underscored the way she used the purchase of the boat as a means of expressing antagonism toward her husband.

In another example, a 16-year-old high-school youth was found in a neighbor's house, dressed in feminine attire, doing his homework on a bed. He declared that he felt like a girl at times. There was no psychotic material. Asked to give five letters, he presented the following:

B—boy—Body build, most usually masculine, and I'm not. I'm so weak. I can't do things like other kids can, like play sports.
F—failure—I'm afraid I'll be a failure in life. Be a bum.
N—Neal—Myself.
O—open—Open the box—you put something in or pull something out of it.
T—top—Top of a mountain—above sea level—usually forests and woods around there.

I was able to follow the first three associations into his relationship with his father; the last two were not pursued, as they presented material he was not ready to cope with.

I find the technique interesting, rich in profusion of material, and direct in approach. Its use is not limited to initial contacts with the patient; it may be applied at any time in therapy. It is a timesaver. The patient cannot claim that nothing comes to mind, as all that has to be done is to give a letter of the alphabet.

Following the end of the interview, I ask the patient—now that I am aware of the information given me—what it is that treatment is expected to accomplish, and a therapeutic goal is set. It is surprising how often the goals set by the patient differ from those presupposed by the therapist.

General personality attributes are important when arriving at a differential diagnosis. For example, if one separates those phobic conditions associated with posttraumatic states and schizoid disorders, one is left almost entirely with patients who display a basic compulsive personality pattern—perfectionism—in varying degrees. These people are, for the most part, neat, systematic, orderly, conscientious, and concerned that everything should be in its right place and convinced that there is indeed a right place for everything. They want to do the good thing and be the good person, to please everyone (except their spouses). They range from the woman—and it is usually a woman—who picks up the ashtray to empty it the moment someone drops a cigarette into it, to the much less frequently seen artist whose studio may be messy but whose concept of his or her work must be perfection.

All of these people have one thing in common: a highly developed conscience that sits heavily on them. The majority have a mother (or, much less frequently a father) who is compulsive and perfectionistic also, and who has dominated them, often to the point of distress.

The phobic symptom is precipitated at a particular time in their lives when they are in a stressful situation and feel particularly helpless. It is important not only to delineate the basic compulsive character structure but to pinpoint the original stressful situation and, if necessary, to desensitize it; it may have been continually reinforced to the present time.

The compulsivity and perfectionism call for a broad array of techniques to help the patient to cope with a stressful environment. These patients often need to be desensitized to feared authoritative figures, and to have the burden of their compulsivity lessened. An important feature of therapy is to help them to a point of not caring so much about what others think of them.

Diagnosis is not limited to the first session; it is an ongoing process. Each time the patient comes for therapy, he or she is asked, "What has occurred since the last session?" Any symptom, old or new, is immediately elaborated on, and its time and setting are specifically described, often with the patient's eyes closed and an attempt to relive the situation as in the present. Then, if the patient cannot state why the symptoms occurred at a particular moment in a particular setting, in its special way, the letter association technique is often able to determine these details.

The sources of reinforcement of the symptom must be dealt with on each occasion. There may be only a repetition of material previously unearthed, but it is important to make patients aware of what it is that keeps them ill. As noted previously, there is extinction of the symptom unless something or someone is keeping it alive, much as a hoop falls down if not given a push from time to time.

Each patient is asked to relate both the good and the bad things that have happened since the previous session. When a patient speaks of several anxiety attacks, each is traced back to its original time of onset and the setting in which it occurred. And if the patient cannot discuss the origin of the attack, the letter association technique is used to quickly pinpoint the source. As an example, a patient opened the session with "Why do I get nervous whenever I think of coming here?" She was asked to sit back in the chair, close her eyes, and become aware of the feeling of nervousness. When she indicated that this feeling was present, she was told to give the first letter that came to her mind. In this instance, it was the letter *F*. The first word she connected with was *fear*. She was then asked to give a letter after thinking, "Fear of what?" This turned out to be "Y—you." Asked to think of the word *because,* she said, "Because I don't know what you're going to do." Further discussion of this point allayed her anxieties.

Ongoing diagnosis is important where there is delay or inability to transfer improvement from office to real life, and it directs attention to motivation in particular. For example, a 20-year-old woman was doing well—in the office—with systematic desensitization of her fears of walking and driving from her home, but she had made no progress at all in the actual situations. Asked to attempt movement in real-life situations, she produced only excuse after excuse during each session explaining why it had been impossible throughout that week. She had an anticipatory fear response, but she would not make the slightest attempt, even with proffered help. Further diagnostic exploration revealed the reason for her lack of progress to be her fear that, if she was free to come and go as she pleased, she would simply go and not return. She had no respect for her husband, yet feared giving up the kind of life that she was leading.

Similarly, a 34-year-old housewife had been doing quite well with her fear of driving away from her home, when her infant child died suddenly under circumstances for which she blamed her pediatrician. Immediately, she relapsed, and no coaxing could get her to drive again until diagnostic exploration revealed her fear that, if she could drive on her own, she might drive to the doctor's office and commit mayhem there. She dreamed of this action and was protected against these effects of her hostility by her inability to drive at all.

Finally, it is worth noting that some patients may appear to suffer a relapse (i.e., the return of the initial symptoms) when, in fact, new organic or different environmental forces are operative. For example, one of the first patients whom I treated with systematic desensitization was a woman in her early 40s. She had been in a phobic state for about 12 years. With systematic desensitization, she progressed to a point where she could travel not only from her home but for great distances. She was a most grateful patient because her husband had always wanted to travel with her and she had held him back. One day, she phoned for an appointment. She was frightened; her symptoms had returned. Diagnostic exploration, however, proved her alarm to be unfounded. She was suffering from some of the symptoms of menopause, had mistaken them for the return of her previous illness, and had developed an anxiety over them. Reassurance and estrogens limited her visits to one, and thereafter, she phoned to say that she was her renewed self again. Another woman who returned for further treatment had developed symptoms about a fear that had not shown itself before because she had had no occasion to encounter similar situations previously. Treatment of this item through desensitization quickly returned her to her previous symptom-free state.

The choice of treatment follows diagnostic evaluation and assessment and is determined by the goals selected, professional training, and experience. Lazarus's multimodal therapy (1986) is a highly eclectic brief approach that pays no specific regard to schools of psychotherapy. He has insisted that an effective therapist must have an armamentarium of scientifically derived skills and techniques to supplement effective interpersonal-relationship skills. Lasting change is, at the very least, an integrated function of techniques, strategies, and modalities. Lazarus described seven interdependent and interactive modalities (his BASIC I.D.) to which attention must be directed for the proper treatment of the patient: Every patient-therapist interaction involves *behavior* (be it lying down on a couch and free-associating or actively role-playing a significant encounter), *affect* (be it the silent joy of nonjudgmental acceptance or the sobbing release of pent-up anger), *sensation* (which covers a wide range of sensory stimuli, from the spontaneous awareness of bodily discomfort to the deliberate cultivation of specific sensual delights), *imagery* (be it the fleeting glimpse of a childhood memory or the contrived perception of a calm-producing scene), and *cognitive* (the insights, philosophies, ideas, and judgments that constitute our fundamental values, attitudes, and beliefs). All of these take place within the context of an *interpersonal* relationship or various interpersonal relationships. An added dimension for many patients is their need for medication, or *drugs* (e.g., phenothiazine derivatives and various antidepressants and mood regulators).

Additionally, I would add to these modalities the use of hypnosis, biofeedback, and other biological treatments. More recently, multimodal therapists have compiled structural profiles, have tracked the "firing order" of complaints, or have subjected the patient to more detailed inquiry with a "second-order BASIC I.D.," the use of a recursive application of the BASIC I.D. to itself to shed new diagnostic light on seemingly recalcitrant problems.

Although there has been much controversy over the use of psychodynamic psychotherapy versus behavior therapy, I find it difficult to disregard the former completely while practicing the latter. The secondary gains derived from symptoms used by the patient have to be further elaborated through a psychodynamic approach. Hypnosis is an excellent adjunct to treating the patient, chemotherapy may be essential, and family therapy is often useful, together with other therapeutic approaches.

SPECIFIC APPLICATION IN AN OUTPATIENT SETTING

The average length of a treatment session remains at the 50-minute level, although there are therapists who give less time and others more. Individual psychotherapy sessions often have to cover much ground, and it is difficult to see how this time can be shortened without depriving the patient of needed care and the strengthening of the therapeutic relationship. For busy psychiatrists in a community clinic, a 15-minute session may seem sufficient to monitor any medication, but in such a setting, psychologists and/or social workers are usually available to take up the slack by way of individual or group sessions.

At the start, the frequency of visits is once or twice a week, mostly weekly, until progress is shown. Then, the interval is gradually extended to biweekly, monthly, or perhaps longer. More frequent sessions are sometimes necessary, particularly if a great deal of anxiety is present or therapy is moving rapidly and the pace must be kept without faltering. The deciding factor is usually economic, depending on whether the patient can afford more frequent sessions. This time schedule, of course, does not refer to psychoanalytic treatment, which has quite different requirements.

Fees are set at community levels. It might be helpful to call around to determine the customary rates. However, third-party payers often set their own limits on fees, and these are rarely altered. Of course, providing reports to third parties is often a requirement for the fee. I have found it helpful to tell the patient my fee when an appointment is made, so that there will be no surprise and no contention at the end of the session. There is nothing unprofessional in discussing the fee before one sees the patient, and it is not likely that you will be seen as "only out for the money and not interested in me." It is all in the businesslike way it is done. Some therapists are embarrassed to ask for money, for fear they may be thought crass. Perhaps a little practice in assertiveness is necessary in such a case.

Except in accepted third-party situations, one should expect to be paid at the completion of the session. This arrangement prevents having to deal with the patient who gets behind in payments, complicating psychotherapy and the patient–therapist relationship. If one wishes to be charitable, a few sessions may be allowed to go by without pay, but the subject should be discussed and a limit drawn so that this state of affairs does not go on too long.

Should you have a waiting room full of patients? I suggest not. Most patients arrive at a predetermined appointment hour, and the flow is generally comfortable.

Is office help necessary? Of course, you need someone to help keep the office clean and someone else to type your reports unless you prefer doing them yourself. Answering the phone yourself so that the patient gets you directly is often preferred. But not every therapist or patient cares for such interruptions. There are answering services and devices, however, to aid the busy practitioner. Benefits lie in the relief patients derive from talking to you directly even if only for 1 or 2 minutes. Further, problems with office help do not arise if there is none!

The preparation of reports for referring sources or third parties is an important professional obligation. It is not only a practical necessity but a self-advertisement and a constant reminder of the therapeutic progress that one is making.

After-hour coverage and handling of emergencies are simply part of the business of treating patients, those who have emotional disorders as well as those with medical problems. Someone must be available to deal with suicidal patients, those in a panic state, and even those with lesser problems who call for help. The therapist may leave various phone numbers where the she or he can be reached. But this means being available 24 hours, day and night. It can be done if the practice is not burdensome. Sooner or later, however, one must have at least one colleague for full coverage.

Middle-of-the-night phone calls are a nuisance, although sometimes a necessity. In an active practice, they are unavoidable and are the price of being in one of the helping professions. Fortunately, emergencies are not as frequent as in a medical practice, and patients are often "thoughtful," waiting to phone the following morning. Such is the nature of the patient–therapist relationship!

The decision to use an answering service or an answering device should not be a difficult one. Devices are mechanical and cold by nature, are not very reassuring, and are best used as a last resort. On the other hand, answering services are not always satisfactory because of delays in answering calls or the placing of an impatient patient on hold. This problem can be ameliorated to a degree by discussion with phone exchange supervisors and by advising patients not to hang up too soon. The problem can be a nuisance, but there appears to be no way out of the dilemma except to choose a service that is not as busy or that has enough phone operators to function smoothly. I find it necessary from time to time to remind my service that patients will sometimes hang up if a call is not answered by the fourth ring. The phone companies suggest seven rings, but because of the nature of their problems, patients are rarely patient.

How long should one talk on the telephone, and should one charge for phone conversations? Added up, the minutes on a phone can take up more time than one can afford in a given practice. I have found it practical to speak from 1 to 2 minutes and then suggest, if needed, that I will call back later when more time is available. If conversations extend much longer, one is privileged to charge for time, again depending on frequency and necessity. Some patients take the therapist's availability for granted, and charges for time should be made if telephoning is abused.

Home phone numbers should rarely be given out. Privacy should be respected. However, provision should be made for emergencies to be passed on to you by an answering service. A good service will see to it that this is done, passing on information quickly either to you at home, or to forwarding numbers, or to a colleague who is covering you. This is just the nature of the practice, and one can be held responsible and accountable for the phone coverage of patients at all times.

It would be ideal if every patient underwent a physical examination before psychotherapy. This is not always practical and sometimes not even necessary. Most patients who come to a therapist have been to their family practitioners or other health specialists, some for years before they arrive at the therapist's door. However, it is professional negligence to ignore physical complaints without a proper physical workup. I bend over backward to avoid the trap of treating as a psychological complaint one that has an organic base.

In any therapeutic alliance, it is of prime importance to reevaluate the complaints of one's patients from time to time and to recommend medical aid where it appears necessary. Table 1 has a review of the systems most likely to go wrong and will alert the therapist to possible physical problems that need to be looked into. The nonmedical therapist should work closely with a medically trained practitioner.

A differential diagnosis has to be made, and if chest pains turn out to be due to angina, epigastric pains to peptic ulcer, headaches to brain tumors, palpitations to thyroid disease, then the therapist is more fully covered by having made a proper diagnosis and the patient is not harmed. The therapist does not have to relinquish a patient under such circumstances, but a consultation with an appropriate specialist should be considered.

The issue of handling sexually provocative patients has received much publicity in the professional and lay press, particularly since Masters and Johnson (1970) directed attention to this topic. They stated, "There is no greater negation of professional responsibility than taking sexual advantage of an essentially defenseless patient; yet this often happens" (p. 389).

Patients may openly proposition their therapists, but there is no therapeutic reason to enter into an intimate relationship, and there are many professional reasons not to do so. When one is propositioned, the simplest answer would be a reminder that the patient is a fine, lovely, and attractive person, but that the relationship is one of therapist and patient and therapeutic gain would be lost in such an involvement. It would be best not to belabor the issue. Romantic countertransference may be dealt with in the context of therapeutic interaction, but no more than other emotional events in the patient's life.

The use of group therapy within an individual practice is a personal matter that depends on background, training, orientation, and how much one values such therapy in treatment. Certainly, it is a worthy alternative or addition to one-to-one therapy and is highly useful in an institutional setting. In my experience, it does not take the place of individual therapy. Further, there are monetary considerations to take into account, that is, how much each participant must contribute to make this a financially sufficient addition to treatment. For therapeutic group sessions, one should allow at least 2 hours.

Office practice is limited when one is dealing with a suicidal patient, a drug addict or abuser, or a floridly psychotic individual. These conditions call for immediate hospitalization both for the protection of the patient and for the institution of more intensive treatment. Where organic complaints are present, one should not hesitate to obtain the aid of either internists or other medical specialists. It is embarrassing to discover that one has neglected or ignored symptoms that are better dealt with by other health professionals.

Solo practitioners rarely practice completely alone. They depend on a network of other consultants and health aides. Psychiatrists may refer to psychologists or social workers, psychologists and social workers to psychiatrists, and both may refer to a variety of medical consultants. They may practice by themselves or in a group, but the latter is more likely to happen in an institutional setting. The network extends to nonmedical groups, such as Alcoholics Anonymous and Narcotics Anonymous; to religious affiliates; to a variety of supportive organizations, including those dealing with vocational rehabilitation; and even to athletic and recreational associations. Practicing alone, one is less likely to be overseen and criticized by others and, therefore, must be more critical of oneself. It sometimes becomes necessary, if therapy is not moving along well, to call on others to help, even to the point of transferring patients to colleagues. In an institutional setting, there is a greater pressure for accountability and the recognition that others may have something to say about one's practice. There is a greater demand for conformity. The choice of working alone or in an institutional setting or both becomes a sensitive issue for each individual.

Confidentiality is important in therapy. Without the written consent of the patient or client, one cannot release information to anyone except under extraordinary circumstances. There are rules of law that protect the patient in confidentiality situations and that also define the conditions under which confidentiality is limited.

It is very difficult to set guidelines for the termination of treatment other than in the broadest possible terms (Canadian Psychiatric Association Position Paper, 1986). Achieving the initial goal or goals is an end point that is not always attainable. The goals are frequently reset as the patient gains insight into his or her condition. There is usually agreement between patient and therapist when it has been determined that what has been achieved is as much as can reasonably be expected in psychotherapy. If this is not apparent, the sessions can be extended according to the patient's needs and desires. In contrast to those therapists who set cutoff points, I find such an extension to be a satisfactory and smooth transition for the patient. The therapist must keep in mind the patient's needs, wishes, and rights. Sometimes, the patient decides that he or she has had enough of therapy or cannot afford to continue and simply does not return. This happens to every therapist at some time or another and must be accepted.

SUMMARY

From my point of view as a board-certified psychiatrist in private practice for some 40 years, I can look back and, with hindsight, determine what has worked, what results in a more comfortable practice, and what leads to a rewarding life.

Psychiatrists, psychologists, and social workers compete with each other, and despite their disparate training, there is an overlap in the type of patient seen. It may be necessary, therefore, to share in the treatment of patients. This sharing has become more important because of the psychopharmacological revolution and the essential part that medication plays in the treatment of many emotional and mental disorders. Further, legal concerns about patients' rights are now gradually returning to a more humanitarian concern about the basic needs of patients and the communities in which they live.

Movement has taken place in the direction of shortening treatment, with an emphasis on symptomatic relief and reeducation toward self-help. Eclectic methods suited to patients' needs appear to be the trend of the future.

Diagnosis and assessment come first, with findings defined through the five axes of the DSM-III. My own history-taking procedure and letter association technique were described, for initial evaluation, ongoing diagnosis, and reinforcement of symptoms. This evaluation is followed by goal setting with the patient and the establishment of therapeutic strategies. A variety of common features are attributed to the therapist, therapy procedures, and the patient, including support factors, learning factors, and action factors. Consideration was given in this chapter to more specifically directed therapies, such as hypnosis and systematic desensitization. Behavioral and multimodal approaches offer certain advantages for diagnostic workup and treatment.

Office therapy was discussed in terms of the length of the treatment sessions; the frequency of visits; setting and collecting fees; patient flow; office help; phone etiquette; confidentiality; emergencies; report preparation; the termination of treatment; the need for physical examinations; health aide networks; sole versus group practice; after-hours coverage; sexually provocative patients; and group therapy.

REFERENCES

Abramovitz, C. M. (1970). Personalistic psychotherapy and the role of technical eclecticism. *Psychological Reports, 26,* 255–263.

American Psychiatric Association. (1980). *Diagnostic and statistical manual of mental disorders* (3rd ed.; DSM-III). Washington, DC: Author.

Annis, A. P. (1967). The autobiography: Its use and value in professional psychology. *Journal of Counseling Psychology, 14,* 9–17.

Bernstein, D. A., & Allen, G. J. (1969). Fear survey schedule, 2. *Behaviour Research and Therapy, 7,* 403–407.

Canadian Psychiatric Association Position Paper. (1986). The role of the psychotherapies in the practice of psychiatry. *Canadian Journal of Psychiatry, 31,* 458–465.

Cautela, J. R., & Kastenbaum, R. (1967). A reinforcement survey schedule for use in therapy, training, and research. *Psychological Reports, 20,* 1115–1130.

Clarke, A. D. B. (1968). Learning and human development. *British Journal of Psychiatry, 114,* 1061–1077.

Davis, R. D. (1958). Clinical problems and experimental researches. *British Journal of Medical Psychology, 31,* 74–82.

Dengrove, E. (1962). A new letter association technique. *Diseases of the Nervous System, 23,* 25–26.

Gantt, W. H. (1964). Autonomic conditioning. In J. Wolpe, A. Salter, & L. J. Reyna (Eds.), *The conditioning therapies* (pp. 51–52). New York: Holt, Rinehart, & Winston.

Lambert, M. J. (1986). Some implications of psychotherapy outcome research of eclectic psychotherapy. *International Journal of Eclectic Psychotherapy, 5,* 16–45.

Lang, P. G. (1964). Experimental studies of desensitization psychotherapy. In J. Wolpe, A. Salter, & L. J. Reyna (Eds.), *The conditioning therapies* (pp. 51–52). New York: Holt, Rinehart, & Winston.

Lanyon, R. I., & Manosevitz, M. (1966). Validity of self-reported fear. *Behaviour Research and Therapy, 4,* 259–263.

Lazarus, A. A. (1966). Broad spectrum behaviour therapy and the treatment of agoraphobia. *Behaviour Research and Therapy, 4,* 95–97.

Lazarus, A. A. (1986). Multimodal psychotherapy: Overview and update. *International Journal of Eclectic Psychotherapy, 5,* 95–103.

Lazarus, A. A., & Serber, M. (1968). Is systematic desensitization being misapplied? *Psychological Reports, 23,* 215–218.

Masters, W. H., & Johnson, V. E. (1970). *Human sexual inadequacy.* Boston: Little, Brown.

Meyer, V., & Crisp, A. H. (1966). Some problems in behaviour therapy. *British Journal of Psychiatry, 112,* 367–381.

Montenegro, H. (1968). Preschool children and separation anxiety. *Journal of Child Psychology and Psychiatry, 9,* 93–103.

Rubin, B. M., Katkin, E. S., Weiss, B. W., & Efran, J. S. (1968). Factor analysis of a fear survey schedule. *Behaviour Research and Therapy, 6,* 65–75.

Rubin, S. E., Lawlis, G. F., Tasto, D. L., & Namenek, T. (1969). Factor analysis of the 122 item fear survey schedule. *Behaviour Research and Therapy, 7,* 381–386.

Scherer, M. W., & Nakamura, C. Y. (1968). A fear survey schedule for children (FSS-FC). *Behaviour Research and Therapy, 6,* 173–182.

Stevenson, I., and Hain, J. H. (1967). On the different meanings of apparently similar symptoms: Illustrated by varieties of barber shop phobia. *American Journal of Psychiatry, 124,* 399–403.

Wolpe, J. (1964). Behavior therapy in complex neurotic states. *British Journal of Psychiatry, 110,* 28–34.

Wolpe, J., & Lang, P. J. (1964). A fear survey schedule for use in behavior therapy. *Behaviour Research and Therapy, 2,* 27–30.

29

Research in Outpatient Clinical Practice

STEVEN C. HAYES AND JOSEPH R. HAAS

INTRODUCTION

Outpatient clinical practice encompasses many activities, but undoubtedly the primary one is this: A clinician is interacting with another individual who is experiencing problems in the natural environment. The nature of the interaction and the interpretation of the client's problem vary widely from clinician to clinician and from one school of thought to another. The purpose, in broad terms, is the same: to help the individual with some aspect of what he or she does (where *doing* includes feeling, thinking, remembering, relating, and so on) as a result of this therapeutic interaction. In this sense, therapy is a form of social influence (Frank, 1973).

In many ways, this fact is the bane of therapy research. All people are immersed in social networks in their own lives. Our personal abilities in such areas as family relationships, child rearing, teaching, managing co-workers, and so on are only rarely informed by research. We learn by doing, by watching others, by word of mouth, and by other such means.

There is considerable evidence that clinicians acquire their techniques in much the same way. Surveys of clinical practitioners show that they base their practices primarily on their experience and on the experiences of others reported in workshops, case conferences, and the like (Cohen, 1979). Notably lacking as primary sources of influence for most clinicians are scientific data developed by the profession. As many as 40% of practitioners believe that *none* of the available research is relevant to practice (Cohen,

STEVEN C. HAYES • Department of Psychology, University of Nevada, Reno, Nevada 89557–0062.
JOSEPH R. HAAS • Department of Psychology, University of North Carolina at Greensboro, Greensboro, North Carolina 27412-5001.

1976). Practicing clinicians generally indicate that their academic training should have included less research training (Garfield & Kurtz, 1976).

As a rule, practicing clinicians neither produce nor consume clinical research (Garfield & Kurtz, 1976; Kelly, Goldberg, Fiske, & Kilkowski, 1978; Levy, 1962). The two sides of this problem may be interrelated. Clinicians can and do accuse clinical researchers of being insensitive to more subtle issues in the therapeutic process (e.g., Lehrer, 1981). It is possible that most existing clinical research may not capture the subtle complexity observed by seasoned clinicians. Practicing clinicians might be more likely to produce research that focuses on this complexity. Therefore, it is possible that practitioners are less likely to consume research results in part because few produce it. As we discuss later, there is good reason to believe that including practitioners in the overall clinical-research enterprise would increase its relevance to the practical environment.

The purpose of this chapter is to examine research in the outpatient setting. We first try to build the case that research in that setting is of critical importance to clinical science and practice. We examine the kind of assessment, intervention, and design considerations involved in research in the outpatient setting. We give some examples of important outpatient research.

WHY SCIENCE?

Science involves the systematic development of descriptions of relations, based on verifiable experience. In clinical science, at least, these descriptions may be evaluated by an increased ability to predict and control the phenomena at hand. Clinical science should help predict our clients' behavior in given situations and point to effective ways of inducing behavioral change.

The need for a scientific analysis of outpatient clinical practice can be readily argued on practical grounds. The patient has a right to expect, in this day and age, that diagnosis and intervention will be based on high scientific standards. Science has unquestionably proved its value in the health fields over the last century. The history of all of the helping professions teaches us that, where the scientific foundation is weak, services are often ultimately shown to be defective. For example, medical practice once included blood letting as an important clinical procedure; today, it would be sufficient cause for a malpractice lawsuit.

A weak scientific base affects the professional as well. The lack of a strong scientific base reduces the independence, standing, and funding of the clinical disciplines. The independent professional status of a health field is not firmly established merely by tradition or by claims of unique professional competence. It is best established on the basis of a distinct knowledge base, and today, that can be credibly accomplished only through scientific theory and research. In outpatient clinical work, one result of a weak scientific base has been the proliferation of professions that purport to train psychotherapists, regardless of the scientific base of the professions.

WHAT DO WE WANT OUTPATIENT RESEARCH TO DO?

Seeing psychotherapy as a complex social interaction directs our attention to the most critical needs of psychotherapy research. We all know from our own lives that some interactions with others produce change and that some do not. The effects of a given interchange seem to depend on exactly what was done, with whom, and under what conditions. No one approach works with everyone, in all circumstances. Thus, what a clinician needs to know is how to interact with this particular client and with this particular problem. Gordon Paul (1969) identified this as the critical question in clinical research more than 20 years ago: "What treatment, by whom, is most effective for this individual with that specific problem, under which set of circumstances, and how does it come about?" (p. 44). An answer to this question is what clinicians want from research. We will refer to Paul's question as the *clinical question*. Research that helps to answer the clinical question has a degree of external validity (Campbell & Stanley, 1963).

If external validity is the ultimate practical reason to do clinical research in the first place, it seems important to understand how best to achieve it. The current model of research practice has clearly failed to provide a convincing source of externally valid information, as the failure of most clinicians to attend to the literature suggests. A brief discussion of external validity is necessary because it provides the major intellectual support for an increased emphasis on research in outpatient practice (see Hayes, 1987, for a more extended analysis of this point).

External Validity

The dominant model of external validity draws from sampling theory and probability theory and is closely related to theories of the internal validity of research. Every beginning researcher learns the model—typically, as a theory of proper research method. Some students even confuse it with the scientific method itself. According to this model, we must randomly select a sample from a known population and randomly assign subjects to groups or conditions. If the variability between subjects is low relative to differences between the groups, we conclude that we have an effect. The effect then should also apply to other random samples from the sample population as a matter of mathematical necessity.

Problems with the Model

This mathematical-necessity model of external validity has a long history and powerful intellectual support. Unfortunately, it is impossible to fully implement the model in the real world of clinical practice. First, *there are few if any "known populations" in outpatient research*. A known population is not just a conceptually specifiable population. It is one thing to talk of "paranoid schizophrenics" (a conceptual population); it is another to have access to all paranoid schizophrenics (where identification and access establish the "known population"). Some individuals may have a problem, but it may not be detected. Others may know that they have a problem but fail to seek treatment. Still others may seek treatment in a manner prohibiting their identification. In the real world, populations are detected by their contact with certain cooperative individuals or institutions. The events producing either the contact or the cooperativeness of the institution may distinguish this population from the conceptual population in important ways.

Second, *true random selection is rarely possible*. In the real world, subjects from a conceptually significant population are selected for practical reasons. For example, a given hospital may allow a researcher access, whereas another may not. Any characteristic leading people to use that particular hospital now also distorts the sample.

Third, *random assignment is difficult to obtain.* Subjects decline assignment to particular conditions. Subjects may drop out of the study more in one condition than in another.

When one puts together these three problems—known populations, random selection, and random assignment—it becomes clear that the mathematical-necessity model of external validity does not exist in the world of clinical research. Ironically, even if it did, the *kind* of external validity such studies would possess is not the kind that would answer the clinical question for practitioners and other consumers of treatment research. If the model were followed, the research results would necessarily apply only to other random samples from the same population. The model can promise no more. The model does not promise that every subgroup in the sample will respond in the same manner as the entire group. A given treatment may work very nicely with the population overall and be iatrogenic with a subpopulation. Clinicians, however, never randomly sample from treatment populations. Patients seek out particular clinicians for all kinds of nonrandom reasons: reputation, location, sex, race, fees, availability, hours, and so on. How are we to know whether the nonrandom characteristics causing an individual to be treated by someone do not also cause her or him to be in a subgroup to whom the overall results will not apply?

Logical Generalization

The mathematical-necessity model is the only one to promise the external validity of a well-designed study. Every other approach to external validity relies on logical generalization (Hersen & Barlow, 1976). The principle of logical generalization is this: If a given treatment is shown to be successful with a given set of behaviors in a given context with a given patient, it is more likely to be successful with the behavior of another patient in another context to the extent that the behaviors, patients, and contexts are similar.

For this principle to work, it is necessary to identify the *individual* successes and failures of treatment. There is wide agreement that this is a critical need in therapy research (e.g., Gendlin, 1986), and as we will attempt to show, it forms the primary basis for an expansion of research in outpatient practice. Unfortunately, most contemporary clinical research is ill suited to the identification of individual treatment successes and failures.

In a typical pre-post group-comparison study, the possible sources of variability are confounded at the level of the individual. If a given person improves from pre- to post-, we cannot say, *for that individual,* whether the improvement is due to inconsistent measurement (false variability), extraneous factors (real variability produced by irrelevant variables), or treatment-related variability of various kinds. It is only at the level of the group that the three types of variability are distinguished. For this reason, research that glosses over individual differences may have limited external validity as applied to the needs of the outpatient practitioner.

Single-Case Designs

At a superficial level, the clinical question seems to demand very complex research designs. The question of what treatment works best for whom seems to lead logically to the use of large multifactorial designs. Such designs are unlikely in outpatient practice. Practitioners are simply not able to gather together large groups of clients with the same disorders, to assign some to control groups, and so on. However, one solution to this problem is to relate individual subject characteristics to treatment-related improvement identified at the level of the individual and to do so many, many times. Based on the principle of logical generalization, the clinical question may then begin to be answered one step at a time, rather than all at once.

One method that promises to do this is the "single-case" experimental design. Since the late 1970s, an explosion of interest has occurred in methodological tools that are built on single-case analysis (e.g., Barlow, Hayes, & Nelson, 1984; Barlow & Hersen, 1984; Chassan, 1979; Hayes, 1981; Hersen & Barlow, 1976; Jayaratne & Levy, 1979; Kazdin, 1980, 1982; Kratchwill, 1978). These tools are not only scientifically defensible, but readily applicable to the clinical environment.

The fundamental idea behind single-case designs is that behavioral variability within an individual across time can, if examined properly, be divided into treatment-related variability, extraneous variability, and measurement error. To the extent that individual treatment successes and failures can be identified one at a time, the clinical question can be approached on the basis of a large series of small *n* designs, not just through a small series of large-number designs. This strategy makes a contribution to the scientific base of the discipline possible for the practitioner. Indeed, if such a strategy is to work, it requires their participation. If multitudes of intensive analyses of individuals can produce the kind of external validity needed by outpatient practitioners, who will produce them? Who has ready access to these cases, other than these same practitioners?

Practitioners are the clinical sciences' greatest resource. The purpose of this chapter is to examine how this resource may be harnessed. What follows is a description of a scientific strategy that is especially tailored to investigations conducted within ongoing outpatient clinical practice.

THE SCIENTIFIC ANALYSIS OF CLINICAL PHENOMENA

It is difficult to know how or where to begin scientific analysis and empirical study in the outpatient environment. The fundamental question is: How do researchers convert their interests and hunches into research questions that lead to sound empirical study and the advancement of science? Although much has been written on the scientific method, little has been written about the preempirical activity of generating research questions. Before experiments can be designed, the phenomena of interest must be described in terms of possible relations among variables. Researchers typically conduct formal or informal analyses in order to identify critical variables and the possible relations between them. Because science is not conducted in a vacuum, the analyses leading to research studies are always a reflection of the implicit and explicit philosophical assumptions of the scientist (Pepper, 1942). These assumptions, implicit or explicit, suggest which causal variables are relevant and which effects are important.

In clinical psychology, it seems helpful to divide this analytical activity into considerations of grand theories (e.g., Freud, Jung, or Skinner), theories and research focusing on specific types of psychopathology (e.g., Craighead's discussion, 1980, of unitary theories of depression), and diverse possible accounts of the dynamics of any given clinical case (see Freud, 1953, and Wolpe & Rachman, 1960, for two different formulations of the case of Little Hans). Each of these areas is discussed here in terms of their contribution to the development of clinical research questions.

The grand theories can provide a rich source of practical techniques and empirical research (Ross, 1985), which can have a great influence on a researcher in the initial phases of formulating a research program. For example, psychoanalytic theory stresses the importance of unconscious conflicts. As this theory is applied to schizophrenia, the conflicts centering on the mother–child relationship are thought to be important. Psychoanalytic research in this area has included the presentation of subliminal stimuli reflective of the symbiotic mother–child relationship in producing the temporary relief of psychotic episodes (Silverman, 1976). The independent variable in this case (symbiotic fantasy stimuli) is suggested by psychoanalytic theory.

In contrast, behavioral theories have focused on the role of the context in establishing and maintaining certain behavioral patterns. With schizophrenia, this theory has led to research on the production and maintenance of adaptive behaviors in psychotic populations, the interpretation of hallucinations based on the analysis of language found in Skinner's 1957 book *Verbal Behavior* (Layng & Andronis, 1984), and similar research. An example of the first effort is the use of token economies designed to help clients become more self-sufficient (Kazdin & Bootzin, 1972). An example of the second effort is the identification of the possible etiology (i.e., significant stressors and maladaptive social relationships) of schizophrenic break, which can be used to guide the therapist in addressing social issues in the client's life.

Thus, grand theories provide an overall structure that guides the development of clinical research questions. It is literally the case that many questions would not even *occur* to researchers without a grand theory to suggest them. Unfortunately, most of these theories are vague, inconsistent, or poorly supported. Thus, they do not directly provide a strong basis for much of what clinicians face: they are more useful as guides than as rulebooks. This fact suggests that outpatient clinicians are less likely to conduct sophisticated research in their practice without maintaining contact with an intellectual tradition to organize that research.

Traditional Research in Psychopathology

Theory and research data on specific forms of psychopathology such as depression or anxiety are also a potential source for generating research questions. Psychology has traditionally followed the medical model in the investigation of psychopathology. In the medical model, pathological syndromes are identified and classified based on the clustering of topographical signs or symptoms. These syndromes are elevated to the level of a disease once they have a known etiology, course, and response to treatment. The value of such a medical model is not fully felt until a disease is discovered: a syndrome is merely a promissory note. Thus, once a syndrome is identified, research on etiology, course, additional characteristics, and treatments begins in order to elevate the syndrome's status to that of a disease.

The scientific method most often used in research driven by the medical model is the standard group-comparison model, as represented in group treatment studies and known-groups descriptive studies. The reason for reliance on this type of research method is that clusters of signs and symptoms are almost always identified across people. Thus, these groups of persons naturally become the unit of analysis (i.e., all the people with *x*, *y*, and *z* signs or symptoms).

In a typical group-comparison treatment study, a population is identified by particular assessment devices. The subjects are randomly divided into treatment and control groups so that one or more treatments may be compared with the control group or to each other. In the known-groups method, subjects within a certain diagnostic category are compared with normals or subjects in another category in terms of the dimensions important to the diagnostic category of interest. In both of these strategies, group inferential statistics tend to be the method of analysis because there are few well-accepted alternative means of summarizing the differences between groups of individuals.

This style of scientific inquiry pushes the focus of science away from the individual. Contemporary diagnostic schemes are based on clusters of topographically similar characteristics across individuals. The identification of such homogeneous groups of individuals does not guarantee that all individuals will show a similar etiology or will respond in the same way to the same intervention. Syndromes are not necessarily diseases. The individuals in the group may be topographically similar but functionally different. This distraction raises concerns that were captured nicely by Sidman (1962):

> Our gross preliminary observations tell us little more than that the patient is not behaving as he should. Perhaps he finds himself involved in a paranoid plot; or walls himself off in autistic silence; or develops an aphasic inability to name objects. Such classifications—paranoia, autism, aphasia—are too general to form a maximally useful diagnostic base. Patients given one label are found to differ among themselves in the etiology of their breakdown, in their response to similar treatments, in their specific patterns of behavior. What is required is a set of general behavioral principles which will serve to regroup behavioral pathologies into classes that may be differentiated in terms of the behavioral processes involved. (p. 197)

Individual Case Analysis

Another source of research ideas is direct contact with clinical cases. This is probably the richest source of research ideas for the outpatient clinician, because it is bound to take up a greater portion of the clinician's time than the other two sources. Ideas that emerge in direct clinical work are more likely to be sophisticated if they are informed by grand theories and research in psychopathology.

The development and testing of ideas drawn from individual cases may proceed together through the use of the individual case study. Popularized in psychoanalytic writing (e.g., Freud's seminal case analyses of Little Hans, the Wolfman, and Anna O), a focus on the individual case has also gained acceptance and use in behavior therapy (Kazdin, 1981; Shapiro, 1957; Turkat, 1986). An example will help clarify what we mean by *individual case analysis* and how it addresses the clinical question.

Wolpe (1979, 1986) provided an elegant description of how case analysis led to the individualized treatment of a 35-year-old woman with a 10-year history of depression and an inability to experience coital orgasm.

An intensive interview and the administration of several instruments (the Willoughby Neuroticism scale and the Fear Survey Schedule) revealed that the client had an intense distrust of the people close to her. Her anxiety in the presence of her husband interfered with her ability to experience organisms and, in turn, resulted in depression. Wolpe supported this hypothesis by appealing to the fact that the woman could experience orgasm only by masturbation if her husband was not in the room. Wolpe also discovered a long history of situations in which significant others had violated her trust (e.g., her father had been very cruel to her when she was a small child). Wolpe treated her fear of trust with systematic desensitization (4 months of weekly sessions), and the client reported no more episodes of depression or orgasmic difficulty during a 12-year follow-up.

If a standard diagnostic assessment had been used, this woman's problem might have been identified as depression and a sexual dysfunction. It would be feasible that to include her in a treatment study for either problem. After diagnosis, the assessor would still have been faced with the traditionally difficult task of deciding which target behavior should be treated and which treatment should be used. A traditional diagnostic approach to this case would not lead to clear-cut treatment choices.

Wolpe's analysis led to a treatment focus that was nonobvious and not readily suggested by the diagnostic categories most obviously applicable to the client. Diagnostic categories are often assumed to represent homogeneous groups of individuals who have problems of similar etiology that respond to similar treatments. Traditional psychiatric diagnoses are almost always, however, mere syndromes, not diseases. They may be useful starting points for an analysis but do not suggest that all individuals in a certain diagnostic category will respond in the same way to the same treatments. Because of assumed homogeneity, the field faces a proliferation of unitary theories that attempt to account for the etiology of the disorder and to suggest a treatment of choice for all group members (Craighead, 1980). Little attention is paid to individual differences between group members. Individual differences that are useful indicators of individual treatment success or failure are missed. The use of group data should be carried out in such a way that the analysis of the individual case will not suffer.

Attention to the unique characteristics of the individual seems common in clinical practice, yet it is rarely reflected in traditional clinical research. Single-subject research is the only analytical method that is designed to be especially sensitive to the nuances of the individual. It seems to be a natural choice for helping outpatient clinicians conduct research on the individual analyses that they do anyway.

In the remainder of this chapter, we provide guidelines that will allow clinicians to carry out this task and, in turn, to make a unique and powerful contribution to science. The areas of psychological assessment, psychological treatment, the interaction between treatment and assessment, and the single-case experimental design form the basis of our suggested outpatient research strategy.

A RESEARCH PROGRAM FOR OUTPATIENT CLINICIANS

The clinical question implies assessment, treatment, and the interaction between the two. Research in outpatient practice starts with assessment and treatment outcome concerns and moves toward selecting the most effective treatment for an individual client.

Psychological Assessment

Clinical assessment is an essential building block for research aimed at the understanding and treatment of psychopathology. As the clinical question indicates, assessment must capture a very complex phenomenon. We have organized our discussion of assessment around three global areas: (1) the identification of specific behaviors or behavior clusters (where by *behavior* we mean thoughts, feelings, actions, memories, attitudes, beliefs, and so on) and their contexts; (2) the identification and measurement of the relevant client characteristics (demographics) that contribute to the understanding of psychopathology, that determine significant predictors of response to treatment, and that suggest new classification schemes; and (3) measurement of the response to treatment as a means of understanding the outcome and processes of various treatments.

Identification of Behavior Clusters and Their Contexts

A major goal of psychological assessment is to describe behaviors and behavior clusters that result in life problems for our clients. In addition, assessment describes the contexts in which these problem behaviors occur. The formal description of problem behaviors and their contexts plays a unique role in single-case analysis—one that is quite different from the role of diagnosis in traditional research strategies. Both approaches acknowledge the need for a careful description of behavior, but they differ radically in the way that the descriptive system is developed and used. In the traditional diagnostic strategy, the codes are devised in an *a priori* fashion, with the goal of detecting topographical similarities. In the single-subject strategy, the development of a code is ongoing, and careful attention is given to the functional utility of the code. This emphasis on functional utility and the ongoing process is underscored by the principle of logical generalization.

The principle of logical generalization suggests that, if a given problem behavior in a given individual, in a given context, responds to a specific treatment, the chances are that a similar client with similar problems in similar contexts will respond the same way. The process of logical generalization depends on the intensive assessment of individuals. In clinical research, it is important to use the assessment devices that best quantify the behaviors and contexts that are presumed to be crucial to the analysis of the individual case. For example, in Wolpe's case, it would be important to measure behavior such as the frequency of orgasms, depression, time spent in the presence of close significant others, anxiety levels in the presence of loved ones, and so on. The assessment of context is particularly difficult for the outpatient clinician because the most relevant contexts often occur outside the therapy situation. Noteworthy contextual factors include the setting in which the client becomes anxious, the environmental precipitants of depression, and the situations that lead to the inability to experience orgasm.

During treatment, new measures are often added, and the case may be reformulated as new data come in. Response to treatment often indicates the utility of the measures that have been selected. After treatment has been concluded, the assessment devices that have been used form the functionally significant "diagnostic system" for that client. In other words, regardless of the formal diagnosis, the principle of logical generalization suggests that clinicians classify clients on the basis of functionally significant descriptive codes. If the treatment is successful, and if this therapy succeeds for another similar client, then the general utility of the descriptive code identifying that similarity is suggested. If the second client does not improve, then the search begins for other factors that account for the differences between these two people. The descriptive code for the second client is expanded, and research may then be carried out on the utility of this new scheme. The following is an example of how a preliminary descriptive code can be developed with a single subject.

In the third edition of the American Psychiatric Association's *Diagnostic and Statistical Manual* (DSM-III; APA, 1980), one of the diagnostic categories for posttraumatic stress disorder includes the "intensification of symptoms by exposure to events that symbolize or resemble the traumatic event'' (p. 238). Fairbanks, Gross, and Keane (1983) presented a single-case analysis concerned with the assessment of a client who met the criteria for posttraumatic stress disorder. Although the client was first identified by means of a standard diagnostic process, this study focused on specific motor behaviors manifested in an individual client and their correlation with contextual factors and other behaviors. Fairbanks *et al.* determined that various motor behaviors indicative of posttraumatic stress disorder (e.g., facial tension, clenching of fists, flailing arms, shouting, and sobbing) occurred when the client was presented with flooding stimuli, and that they did not tend to occur when the client was presented with relaxation cues. The measures also changed in response to treatment. Similarly, these behaviors correlated with a decrease in depression, nightmares of the traumatic event, and the degree of emotional disturbance elicited by recollection of the traumatic event. Covariation of these behaviors with such contextual factors and other problem behaviors confirmed the notion that they were functionally related to the client's overall problems. This study yielded promising data that may aid in both the identification of posttraumatic stress disorder and the assessment of treatment outcome. Its ultimate utility will be demonstrated if further research can show that this specific code helps to identify other functionally similar subjects.

Demographics

Demographics is a term that refers to general client characteristics beyond the problem behavior itself that could relate to the response of this specific problem behavior to treatment. The DSM-III provides several categories that summarize the types of demographic information that may be important to consider for each disorder of interest. These categories include associated features, age at onset, course, impairment, complications, predisposing factors, prevalence, sex ratio, familial patterns, and differential diagnosis. The DSM-III includes a brief section on each of these categories in its discussion of each disorder.

An example illustrates how the identification of demographic features leads to the illumination of idiosyncratic results. Rossiter and Wilson (1984) treated four bulimics with exposure and cognitive therapy. One of these patients did not show strong signs of recovery and began to cancel appointments. Monitoring of scores on the Beck Depression Inventory demonstrated that this person differed from the other three, in that she had shown an extreme increase in depression during treatment. This characteristic suggests a possible individual difference that could help predict the response of other bulimics to treatment. The measurement of depression may be incorporated into subsequent research so that its interaction with treatment can be measured in a preplanned manner.

Studying the assessment of demographic features and their relationship to specific behavior problems seems both important and well within the grasp of the scientist-practitioner. It also fits nicely into the process of logical generalization.

Assessment of Response to Treatment

Our discussion thus far has focused on assessing clusters of maladaptive behaviors and their contexts, and on important associated features that correlate with these clusters.

The backbone of a practical clinical research program, however, is to assess the response of these behaviors to specific interventions. Assessment can identify basic changes in behavior patterns (perhaps a goal of all therapies) as well as changes in dimensions that are relevant to the specific process through which the treatment is said to work. The inclusion of both outcome and process measures is very important to the development of clinical knowledge. It ensures that the assessment data will reflect the complex mechanisms behind psychopathology as well as the way in which treatment interacts with pathology.

Last, Barlow, and O'Brien (1984a,b) provided an excellent example of a research program focusing on process. They reported a series of single-case analyses designed to study the role of negative and positive cognitions in agoraphobics undergoing exposure-based treatments and cognitive therapy. The underlying theoretical goal was to determine the mechanism through which exposure and cognitive therapy reduce phobic avoidance. These authors were specifically interested in determining whether exposure works by effecting cognitive changes and whether cognitive therapy actually reduces negative beliefs.

The basic methodology involved the use of two measures of the quality of cognitions occurring during and after each treatment session. Behavioral, self-report, and physiological measures were also taken. Seven subjects were examined across the two studies. Taken together, these studies indicate that cognitive change (increases in positive cognitions and decreases in negative cognitions) was inconsistent across the subjects, whether they were treated with exposure or cognitive therapy.

The finding that subjects vary on this dimension is an important first step. Subsequent research might focus on characteristics that are common to subjects who show cognitive change and those who do not. The study of this important question required both process and outcome measures of response to treatment.

Throughout the sections on assessment we have implied an interface between assessment and treatment. Before this interface can be made clear, specific treatment concerns must be discussed.

Psychological Treatment

Practitioners are primarily interested in data that are related to the effectiveness of the treatments that are available. Single-subject methodology can be used to answer questions such as: Does this treatment work? The scope of the problems and treatments that are amenable to outpatient research is impressive. Single-case studies conducted with outpatients have dealt with the treatment of agoraphobia with self-exposure (Frame, Turner, Jacob, & Szekely, 1984) and self-help manuals (Hoden, O'Brien, Barlow, Stetson, & Infantino, 1983); the treatment of depression with self-control and social-skills treatment (Heiby, 1986) and aerobic exercise (Doyne, Chambless, & Beutler, 1983); the treatment of insomnia with paradoxical intention (Espie & Lindsay, 1985); the treatment of an incest victim with implosive therapy (Rychtarik, Silverman, Van Landingham, & Prue, 1984); the treatment of hypochondriasis with cognitive-behavioral therapy (Salkovskis & Warwick, 1986); and the treatment of bulimia with cognitive therapy and exposure (Rossiter & Wilson, 1984). Many of these studies address specific outcome questions. Together, they can also be incorporated into a strategy of extreme importance to outpatient clinical research: clinical replication.

An effective strategy for the study of treatment effectiveness in outpatient settings is clinical replication (Hersen & Barlow, 1976; Barlow *et al.*, 1984). Clinical replication was defined by Barlow *et al.* (1984) as

> a process wherein practitioners using a clearly defined set of procedures or "treatment" intervene with a series of cases that have a well-specified and measured problem often encountered in applied settings such as depression in adults or attention deficit disorder in children. In the course of this series, the practitioner observes and records successes and failures, analyzing, where able, the reasons for the individual variations (or intersubject variability). (p. 58)

Barlow *et al.* (1984, p. 291) discussed four treatment-related questions that can be asked by a clinical replication series: (1) "Using a well-defined, clinically significant criterion of improvement and applying an intervention in its most powerful form, how many of a series of clients improve?" (2) "How many clients show limited improvement that would not be judged clinically significant by practitioners, who would then be forced to consider additional or alternative interventions?" (3) "How many people fail to improve or perhaps even deteriorate during administration of the intervention?" (4) "What are the reasons for limited improvement or deterioration?" (5) Question 5 is related to Question 4: "If failures or limited success is observed, what subsequent treatment will result in improvement?"

The definition of clinical replication and these five major questions come very close to a research program that addresses the complexity of the clinical question. The treatment research strategy presented here involves the study of how specific treatments interact with the unique complexity of each client. It is the hope that functionally similar groups of clients will eventually be identified, so that general prescriptions can be passed on to help practicing clinicians choose the right treatment for the right client.

Clinical replication series are still relatively rare. There are, however, several examples of studies, not actually part of a clinical replication series, that can be analyzed with an eye to the questions discussed above.

The outcome of specific treatments for clearly defined problems must be assessed in a way that reflects the clinical significance of the treatment result. Franco, Christoff, Crimmins, and Kelly (1983) demonstrated how empirical and clinical significance can be combined in a study involving social skills training for a single male subject. Not only did they monitor change in the behaviors targeted for treatment, but they went on to include parent reports of dating and involvement in friendships, ratings of the subject's behavior by other popular adolescents, and reports by teachers at school. These latter ratings are examples that clinicians might use informally in their own practice, especially reports of relevant life changes and reports from significant others. Their inclusion in clinical replication studies will help to decrease the gap between statistical and clinical significance.

In clinical replication, it is always important to monitor failures and the possible reasons for failures. The previously discussed studies conducted by Last *et al.* (1984a,b) were quite open in analyzing failures in the use of exposure and cognitive therapy to treat agoraphobia. Other studies from this laboratory have attempted to pinpoint specific predictors of relapse in agoraphobia after treatment. Barlow and Mavisikalian (1981) discussed data that indicate that the presence of high posttreatment physiological arousal, combined with less avoidance and the report of no significant anxiety, may be a strong predictor of relapse in agoraphobics.

It is also possible to follow up on failures with other treatments that might be suggested by the data. Espie and Lindsay (1985) provided an interesting example in their study of the effects of paradoxical intention in treating insomnia. They treated six subjects, three of whom showed rapid reduction of sleep onset latency, one who showed eventual reduction, and two who did not improve at all. These latter subjects were then treated successfully by relaxation training; this success suggests the possibility of two types of insomniacs, who respond differently to popular treatments. The discovery of the etiological variables that lead to these different types of insomnia may provide useful predictors that will aid in treatment selection.

The aforementioned examples suggest a strategy of conducting clinical research that addresses the complexity of the clinical question. This complexity is further understood when the interaction of assessment and treatment is examined.

The Interaction of Assessment and Treatment

Assessment and treatment should be inextricably linked to each other. Assessment research should be concerned not only with developing a taxonomy of psychopathology, and treatment research should be concerned not only with pure outcome questions. A focus on these questions alone leads to an analysis that is too simple and of limited utility.

An adequate level of complexity is captured by the question: How does assessment contribute to treatment? This question involves what has been termed the *treatment utility* of assessment (Hayes, Nelson, & Jarret, 1986; Nelson & Hayes, 1979, 1981). Treatment utility suggests that assessment systems should be judged by their utility in leading to successful treatment outcomes.

Treatment utility is a fundamental component of clinical replication. The careful specification of problem behaviors in individuals is designed to lead to the identification of a group of subjects uniquely responsive to certain treatments.

The interaction of assessment and treatment is highlighted by the analysis of specific failures. When a particular subject shows an idiosyncratic response to treatment, the researcher must search all the available assessment information to determine if this subject is different from others along a certain unique dimension. The issues discussed in the section on assessment become very important here. Data collected before the experiment may be correlated with differential outcomes for individual subjects. Subsequent research may then select subjects for this dimension and examine treatment and modifications that will bring the responding of these types of subjects in line with the data from subjects who are successfully treated.

An example of this endeavor can be found in the depression literature. For a long time, depression has been viewed as a unitary phenomena (Craighead, 1980). One assumption of this view is that all people who are identified as depressed should show a uniform response to an effective treatment for depression. Recent research has indicated that there may be several subtypes of depression that are differentially responsive to existing popular therapies (Heiby, 1986; McKnight, Nelson, Hayes, & Jarrett, 1984; Wolpe, 1986). Heiby (1986) identified two subgroups of depressives: depressives with social skills deficits and depressives with self-control problems. Her subsequent study demonstrated that depressives identified as having self-control problems responded to treatment designed to enhance self-control and were not responsive to social skills training. The converse held true for subjects identified as having social skills problems. In the past, social skills deficits and self-control problems have been a fundamental component of separate unitary theories of depression. Outcomes studies have examined the effects of these therapies on generic depressive populations. However, the outcome of Heiby's and other treatment-utility studies suggests that the presence or absence of specific problems dictates very different treatment procedures.

Thus far, we have discussed a conceptual system for formulating researchable questions relevant to outpatient practice. The discussion has focused on single-subject analysis of the "clinical question." Our main concern has been with the external validity of the research program. We now turn to the issue of experimental design, which allows our conceptual system to be converted to empirical demonstrations.

Experimental Design for the Practicing Clinician

The preceding discussion has focused on external validity as a guide to generating effective clinical research. Design issues are specifically concerned with internal validity (Campbell & Stanley, 1963). *Internal validity* refers to the extent to which an experimental design allows the researcher to attribute a change in the dependent variable to the manipulation of the independent variable. Traditional research strategies (between-groups comparison) typically use a control group who are identical to the treatment group in all ways except their not being exposed to the independent variable. If the treatment group changes and the control group does not, then the independent variable can be held responsible for the changes observed.

In single-subject research, the problem of internal validity is solved by allowing for each subject to serve as his or her own control. There are many types of single-case designs (Barlow *et al.*, 1984; Hayes, 1981; Hersen & Barlow, 1976), but three specific types are discussed briefly below. Examples are drawn from the literature to demonstrate the use of this methodology in outpatient clinical settings.

A common strategy in single-subject research is to use a within-series phase change (Barlow *et al.*, 1984). This strategy entails establishing the degree of variability, the level, and the trend in a series of data points across time, collected under similar conditions. These conditions are then changed, and changes in the data are examined. For example, a baseline phase might be implemented to determine the pretreatment levels of the behavior of interest. After a stable baseline is recorded, the phase is changed by implementing a treatment. If a treatment affects the behavior in question, one might expect the behavior to change shortly after the implementation of treatment. After a stable response to treatment has been documented, a return to baseline is typically implemented, and changes in behavior are once again examined.

The resultant "ABA" design demonstrates internal validity by showing that the dependent variable reliably changes in response to the presentation and withdrawal of the independent variable. The strength of the behavior change and its subsequent replication provide strong evidence that the observed effect was due to the independent variable and not to other sources of control. This is true because the chances are slim that competing sources of control would exert their impact only at the point of phase changes. Therefore, the internal validity increases as the number of effective reversal or phase changes increases.

Dubbert, Martin, Zimering, Burkett, Lake, and Cushman (1984) used a reversal design to examine the effects of aerobic exercise on mild hypertension. The concrete treatment and the clearly defined response made a phase-change design a good choice for examining this problem. In this study, the authors took baseline measures of diastolic blood pressure and a scale designed to assess the amount of aerobic exercise. Two subjects were examined.

The first subject showed moderately high diastolic pressure during 4 weeks of no-exercise baseline. When aerobic exercise was introduced, the blood pressure was reduced to a healthy range. When exercise was stopped for 10 weeks, the blood pressure rose to near baseline measures. Exercise was reintroduced again (a substantial reduction in blood pressure resulted) and was then terminated again (a substantial increase in blood pressure resulted). Such replication of the phase change produced much higher internal validity for the conclusion that the aerobic exercise resulted in changes in blood pressure. The internal validity was further increased when the same pattern of results was demonstrated in another subject. This subject underwent one reversal and ended the experiment in the exercise phase, which resulted in the maintenance of healthy diastolic pressure.

Often, the treatment phase results in a stable change in the dependent variable, which is resistant to change when faced with a reversal to baseline. In this case, several replications of the effect across subjects increases the probability that the observed change is due to the treatment. The larger the number of subjects who show identical responses to the same phase change, the more likely it is that the specific phase change actually produced the change in the dependent measure. Such logic is encompassed in the multiple-baseline design. The multiple-baseline design is composed of a phase change implemented across several persons (or several behaviors or situations within a single person), in which the phase change occurs at different points in real time and after different phase lengths. For example, if a researcher is interested in the effect of Treatment X on Behavior Y, he or she might arrange to test the effects of Treatment X on three subjects who exhibit Behavior Y. The baseline might be taken for 3 weeks for Subject 1, 5 weeks for Subject 2, and 7 weeks for Subject 3. If Treatment X effects a change across all subjects and this change is shown only at the point where Treatment X is introduced, then internal validity is preserved.

Franco *et al.* (1983) presented a multiple-baseline design evaluating the effects of social skills training across four separate skills on a 14-year-old male. Videotaped conversations indicated that this subject emitted very few questions directed at conversational partners, was deficient in the number of acknowledgments given to conversational partners, showed poor eye contact, and showed little affective warmth. The assessment sessions were comprised of free-flowing conversations with new partners to maximize generalization. The treatment focused on one skill at a time, and baseline measures were recorded for all behaviors that were yet to be treated. The results showed that each skill remained at stable baseline until targeted for treatment. When each skill was targeted in treatment, the frequency of the targeted behavior increased significantly. In addition, these authors also used measures of social validity that included ratings by parents and teachers and ratings by popular adolescents who viewed tapes at different treatment intervals. The subject's parents also reported that friends had begun to pay visits to the subject's home and that the subject had started dating. This study provides an excellent example of how formal designs may be augmented by less formal measures as a means of conducting a wide-range assessment of the response to treatment.

The final design to be discussed is the alternating-treatments design (ATD; Barlow & Hayes, 1979). This design is especially useful in comparison of the effectiveness of two or more treatments. This design involves rapidly alternating the treatments and monitoring the effects of each on the behavior or behaviors in question. The dependent measure is usually graphed separately for each treatment. For example, if Treatment X is administered in Weeks 1, 3, 4, 6, and 9, the data points for these weeks would constitute one series (i.e., they would be graphically connected with one line). In turn, the data for Treatment Y, administered in Weeks 2, 5, 7, 8, and 10, would constitute another series. Separations between the series indicate functional differences between the treatments.

An example of an ATD that reflects its complexity was presented by McKnight, Nelson, Hayes, and Jarrett (1984). These authors examined the utility of assessing social skills deficits and irrational beliefs in generating specific treatment for nine depressed clients. Three clients were selected who demonstrated social skills deficits without high levels of irrational cognitions, three were selected who had no social skills problems but significant amounts of irrational cognitions, and three clients were selected who showed both social skills deficits and high levels of irrational cognitions. Again, the purpose was to determine the treatment utility of this categorization. The authors predicted that subjects in the social-skills-only group would show a greater decrease in depression after social skills training than after cognitive treatment; that the reverse would hold true for clients who were high in irrational cognitions; and that subjects who demonstrated both problems would respond equally to both treatments.

After a baseline period, each subject was exposed to four sessions of social skills training and four sessions of cognitive therapy presented in a random order. Assessments were conducted before each session and were presumed to reflect changes produced by the treatment administered in the preceding session. The results confirm the predictions: treatments that matched the clients' identified deficiency were more successful.

The preceding has been only a brief summary of single-subject designs with some concrete examples of their use in clinical practice. The use of these designs is limited only by the researcher's own creativity, and they seem to be a useful and viable technique for answering clinically significant questions.

There are a few special considerations when one is conducting such research on outpatients as opposed to inpatients. First, it is important to assess change in the client's environment outside the therapy setting. In traditional 1-hour-per-week outpatient work, 167 hours are lived outside the therapy setting for every 1 hour in it. What goes on during this time can have as much impact as the therapy itself—or more impact. Second, it is not always clear when a client is in a given therapeutic condition and when the client is not. Are the 167 hours outside therapy "treatment" or "baseline"? The answer is not always clear-cut. Thus, more flexibility may be needed in the outpatient setting regarding such issues as when a treatment phase begins or ends, or when a behavior change should be expected.

The preceding discussion highlights research designs that can be readily used in outpatient practice. Most of the examples were conducted with a minimal number of subjects and in an outpatient setting. Each design can be implemented in ways that do not interfere with the quality of the treatment that a paying client receives. They also provide a sophisticated way of ensuring the internal validity of research that is designed to address the subtleties of the clinical question.

SUMMARY

The outpatient clinic has been largely ignored as a setting for the development of scientifically valid clinical information. Ironically, answers to the clinical question are both most demanded in that setting and most likely to emerge from it. This chapter was designed to present the outline of an approach to the clinical question that can be taken in the outpatient setting. Without harnessing the work of outpatient practitioners to the development of clinical science, it is hard to see how that science can rapidly progress.

REFERENCES

American Psychiatric Association (1980). *Diagnostic and Statistical Manual of Mental Disorders (3rd ed.; DSM-III)*. Washington, DC: Author.

Barlow, D. H., & Hayes, S. C. (1979). Alternating treatments design: One strategy for comparing the effects of two treatments in a single subject. *Journal of Applied Behavior Analysis, 12,* 199–210.

Barlow, d. H., & Hersen, M. (1985). *Single-case experimental designs: Strategies for studying behavior changes* (2nd ed.). New York: Pergamon Press.

Barlow, D. H., & Mavissakalian, M. (1981). Directions in the assessment and treatment of phobia: The next decade. In D. H. Barlow & M. Mavissakalian (Eds.), *Phobia: Psychological and pharmacological treatment* (pp. 199–245). New York: Guilford Press.

Barlow, D. H., Hayes, S. C., & Nelson, R. O. (1984). *The scientist-practitioner: Research and accountability in clinical and educational settings*. New York: Pergamon Press.

Campbell, D. T., & Stanley, J. C. (1963). *Experimental and quasi-experimental designs for research*. Chicago: Rand-McNally.

Chassan, J. B. (1979). *Research design in clinical psychology and psychiatry* (2nd ed.). New York: Irvington.

Cohen, L. H. (1976). Clinician's utilization of research findings. *JSAS Catalog of Selected Documents in Psychology, 6,* 116.

Cohen, L. H. (1979). The research leadership and information source reliance of clinical psychologists. *Professional Psychology, 10,* 780–786.

Craighead, W. E. (1980). Away froma unitary model of depression. *Behavior Therapy, 11,* 122–128.

Doyne, E. J., Chambless, D. L., & Beutler, L. E. (1983). Aerobic exercise as a treatment for depression in women. *Behavior Therapy, 14,* 434–440.

Dubbert, P. M., Martin, J. E., Zimering, R. T., Burkett, P. A., Lake, M., & Cushman, W. C. (1984). Behavioral control of mild hypertension with aerobic exercise: Two case studies. *Behavior Therapy, 15,* 373–380.

Espie, C. A., & Lindsay, W. R. (1985). Parodoxical intention in the treatment of chronic insomnia: Six case studies illustrating variability in therapeutic response. *Behaviour Research and Therapy, 23,* 702–709.

Fairbanks, J. A., Gross, R. T., & Keane, T. M. (1983). Treatment of posttraumatic stress disorder: Evaluating outcome with a behavioral code. *Behavior Modification, 7,* 557–568.

Frame, C. L., Turner, S. M., Jacob, R. G., & Szekely, B. (1984). Self-exposure treatment of agoraphobia. *Behavior Modification, 8,* 115–122.

Franco, D. P., Christoff, K. A., Crimmins, D. B., & Kelly, J. A. (1983). Social skills training for and extremely shy young adolescent: An empirical case study. *Behavior Therapy, 14,* 568–575.

Frank, J. D. (1973). *Persuasion and healing*. Baltimore: Johns Hopkins University Press.

Freud, S. (1953). *Collected Papers* (Vol. 3). London: Hogarth Press.

Garfield, S. L., & Kurtz, R. M. (1976). Clinical psychologists in the 1970s. *American Psychologist, 31,* 1–9.

Gendlin, E. T. (1986). What comes after traditional psychotherapy research? *American Psychologist, 41,* 131–136.

Hall, C. S., & Lindzey, G. (1978). *Theories of personality* (3rd ed.). New York: Wiley.

Hayes, S. C. (1981). Single-case experimental designs and empirical clinical practice. *Journal of Consulting and Clinical Psychology, 49,* 193–211.

Hayes, S. C. (1987). The implications of external validity for strategies of treatment research. In J. Grabowski & E. Ruckert (Eds.), *Adolescent drug abuse: Analyses of treatment research*. Washington, DC: National Institute on Drug Abuse.

Hayes, S. C., Nelson, R. O., & Jarret, R. B. (1986). Evaluating the quality of behavioral assessment. In R. O. Nelson & S. C. Hayes (Eds.), *The conceptual foundations of behavioral assessment* (pp. 463–503). New York: Guilford Press.

Heiby, E. M. (1986). Social versus self-control skills deficits in four cases of depression. *Behavior Therapy, 17,* 158–169.

Hersen, M., & Barlow, D. H. (1976). *Single case experimental design: Strategies for studying behavior therapy*. New York: Pergamon Press.

Holden, A. E., O'Brien, G. T., Barlow, D. H., Stetson, D., & Infantino, A. (1983). Self-help manual for agoraphobia: A preliminary report of effectiveness. *Behavior Therapy, 14,* 545–556.

Jayaratne, S., & Levy, R. L. (1979). *Empirical clinical practice.* New York: Columbia University Press.

Kazdin, A. E. (1980). *Research design in clinical psychology,* New York: Harper & Row.

Kazdin, A. E. (1981). Drawing valid inferences from case studies. *Journal of Consulting and Clinical Psychology, 49,* 183–192.

Kazdin, A. E. (1982). *Single-case research designs: Methods for clinical and applied settings.* New York: Oxford University Press.

Kazdin, A. E., & Bootzin, R. (1972). The token economy: An evaluative review. *Journal of Applied Behavior Analysis, 5,* 343–372.

Kelly, E. L., Goldberg, L. R., Fiske, D. W., & Kilkowski, J. M. (1978). Twenty-five years later. *American Psychologist, 33,* 746–755.

Kratochwill, T. F. (1978). *Single subject research: Strategies for evaluating change.* New York: Academic Press.

Last, C. G., Barlow, D. H., & O'Brien, G. T. (1984a). Cognitive changes during in vivo exposure in an agoraphobic. *Behavior Modification, 8,* 93–113.

Last, C. G., Barlow, D. H., & O'Brien, G. T. (1984b). Cognitive change during treatment of agoraphobia: Cognitive-behavioral approaches. *Behavior Modification, 8,* 181–210.

Layng, T. V., & Andronis, P. T. (1984). Toward a functional analysis of delusional speach and hallucinatory behavior. *The Behavior Analyst, 7,* 139–156.

Lehrer, A. (1981). Not a science. *APA Monitor, 12,* 42.

Levy, L. H. (1962). The skew in clinical psychology. *American Psychologist, 17,* 244–249.

McKnight, D. L., Nelson, R. O., Hayes, S. C., & Jarrett, R. B. (1984). Importance of treating individually-assessed response classes in the amelioration of depression. *Behavior Therapy, 15,* 315–335.

Nelson, R. O., & Hayes, S. C. (1979). Some current dimensions of behavioral assessment. *Behavioral Assessment, 1,* 1–16.

Nelson, R. O., & Hayes, S. C. (1981). Nature of behavioral assessment. In M. Hersen & A. Bellack (Eds.), *Behavioral assessment: A practical handbook* (pp. 3–37). New York: Pergamon Press.

Paul, G. L. (1969). Behavior modification research: Design and tactics. In C. M. Franks (Ed.), *Behavior therapy: Appraisal and status* (pp. 29–62). New York: McGraw-Hill.

Pepper, S. C. (1942). *World hypotheses: A study in evidence.* Berkeley: University of California Press.

Ross, A. O. (1985). To form a more perfect uinion: It is time to stop standing still. *Behavior Therapy, 16,* 195–204.

Rossiter, E. M., & Wilson, G. T. (1984). Cognitive restructuring and response prevention in the treatment of bulemia nervosa. *Behaviour Research and Therpay, 23,* 349–359.

Rychtarik, R. G., Silverman, W. K., Van Landingham, W. P., & Prue, D. M. (1984). Treatment of an incest victim with implosive therapy: A case study. *Behavior Therapy, 15,* 410–420.

Salkovskis, P. M., & Warwick, H. M. C. (1986). Morbid preoccupations, health anxiety, and reassurance: A cognitive-behavioral approach to hypochondriasis. *Behaviour Research and Therapy, 24,* 597–602.

Shapiro, M. B. (1957). Experimental method in the psychological description of the individual psychiatric patient. *International Journal of Social Psychiatry, 1,* 89–102.

Sidman, M. (1962). Operant techniques. In A. J. Bachrach (Ed.), *Experimental foundations of clinical psychology* (pp. 170–210). New York: Basic Books.

Silverman, L. H. (1976). Psychoanalytic theory: "The reports of my death are greatly exaggerated." *American Psychologist, 31,* 621–637.

Skinner, B. F. (1957). *Verbal behavior.* Englewood Cliffs, NJ: Prentice-Hall.

Turkat, I. D. (1986). The behavioral interview. In A. R. Ciminero, K. S. Calhoun, & H. E. Adams (Eds.), *Handbook of behavioral assessment* (pp. 109–149). New York: Wiley.

Wolpe, J. (1979). The experimental model and treatment of neurotic depression. *Behaviour Research and Therapy, 17,* 555–565.

Wolpe, J. (1986). The positive diagnosis of neurotic depression as an etiological category. *Comprehensive Psychiatry, 27,* 449–460.

Wolpe, J., & Rachman, S. (1960). Psychoanalytic "evidence": A critique based on Freud's case of Little Hans. *Journal of Nervous and Mental Disease, 130,* 136–148.

Index